T0176619

High-Quality, High-Volume Spay and Neuter and Other Shelter Surgeries

High-Quality, High-Volume Spay and Neuter and Other Shelter Surgeries

Edited by Sara White

Executive Director and Veterinarian, Spay ASAP Inc.
Founder, ergovet
Member, 2008 and 2016 ASV Veterinary Task Force to Advance Spay-Neuter

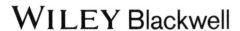

Registered Office
John Wiley & Sons, Inc., 111 River Street, Hoboken, NJ 07030, USA

Editorial Office
111 River Street, Hoboken, NJ 07030, USA

For details of our global editorial offices, customer services, and more information about Wiley products visit us at www.wiley.com.

Wiley also publishes its books in a variety of electronic formats and by print-on-demand. Some content that appears in standard print versions of this book may not be available in other formats.

Library of Congress Cataloging-in-Publication Data

Names: White, Sara, 1972– editor.
Title: High-quality, high-volume spay and neuter and other shelter
    surgeries / edited by Sara White.
Description: Hoboken, NJ: Wiley-Blackwell, 2020. | Includes
    bibliographical references and index.
Identifiers: LCCN 2019039394 (print) | LCCN 2019039395 (ebook) | ISBN
    9781118517208 (paperback) | ISBN 9781118810927 (adobe pdf) | ISBN
9781118810873 (epub)
Subjects: MESH: Surgery, Veterinary–methods | Sterilization,
    Reproductive–veterinary | Animal welfare
Classification: LCC SF911 (print) | LCC SF911 (ebook) | NLM SF 911 | DDC
    636.089/7–dc23
LC record available at https://lccn.loc.gov/2019039394
LC ebook record available at https://lccn.loc.gov/2019039395

Cover Design: Wiley
Cover Image: © Cat ovary Photo credit Intraoperative picture Philip Bushby, © Rabbit intubation Photo credit – Ramiro Isaza, © Feral cat Photo credit – Brenda Griffin, © Puppy in sock Photo credit – Pamela Krausz

Set in 9.5/12.5pt STIXTwoText by SPi Global, Pondicherry, India

Contents

List of Contributors

Mark W. Bohling, DVM, PhD, DACVS
Staff Surgeon
Animal Emergency and Specialty Center
Knoxville, TN, USA
Member, 2008 and 2016 ASV Veterinary Task
Force to Advance Spay-Neuter

Karla Brestle, DVM
Senior Director – Strategic Medical
Operations
ASPCA Spay/Neuter Alliance
Asheville, NC, USA
Member, 2008 and 2016 ASV
Veterinary Task Force to Advance
Spay-Neuter

Amber Burton, DVM, MBA
Founder and Executive Director
Wolf Trap Animal Rescue
Merrifield, VA, USA

Philip Bushby, DVM, MS, ACVS
Professor Emeritus
Marcia Lane Endowed Chair of Humane
Ethics and Animal Welfare
Department of Clinical Sciences
Mississippi State University College of
Veterinary Medicine
Mississippi State, MS, USA
Member, 2008 and 2016 ASV Veterinary Task
Force to Advance Spay-Neuter

Brian A. DiGangi, DVM, MS, DABVP (Canine & Feline Practice, Shelter Medicine Practice)
Senior Director, Shelter Medicine
Shelter Outreach
ASPCA
Gainesville, FL, USA

Diana L. Eubanks, DVM, MS, DABVP (canine and feline), Fellow Academy of Veterinary Dentistry
Clinical Professor
Service Chief, Community Veterinary Services
Department of Clinical Sciences
Mississippi State University College of
Veterinary Medicine
Mississippi State, MS, USA

Brenda Griffin, DVM, MS, DACVIM
Adjunct Associate Professor of Shelter
Medicine
Department of Small Animal Clinical
Sciences
College of Veterinary Medicine
University of Florida
Gainesville, FL, USA
Member, 2008 and 2016 ASV Veterinary Task
Force to Advance Spay-Neuter

Jessica Hekman, DVM, PhD
Post-doctoral Associate
The Broad Institute of MIT and Harvard
Cambridge, MA, USA

Natalie Isaza, DVM, DACVPM
Clinical Professor – Shelter Medicine
Veterinary Community Outreach Program
College of Veterinary Medicine
University of Florida
Gainesville, FL, USA

Ramiro Isaza, DVM, MS, DACZM, MPH
Professor – Zoological Medicine
Department of Small Animal Clinical Sciences
College of Veterinary Medicine
University of Florida
Gainesville, FL, USA

**Stephanie Janeczko, DVM, MS, DABVP
(Canine & Feline Practice, Shelter Medicine
Practice), CAWA**
Vice President, Shelter Medicine Services
Shelter & Veterinary Services
ASPCA
New York, NY, USA

Lydia Love, DVM, DACVAA
Clinical Assistant Professor of Anesthesiology
College of Veterinary Medicine
North Carolina State University
Raleigh, NC, USA

**Kathleen V. Makolinski, DVM, DABVP
(Shelter Medicine Practice)**
Lincoln Memorial University, College of
Veterinary Medicine
Harrogate, TN, USA
Member, 2016 ASV Veterinary Task Force to
Advance Spay-Neuter

Emily McCobb, DVM, MS, DACVAA
Director, Shelter Medicine Program and
Lerner Clinic
Clinical Associate Professor, Anesthesiology
Cummings School of Veterinary Medicine at
Tufts University
North Grafton, MA, USA
Member, 2016 ASV Veterinary Task Force to
Advance Spay-Neuter

Susan Nelms, DVM, MS, DACVO
Veterinary Eye Care
Bessemer, AL, USA

Luisito S. Pablo, DVM, MS, DACVA
Clinical Professor, Anesthesiology and Pain
Management
Department of Comparative, Diagnostic &
Population Medicine
College of Veterinary Medicine
University of Florida
Gainesville, FL, USA

**Sheilah Robertson, BVMS (Hons), PhD, DACVAA,
DECVAA, DACAW, DECAWBM (WSEL),
CVA, MRCVS**
Senior Medical Director
Lap of Love Veterinary Hospice
Member, 2016 ASV Veterinary Task Force to
Advance Spay-Neuter

BJ Rogers, CAWA, CDET
Chief Communication Officer
Emancipet
Austin, TX, USA

Margaret V. Root Kustritz, DVM, PhD, DACT
Assistant Dean of Education, Department of
Veterinary Clinical Sciences
College of Veterinary Medicine
University of Minnesota
Minneapolis, MN, USA

Margaret Slater, DVM, PhD
Senior Director, Research
Strategy & Research
ASPCA
New York, NY, USA

Ruth Steinberger
Executive Director
Spay FIRST!
Oklahoma City, OK, USA

G. Robert Weedon, DVM, MPH
Retired Clinical Assistant Professor &
Service Head
Shelter Medicine
College of Veterinary Medicine
University of Illinois
Urbana, IL, USA

James Weedon, DVM, MPH, BVSc, DACPVM
San Antonio, TX, USA
Member, 2008 ASV Veterinary Task Force to
Advance Spay-Neuter

Joseph P. Weigel, DVM, MS, DACVS
Associate Professor, Small Animal Clinical
Sciences
University of Tennessee College of Veterinary
Medicine
Knoxville, TV, USA

Emily Weiss, PhD, CAAB
Vice President, Equine Welfare
ASPCA
New York, NY, USA

Sara White, DVM, MSc
Executive Director and Veterinarian,
Spay ASAP Inc.
Founder, ergovet
Hartland, VT, USA
Member, 2008 and 2016 ASV
Veterinary Task Force to Advance
Spay-Neuter

Christine Wilford, DVM
Feral Cat Spay/Neuter Project, Founder
Staff Veterinarian
Island Cats Veterinary Hospital
Mercer Island, WA, USA
Member, 2008 and 2016 ASV Veterinary Task
Force to Advance Spay-Neuter

**Kimberly Woodruff, DVM, MS, DACVPM
(Epidemiology)**
Assistant Clinical Professor
Service Chief, Shelter Medicine
Mississippi State University College of
Veterinary Medicine
Mississippi State, MS, USA

Preface

Why do we need a spay and neuter textbook?

Spaying and neutering are often the first (and in some cases, the only) surgeries that students learn in veterinary school, and are expected skills for every new graduate in general small- or mixed-animal practice. It can be tempting to dismiss them as "beginner surgeries," the easily trivialized but sometimes terrifying rites of passage into the veterinary profession. Perhaps because spaying and neutering are skills learned so early and repeated so often in a general practitioner's veterinary career, they are rarely the subject of continuing education seminars and articles, and general practitioners may go their entire career without modifying or even questioning the techniques for spaying and neutering that they learned as third-year veterinary students.

At the same time, spaying and neutering have been central to efforts to reduce the overpopulation and euthanasia of unwanted and unowned cats and dogs. The spay–neuter clinics and programs that have arisen over the past several decades recognized the need for minimally invasive, efficient techniques that would shorten surgical times and improve patient recovery. This textbook pulls together many of the surgical, anesthetic, peri-operative, and operational techniques discovered, developed, and popularized over the decades by these innovative spay–neuter pioneers.

As the field of spay–neuter developed, practitioners recognized the need for greater acceptance and clarity. In 2006, a task force was convened that developed the first guidelines for medical care in spay–neuter programs; this document was published in JAVMA in 2008 as "The Association of Shelter Veterinarians' veterinary medical care guidelines for spay-neuter programs" (Looney et al. 2008). The goals of these guidelines were to promote acceptance of spay–neuter practice by the veterinary profession and the public, as well as to provide guidance for veterinarians and spay–neuter programs regarding standards of care and practices based on scientific evidence and expert opinion. The ASV Spay Neuter Task Force reconvened in 2014 to update and expand the document, resulting in "The Association of Shelter Veterinarians' 2016 Veterinary Medical Care Guidelines for Spay-Neuter Programs" (Griffin et al. 2016).

High-quality, high-volume spay–neuter (or HQHVSN, the awkward but now widely used acronym adopted by the first Spay Neuter Task Force) is the field of veterinary medicine that began with the efforts of spay–neuter pioneers in the 1970s through the 1990s, and became firmly established and advanced by the publication of the 2008 and 2016 spay–neuter guidelines. HQHVSN is defined as "efficient surgical initiatives that meet or exceed veterinary medical standards of care in providing accessible, targeted sterilization of large numbers of cats and dogs to reduce their overpopulation and subsequent euthanasia" (Griffin et al. 2016).

Until now, practitioners new to HQHVSN or isolated in their practice have had no single place to turn to find out about HQHVSN techniques and protocols and the evidence supporting them, or about spay–neuter program types, their implementation and staffing, and their effects on animal populations and individual animal health. Many of the techniques used in HQHVSN have been taught at conferences and mentorship programs and shared and spread between practitioners, and many have been subjects of peer-reviewed research; however, few appear in textbooks. Nevertheless, the medical, surgical, and peri-operative care described in this book need not be limited to high-volume or shelter settings – it is applicable wherever veterinary surgery is performed.

This book is divided into two parts, and each of those parts is divided into several sections. Part One, Clinical Techniques and Patient Care, is concerned with evidence-based clinical knowledge and skills, including peri-operative, anesthetic, and surgical techniques. Part Two, Fundamentals of HQHVSN, introduces the high-volume surgical setting and the special organizational, logistical, and epidemiologic challenges that arise when striving to optimize a clinic's operations and impact.

The book is intended for a range of audiences: from the veterinary student to the experienced HQHVSN practitioner, and from the veterinary technician to the aspiring spay–neuter clinic founder. Part One begins with chapters on the determination of patient sex and neuter status, reproductive anomalies and pathologies, the selection of surgical instruments and suture, infectious disease control, asepsis, and stress reduction in the clinic. The sections on anesthesia and surgery cover general principles as well as specific techniques and protocols, including chapters on avoiding and managing both anesthetic and surgical complications, and a chapter on anesthetic and surgical techniques in rabbits and other small mammals.

While many of the techniques covered in Part One are well known to experienced HQHVSN surgeons, some of the anomalies, complications, and complicated presentations are unusual and may be once-in-a-lifetime cases for some. Experienced practitioners may also learn of useful variations on or alternatives to their accustomed techniques, or discover new ways of preventing or addressing frustrating complications.

Part One concludes with a section on other common shelter surgeries and associated anesthetic procedures, and can serve as a reference for shelter surgeons with a variety of levels of experience. This section includes amputations, eye surgeries, vulvar or rectal prolapse treatment, and dental extractions.

Part Two of this book moves away from the clinical care of individual patients and into the structures and systems fundamental to HQHVSN, with sections on population medicine, human resources and wellbeing, and HQHVSN program models. Optimizing the potential of HQHVSN requires more than just proficiency in the clinical care (anesthesia and surgery) of individual patients. Effective HQHVSN programs must understand the effects of their interventions on animal populations and individuals; they must combine their clinical skills with appropriate staffing and facilities to allow an efficient and streamlined workflow; they must institute systems that are financially, physically, and emotionally sustainable. Chapter 23 serves as an introduction and roadmap to the second half of this book. The material here should be of interest to anyone seeking to establish a new HQHVSN program or improve an existing one.

References

Griffin, B., Bushby, P.A., McCobb, E. et al. (2016). The Association of Shelter Veterinarians' 2016 veterinary medical care guidelines for spay-neuter programs. *JAVMA* 249: 165–188.

Looney, A.L., Bohling, M.W., Bushby, P.A. et al. (2008). The Association of Shelter Veterinarians' veterinary medical care guidelines for spay-neuter programs. *JAVMA* 233: 74–86.

Acknowledgments

First, I want to thank the original four editors of the book: Brenda Griffin, Karla Brestle, Philip Bushby, and Mark Bohling. These four veterinarians have been instrumental in establishing and promoting the field of HQHVSN; this book would not have existed without them. I have had the privilege of working with all four of these people in different capacities over the past decade and a half: as teammates on the ASV Spay Neuter Task Force and co-authors on the 2008 and 2016 Guidelines, as co-teachers in pediatric spay–neuter wet labs, and finally as contributing authors to this textbook. Thank you for being my mentors and colleagues, and for believing I could do this. Thanks especially to Brenda, who during my editorship has been my cheerleader and sounding board, my informant and historian, and a bridge between the original vision for this book and its evolution and re/vision. The encouragement, context, and friendship you have offered throughout this process have supported and inspired me.

I also want to thank all the HQHVSN and shelter veterinarians I have met over the years in person and online. My early teachers in this field were all virtual (but real!) colleagues who took the time to explain and describe surgical techniques in words, back in the days of dial-up internet, before YouTube. From the sheltervet electronic mailing list that I joined in 2001 to today's shelter veterinary and spay neuter Facebook communities and hqhvsnvets online group, you have been and continue to be my mentors and my inspiration. Thank you also to my online colleagues who contributed photos for this textbook – your eagerness, openness, and surgical and photographic skills have made this book better.

And a huge thank-you to all the authors who have contributed chapters to this textbook. It is your expertise that has driven the field of HQHVSN forward and that makes this book all that it is. This book is a first edition, but it is also a revision: by the time I signed on as editor in early 2018, many of the submitted manuscripts had become dated. I want to thank the authors for their patience and willingness to revise or even overhaul these chapters in order to make the materials as relevant, timely, and useful as possible.

And finally, thanks to my wife Tina, who kept the refrigerator full and the woodstove stoked during my many long hours of writing and editing.

Part One

Clinical Techniques and Patient Care

Section One

Peri-operative Care Associated with Spay and Neuter

1

Determination of Patient Sex and Spay–Neuter Status

Brenda Griffin

Sex Determination

Physical examination should always include determination or verification of each patient's sex. Obviously, this is essential in the context of spay–neuter programs. Wise clinicians never assume a patient is the sex they have been told, but instead always make that determination for themselves prior to performing surgery. Verifying the animal's sex, as well as assessing their reproductive status, informs and prepares the surgeon for the appropriate procedure. It may also prevent him/her from attempting to spay a male calico cat.

Sexing Dogs

Determining the sex of a dog is generally straightforward and can almost always be quickly accomplished through physical examination, including simple visual inspection of the external genitalia. In this species, the male and female anatomy are distinct and easy to identify, even in the case of very young patients. In female dogs of all ages, the vulva is readily identified on the ventral midline in the caudal inguinal area between the hind limbs (Figure 1.1a and b). It consists of two thick folds of tissue (called the *labia pudenda* or vulvar lips), which form a rounded commissure dorsally and a pointed commissure ventrally, producing a tear-drop shape. The vertical slit-like

opening between the two labia (known as the vulvar cleft) marks the external orifice of the urogenital tract. Of note is that a fold of skin surrounds the canine vulva. In young puppies, the vulva is small and somewhat recessed in this fold (referred to as an "infantile" or "juvenile" vulva), but becomes increasingly prominent as the pup develops and attains puberty.

In male dogs, both the penis and the scrotum are readily identified on the ventral midline. The penis, encased in its prepuce or sheath, is located in the mid abdominal region caudal to the umbilicus, while the scrotum lies in the caudal inguinal area between the hind limbs (Figure 1.2a and b). Although minimal hair is present in the inguinal region of young puppies, within a few months the prepuce generally becomes well covered by hair, while the scrotum becomes increasingly pendulous. In puppies the testicles descend into the scrotum very soon after birth, usually within the first several days, and are typically palpable by two to four weeks of age depending on the pup's size (Ley et al. 2003). By the time a male puppy is presented for castration (i.e. at six weeks of age or older) both testes should be present in the scrotum and, if not, a tentative diagnosis of cryptorchidism should be made. Although relatively uncommon, testicular descent is sometimes delayed. Later descent is possible because the inguinal canals do not close until the time of puberty, usually around 5–10 months of age

(a)

(b)

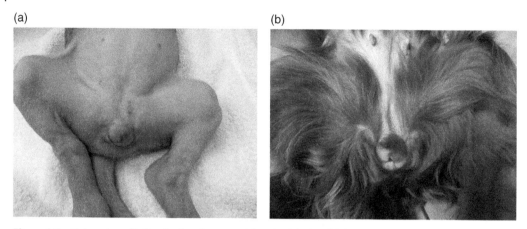

Figure 1.1 External genitalia of a female puppy (a) and adult dog (b). Note the tear-drop shape of the vulva, which is located in the caudal inguinal area between the hind limbs.

(a)

(b)

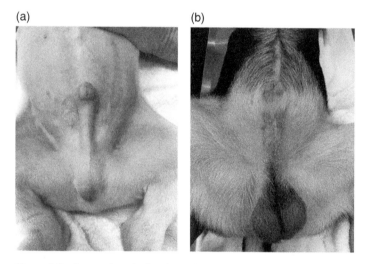

Figure 1.2 External genitalia of a male puppy (a) and adult dog (b). The penis is encased in a sheath (called the prepuce) and the testicles lie within the scrotum. Note that the adult dog's prepuce is well covered with hair and the scrotum is much more pendulous than that of the male puppy.

depending on the individual dog. Although late descent of one or both testicles is possible during this time frame, it may not be desirable to postpone castration (Griffin et al. 2016).

In dogs, the reported prevalence of cryptorchidism ranges from 0.8 to 10%, with the highest rates often occurring in certain breeds, including Chihuahuas, miniature schnauzers, Pomeranians, toy and miniature poodles, Shetland sheepdogs, Yorkshire terriers, boxers, and German shepherd dogs (Yates et al. 2003; Birchard and Nappier 2008). Despite the

fact that cryptorchidism is one of the most frequently recognized congenital defects in small animal practice, it is not necessarily the most common reason that one or both testicles are not readily palpable in the scrotum of young puppies. In fact, a more common reason might be temporary retraction into the inguinal area. Indeed, when the testicles are not readily palpable in the scrotum, it may not indicate that a puppy is truly cryptorchid; rather, it may simply be a function of the fact that small, slippery testicles can easily escape detection during examination because they sometimes retract into the inguinal area when digital pressure is applied. Furthermore, it is possible for one or both testicles to slip back through its respective external inguinal ring into the canal or abdomen. This can occur in awake patients, and in the author's experience it occurs even more commonly when a pediatric puppy is anesthetized and placed in dorsal recumbency. If the testicles are absent from the scrotum on palpation, lifting the patient into an upright position often allows the "missing" testicle(s) to descend back into its proper anatomic location in the scrotum. This can be done by holding the puppy gently around the chest to support its body weight, taking care to support the head and neck if needed, while allowing the hind limbs to gently hang down (Figure 1.3a–c). Alternatively, with the puppy in dorsal recumbency, gentle continuous digital pressure may be applied to "smooth" down the soft tissue of the groin, beginning in the area of the inguinal rings and continuing caudally toward the scrotum; this action will usually push the missing testicle(s) back into the scrotal sac (Figure 1.4a–c). These techniques can be used to locate testicles that "disappear" from the scrotum and help the surgeon avoid unnecessary exploration for the gonads. Whenever possible, the goal should be to verify that both testicles are present in the scrotum prior to surgery, so that the surgeon can plan accordingly if cryptorchidism truly exists. For information on surgical castration of cryptorchid dogs, see Chapter 14.

Sexing Cats

In contrast to dogs, determining the sex of cats can be more challenging, particularly in the case of small kittens. Unlike dogs, where the external genitalia of both sexes are readily visible in the inguinal (groin) area, the external genitalia of male and female cats are located in the perineal region beneath the tail. The small size of the species' penis and vulva, combined with the fact that these structures are generally well covered by hair, further complicates their identification. Upon inspection, the penis is not visually obvious in tomcats at any age and, prior to weaning age, the presence of the testicles in the scrotum is usually not visually apparent either. Although present in the scrotum at or within a few days of birth, the testes are simply too small to be either visually apparent or easily

(a) (b) (c)

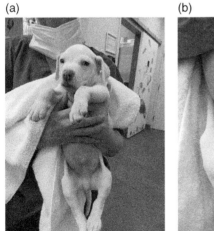 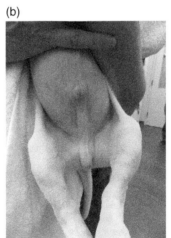 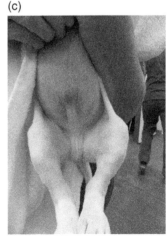

Figure 1.3 (a–c) Holding a puppy upright in this position with the hind limbs hanging down may allow the testicles to descend back into their proper anatomic location within the scrotal sac (a). Initially, the left testicle was retracted back into the inguinal area proximal to the scrotum (b), but it quickly reappeared in the scrotum when the puppy was held in this position (c).

(a)

(b)

(c)

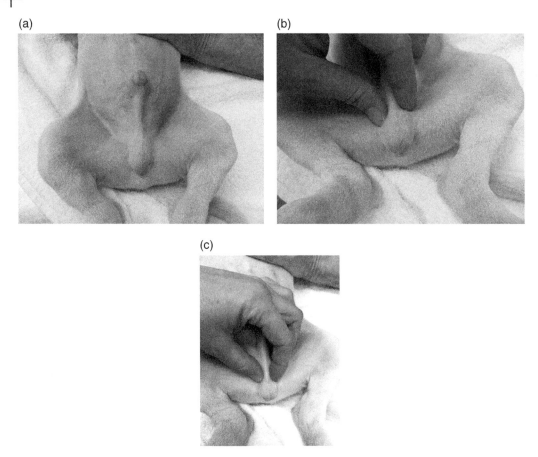

Figure 1.4   (a–c) With the puppy in dorsal recumbency, the soft tissue of the groin can be digitally "smoothed" down from the area of the inguinal rings toward the scrotum in order to gently push the testicles back into the scrotal sac.

palpable in the first few weeks of life. Although the feline penis never becomes visually obvious, the testes do quickly become larger as kittens grow and are increasingly readily visible beneath the anus by six to eight weeks of age. Usually by the time of a kitten's first veterinary visit, the testicles are readily palpable in the scrotum (Griffin 2006). If one or both testicles is absent, a diagnosis of cryptorchidism is highly likely: delayed or late testicular descent is possible but very uncommon in cats. The reported prevalence of cryptorchidism is relatively low in cats (<2%), although much higher rates have been reported in the Persian breed (Millis et al. 1992). As is the case in pediatric puppies, care must be taken to ensure accurate examination, because gentle digital pressure applied during

scrotal palpation may cause small testicles to temporarily slip into the inguinal region, where they may elude detection. The techniques previously described for returning such testicles to their proper anatomic location in the scrotum can be used for kittens as well as puppies. Notably, the absence of testicles following neutering can also make sexual determination of a tomcat difficult for untrained observers.

Careful inspection of the perineal area is necessary in order to determine the sex of a cat or kitten. For adults, an individual's overall body type and/or appearance may sometimes suggest the cat's sex. For example, many male cats are larger in stature with heavier bones than female cats, and most calico cats are females (Figure 1.5). That said, such characteristics

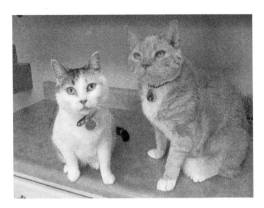

Figure 1.5   The body appearance and coat color of the cat on the left suggest that she is a female, while the large size and masculine features of the cat on the right suggest that he is a male. In this case, the visual appearance of these cats does accurately reflect their sex. However, a wise clinician never assumes the sex of a cat based on general appearance alone; careful inspection of the perineal region is essential for accurate assessment.

should never be used to determine sex without concurrent inspection of the perineal area. When there are no obvious testicles present, visual inspection of the perineum focuses on evaluating the distance between the anus and genital opening, as well as the shape of the genital opening itself. This is accomplished by gently lifting the tail, or by stroking the dorsal rump, which often stimulates the cat to lift its tail, allowing visual inspection of this area.

In female cats, the anus and opening to the vulva are spaced very close together, such that the vulva lies just beneath the anus. Furthermore, the opening to the vulva (vulvar cleft) is shaped like a small slit or comma. As such, the female's anogenital anatomy is sometimes described as having the appearance of a semicolon (;). Figure 1.6a illustrates the anogenital anatomy of a young female kitten. In contrast, a tomcat's anus and penile opening are spaced relatively far apart since the scrotum lies between them, while the opening is shaped like a small dot or period. For this reason, the male's anogenital anatomy is sometimes described as having the appearance of a colon (:). Figure 1.6b illustrates the anogenital anatomy of a young male kitten.

The anatomy is smaller and more difficult to visualize in young kittens compared to adults, but the same rules for identification apply regardless. Thus, the anogenital anatomy of a mature female cat can also be described as a semicolon (Figure 1.7). Older intact tomcats are much easier to distinguish because the testicles, which are well covered by hair, are obvious (Figure 1.8). In contrast, neutered tomcats are commonly misidentified as female

(a)

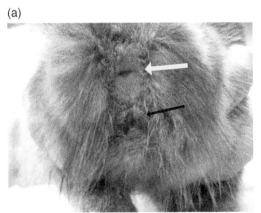

(b)

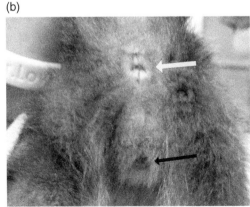

Figure 1.6   (a) Anogenital anatomy of a female kitten. White arrow: anus. Black arrow: small slit-like opening of vulva. Note the relatively small distance between the anal and genital openings. (b) Anogenital anatomy of a male kitten. White arrow: anus. Black arrow: small dot-like opening of penis. Note the relatively large distance between the anal and genital openings.

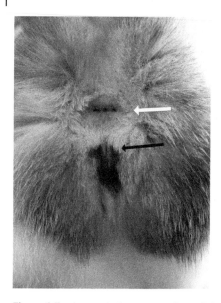

Figure 1.7 Anogenital anatomy of an adult female cat. White arrow: anus. Black arrow: small slit-like opening of vulva. Note the relatively small distance between the anal and genital openings. The anatomy is larger and easier to visualize in adult cats compared to kittens.

cats – the key to their identification is careful visual evaluation of the distance between the anus and genital opening, as well as the shape of the genital opening. Once again, the same rules apply: a neutered male looks like a widely spaced colon (Figure 1.9). That said, the absence of testes in the scrotum does not always indicate that a male cat (or dog) has been neutered.

It is also possible, albeit rare, for a male cat to present without a penis. This occurs in the case of previous perineal urethrostomy surgery. Perineal urethrostomy is a surgical treatment for tomcats with recurrent or complicated lower urinary tract obstruction. The procedure entails removal of both the penis and scrotum and creation of a urethral stoma in the perineal area immediately ventral to the anus for voiding urine. In this case, careful examination of the patient's perineal anatomy will enable the clinician to correctly identify the sex of such a patient (Figure 1.10a and b).

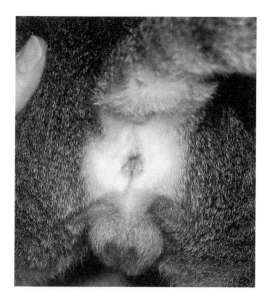

Figure 1.8 Anogenital anatomy of a sexually intact adult tomcat. The hair-covered testicles are readily identifiable beneath the anus. The opening to the penis is not seen because it is obscured from view by the testicles.

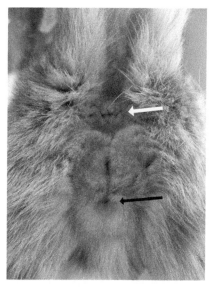

Figure 1.9 Anogenital anatomy of a neutered male adult cat. White arrow: anus. Black arrow: small dot-like opening of penis. Note the relatively large distance between the anal and genital openings. The empty hair-covered scrotum lies in between.

(a)   (b)

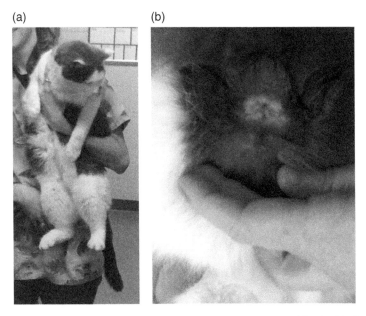

Figure 1.10   (a and b) The large size of this mature cat combined with the lack of facial jowls suggest a neutered male cat; however, inspection of his anogenital region reveals a punctate opening immediately ventral to the anus – somewhat resembling the anogenital anatomy of a female cat. Shaving the area around the urethral stoma revealed scarring from previous suture lines and careful palpation revealed the absence of either a penis or a vulva. This cat was therefore determined to be a neutered male cat that had undergone previous perineal urethrostomy surgery. *Source:* Photo courtesy of Sara White.

On rare occasions, a patient may present with a combination of both male and female sex organs. Chapter 2 includes information about male and female pseudohermaphroditism and other atypical sexual genotypes and phenotypes in dogs and cats.

Distinguishing between Sexually Intact and Previously Altered Dogs and Cats

In preparation for spay–neuter surgery, it is not only important to determine the correct sex of a dog or cat, but one should also make an attempt to determine if the animal has been previously spayed or neutered. This can be surprisingly difficult in some cases, and it behooves the clinician to approach this task carefully and cautiously, especially in the context of a spay–neuter program where the opportunity to neuter any individual animal

may not present itself again in the future. Although no one wants an animal to undergo unnecessary anesthesia and surgery, this will sometimes be necessary to ensure that an animal leaves the spay–neuter clinic without the possibility of reproducing in the future. Provided there is no compelling medical reason not to proceed with such surgery, the benefits will likely outweigh the risks for the vast majority of patients when spay–neuter status remains uncertain.

That said, there will be a number of cases where the clinician can verify the spay–neuter status of the patient without surgery. First and foremost, each patient should be carefully inspected for the presence of a standard identification mark indicating previous surgical sterilization. The Association of Shelter Veterinarians (ASV) recommends the use of permanent, visibly distinct identifying marks to indicate that an animal has been spayed or neutered: a green linear tattoo should be used to identify all neutered pet animals and ear tipping should be used to identify all community cats (Griffin et al. 2016; Figures 1.11 and 1.12). Table 1.1 describes the recommended standard locations for the placement of green linear tattoos. Note that removal of the hair from the ventral abdomen will sometimes be necessary to ensure discovery of green linear tattoos,

Table 1.1 Association of Shelter Veterinarians (ASV) recommendations for standard placement of green linear tattoos for identification of neutered dogs and cats (Griffin et al. 2016).

Sex and species	Location of green linear tattoo
Female dogs and cats	On or immediately lateral to the ventral midline incision; if a flank approach is used to spay a female patient, the tattoo should be placed in the area where a ventral midline spay incision would have been placed
Male dogs	At the caudal aspect of the abdomen in the pre-scrotal incision or pre-scrotal area immediately lateral to the prepuce
Male cats	In the area where a ventral midline spay incision would typically be placed

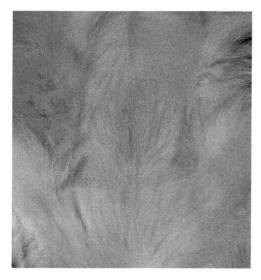

Figure 1.11 Green linear tattoo on the abdomen of a cat. The Association of Shelter Veterinarians (ASV) recommends the use of green linear tattoos to identify all spayed or neutered pet cats and dogs.

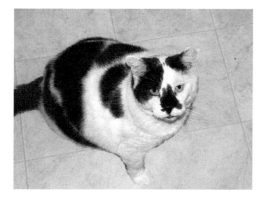

Figure 1.12 Ear-tipped cat. The Association of Shelter Veterinarians (ASV) recommends the use of ear tipping to identify all spayed/neutered community cats.

while the presence of a "tipped" ear in a cat should be visually obvious. Surgical removal of the distal tip of one pinna is the universal symbol for denoting a neutered free-roaming cat. In contrast, ear notching is not recommended, because earflap injuries are common and easily mistaken for surgically notched ears. Caution must be taken not to mistake frostbite of the ear for a surgically tipped ear. Chapter 16 contains detailed information on techniques for identification of neutered animals. Obviously, the presence of a distinct standard mark will greatly facilitate the clinician's assessment. In animals with a distinct mark indicative of previous sterilization, no further action will be necessary.

In addition to inspection of the ventral abdomen for a green linear tattoo and the pinna for tipping, patients should also be scanned for a microchip using a universal scanner. If a microchip is identified, it may be linked through a registry to a known owner and/or medical record, which might provide definitive information regarding the pet's spay–neuter status. Importantly, the discovery of a microchip might also result in pet–owner reunification.

For those animals whose spay–neuter status remains undetermined, a thorough and systematic clinical evaluation should follow. To avoid incorrect or invalid determinations, the clinician's assessment should be based on objective findings rather than subjective impressions whenever possible.

Male Dogs and Tomcats: Reproductively Intact, Cryptorchid, or Neutered?

Most male patients that present without the presence of scrotal testicles have been previously neutered. However, a few male patients will lack scrotal testes because of either bilateral cryptorchidism or unilateral cryptorchidism, where surgical removal of the scrotal testicle was previously performed. Distinguishing these animals and ensuring that they are properly sterilized will likely have major positive impacts on their future health and wellbeing.

Definitions

As previously described, cryptorchidism is a congenital defect in which one or both of the testes do not descend into the scrotum at the appropriate time (see also Chapter 2 on common reproductive anomalies). Although unilateral cryptorchidism is more common, bilateral cryptorchidism also occurs. In either case, the testicles may be retained anywhere along their normal path of descent from the abdomen: in the abdomen, inguinal ring, or subcutaneous tissue of the groin between the inguinal ring and scrotum. Monorchidism, which is defined as the presence of only a single testicle, is exceedingly rare in both dogs and cats. For this reason, dogs and cats presenting with only one testicle should be considered cryptorchid until proven otherwise (Ley et al. 2003).

Clinical Signs

Retained testes do not produce spermatozoa, but do produce testosterone (Ley et al. 2003).

Thus, the absence of scrotal testicles causes infertility; however, it does not prevent the development of androgen-dependent behaviors. For this reason, cryptorchid dogs and cats may present with a history of urine marking or spraying, fighting, attraction to females, mounting, and in the case of tomcats, urine odor (Millis et al. 1992). This is especially significant in the case of tomcats because urine spraying is a leading reason for relinquishment of pet cats by their owners (Salman et al. 2000). Cryptorchidism is an important differential diagnosis to consider, especially in adolescent or young adult tomcats, since this is the expected time for puberty and the onset of such behavioral effects of testosterone. Although relatively uncommon, this cause of spraying is associated with an excellent prognosis, since removing the retained testicle(s) most often results in resolution of spraying (Griffin 2006).

In dogs, cryptorchidism may be associated with clinical signs of feminization, including gynecomastia (mammary enlargement) and alopecia in affected dogs. This is because abdominally retained testes are at increased risk for development of Sertoli cell tumors, especially in older dogs. Retained testicles are also at increased risk of spermatic cord torsion, which can result in signs of an acute abdomen (Ley et al. 2003).

Diagnosis

In addition to obtaining any available clinical history, diagnostic evaluation should include physical examination. In the case of tomcats, physical examination alone is a highly reliable means of diagnostic determination of neuter status. Unfortunately, the same is not true for dogs and other means of diagnosis such as ultrasound and hormonal evaluation, when available, are often required.

History   If history is available, it can be very helpful to the clinician tasked with determining the animal's true neuter status. Even with a history of previous castration, the possibility of cryptorchidism should not be discounted, since it is conceivable that the surgeon may have removed only a single testicle in a unilaterally cryptorchid animal.

As previously described, cryptorchid dogs and cats may present with a history of undesirable male behaviors. Owners should be questioned carefully regarding the potential for exposure to exogenous hormones, including hormone replacement therapies and anabolic steroids, which could result in such behaviors. Use of therapeutic creams for hormone replacement is common in people and repeated exposure of pets (especially dogs) can occur as a result of licking an owner's contaminated hands (Griffin 2006; Birchard and Nappier 2008).

Physical Examination A complete physical examination should be performed, including careful inspection of the penis and palpation of the inguinal area. In cats, penile spines are reliable external indicators of the presence of testosterone, and are present in unilateral and bilateral cryptorchid cats. Penile spines begin to appear in kittens as early as 12 weeks of age and are obvious by 6 months of age (Aronson and Cooper 1967). They regress within six weeks following castration, and the mucosal surface of the penis becomes flat and

smooth. Although it is theoretically possible for a neutered tomcat to develop penile spines as a result of chronic exogenous hormone exposure, this is seldom seen in cats. Thus, it is entirely reasonable for a clinician to consider the presence of penile spines as diagnostic for the presence of a testicle in a tomcat (Richardson and Mullen 1993; Johnston et al. 1996; Griffin 2006; Figure 1.13a). Likewise, the absence of penile spines in an adult tomcat is an objective finding that verifies previous neutering (Figure 1.13b). The absence of penile spines in cats less than six months of age, however, is equivocal, neither supporting nor refuting previous neutering.

Fully extruding the penis of a cat to examine its mucosal surface for the presence of penile spines can be challenging in awake patients (Figure 1.14a–c). If the penis cannot be fully extruded, heavy sedation is required to ensure a thorough examination. Even with heavy sedation, full extrusion of the penis will not be possible in some cats simply as a function of their anatomy. In kittens, the balanopreputial fold connects the penis to the prepuce and prevents full penile extrusion. Its dissolution is an androgen-dependent event, occurring as tomcats mature (Johnston et al. 1996). Tomcats are routinely neutered prior to puberty (which typically occurs between 8 and 13 months of

(a)

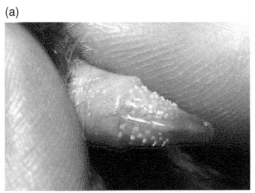

(b)

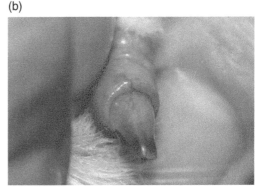

Figure 1.13   (a) The presence of penile spines in a male cat as seen in this photo is diagnostic for the presence of a testicle. (b) The absence of penile spines in an adult tomcat as seen in this photo verifies previous neutering. Within a few weeks of castration, penile spines atrophy and the penile mucosa becomes smooth and flat in appearance.

(a)

(b)

(c)

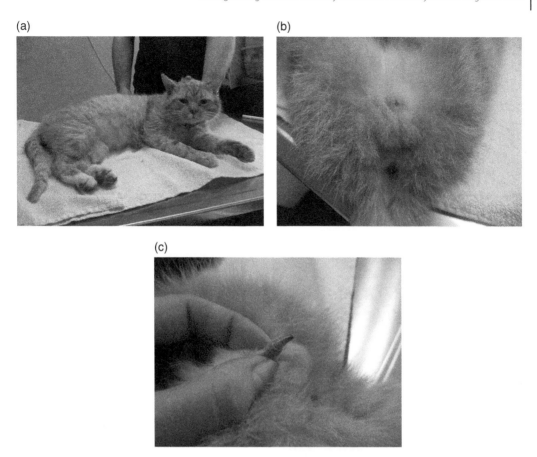

Figure 1.14   (a) This male cat, who was believed to be neutered, presented with a history of undesirable male behaviors including spraying, fighting, and breeding behavior. In this photo he has been sedated for examination. Note the presence of jowls. (b) Examination revealed the absence of scrotal testicles. Note that the anus is at the bottom of the photo in this picture. (c) Examination also revealed the presence of penile spines with full penile extrusion. This cat was a bilateral cryptorchid and both testicles were found in the abdomen at the time of surgery. Following surgery, the cat recovered uneventfully and all of the previously displayed undesirable behaviors ceased.

age) in order to prevent the development of undesired male behaviors. In many tomcats neutered prior to puberty, the balanopreputial fold remains intact and complete penile extrusion is not possible (Root et al. 1996b). Thus, if the balanopreputial fold is intact in an adult cat, this objective finding is consistent with previous neutering (Figure 1.15). In other words, the inability to fully extrude the penis of an anesthetized adult cat can be considered equally reliable as the absence of penile spines for verification of neuter status. Of note is that failure of the balanopreputial fold to regress

has not been shown to be clinically significant, though it can be more difficult to exteriorize the penis for catheterization in the event the patient requires a urinary catheter (Herron 1972; Stubbs and Bloomberg 1995; Stubbs et al. 1996; Howe et al. 2000; Spain et al. 2004).

In contrast, penile barbs are not part of the anatomy of male dogs: the penile mucosa appears flat and smooth in both intact and neutered males of this species. Although dogs lack penile spines, there are some physical characteristics of their external genitalia that are consistently observable depending on the age at which

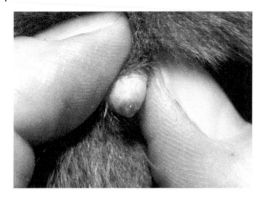

Figure 1.15 The balanopreputial fold of this neutered male cat remains intact, preventing complete extrusion of the penis. Presence of the balanopreputial fold in a post-pubertal male cat indicates previous castration.

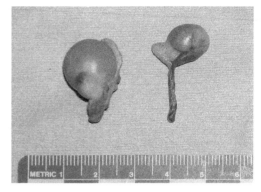

Figure 1.17 Comparison of scrotal testicle (left) and retained testicle (right) from a cryptorchid tomcat. Retained testicles are generally smaller than scrotal testicles. The retained testicle pictured here was removed from the inguinal ring and palpation was not possible through the large inguinal fat pad of this cat.

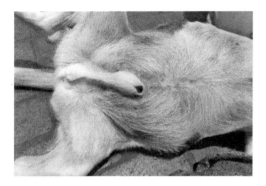

Figure 1.16 The infantile appearance of the penis and prepuce of this mature adult beagle is strong evidence that he was neutered at an early age.

an individual dog is neutered. When dogs are neutered as very young puppies (i.e. <12 weeks of age), the penis, *os penis*, and prepuce remain infantile in their appearance compared to those neutered at a more traditional age or as mature adults (Olson 2003). Thus, the presence of an infantile penis and prepuce in an adult dog without testicles is an objective finding that supports previous castration (Figure 1.16).

Physical examination should also include careful palpation of the entire inguinal region (i.e. from the level of the inguinal rings to the scrotum). When compared to scrotal testicles, retained testicles are generally grossly smaller (Ley et al. 2003; Figure 1.17). Testicles located

in the inguinal region are often difficult to palpate and may be obscured by inguinal fat. In some instances, irregular deposits of fat may be mistaken for retained testicles. Abdominally retained testicles are generally too small to palpate, except in the case of Sertoli cell tumors in dogs, which are frequently quite large. In this case, signs of feminization may also be apparent on physical examination. In dogs, the presence of an obvious pre-scrotal scar may suggest previous neutering, but should be interpreted with some skepticism, since scars may also result from unrelated skin trauma.

Both dogs and cats develop secondary sex characteristics as they mature to puberty. Androgen-dependent physical changes tend to be more consistent and dramatic in tomcats compared to male dogs. For cats, these features include the formation of jowls, widening of the neck, and thickening of the skin (Figure 1.18). Although most tomcats do not develop distinct jowls before two years of age, their skin may subjectively appear "tougher" or more difficult to puncture with a hypodermic needle. In dogs, secondary sex characteristics may be less obvious and vary considerably among breeds. This is not surprising, given that dogs possess more physical diversity than any other species. In general, intact male dogs tend to be more

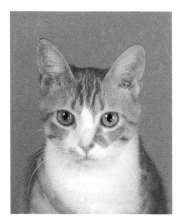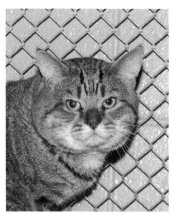

Figure 1.18 Comparison of facial features of a neutered male cat (left) and an intact tomcat (right). Note the thick neck and the presence of large jowls in the intact tomcat.

massive and muscular compared to neutered males, and changes in the hair coat may occur following neutering. That said, such changes are highly subjective, influenced by many factors besides neuter status, and often go unrecognized except by those who are extremely familiar with a specific breed.

Diagnostic Imaging When available, ultrasonographic examination of the abdomen and inguinal area may allow visualization of retained testicles. Although this may provide the clinician with additional useful information, it is not required, nor is it necessarily definitive for determination of neuter status in dogs and cats. This modality can be particularly helpful for diagnosing testicular tumors and torsion in dogs. Likewise, radiography can also be a useful diagnostic tool in such cases. However, radiography is otherwise unrewarding for detection of retained testicles because of their small size and indistinct radiodensity.

Hormonal Evaluation In dogs, hormonal evaluation is the most definitive pre-surgical diagnostic test available for determination of neuter status. Hormonal evaluation can also be used for diagnosis of retained testicle(s) in the cat, but is not necessary because the presence of penile spines serves as a reliable "bioassay"

for testosterone in this species. In both dogs and cats, testosterone is secreted in an episodic, pulsatile fashion throughout the day. As such, a single resting sample where no detectable testosterone is measured does not rule out the presence of a testicle (Johnston et al. 1996). In contrast, a hormone stimulation test is a highly reliable indicator of testosterone production. Stimulation of testosterone secretion can be accomplished by the administration of human chorionic gonadotropin (hCG) or gonadotropin-releasing hormone (GnRH). Baseline serum samples are collected prior to administration and again at one or more intervals following administration. Various protocols are available from diagnostic laboratories. An increase in serum testosterone is diagnostic for the presence of a testis (Memon et al. 1992; Johnston et al. 1996).

More recently, tests for measuring serum concentrations of luteinizing hormone (LH) and anti-Mullerian hormone (AMH) have been investigated as diagnostic aids for determining neuter status in dogs and cats (Olson et al. 1992; Gunzel-Apel et al. 2009; Wheeler and Kutzler 2010; Place et al. 2011; Axner and Strom-Holst 2015; Themmen et al. 2016; Alm and Holst 2018; Krecic et al. 2018; Morrow et al. 2018). In the reproductively intact male, testosterone production by the testes inhibits hypothalamic production of GnRH, in turn inhibiting pituitary production of follicle-stimulating hormone and LH. Following castration, serum concentrations of these reproductive cascade hormones increase as a result of the lack of negative feedback from the gonads. A commercially available point-of-care LH test (Witness[®] LS, Zoetis, Parsippany, NJ, USA), which was originally developed as a means of determining ovulation timing in dogs, has been used as a diagnostic aid to elucidate neuter status (Figure 1.19). A "positive" test is consistent with previous neutering, while a negative result supports the need for surgery. In a study of 53 male cats, the reported sensitivity and specificity were 85 and 95%, respectively (Krecic et al. 2018). In a study of 10 dogs, the reported sensitivity and specificity were 100% (Wheeler and Kutzler 2010). Point-of-care tests have the obvious advantages of being very convenient and providing rapid, same-day results. As more data from field studies becomes available to evaluate the performance of this patient-side test in dogs, its use may become an increasingly attractive option for determination of neuter status.

A final diagnostic option is measurement of serum concentrations of AMH through a reference laboratory. AMH is continuously produced by the Sertoli cells of the testes in post-pubescent male dogs and tomcats, and production continues throughout an animal's reproductive life. Thus, positive test results in a post-pubertal patient are consistent with the need for surgery. In contrast, negative test results suggest previous neutering (Axner and Strom-Holst 2015; Themmen et al. 2016). Reported sensitivities and specificities of AMH assays vary: in a study of 27 male cats, the reported sensitivity and specificity were 100% (Axner and Strom-Holst 2015), whereas in a study of 98 male dogs, the sensitivity and specificity were 76 and 100%, respectively (Themmen et al. 2016). In the latter study, AMH testing correctly identified all neutered male dogs, but unfortunately failed to correctly identify a significant number of intact male dogs.

Assessment and Follow-Up

Spay–neuter programs should have policies and protocols in place to optimize identification of previously neutered male dogs and cats and to ensure proper sterilization of cryptorchid animals.

Verification of previous castration is generally much easier in cats, since examination of the penis allows for an accurate assessment in the majority of cases. Only in very young kittens and very recently neutered cats may findings be equivocal. When penile spines are present, surgery is indicated. Conversely, if the cat is verified to be neutered based on the absence of penile spines or an intact balano-prepucial fold in an adult cat, then marking the cat in accordance with the ASV guidelines for identification of neutered cats is indicated. No one will ever have to wonder again!

In dogs, verification of neuter status is frequently more challenging. The one exception might be an adult dog with an infantile penis. In this case, it is probably safe to assume the patient has been previously castrated. In the absence of such a finding, hormonal testing will be necessary for diagnostic confirmation, unless a testicle is readily palpable in the inguinal area or a Sertoli cell tumor is diagnosed. Point-of-care LH test kits are a convenient and promising option. When such hormonal testing is not an option due to lack of resources, assessment of neuter status should be based on

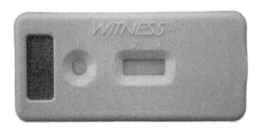

Figure 1.19 Witness LH test device. A commercially available point-of-care LH test (Witness LS, Zoetis, Parsippany, NJ, USA) may be used to distinguish reproductively intact and spayed dogs and cats. This test is simple to use and requires only four drops of serum.

a subjective clinical judgment considering all available information. The decision as to whether or not to pursue additional diagnostics or surgery should take into account the dog's breed, since there are significant known breed predilections for cryptorchidism. Considering all of the information available, if the clinical suspicion for cryptorchidism remains low, it is reasonable to assume that the dog has been previously neutered. However, without definitive determination, neuter identification marking should not be performed. Owners can be advised to watch for signs such as excessive urine marking or attraction to females that could alert them to the need for additional assessment.

Bitches and Queens: Reproductively Intact or Spayed?

The accurate identification of female dogs and cats that have been previously spayed poses a longstanding clinical dilemma. Bitches and queens with unknown histories are commonly presented to veterinarians and animal shelters. Some of these animals undergo anesthesia and surgery, only to reveal that previous ovariohysterectomy has been performed. This can translate into trauma for the animal, expense for the owner, and frustration for the attending veterinarian. It is important to recognize, however, that in the context of most spay–neuter programs, it may not be possible to make a definitive determination of spay status in many cases. As such, surgical exploration will often be the best course of action. Not only is it diagnostic, it will ensure that no female patient leaves without the benefit of an ovariohysterectomy. That said, in some cases surgery can be avoided. Avoiding surgery is especially important for patients that are assessed as potentially "high risk" for anesthesia, such as morbidly obese and brachycephalic animals.

Diagnosis

In addition to obtaining any available clinical history, diagnostic evaluation should also include a thorough physical examination. Imaging may be useful in some cases, but hormonal evaluation, when available, will provide the most definitive diagnostic information without surgery.

History and Clinical Signs

If history is available, it can be very helpful to the clinician tasked with determining the animal's true spay status. Even with a history of previous spaying, the possibility of ovarian remnant syndrome should not be discounted, especially in cats, since it has been reported to occur more frequently in this species compared to dogs (Wallace 1991; Miller 1995). Owners should always be questioned carefully regarding possible displays of estrus behavior or attraction of males. Cat owners may note vocalization, rubbing, and "friendly" behavior. Many estrual queens stretch, squirm, and roll in lateral recumbency, opening and closing their paws. They may also crouch and assume a lordosis stance while treading in place with their hind limbs and deflecting their tail laterally (Figure 1.20). Most cats experience winter anestrus, therefore time of year should be considered when assessing the presence of estrus signs. Cat owners may confuse normal affiliative or greeting behaviors such as head rubbing or tail waving with signs of estrus. Lordosis and treading can usually be induced in estrual queens by stroking the back or dorsal rump. This can be done during the course of an exam

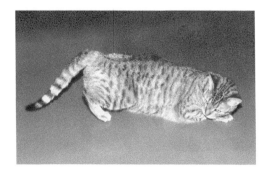

Figure 1.20   Cat in heat. An estrual queen exhibits a typical display of lordosis and tail deflection.

to help verify the presence of behavioral signs of estrus (Griffin 2001, 2006).

In the bitch, estrus is accompanied by dramatic physical changes, including marked enlargement of the vulva and bloody discharge, which are easy to recognize (Figure 1.21). In contrast, physical changes accompanying estrus are very subtle in cats. The queen's vulva becomes only slightly edematous and hyperemic, but remains so small and well covered by hair that changes are rarely noticed. Furthermore, vulvar discharge is scant, and because of the fastidious grooming habits of the queen, rarely noted (Griffin 2001). In cases where the presence of behavioral estrus is present or suspected at the time of examination, vaginal cytology to look for the presence of cornified vaginal epithelial cells can be performed for confirmation. Owners should also be questioned carefully regarding potential exposure to exogenous hormones, such as hormone replacement therapy, that could account for clinical signs (Griffin 2006).

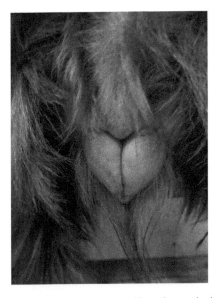

Figure 1.21 Dog in heat. Note the marked swelling of the labia and the presence of bloody discharge.

Physical Examination A complete physical examination should be performed. The overall body condition should be noted. Metabolic rate has been shown to significantly decrease and a tendency toward obesity has been well documented in spayed cats compared to reproductively intact queens (Flynn et al. 1996; Root et al. 1996a). If a cat is very overweight, a clinical suspicion that she has been previously spayed is warranted. In contrast, changes in metabolic rate following ovariohysterectomy have not been as well defined in bitches. These findings are consistent with the common clinical experiences of many surgeons, who find themselves regularly performing "big fat dog spays" but rarely performing ovariohysterectomies in highly obese feline patients.

To facilitate examination, the ventral abdomen should be shaved from the umbilicus to the pubis, and the skin of the midline carefully inspected for the presence of a scar. In some cases, sedation will be necessary for hair removal and thorough examination. Using a good light source to aid in inspection of the area is often rewarding. Applying a small amount of isopropyl alcohol to the skin may aid in visualization of linear scars that may otherwise remain undetected. In the author's experience, palpation is not a reliable indicator of the presence of a spay scar. Some intact females have a prominent linea alba that may be mistaken for a scar, and spayed cats and dogs frequently have scars that are not readily palpable, yet may be visualized once the overlying hair is removed. Although looking for a ventral abdominal scar is recommended, discovery of a scar does not verify that an animal has been previously spayed with certainty and should never be used as the sole criterion for assessment. The clinician must interpret this finding cautiously and in context with all other findings (e.g. history, body condition score, mammary development, etc.) in order to make the best possible assessment. In some cases, scars may be the result of other abdominal procedures such as C-section (Figure 1.22). In addition, previously spayed

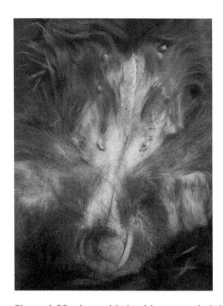

Figure 1.22 Intact bitch with a ventral abdominal scar from previous C-section. Note the well-developed mammary glands and vulva. Although looking for a ventral abdominal scar is recommended, discovery of a scar does not verify with certainty that an animal has been previously spayed and should never be used as the sole criterion for assessment.

animals may lack any such evidence of an abdominal incision, particularly if the animal was spayed at a very young age or if a flank approach was used (Griffin 2006).

Careful inspection of the mammary glands should also be performed. Spayed cats and dogs typically have atrophied mammary glands and very small teats subjectively, compared to the well-developed glands and prominent teats of intact females (Figure 1.22). In particular, the teats of cats spayed at very young ages remain underdeveloped and appear as tiny specks (Figure 1.23). Finally, examination of the vulva is indicated in bitches: when ovario-hysterectomy is performed prior to puberty, the vulva generally remains small and under-developed compared to intact females. When spayed following maturity, well-developed bitches typically experience some vulvar atrophy, but the vulva is unlikely to appear infantile (Olson 2003). That said, dogs can be very diverse physically and the vulva of some intact bitches will appear very small during anestrus, and some well-developed bitches will experience dramatic vulvar atrophy following ovario-hysterectomy (Figure 1.24a and b). Although

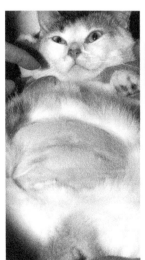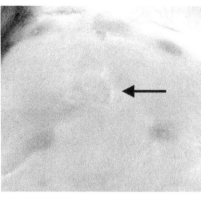

Figure 1.23 The shaved abdomen of a spayed cat. Careful inspection of the mammary glands may be helpful in distinguishing reproductively intact and spayed queens, since the mammary glands of spayed cats are generally underdeveloped or atrophic. Note the presence of a "spay scar" (arrow). This cat's body condition with ample abdominal fat also suggests that she is spayed.

(a)

(b)

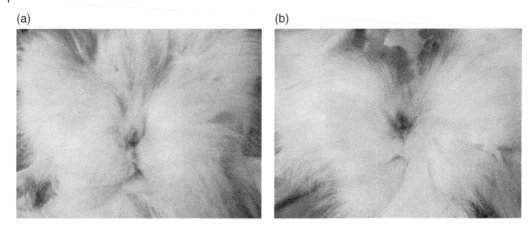

Figure 1.24   Clinicians should never use small vulvar size as a singular means of assessing spay status. In each photo, the vulva appears relatively small and underdeveloped, yet the reproductive status and history of these two bitches are very different. (a) Vulva of a three-year-old intact Great Pyrenees bitch. She whelped a litter six months prior to this photograph being taken. (b) Vulva of an eight-year-old spayed female Great Pyrenees bitch. She was spayed one year prior to this photo being taken.

examination of the external genitalia is recommended, neither mammary development nor vulvar size should be used as the sole criterion for assessment. As always, the clinician must interpret findings cautiously and in context with all other findings.

Diagnostic Imaging   When available, diagnostic imaging may be useful in some cases. If uterine enlargement or other pathology is present, radiography can sometimes be helpful, but otherwise this imaging modality is generally unrewarding for confirming or refuting the presence of the ovaries and uterus because of their indistinct radiodensity. In contrast, a highly skilled ultrasonographer with quality equipment should be able to identify the female reproductive tract in a cooperative patient. Practically speaking, however, this technique is infrequently used to assess spay status.

Hormonal Evaluation   If reproductive status cannot be determined based on physical examination, hormonal evaluation is ideally recommended prior to consideration of exploratory surgery. In some cases, owners may elect to wait and see if signs of behavioral estrus appear. Whenever possible, definitive

determination of reproductive status should be made.

Numerous studies have evaluated the diagnostic usefulness of LH and AMH tests for determination of spay status in female dogs and cats (Lofstedt and VanLeeuwen 2002; Place et al. 2011; Axner and Strom-Holst 2015; Themmen et al. 2016; Alm and Holst 2018; Krecic et al. 2018; Morrow et al. 2018). Serum concentrations of LH increase after ovarian removal as a result of the lack of negative feedback from the gonads. In reproductively intact females, the normal sequence of endocrinological events is such that LH concentrations remain at low basal concentrations, except for very brief periods when ovulation occurs and gonadotropin-releasing hormone stimulates LH release. After this sudden spike, LH returns to basal concentrations, usually within 24 hours. Negative feedback control of LH results from ovarian estradiol secretion and maintains LH at basal concentrations. Following ovariohysterectomy, this negative feedback control is removed, and LH concentrations remain increased indefinitely. Commercially available LH test kits will be "positive" in spayed animals, while negative results are consistent with the need for surgery. Patients should not be tested when signs of estrus are present to avoid false positive test results which occur during the LH surge. A study of 216 female cats revealed a 91% specificity and a 92% sensitivity using the Witness LH test (Krecic et al. 2018). In this study, it was unknown whether cats were displaying signs of estrus at the time of presentation for ovariohysterectomy. A study of 236 cats revealed a sensitivity of 69% and a specificity of 100% using the same test (Morrow et al. 2018). In other words, the test correctly detected all intact queens, and importantly there were no false positive results that would have incorrectly identified an intact cat as previously spayed. For cats without signs of heat, the point-of-care Witness LH test appears to be a highly useful means of distinguishing intact and spayed cats, while avoiding the need always to perform surgery to confirm spay status.

Alternatively, tests for measuring AMH may be used to distinguish spayed and sexually intact animals, since serum concentrations of AMH are only present in intact animals. AMH is continuously produced by the ovaries in post-pubescent queens and bitches, and production continues throughout the animal's reproductive life. AMH tests are positive in mature intact animals, while negative results are consistent with previous ovariohysterectomy (Place et al. 2011; Axner and Strom-Holst 2015; Themmen et al. 2016; Alm and Holst 2018). When using this test, is important to recognize that negative results may also be seen in intact females tested before reproductive maturity or after reproductive senescence. In one study of 31 female cats, AMH testing had 100% sensitivity and specificity (Axner and Strom-Holst 2015).

A recent study of 125 dogs utilized both AMH and LH testing for spay status determination (Alm and Holst 2018). Excluding bitches in heat, LH testing identified 100% of intact bitches compared to 88% correctly identified by AMH testing. In some instances, low concentrations of AMH were obtained in intact bitches, leading to incorrect classifica-

tion. The convenience of a point-of-care test and the diagnostic accuracy reported to date make the Witness LH test an especially desirable option for spay status determination. Both LH and AMH testing may also be helpful in the diagnosis of ovarian remnant syndrome in dogs and cats. For more information on diagnosis of ovarian remnant syndrome, see Chapter 18.

Assessment and Follow-Up

Spay–neuter programs should have policies and protocols in place to optimize identification of previously spayed female dogs and cats and to ensure that all patients are ultimately spayed. Ensuring that ovariohysterectomy is complete will not only prevent unwanted estrus behavior and pregnancies, it will also safeguard the health and welfare of the individual. Verification of previous spaying with absolute certainty is sometimes difficult and resources to perform hormonal testing may not be available. In some cases, the clinician will be able to make a confident assessment based on multiple findings consistent with a previously spayed animal. For example, it is reasonable to assume that an obese adult cat with a ventral midline scar and underdeveloped mammary glands has been previously spayed. In the event of available testing, it is also very reasonable to assume that dogs and cats with positive LH test results have been spayed, provided they are not tested while in heat.

Exploratory surgery is the final and most definitive diagnostic option for assessing spay status. Many surgeons will not "mark" a female animal as spayed unless they have either personally removed the ovaries or performed a negative exploratory laparotomy themselves. This approach is indeed wise and recommended, given how good the girls can be at fooling us sometimes.

References

Alm, H. and Holst, B.S. (2018). Identifying ovarian tissue in the bitch using anti-Mullerian hormone or luteinizing hormone. *Theriogenology* 106: 15–20.

Aronson, L.R. and Cooper, M.L. (1967). Penile spines of the domestic cat: their endocrine-behavior relations. *Anat. Rec.* 157: 71–78.

Axner, E. and Strom-Holst, B. (2015). Concentrations of anti-Mullerian hormone in the domestic cat: relation with spay or neuter status and serum estradiol. *Theriogenology* 83: 817–821.

Birchard, S.J. and Nappier, M. (2008). Cryptorchidism. *Compend. Contin. Educ. Pract. Vet.* 30: 325–337.

Flynn, M.F., Hardie, E.M., and Armstrong, P.J. (1996). Effect of ovariohysterectomy on maintenance energy requirement in cats. *JAVMA* 209: 1572–1581.

Griffin, B. (2001). Prolific cats: the estrous cycle. *Compend. Contin. Educ. Pract. Vet.* 23: 1049–1056.

Griffin, B. (2006). Feline reproductive hormones: diagnostic usefulness and clinical syndromes. In: *Consultations in Feline Internal Medicine V* (ed. J.R. August), 217–226. St Louis, MO: Elsevier Saunders.

Griffin, B., Bushby, P.A., McCobb, E. et al. (2016). The Association of Shelter Veterinarians' 2016 veterinary medical care guidelines for spay–neuter programs. *JAVMA* 249 (2): 165–188.

Gunzel-Apel, A.R., Seefeldt, A., Eschricht, F.M. et al. (2009). Effects of gonadectomy on prolactin and LH secretion and the pituitary thyroid axis in male dogs. *Theriogenology* 71: 746–753.

Herron, M.A. (1972). The effect of prepubertal castration on the penile urethra of the cat. *JAVMA* 160: 208–211.

Howe, L.M., Slater, M.R., Boothe, H.W. et al. (2000). Long-term outcome of gonadectomy performed at early age or traditional age in cats. *JAVMA* 217: 1661–1665.

Johnston, S.D., Root, M.V., and Olson, P.N.S. (1996). Ovarian and testicular function in the domestic cat: clinical management of spontaneous reproductive disease. *Anim. Reprod. Sci.* 42: 261–274.

Krecic, M.R., DiGangi, B.A., and Griffin, B. (2018). Accuracy of a point-of-care luteinizing hormone test for help in distinguishing between sexually intact and ovariectomized or castrated domestic cats. *J. Feline Med. Surg.* 20 (10): 955–961.

Ley, W.B., Holyoak, G.R., Digrassie, W.A. et al. (2003). Testicular and epididymal disorders. In: *The Practical Veterinarian: Small Animal Theriogenology* (ed. M.R. Kustritz), 457–491. St. Louis, MO: Elsevier Science.

Lofstedt, R.M. and VanLeeuwen, J.A. (2002). Evaluation of a commercially available luteinizing hormone test for its ability to distinguish between ovariectomized and sexually intact bitches. *JAVMA* 220: 1331–1335.

Memon, M.A., Ganjam, V.K., Pavletic, M.M. et al. (1992). Use of human chorionic gonadotropin stimulation test to detect a retained testis in a cat. *JAVMA* 201: 1602.

Miller, D.M. (1995). Ovarian remnant syndrome in dogs and cats: 46 cases (1988–1992). *J. Vet. Diagn. Investig.* 7: 572–574.

Millis, D.L., Hauptman, J.G., and Johnson, C.A. (1992). Cryptorchidism and monorchism in cats: 25 cases (1980–1989). *JAVMA* 200: 1128–1130.

Morrow, L.D., Gruffydd-Jones, T.J., Skillings, E. et al. (2018). Field study assessing the performance of a patient-side blood test to determine neuter status in female cats based on detection of luteinising hormone. *J. Feline Med. Surg.* 21: 553–558.

Olson, P.N. (2003). Prepuberal gonadectomy (early age neutering) in dogs and cats. In: *The ractical Veterinarian: Small Animal Theriogenology* (ed. M.R. Kustritz), 165–181. St. Louis, MO: Elsevier Science.

Olson, P.N., Mulnix, J.A., and Nett, T.M. (1992 May). Concentrations of luteinizing hormone and follicle-stimulating hormone in the serum of sexually intact and neutered dogs. *Am. J. Vet. Res.* 53 (5): 762–766.

Place, N.J., Hansen, B.S., Cheraskin, J. et al. (2011). Measurement of serum anti-Mullerian hormone concentration in female dogs and cats before and after ovariohysterectomy. *J. Vet. Diagn. Investig.* 23 (3): 524–527.

Richardson, E.F. and Mullen, H. (1993). Cryptorchidism in cats. *Compend. Contin. Educ. Pract. Vet.* 15: 1342–1345.

Root, M.V., Johnston, S.D., and Olson, P.N. (1996a). The effect of prepubertal and postpubertal gonadectomy on heat production measured by indirect calorimetry in male and female domestic cats. *Am. J. Vet. Res.* 57: 371–374.

Root, M.V., Johnston, S.D., and Olson, P.N. (1996b). The effect of prepubertal and postpubertal gonadectomy on penile extrusion and urethral diameter in the domestic cat. *Vet. Radiol. Ultrasound* 37: 363–366.

Salman, M.D., Hutchison, J., Ruch-Gallie, R. et al. (2000). Behavioral reasons for relinquishment of dogs and cats to 12 shelters. *J. Appl. Anim. Welf. Sci.* 2: 93–106.

Spain, C.V., Scarlett, J.M., and Houpt, K.A. (2004). Long-term risks and benefits of early-age gonadectomy in cats. *JAVMA* 224: 380–387.

Stubbs, W.P. and Bloomberg, M.S. (1995). Implications of early neutering in the dog and cat. *Semin. Vet. Med. Surg.* 10: 8–12.

Stubbs, W.P., Bloomberg, M.S., Scruggs, S.L. et al. (1996). Effects of prepubertal and postpubertal gonadectomy on physical and behavioral development in cats. *JAVMA* 209: 1864–1871.

Themmen, A.P.N., Kalra, B., Visser, J.A. et al. (2016). The use of anti-Mullerian hormone as a diagnostic for gonadectomy status in dogs. *Theriogenology* 86: 1467–1474.

Wallace, M.S. (1991). The ovarian remnant syndrome in the bitch and queen. *Vet. Clin. North Am. Small Anim. Pract.* 21: 501–517.

Wheeler, R. and Kutzler, M. (2010). LH testing is accurate for diagnosing the presence or absence of testicular tissue and dogs [abstract]. *Clin. Theriogenol.* 2: 382.

Yates, D., Hayes, G., Heffernan, M., and Beynon, R. (2003). Incidence of cryptorchidism in dogs and cats. *Vet. Rec.* 152 (16): 502–504.

2

Disorders of Sexual Development and Common Reproductive Pathologies

Brenda Griffin, Sara White, and Margaret V. Root Kustritz

Over the course of their practice, the high-quality high-volume spay–neuter (HQHVSN) surgeon can expect to see a number of unusual presentations of patient sex resulting from various disorders of sexual development (DSDs), as well as a variety of reproductive tract pathologies that may also be discovered at the time of spay–neuter surgery. This chapter reviews the embryonic process of sexual determination and differentiation and discusses the clinical findings associated with various DSDs. Notable reproductive pathologies (such as pyometra, ovarian cysts, mammary hyperplasia, and ectopic fetuses) that may be seen at the time of spay–neuter surgery are also briefly reviewed.

Embryology of Sexual Development

Normal embryologic development of the canine and feline reproductive tracts is briefly reviewed here for the purpose of informing the reader's understanding of normal versus anomalous development (Figure 2.1). For more detailed information, readers are referred to comprehensive reviews of embryology of the dog and cat, which are readily available elsewhere in the veterinary literature (McGeady et al. 2006; Fletcher and Weber 2012).

During embryologic development, sexual differentiation occurs in three sequential steps.

First, chromosomal sex (XX or XY) is established at fertilization. Next, gonadal differentiation is determined by the sex chromosomes of the individual – the development of ovaries confers the gonadal sex of females, while the development of testes confers that of males. Ultimately, phenotypic sexual development (internal and external genitalia) occurs in response to gene expression which prompts the production of various chemical substances and ultimately the male and female hormones. Current knowledge and understanding of these processes suggest that an active interplay of testis-producing versus ovary-producing products is responsible for normal development. This is in contrast to the traditional or historical view that deemed ovarian development a default that occurred in the absence of a Y chromosome. This current knowledge of normal development makes it easier to understand how anomalous development can occur.

In the developing embryo, mesodermal tissue forms the urogenital ridge, which splits into the nephrogenic cord (which goes on to form the urinary tract) and the genital ridge. Primordial germ cells from the yolk sac migrate in the developing embryo to the genital ridge in the first trimester of pregnancy. These cells must be present for formation of the gonads to occur, and it is the formation of a specific type of gonad (i.e. male or female) that directs all further development. The initial undifferentiated, or

High-Quality, High-Volume Spay and Neuter and Other Shelter Surgeries, First Edition. Edited by Sara White.
© 2020 John Wiley & Sons, Inc. Published 2020 by John Wiley & Sons, Inc.

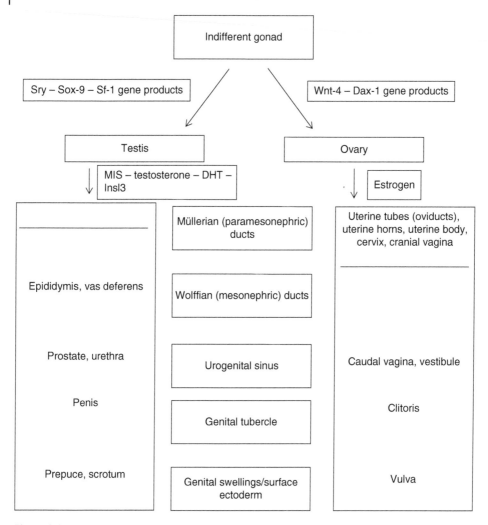

Figure 2.1 Normal embryologic development of the canine and feline reproductive tract. DHT, dihydrotestosterone; Insl3, insulin-like peptide 3; MIS, müllerian-inhibiting substance.

indifferent, gonad is stimulated to form either an ovary or a testis by virtue of the chromosome complement of the developing embryo. In the presence of the indifferent gonad, both the wolffian ducts (also known as the mesonephric ducts) and the müllerian ducts (also known as the paramesonephric ducts) are present. These ducts go on to form the internal male and female reproductive tracts, respectively.

A region of the Y chromosome, the Sry or sex-determining region, contains genes that express products directing formation of cords of tissue enclosing the primordial germ cells to

form early seminiferous tubules. Genes and their products associated with formation of the testis include Sox-9 and Sf-1, which stimulate development of Sertoli cells and Leydig cells (also known as interstitial cells). The fetal testes secrete testosterone during gestation (Arrighi et al. 2010).

Three secretory products from the fetal testes guide development of the male tubular tract and external genitalia. Sertoli cells secrete müllerian-inhibiting substance (MIS; also known as anti-müllerian factor or anti-müllerian hormone), which inhibits continuing development of the female ductal tract. Leydig cells secrete testosterone and insulin-like peptide 3 (Insl-3). Testosterone and its metabolite, dihydrotestosterone, promote development of the male ductal tract and external genitalia. Insl-3 plays a role in mediation of the process of testicular descent (Nef and Parada 2000; Cassata et al. 2008; Arrighi et al. 2010).

Testicular descent occurs in three stages and requires the presence of hormonally active testes and gubernacula – embryonic structures that attach to the caudal pole of each gonad (Baumans et al. 1982, 1983). Each embryonal testis is held caudal to the respective kidney by the cranial suspensory ligament, while the caudal pole of the testis is attached to the external inguinal ring by its gubernaculum. The first stage of testicular descent, abdominal translocation, is characterized by maintenance of the testes at the internal inguinal rings as the body lengthens and the gubernacula stretch and thin (Amann and Veeramachaneni 2007). This stage is mediated by Insl-3 (Christensen 2012). The second stage, transinguinal migration, is associated with increase in size of the gubernacula due to increased intracellular fluid, with subsequent dilation of the inguinal canals. This, coupled with increasing intraabdominal pressure and contraction of the internal inguinal rings and abdominal oblique muscles, pushes the testes through the inguinal canals. This stage is testosterone dependent. In the final stage of testicular descent, inguinoscrotal descent (which is also testosterone dependent), the gubernacula decrease in size and migrate to the scrotum, ultimately pulling the testes into the scrotal sac (Nef and Parada 2000; Christensen 2012). A final factor contributing to translocation of the testis into the scrotum is release of the chemoattractant calcitonin gene-related peptide from the genitofemoral nerve, which innervates the distal quarter of the scrotum (Kitchell et al. 1988; Amann and Veeramachaneni 2007).

The male tubular tract (i.e. the epididymis and vas deferens) forms from the wolffian ducts under the influence of testosterone and dihydrotestosterone. Secretion of MIS from the fetal testis causes regression of the müllerian ducts. Under the influence of dihydrotestosterone, the urethra and prostate form from the urogenital sinus, the penis from the genital tubercle, and the prepuce and scrotum from the genital swellings and surface ectoderm.

In the absence of a Y chromosome, a conflicting set of gene products guides gonad development. Wnt-4 promotes development of the ovary by inhibiting formation of Leydig cells and stimulating mesothelial cells surrounding primordial germ cells to form sex cords that break apart into primordial follicles (Nef and Parada 2000). Wnt-4 is also present and active in the fetal male prior to sex differentiation, but is repressed by Sox-9 (Carlson 2018). Wnt-4 also upregulates expression of Dax-1, which inhibits Sf-1 by downregulating Sox-9, and subsequently inhibits male development (Nef and Parada 2000; Christensen 2012). The fetal ovaries secrete estrogen.

The female tubular tract forms from the müllerian ducts. The müllerian ducts form the uterine tubes (oviducts), uterine horns, uterine body, cervix, and cranial vagina. Under the influence of estrogen, the caudal vagina and vestibule form from the urogenital sinus, the clitoris from the genital tubercle, and the vulva from the genital swellings and surface ectoderm.

Disorders of Sexual Development

DSDs are present at birth, but are often not identified until affected individuals with abnormal genitalia are presented for spay–neuter surgery. DSDs include abnormalities of chromosomal sex, abnormalities of gonadal sex (the gonads do not correspond to the chromosomal sex), and abnormalities of phenotypic sex (internal or external genitalia do not agree with the gonads and sex chromosome complement). In all cases, gonadectomy is recommended for affected individuals. In rare cases, affected individuals may have concurrent signs of urinary tract abnormalities, in which case additional medical evaluation is warranted, ideally prior to spay–neuter surgery.

Nomenclature

Nomenclature in veterinary medicine to describe the abnormalities is changing to better incorporate findings of molecular diagnosis and to match that used in the human literature. Historically, the term "intersex" was used to describe any condition in which the animal has characteristics of both sexes and encompassed both pseudohermaphrodites and true hermaphrodites (Howard and Bjorling 1989). Currently, the term "intersex" is being replaced with "disorder of sexual development" and divided into three main categories: sex chromosome DSD, XX DSD, and XY DSD. Sex chromosome DSD is any abnormality of sex chromosome number associated with a DSD. Examples include Klinefelter's syndrome (XXY) and Turner's syndrome (XO), both of which are associated with underdeveloped internal and external genitalia and abnormal cycling or infertility. XY DSD describes any abnormality of gonads, or internal or external genitalia, in an individual with one X and one Y chromosome, while XX DSD describes any such abnormality in an individual with two X chromosomes (Meyers-Wallen 2012a).

The terms hermaphrodite and pseudohermaphrodite have been phased out and replaced in human healthcare, but are still commonly used in veterinary settings and veterinary publications and may be most familiar to readers. These DSDs represent discordance between gonadal and phenotypic sex (i.e. errors in the sex differentiation processes). In short, a female pseudohermaphrodite has ovaries and XX chromosomes, but the external genitals appear masculine, resulting in some mixture or blurring of sexual anatomy. The degree of masculinization ranges from a normal vulva with mild clitoral enlargement to a somewhat normal penis and prepuce with an internal prostate. A male pseudohermaphrodite has

testes and XY chromosomes, but external genitals appear feminine, resulting in some mixture or blurring of sexual anatomy. The degree of feminization varies – a penis may be present or, more often, a vulva with an enlarged clitoris. The testes may be located in the abdomen, scrotum, or lateral to the vulva, and internally vestigial oviducts and a uterus may be present. A true hermaphrodite (Figure 2.2) has at least one ovary and at least one testis, or at least one ovotestis, regardless of chromosomal (XX or XY) or phenotypic sex (Dreger et al. 2005). Finally, the term "sex reversal" is sometimes used to denote abnormalities of gonadal sex. In this case, the gonads present do not match the individual's karyotype (i.e. XX males, XX true hermaphrodites, XY females, XY true hermaphrodites).

In most cases, the HQHVSN or shelter veterinarian presented with a patient with ambiguous or mixed sex characteristics will have no idea of the chromosomal sex, the true gonadal sex or the genetic origins of the particular DSD (Figure 2.3). Whether using new or old nomenclature, the correct categorization of the

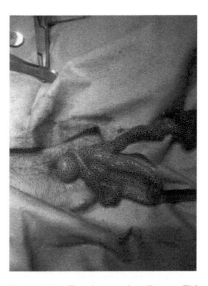

Figure 2.2   True hermaphrodite cat. This cat appeared to be unilaterally cryptorchid, but upon exploration for the abdominal testicle, a uterus and ovaries, as well as the abdominal testicle, were found. *Source:* Photo courtesy of Kristin Budinich.

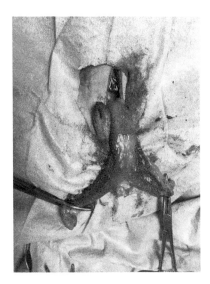

Figure 2.3 Dog who appeared to be a cryptorchid male, but upon abdominal exploration a uterus and ovaries were found. *Source:* Photo courtesy of Alana Canupp.

individual patient may be impossible (especially prior to surgery), since different developmental pathways can result in similar external appearances. For example, an externally female dog with an enlarged clitoris (Figure 2.4) may have (i) an XY genotype, testes, and male tubular structures (a male pseudohermaphrodite); (ii) an XX genotype and ovaries (a female pseudohermaphrodite); (iii) an XY genotype with ovary and testis or ovotestes

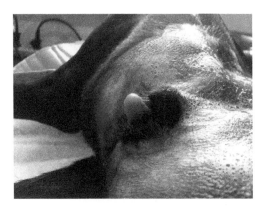

Figure 2.4 Dog presenting as a female with an enlarged clitoris. During surgery, this dog was found to have two testes. *Source:* Photo courtesy of Sara White.

(a true hermaphrodite); or (iv) an XX genotype with ovotestes (also a true hermaphrodite; Sumner et al. 2018). When approaching surgery on these patients, the goal is to remove the gonads. Fortunately for the surgeon, the approach is familiar and is similar to the approach to cryptorchid surgery: the gonads and their tubular structures are located somewhere between the caudal pole of the kidneys, the inguinal area, and the perineum (see Chapter 14 for more details). After gonadectomy, a more specific diagnosis or description of the disorder may be evident based on the physical appearance of the gonads and genitalia. However, karyotyping is necessary to define chromosomal abnormalities (check laboratory instructions online for sample collection instructions), and gross descriptions of both external and internal genitalia combined with histopathology of the gonads and tubular tracts are required for definitive characterization of the given disorder. Although histologic examination of the gonads and tubular structures could be pursued, it is not necessary for the patient's care in most cases. Some patients, such as female dogs with an enlarged clitoris, may require additional surgery such as clitoridectomy to relieve chronic urinary tract infections and local irritation (Sumner et al. 2018). Similarly, patients with hypospadias may require urinary tract surgery due to urine scald or urinary incontinence.

Sex Chromosome Disorders of Sexual Development

Abnormalities of chromosomal sex are those in which the karyotype does not match the gonads, tubular tract, or external genitalia, and often are errors of gamete formation such that too many or too few sex chromosomes are present (Poth et al. 2010). Disorders of sex chromosomes occur randomly during gamete formation or early development, therefore it is possible for them to occur in dogs and cats of any breed. Klinefelter's syndrome (XXY) is the most commonly reported sex chromosome abnormality in dogs and cats. Affected individuals typically have hypoplastic testes and are infertile. Other examples of abnormalities of chromosomal sex include XO syndrome (monosomy X, known as Turner's syndrome in humans) and XXX syndrome (trisomy X; O'Connor et al. 2011). Both are very rarely reported in the veterinary literature and are typically associated with underdeveloped internal and external genitalia and infertility. Finally, chimeras or mosaics (XX/XY and XY/XY) represent another possible abnormality in chromosomal development. These animals may have a variety of different presentations, ranging from those with normal sexual development to true hermaphrodites (Strain et al. 1998).

Male Calico Cats

One specific example of an abnormality of chromosomal sex is the calico or tortoiseshell male cat (Figure 2.5a and b), which is almost always related to a sex chromosome DSD. In cats, white coat color is carried on an autosome. Orange and non-orange (black) are alleles on the X chromosome (Chastain et al. 1988). For a male cat to exhibit both orange and non-orange, he must have two different X chromosomes. This can be due to a simple increase in the number of sex chromosomes from nondisjunction errors during gamete

formation, or may be due to the presence of multiple cell lines, either as a chimera (two cell lines derived from two zygotes) or as a mosaic (two cell lines derived from one zygote). Male calico or tortoiseshell cats with XY/XY or XX/XY karyotypes may be fertile, but many affected male cats have karyotypes with abnormal cell lines (for example XY/XXY) and are infertile (Malouf et al. 1967; Loughman et al. 1970; Loughman and Frye 1974; Hageltorn and Gustavsson 1981; Long et al. 1981). Male calico cats with XXY genotype (Klinefelter's syndrome) are infertile (Meyers-Wallen 2012b). Regardless of their fertility status, bilateral scrotal testes are often present in tomcats with any of these sex chromosome abnormalities. For those tomcats that are infertile, the testes may appear relatively small.

Sex chromosome DSD is not the only way that a calico cat can present as a male, although it appears to be by far the most common. There is a report of a single calico cat with male external genitalia who presented bilaterally cryptorchid, but who had an XX karyotype accompanied by an adrenal enzyme deficiency causing androgen excess (Meyers-Wallen 2012b). Two other case reports describe an SRY-negative, testicular XX tortoiseshell cat with apparently normal scrotal testes (De Lorenzi et al. 2017) and an SRY-positive XX

(a)

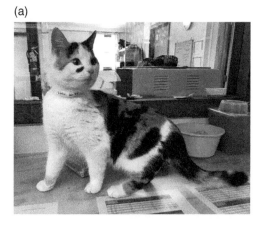

(b)

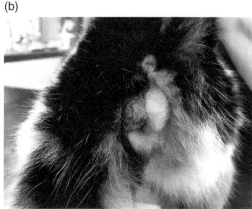

Figure 2.5 (a and b) Male calico cat neutered at a HQHVSN clinic. Both testicles were in the scrotum, and the cat had penile spines. *Source:* Photo courtesy of Pamela Krausz.

tortoiseshell cat with a juvenile penis without spines, two vas deferens, no scrotum, and no detectable gonads (Szczerbal et al. 2015).

When presented with a male calico cat for neutering, the spay–neuter veterinarian is unlikely to know the genetic and/or hormonal mechanism behind the cat's unusual presentation. Fortunately, these cats can be approached like any other cat castration. If a male calico has scrotal testes, he should be neutered routinely without abdominal exploration for additional gonads. If the cat appears cryptorchid, then abdominal surgery is obviously required, and the gonads and tubular system may be those of a male, female, or true hermaphrodite. While there is a small chance that a calico male with two scrotal testes could also have internal vestigial female tubular structures, these may cause no future problems, and routine abdominal exploration of these cats is not warranted unless clinical problems are evident.

XY Disorders of Sexual Development

As previously stated, XY DSD describes any abnormality of gonads, or internal or external genitalia, in an individual with one X and one Y chromosome. These include XY males with failure of the müllerian ducts to regress, as well as individuals with defects in androgen-dependent masculinization. The XY DSD classification therefore encompasses both male pseudohermaphrodites and true hermaphrodites (also known as ovotesticular DSD).

Persistent Müllerian Duct Syndrome
Persistent müllerian duct syndrome (PMDS) is a hereditary condition of miniature Schnauzers in the United States and of basset hounds in Europe, and has been reported in other breeds as well. Affected dogs possess male external genitalia, but develop both male and female internal tubular structures (i.e. they develop a uterus). In addition, many affected dogs are cryptorchid (Nickel et al. 1992; Meyers-Wallen

2009). Affected dogs may be asymptomatic or may present with clinical signs of hyperestrogenism due to neoplasia of retained testes, including gynecomastia, pendulous preputial sheath, symmetrical nonpruritic alopecia, and attraction of male dogs; pyometra; urinary tract disease; abdominal pain; or prostate disease (Brown et al. 1976; Nickel et al. 1992; Wu et al. 2009; Christensen 2012). Dogs with this condition with at least one scrotal testicle are fertile (Meyers-Wallen 2012b). Similar abnormalities are likely in cats, but have not been confirmed (Meyers-Wallen 2012b). Surgical removal of gonads and all tubular reproductive structures is indicated.

Defects in Androgen-Dependent Masculinization
In this case, XY males develop bilateral testes and no müllerian duct derivatives, but experience incomplete masculinization of the internal and external genitalia. A variety of defects in androgen-dependent masculinization are possible and can result in abnormal phenotypes ranging from mild to severe. Examples of defects include insufficient androgen production, androgen resistance, and deficiencies in androgen receptors. Affected individuals may have poorly developed or ambiguous external genitalia (as in a male pseudohermaphrodite). In particular, one such defect results in "testicular feminization syndrome," where an animal has testes, usually is cryptorchid, and is a phenotypic female (Meyers-Wallen et al. 1989; Peter et al. 1993). The fault in development is due to defective androgen receptor function and the condition may be hereditary in dogs and cats (Meyers-Wallen et al. 1989; Peter et al. 1993). The testes are present in affected animals and secrete normal amounts of testosterone and MIS, therefore müllerian duct derivatives are absent. However, masculinization is absent or incomplete as a result of the defect in the androgen receptor gene. Other clinical presentations associated with defects in androgen-dependent masculinization include

cryptorchid animals, hypospadias, and other abnormalities of the penis and/or prepuce.

Cryptorchidism Cryptorchidism (Figure 2.6) is characterized by failure in the descent of one (unilateral) or both (bilateral) testis from the abdominal cavity to the scrotum (Burke 1986). Undescended or incompletely descended testes may be located in the abdomen, in the inguinal canal, or in the subcutaneous tissue between the inguinal canal and the scrotum. Testes should be descended into the scrotum in most dogs and cats by 5 days of age, and one-fourth of those not descended by 10 days of age will descend by 14 weeks of age (Dunn et al. 1968). In one study of 1494 cryptorchid dogs, testicular descent occurred in 24.5% by six months of age, with descent of testes more common in dogs with unilateral cryptorchidism than in those with bilateral cryptorchidism (Dunn et al. 1968). By six months of age on average, the inguinal canal is closed in dogs and further testicular descent is not likely.

Genetic, epigenetic, and environmental factors contribute to abnormal testicular descent (Amann and Veeramachaneni 2007). The mode of inheritance is not defined, but is most likely polygenic recessive (Amann and Veeramachaneni 2007). Heritability, defined as the amount of variation in the population due to genetic factors, is reported to vary by breed, with a range from 0.23 in boxers to 0.75 in German shepherd dogs (Neilen et al. 2001; Dolf et al. 2010). Although cryptorchidism can only be exhibited in male dogs (sex-limited trait), bitches can carry genes for abnormal testicular descent and carriers bred to carriers will produce affected pups (Gubbels et al. 2009). Breeding of carriers also is associated with increased litter size and increased number of males in the litter, suggesting that selection for those desirable traits may contribute to the persistence of cryptorchidism in a breeding population (Turba and Willer 1988; Gubbels et al. 2009).

Cryptorchidism is more prevalent in purebred animals than in crossbred animals, in some specific breeds of dog and cat, and in smaller variants of a given type of breed, for example toy poodles compared to standard poodles (Hayes et al. 1985; Millis et al. 1992). The reported incidence is 1.2–12.9% in dogs and 0.007–1.7% in cats (Priester et al. 1970; Kawakami et al. 1984; Millis et al. 1992; Ruble and Hird 1993). Cryptorchidism may be unilateral or bilateral, with unilateral cryptorchidism more common (Millis et al. 1992). There is no difference in incidence between right unilateral and left unilateral cryptorchidism (Kawakami et al. 1984; Millis et al. 1992; Nelson and Couto 1994), although one report (Mattos et al. 2000) indicates that the lack of descent in dogs is found twice as often on the right side as on the left.

Abnormalities associated with cryptorchidism in dogs include PMDS, umbilical hernias, hypospadias, micropenis, and phimosis (Brown et al. 1976; Pope and Swaim 1985; Nickel et al. 1992; Switonski et al. 2012). Concurrent abnormalities reported in cats include cardiac murmurs, microphthalmia and upper eyelid agenesis, patellar luxation, tarsal defect, and shortened tail (Richardson and Mullen 1993).

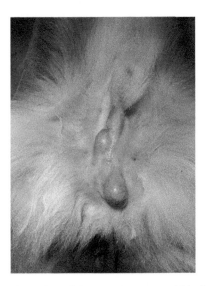

Figure 2.6 Subcutaneous cryptorchid adult dog. The cryptorchid testis is evident just lateral to the prepuce. *Source:* Photo courtesy of Sara White.

Veterinarians occasionally are presented with an animal with no scrotal testes who is assumed to have been previously castrated, but who is showing male behaviors or physiologic changes suggesting the presence of one or more retained testes. Detection of intraabdominal testes by imaging techniques is difficult, because retained testes are smaller than descended testes and they may be anywhere in the inguinal area or abdomen (Cox et al. 1978; Batista Arteaga et al. 2000). In cats, presence of penile spines is a good bioassay for presence of elevated serum testosterone concentration and indicates that one or both testicles are retained. Penile spines begin to form by 12 weeks of age and are fully developed by 6 months of age (Aronson and Cooper 1967) (see Chapter 1). If blood testing is done, the pulsatile release of testosterone requires challenge testing. A reported regimen in dogs is administration of 1–2 mcg/kg gonadotropin-releasing hormone (GnRH) intramuscularly (IM) with blood drawn 60 minutes later; any value greater than 3 ng/ml is indicative of testicular tissue (Meyers-Wallen 1991). A reported regimen in cats is administration of 500 IU of human chorionic gonadotropin (hCG) intravenously (IV) with blood drawn at baseline, 30 minutes, and 2 hours later; rising values are indicative of testicular tissue (Memon et al. 1992). See Chapter 1 for more information on testing to determine neuter status.

Bilateral castration is recommended for all cryptorchid dogs and cats. Retained testes do not produce spermatozoa but do produce testosterone, leaving the animal exposed to risk for androgen-dependent disease (Batista Arteaga et al. 2000). In dogs, retained testes are 9.2–13.6 times more likely to become neoplastic than are descended testes and testicular neoplasia develops earlier in life in retained than in descended testes (Reif and Brodey 1969; Neilsen and Lein 1974; Pendergrass and Hayes 1975; Hayes and Pendergrass 1976; Hayes et al. 1985). Neoplasia, most often Sertoli cell tumors and seminomas, occurs in the ectopic testis more frequently than in the eutopic, and generally appears in animals of 6–10 years of age (Mattos et al. 2000).

Monorchidism (one testis) and polyorchidism (three testes) are described in dogs and cats, but are exceedingly rare events (Millis et al. 1992; Atkinson 1998). Individuals that present with only one scrotal testicle should be considered cryptorchid until proven otherwise (see Chapter 1 for more information).

Hypospadias Hypospadias is abnormal ventral closure of the penis and in some cases the prepuce, with subsequent abnormal translocation of the urethral opening ventral and posterior to the location of the normal urethral orifice (Figures 2.7a and b and 2.8a–c). Hypospadias may be glandular, with the opening just proximal to the normal urethral orifice; penile, with the opening on the shaft of the penis; scrotal, with the opening near the body of the penis; or perineal.

Reported associated conditions include cryptorchidism, penile frenulum, micropenis, intersex states, monorchidism, recurrent urinary tract infections, and anorectal defects (Kipnis 1974; Hayes and Wilson 1986; Galanty et al. 2008; Jurka et al. 2009; Switonski et al. 2012; Guimaraes et al. 2013). Reported clinical manifestations include inability to achieve a normal stream during voluntary micturition, stranguria, hematuria, urinary incontinence, recurrent urinary tract infections, licking of the penis/prepuce, periurethral dermatitis, urine scald dermatitis of the inguinal area, and medial hindlimbs (Root Kustritz 2001; Pavletic 2007; Adelsberger and Smeak 2009; Jurka et al. 2009; Guimaraes et al. 2013). Some dogs are asymptomatic and there is one report of hypospadias as an incidental finding in a dog that had successfully bred a bitch (Ader and Hobson 1978; Hardy and Root Kustritz 2005).

Diagnosis is by inspection. If the abnormal urethral opening is near the penile tip, it may not require surgery; in other cases reconstruction is recommended (Guimaraes et al. 2013). Surgical repair of glandular or penile hypospadias may be as simple as recreation of a patent

(a) (b)

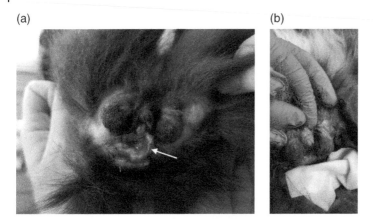

Figure 2.7 Hypospadias in two tomcats. In both photos the cats have been anesthetized, prepped, and positioned in dorsal recumbency for castration. In both cases, two scrotal testicles are present. In the absence of clinical signs of urinary problems, castration can be surgically approached as for any other tomcat. (a) This cat's urethral opening is large (white arrow) and his prepuce has not formed completely, so that his penis could be mistaken for an enlarged clitoris. *Source:* Photo courtesy of BobbieJean Baker. (b) This cat is similar to the first, but the prepuce has been partially reflected to expose the tip of the penis. Note that penile spines are evident. In this photo, the anus is covered by a gauze sponge. *Source:* Photo courtesy of Rebecca Trejo.

(a) (b) (c)

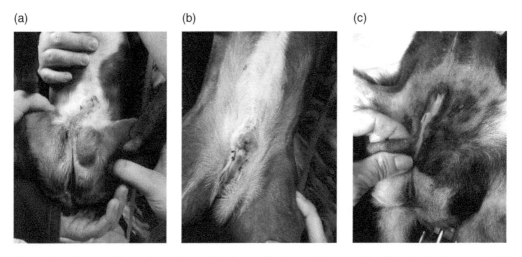

Figure 2.8 Hypospadias in dogs. (a) An adult Boston Terrier with hypospadias. This dog is also cryptorchid. Location and evaluation of the urethral orifice are needed in order to determine the appropriate surgical management necessary for this patient in addition to castration. In cases of hypospadias, the orifice may be located anywhere along the ventrum of the glans penis to the perineum. (b) The prepuce of the same Boston Terrier as in (a). The dog had openings on each side of the partially formed prepuce that resembled a vulva with smegma-like discharge. *Source:* Photos courtesy of Brooke Groskopf. (c) Hypospadias in a puppy. Testicles are present caudally on each side of the urethra. *Source:* Photo courtesy of Alana Canupp.

urethra by appropriate apposition of mucosal and serosal tissues. Surgical repair is more complicated in cases of scrotal or perineal hernia; in the most extreme cases, penile amputation and perineal urethrostomy may be required.

Penile Frenulum The balanopreputial fold is an androgen-dependent piece of tissue that binds the penis to the prepuce ventrally during development and is normally dissolved by the time of puberty or even earlier in dogs and cats

(Howard and Bjorling 1989; Root et al. 1996). Persistence of a portion of this fold usually is seen as a band of tissue connecting the glans penis to the shaft of the penis or to the preputial mucosa (see Chapter 1, Figure 1.14). Dogs may be asymptomatic or may have clinical manifestations including dysuria, discomfort or inability to breed by natural service or have semen collected by manual ejaculation, licking of the penis/prepuce, phallocampsis (curvature of the erect penis), and urine scald dermatitis of the inguinal area and medial hindlimbs (Belkin 1969; Hutchison 1973; Ryer 1979; Balke 1981; Pugh et al. 1987; Sahay et al. 1987; Olsen and Salwei 2001). Diagnosis is by inspection and surgical repair involves simple transection of the frenulum, which usually is avascular.

Micropenis   Micropenis, or infantile penis, is an unusually small penis relative to the size of the dog. This condition may be associated with cryptorchidism, phimosis, or intersex states (Proescholdt and DeYoung 1977; Root Kustritz 2001). Clinical manifestations include dripping of urine, hematuria, dysuria, and balanoposthitis (Proescholdt and DeYoung 1977).

Phimosis   Phimosis is inability to extrude the penis. Congenital phimosis usually is associated with a stenotic preputial orifice such that the urine stream is very small and the prepuce may fill with urine (Papazoglou and Kazakos 2002). The penis may or may not be normal and other abnormalities may be present, such as cryptorchidism (Jacobs and Baughman 1977; Pope and Swaim 1985). The condition may be congenital or acquired. The most common causes of acquired phimosis are scarring from lacerations following trauma, sucking of the puppy's or kitten's prepuce by littermates, and licking from the dam. Neoplasia in this area may also narrow the preputial orifice (Papazoglou and Kazakos 2002). Surgical repair involves recreation of a preputial orifice.

XX Disorders of Sexual Development

As previously stated, XX DSD describes any abnormality of gonads, or internal or external genitalia, in an individual with two X chromosomes. The XX DSD classification therefore encompasses both female pseudohermaphrodites and true hermaphrodites. The degree of phenotypic masculinization has been correlated to the proportion of testicular tissue present in a given individual (Meyers-Wallen 2012a). Clinical presentations range from a normal vulva with mild clitoral enlargement to a somewhat normal penis and prepuce with an internal prostate.

XX sex reversal has been well documented in dogs, although it has not been reported in cats. Affected dogs can either have both ovarian and testicular tissue (true hermaphrodites or ovotesticular DSD) or only testicular tissue (pseudohermaphrodites or testicular DSD; Meyers-Wallen 2012a). Individuals with XX sex reversal have an XX karyotype, testes or ovotestes, and abnormal male genitalia, such as a small or caudally displaced penis, or ambiguous female genitalia, such as a prepuce-like vulva (Figure 2.9; Hare et al. 1974; Sommer and Meyers-Wallen 1991). Clinical presentations range from true hermaphrodites – partially masculinized females with ovotestes – to XX males with malformed male external genitalia and cryptorchid aspermatogenic testes. This condition is inherited as an autosomal recessive trait in American cocker spaniels. Other breeds, including English cocker spaniels, beagles, Weimaraners, pugs, and German shorthaired pointers, have also been reported to have a hereditary predisposition (Stewart et al. 1972; Hare et al. 1974; Christensen 2012).

Other less dramatic abnormalities of the female reproductive tract can also result from variations in development. These may involve the ovaries, uterus, vagina, and/or vulva. In many cases, these abnormalities will be clinically insignificant, although some may require special treatment. Additionally, a number of reproductive pathologies may be seen in

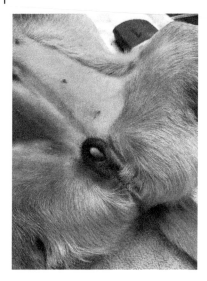

Figure 2.9   Dog with a prepuce-like vulva. This dog had a uterus and intraabdominal gonads that were removed at surgery. *Source:* Photo courtesy of Sara Cooper.

female patients undergoing spay surgery, and the most notable of these are described in this section as well.

Abnormalities of the Ovaries

Agenesis   Ovarian agenesis is rare. If absence of a uterine horn or a kidney is noted during surgery, a concerted effort should still be made to find an ovary on that side. Ovarian

dysgenesis has been reported in cats with XO/XXX and XO/XX mosaicism; these cats had normal ovarian tissue on one side and nodular tissue at the site where the ovary should have been on the other side (Dybdahl Thomsen et al. 1987).

Cysts   Ovarian cysts (Figure 2.10a–c) are acquired (not congenital) abnormalities that can occur in both dogs and cats (Gelberg et al. 1984; Arlt and Haimerl 2016; Eissa et al. 2017). Ovarian cysts are fluid-filled structures that may originate from various tissues and include hormonally active stromal (follicular and luteal) cysts (Marino et al. 2010), as well as hormonally inactive cystic rete ovarii and paraovarian (or extraovarian) cysts (Arlt and Haimerl 2016). Prevalence estimates of the different types of cysts vary between studies and between species. Follicular cysts are most likely to appear lobular, whereas cystic rete ovarii may have a single, large, fluid-filled cyst compressing the stroma of the ovary (Eissa et al. 2017). The hormonally active stromal cysts may result in signs of persistent estrus or signs related to chronically elevated estrogen concentrations (Arlt and Haimerl 2016). Both stromal and rete ovarii cysts, when large, can compress ovarian stroma and cause infertility. Paraovarian cysts (Figure 2.11) are more

(a)

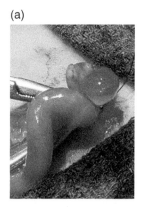

(b)

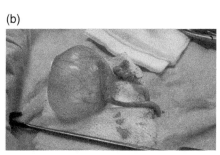

(c)

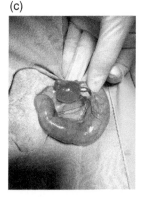

Figure 2.10   Ovarian cysts. (a) Ovarian cyst in a cat. Cyst measuring approximately 1 cm is to the right above the hemostat tip, and actively cycling ovary with corpora hemorrhagica is to the left above the hemostat. *Source:* Photo courtesy of Jaime Feroli Giunta. (b) Very large ovarian cyst from a cat. No normal ovarian tissue is visible. *Source:* Photo courtesy of Faith Perrin. (c) Cat with large ovarian cyst and pyometra. *Source:* Photo courtesy of Catherine Malgieri.

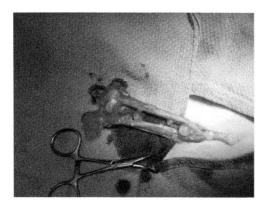

Figure 2.11 Paraovarian cysts in a cat. *Source:* Photo courtesy of Brenda Griffin.

common in cats but also occur commonly in dogs, and are most often an incidental finding during spay in an otherwise "normal" healthy female. They originate from the embryonic remains of the mesonephric and paramesonephric ducts and tubules. Paraovarian cysts usually do not produce hormones or cause any clinical signs, nor do they disrupt the structure of the ovaries. In all cases of ovarian cysts, spaying is curative.

Accessory or Duplicate Ovarian Tissue It is unclear how commonly accessory or duplicate

ovarian tissue occurs in cats and dogs, although it appears to be much rarer than has been previously assumed. In cats, it is not uncommon to see nodules associated with the ovarian pedicle (Figure 2.12a and b), and many veterinarians assume these nodules are ovarian in origin. However, published research examining 17 such nodules found that they were adrenal cortical tissue, not ovarian tissue (Altera and Miller 1986). More recent research on 73 samples found that 70% were ectopic adrenal tissue and 24% were mesonephric remnants, with no ovarian tissue found in any sample (Haase-Berglund et al. 2019). Early reports of accessory ovarian tissue in cats describe just two cases – a duplicate ovary and an extraovarian granulosa cell tumor – and may not have been referring to these commonly encountered pedicle nodules (McEntee 1990). Similar ectopic adrenal tissues may be discovered on the spermatic cord during castration. When such nodules are discovered on an ovarian pedicle or spermatic cord, removal is recommended when feasible. Since reports describe some instances of bilateral nodules, inspection of the contralateral pedicle is recommended when these nodules are found.

(a)

(b)

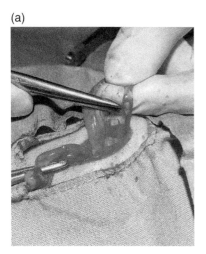 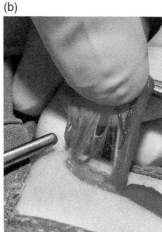

Figure 2.12 Ovarian pedicle nodules in a cat can be (a) adhered to the ovarian vessels or (b) located in the suspensory ligament. Despite their proximity to the ovary, these nodules are not accessory ovarian tissue, but are adrenal cortical tissue or mesonephric remnants. *Source:* Photos courtesy of Kim Culbertson.

Uterus

Uterine abnormalities are uncommonly encountered in veterinary medicine, but have been identified in many species, including cats and dogs. Prevalence of congenital uterine abnormalities in cats has been estimated to be 0.09%, and include uterus unicornis, segmental agenesis of one uterine horn, and uterine horn hypoplasia (Brookshire et al. 2017).

Uterus Unicornis Uterus unicornis, or incomplete formation of one uterine horn, has been reported in dogs and cats (Figure 2.13a and b). One study (McIntyre et al. 2010) reported an incidence of less than 0.06% in cats and 0.03% in dogs. Absence of the ipsilateral ovary is rare and a concerted effort should be made to find that ovary to prevent development of ovarian remnant syndrome. In contrast, absence of the ipsilateral kidney is not uncommon (Robinson 1965; Marcella et al. 1985; Chang et al. 2008; Goo et al. 2009), and occurred in 29.4% of cats and 50.0% of dogs evaluated in one large study (McIntyre et al. 2010). There are two reports of cats with unilateral agenesis of a uterine horn and pregnancy in the other horn (Reis 1966; Brookshire et al. 2017).

Segmental Aplasia Segmental aplasia of one or both uterine horns has also been reported, but is even less common (Figure 2.14a and b). There may be cystic dilation with accumulation of estrous secretions in the portion of the uterine horn carnial to the stricture if there is no outflow to the vagina, urinary bladder, or associated structures (Rousset et al. 2011). There are reports of bitches and queens with unilateral uterine horn aplasia presenting for asymptomatic intermittent abdominal distension or for cystic endometrial hyperplasia (CEH) with mucometra or pyometra in the contralateral horn (Marcella et al. 1985; Laznicka et al. 1997; Prestes et al. 1997; Schulman and Bolton 1997).

Hydrometra/Mucometra/Pyometra While not congenital anomalies, hydrometra, mucometra, and pyometra are common abnormal findings during spay surgery. Each of these pathologies can occur in dogs, cats, and rabbits, and each is characterized by an enlarged, fluid-filled uterus. These conditions are often associated with CEH, in which endometrial glands proliferate and form cysts, leading in some cases to fluid accumulation (Hagman 2014).

In hydrometra (Figure 2.15a), the fluid is watery or serous, and in mucometra, the fluid

(a) 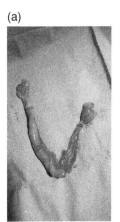 (b)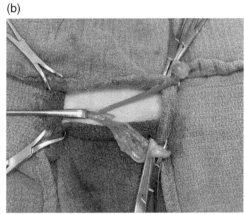

Figure 2.13 Uterus unicornis. (a) In this cat uterus, the uterine horn on the left is normal and the horn on the right is hypoplastic. Ovaries are present on each side. *Source:* Photo courtesy of Faith Perrin. (b) Uterus unicornis in a puppy. The uterine horn at the top of the photo is normally developed, while the one at the bottom of the photo has not developed. Both ovaries are present. *Source:* Photo courtesy of Brenda Griffin.

(a)

(b)

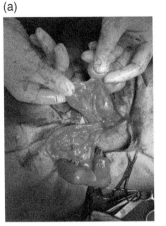
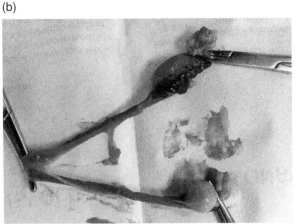

Figure 2.14 Segmental aplasia of the uterus. (a) This dog has segmental aplasia with dilation of the uterine segments proximal to the aplastic segments. *Source:* Photo courtesy of Robyn Barton. (b) This cat with segmental aplasia has normally developed uterine horns only at the tips near the ovaries. The tissue is not dilated or fluid filled, only enlarged due to the cat's active cycling. *Source:* Photo courtesy of Sara White.

is sero-mucoid to mucoid. Bacterial infection is not a component of either of these conditions (von Reitzenstein et al. 2000). Hydrometra and mucometra are generally incidental findings, as they may not cause any clinical signs other than decreased fertility (Hagman 2014). In cats, CEH is frequent in nulliparous queens over three years of age and in any queen over five years of age (Agudelo 2005), and it is common to see some degree of hydrometra in older cat spays.

Pyometra (Figure 2.15b and c) is the accumulation of purulent material in the uterus due to bacterial infection. It is a luteal phase disease, meaning it occurs following estrus once estrogen concentrations have peaked and declined and progesterone concentrations are elevated. The influence of these hormones is believed to be an integral part of the pathogenesis of this potentially life-threatening disease. The combination of opportunistic bacteria ascending from the vagina into the uterus combined with an abnormal endometrium due to CEH appears to further predispose animals to pyometra (von Reitzenstein et al. 2000). Pyometra is generally thought of as an emergency (von Reitzenstein et al. 2000; Hagman 2014), although many patients

(especially cats) show no signs of illness and are diagnosed with pyometra incidentally at the time of spay surgery. Techniques and considerations for spaying a cat or dog with pyometra are described in Chapter 12.

Ectopic Fetuses The presence of one or more extrauterine fetuses is another pathology that may be an incidental finding at the time of routine spay surgery (Figure 2.16a–f). Ectopic fetuses have been reported in both cats and dogs, though their occurrence is considered very rare (Nack 2000; Rosset et al. 2011; Eddey 2012; Chong 2017). Although a palpable abdominal mass would be evident on physical examination, affected cats and dogs often display no overt clinical signs. For this reason, ectopic fetuses may remain undiscovered for weeks, months, or even years. In some cases, affected animals do present with nonspecific signs such as fever, lethargy, inappetence, and/ or vomiting, although there is no clear association between duration of the ectopic fetus and the onset of such signs. Ectopic fetuses have been discovered in both sexually intact and previously spayed patients.

Ectopic pregnancies (i.e. pregnancies that occur outside of the uterus) are well known in

(a)

(b)

(c)

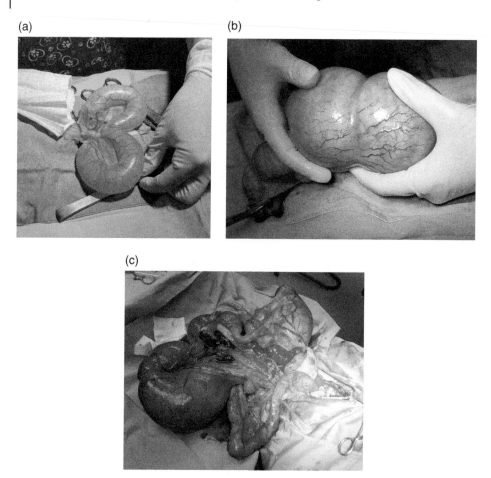

Figure 2.15   (a) Hydrometra in a cat. *Source:* Photo courtesy of Debbie Statland. (b and c) Pyometra in a dog. Pyometras can become greatly enlarged. *Source:* Photos courtesy of Sherri Therrien.

Figure 2.16   Ectopic fetuses. (a) This recently acquired, otherwise healthy-appearing stray dog was presented for spay surgery and removal of a large, firm, nonmovable mass from the ventral abdominal wall noted by the owner. (b) On pre-surgical physical examination, a second large, firm mass was palpated in the caudal abdomen. This mass, which is visible through the abdominal incision, was removed. (c) Once removed, the membranous outer covering of the mass was resected, revealing a well-developed fetal puppy. (d) Next, the uterus was exteriorized and a large omental adhesion (left) was discovered on the uterine horn, presumably at the site of a previous rupture. This adhesion was attached to both the spleen and abdominal wall, creating the mass effect that the owner had originally noted. *Source:* Photos courtesy of Janice Ramirez and Coco's Animal Welfare, and surgeon Karina Valenti. (e) Ectopic fetus discovered during ovariohysterectomy of a feral cat. In this photo, both uterine horns are visible, with scarring from previous uterine rupture visible near the bifurcation. The grayish-green mass attached to the omentum on the right is an encapsulated fetus. *Source:* Photo courtesy of Alexandra Devine. (f) Ectopic fetuses have also been reported in rabbits (Segura Gil et al. 2004). These three ectopic fetuses of varying sizes were discovered incidentally during ovariohysterectomy of a clinically normal rabbit. Note the normal appearance of the uterus. *Source:* Photo courtesy of Erin Doyle

(a)

(b)

(c)

(d)

(e)

(f)

humans and are typically classified as either tubal or abdominal, depending on the site of implantation (Nack 2000; Rosset et al. 2011; Eddey 2012; Chong 2017). Tubal pregnancies have not been reported in dogs and cats. Abdominal ectopic pregnancies are classified as either primary or secondary. In the case of a primary abdominal ectopic pregnancy, a fertilized ovum is expelled into the abdomen prior to implantation and develops a "placental relationship" with a peritoneal or omental surface. In contrast, secondary abdominal ectopic pregnancy occurs when a fetus initially gestates in the uterus and then later enters the abdomen as a result of uterine wall rupture. The vast majority (if not all) of the cases of ectopic pregnancies in cats and dogs are secondary, and are perhaps better termed ectopic fetuses, rather than pregnancies, since these fetuses do not remain viable in extrauterine locations.

Ectopic fetuses in dogs and cats typically result from uterine rupture during pregnancy. Uterine wall rupture can occur as a result of external trauma or during parturition, especially when signs of dystocia are present. A history of trauma, evidence of uterine trauma, and gross findings of mummified fetuses in the abdomen without evidence of implantation or a placental relationship with abdominal organs are all consistent with the diagnosis of ectopic fetus. However, evidence of trauma may be

lacking, since the presence of ectopic fetuses may not be discovered for months or years. Abdominal radiographs and/or ultrasound findings are consistent with the presence of a tightly curled fetus in an extrauterine location, with or without the presence of free abdominal fluid. Exploratory surgery is both diagnostic and therapeutic. The number and location of extrauterine fetuses may vary. One or more fetuses may be present, and they may be located in the omentum surrounding the intestines, mesentery, broad ligament of the uterus, ovary, and/or body wall. In some cases, extensive dissection will be required for removal. Nonetheless, the prognosis is considered excellent: in all reported cases affected patients recovered well from surgery (Nack 2000; Rosset et al. 2011; Eddey 2012; Chong 2017).

Vagina/Vulva

Clitoral Hypertrophy/Os Clitoris Clitoral hypertrophy, with or without presence of a cartilaginous or bony internal structure, is often the first physical evidence of true hermaphroditism or pseudohermaphroditism noted by owners or veterinarians (Figure 2.17a and b). The structure is sensitive and its presence is frequently associated with vulvar licking, urinary incontinence, and/or recurrent vaginitis (Tangner et al. 1982; Mantri and Vishwasrao 1994). Removal of the gonads may

(a)   (b)

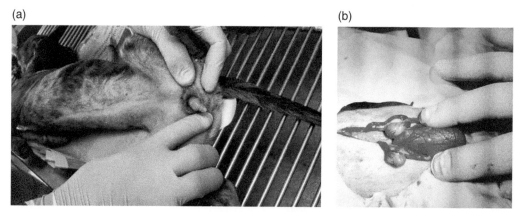

Figure 2.17 (a) Clitoral hyperplasia in a puppy and (b) abdominal testicles and uterus were located during surgery. *Source:* Photo courtesy of Maroqui Serrano.

or may not cause decrease in size of the clitoral tissue. Before surgical removal of the clitoris is attempted, passage of a urinary catheter and/or radiographic contrast studies to define placement of the urethra within or around related structures are strongly recommended.

Clitoral hypertrophy may also occur in otherwise normally developed female dogs as a result of exogenous exposure to androgens. Perhaps the most common example of this is in racing greyhounds, because the drug mibolerone is commonly used for estrus suppression. Withdrawal of the drug and removal of the gonads may result in partial reversal. If associated clinical signs are present, surgery may be indicated in these cases as well.

Vestibulovaginal Malformations Various vestibulovaginal malformations have been reported in dogs, including an imperforate or persistent hymen, vestibulovaginal stenosis, vaginal segmental hypoplasia or aplasia, persistent paramesonephric septal remnant, vaginal septa, and dual vaginas (Capel-Edwards 1977; Holt and Sayle 1981; Wykes and Soderberg 1983; Root et al. 1995; Kyles et al. 1996; Nomura et al. 1997; Burdick et al. 2014). Septa and strictures most often form at the vestibulovaginal junction, because that is where the paramesonephric ducts and urogenital sinus join during embryologic development. There may be cystic dilation with accumulation of estrous secretions if there is no outflow to the caudal vagina (Nomura et al. 1997; Baines et al. 1999; Tsumagari et al. 2001; Viehoff and Sjollema 2003). Failure of closure of the dorsal commissure of the vulva and complete vulvar agenesis have also been reported in dogs, as have rectovaginal and rectovestibular fistulas (Burke and Smith 1975; Capel-Edwards 1977; Meij et al. 1990; Tivers and Baines 2010). There are no reported genetic or breed predispositions for any of these malformations, and their prevalence is unknown (Burdick et al. 2014).

In some individuals vestibulovaginal malformations are incidental findings, whereas in others they may be underlying causes or contributing factors to a wide variety of clinical problems, ranging from urinary incontinence, vaginal pooling of urine, recurrent urinary tract infection, recurrent vaginitis, and infertility to inability to breed or whelp naturally (Burdick et al. 2014). When clinical signs are present, correction of the malformation may be warranted to treat the underlying condition. Among the various vestibulovaginal malformations, a persistent or imperforate hymen is generally the easiest to treat, because these can usually be broken down digitally. For the remainder of these conditions, invasive surgery has historically been performed for correction, including vaginectomy, vaginoplasty, and vaginal resection and anastomosis, among others – all of which are associated with potentially serious risks and complications (Kyles et al. 1996; Kieves et al. 2011). More recently, endoscopic-guided laser ablation has been described as a noninvasive diagnostic and therapeutic option. This technique provides an effective, safe, and minimally invasive treatment option for dogs with various vaginal malformations, avoiding the need for more invasive surgery (Burdick et al. 2014).

Mammary Hyperplasia

Another reproductive pathology that the spay–neuter surgeon may encounter is mammary hyperplasia, a non-neoplastic enlargement of one or more mammary glands in cats (Figure 2.18). It most often occurs in sexually intact young queens that are actively cycling (Little 2011), although it may occur in intact queens of any age, as well as in female or male cats receiving progestin treatment (Payan-Carreira 2013). The benign fibroglandular proliferation of the mammary glands occurs under the influence of progesterone. As such, it occurs during the luteal phase of the estrous cycle and may also occur during pregnancy. Although cats are considered induced ovulators, affected cats need not have been bred to develop the condition, because ovulation can occur as a result of noncopulatory stimulation. Anywhere from one to all mammary glands

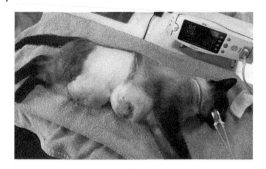

Figure 2.18 Severe mammary hyperplasia in a cat. Although many affected cats present with only mild mammary enlargement, the severe changes in this case warranted a flank approach for spay surgery. A nonviable pregnancy was discovered at surgery; while many cats with mammary hyperplasia are not pregnant, the elevated concentrations of progesterone present during gestation can trigger hyperplasia. *Source:* Photo courtesy of Sara White.

may be affected and typically undergo diffuse enlargement over two to four weeks. In most cases the glands are firm, and a small amount of brown milk may sometimes be expressed from them. In severe cases massive rapid enlargement can result in areas of ulcerative necrosis of the overlying skin (Little 2011). Mammary gland hyperplasia spontaneously resolves after progesterone concentrations

decline, although resolution may take several weeks. Surgical removal of the affected glands is not recommended; in cases where ulceration or abscessation of the glands has occurred, debridement and treatment with antibiotics have been successful (Burstyn 2010). Recovery is hastened by spaying, which also prevents recurrence. A flank approach to spay is generally recommended for cats with mammary hyperplasia (see Chapter 12). In contrast, mammary neoplasia is generally a condition of older bitches and queens, and is not associated with a particular stage of estrous. It usually presents as nodular masses rather than diffuse enlargement.

Conclusion

Experienced HQHVSN surgeons probably see more DSDs and reproductive pathologies than most practicing veterinarians. Indeed, mother nature has a way of providing periodic "spay–neuter surprises" to even the most seasoned of surgeons. Fortunately, to cut is to cure! Spay–neuter surgery is the treatment of choice and often the only treatment necessary for these conditions in the vast majority of patients.

References

Adelsberger, M.E. and Smeak, D.D. (2009). Repair of extensive perineal hypospadias in a Boston terrier using tubularized incised plate urethroplasty. *Can. Vet. J.* 50: 937–942.

Ader, P.L. and Hobson, H.P. (1978). Hypospadias: a review of the veterinary literature and a report of three cases in the dog. *J. Am. Anim. Hosp. Assoc.* 14: 721–727.

Agudelo, C. (2005). Cystic endometrial hyperplasia-pyometra complex in cats. A review. *Vet. Quart.* 27: 173–182.

Altera, K. and Miller, L. (1986). Recognition of feline parovarian nodules as ectopic adrenocortical tissue. *JAVMA* 189: 71–72.

Amann, R.P. and Veeramachaneni, D.N.R. (2007). Cryptorchidism in common eutherian mammals. *Reproduction* 133: 541–561.

Arlt, S.P. and Haimerl, P. (2016). Cystic ovaries and ovarian neoplasia in the female dog – a systematic review. *Reprod. Domest. Anim* 51 (Suppl 1): 3–11.

Aronson, L.R. and Cooper, M.L. (1967). Penile spines of the domestic cat: their endocrine-behavior relations. *Anat. Rec. (Hoboken)* 157: 71–78.

Arrighi, S., Bosi, G., Groppetti, D. et al. (2010). An insight into testis and gubernaculum dynamics of Insl3-RXFP2 signalling during testicular descent in the dog. *Reprod. Fertil. Dev.* 22: 751–760.

Atkinson, M.C. (1998). Polyorchidism in a dog. *Vet. Rec.* 143: 684–685.

Baines, S.J., Speakman, A.J., Williams, J.M. et al. (1999). Genitourinary dysplasia in a cat. *J. Sm. Anim. Pract.* 40: 286–290.

Balke, J. (1981). Persistent penile frenulum in a cocker spaniel. *Vet. Med. Sm. Anim. Clin.* 76: 988–990.

Batista Arteaga, M., Gonzalez Valle, F., Cabrera Martin, F. et al. (2000). Morphologic and endocrinological characteristics of retained canine testes. *Canine Pract.* 25: 12–15.

Baumans, V., Dikjstra, G., and Wensing, C.J.G. (1982). The effect of orchiectomy on gubernacular outgrowth and regression in the dog. *Int. J. Androl.* 5: 387–400.

Baumans, V., Dijkstra, G., and Wensing, C.J.G. (1983). The role of a non-androgenic testicular factor in the process of testicular descent in the dog. *Int. J. Androl.* 6: 541–552.

Belkin, P.B. (1969). Persistence of a penile frenulum in a dog. *Mod. Vet. Pract.* 50: 80.

Brookshire, W.C., Shivley, J., Woodruff, K. et al. (2017). Uterus unicornis and pregnancy in two feline littermates. *J. Feline Med. Surg. Open Rep* 3 (2): 1–5. https://doi.org/10.1177/2055116917743614.

Brown, T.T., Burek, J.D., and McEntee, K. (1976). Male pseudohermaphroditism, cryptorchism, and Sertoli cell neoplasia in three miniature schnauzers. *JAVMA* 169: 821–825.

Burdick, S., Berent, A.C., Weisse, C., and Langston, C. (2014). Endoscopic-guided laser ablation of vestibulovaginal septal remnants in dogs: 36 cases (2007–2011). *JAVMA* 244: 944–949.

Burke, T.J. (1986). Causes of infertility. In: *Small Animal Reproduction and Infertility* (ed. T.J. Burke), 233–235. Philadelphia, PA: Lea & Febiger.

Burke, T.J. and Smith, C.W. (1975). Vulvo-vaginal cleft in a dog. *J. Am. Anim. Hosp. Assoc.* 11: 774–777.

Burstyn, U. (2010). Management of mastitis and abscessation of mammary glands secondary to fibroadenomatous hyperplasia in a primiparturient cat. *JAVMA* 236: 326–329.

Capel-Edwards, K. (1977). Double vagina with perineal agenesis in a bitch. *Vet. Rec.* 101: 57.

Carlson, B.M. (2018). *Human Embryology and Developmental Biology*. St Louis, MO: Elsevier.

Cassata, R., Iannuzzi, A., Parma, P. et al. (2008). Clinical, cytogenetic and molecular evaluation in a dog with bilateral cryptorchidism and hypospadias. *Cytogenet. Genome Res.* 120: 140–143.

Chang, J., Jung, J.-H., Yoon, J. et al. (2008). Segmental aplasia of the uterine horn with ipsilateral renal agenesis in a cat. *J. Vet. Med. Sci.* 70: 641–643.

Chastain, C.B., Guilford, W.G., and Schmidt, D. (1988). The 38,XX/39,SSY genotype in cats. *Comp. Cont. Educ. Pract.* 10: 18–22.

Chong, A. (2017). A case of feline ectopic abdominal fetuses secondary to trauma. *Can. Vet. J.* 58: 400.

Christensen, B.W. (2012). Disorders of sexual development in dogs and cats. *Vet. Clin. N. Am. Sm. Anim. Pract.* 42: 515–526.

Cox, V.S., Wallace, L.J., and Jessen, C.R. (1978). An anatomic and genetic study of canine cryptorchidism. *Teratology* 18: 233–240.

De Lorenzi, L., Banco, B., Previderè, C. et al. (2017). Testicular XX (*SRY* -negative) disorder of sex development in cat. *Sex. Dev.* 11: 210–216.

Dolf, G., Holle, D., Gaillard, C. et al. (2010). Heritabilities for abdominal cryptorchidism and umbilical hernia in dog. World Congress on Genetics Applied to Livestock Production, Leipzig. Germany. http://www.wcgalp.org/system/files/proceedings/2010/heritabilities-abdominal-cryptorchidism-and-umbilical-hernia-dog.pdf (accessed 3 August 2019).

Dreger, A.D., Chase, C., Sousa, A. et al. (2005). Changing the nomenclature/taxonomy for intersex: a scientific and clinical rationale. *J. Pediatr. Endocrinol. Metabol.* 18: 729–734.

Dunn, M., Foster, W., and Goddard, K. (1968). Cryptorchidism in dogs: a clinical survey. *J. Am. Anim. Hosp. Assoc.* 4: 180–182.

Dybdahl Thomsen, P., Byskov, A.G., and Basse, A. (1987). Fertility in two cats with X-chromosome mosaicism and unilateral ovarian dysgenesis. *J. Reprod. Fertil.* 80: 43–47.

Eddey, P.D. (2012). Ectopic pregnancy in an apparently healthy bitch. *J. Am. Anim. Hosp. Assoc.* 48: 194–197.

Eissa, H., Farghali, H., and Osman, A. (2017). Persian queens: pathological and ultrasonography evaluation of ovarian affections in Egypt. *J. Anim. Health Behav. Sci.* 1: 2.

Fletcher, T.F. and Weber, A.F. (2013). Veterinary developmental anatomy. http://vanat.cvm. umn.edu/vanatpdf/embryolectnotes.pdf (accessed 3 August 2019).

Galanty, M., Jurka, P., and Zielinska, P. (2008). Surgical treatment of hypospadias: techniques and results in six dogs. *Pol. J. Vet. Sci.* 11: 235–243.

Gelberg, H., McEntee, K., and Heath, E. (1984). Feline cystic rete ovarii. *Vet. Pathol.* 21: 304–307.

Goo, M.-J., Williams, B.H., Hong, I.-H. et al. (2009). Multiple urogenital abnormalities in a Persian cat. *J. Feline Med. Surg.* 11: 153–155.

Gubbels, E.D.G., Scholten, J., Janns, L. et al. (2009). Relationship of cryptorchidism with sex ratios and litter sizes in 12 dog breeds. *Anim. Reprod. Sci.* 113: 187–195.

Guimaraes, L.D., Bourguignon, E., Santos, L.C. et al. (2013). Canine perineal hypospadias. *Arq. Bras. Med. Vet. Zootec.* 65 (6): 1647–1650.

Haase-Berglund, M.L., Yang, C., and Premanandan, C.L. (2019). Histologic evaluation of parovarian nodules in the cat. *J. Feline Med. Surg.* https://doi.org/10.1177/1098 612X19867166.

Hageltorn, M. and Gustavsson, I. (1981). XXY-trisomy identified by banding techniques in a male tortoiseshell cat. *J. Hered.* 72: 132–134.

Hagman, R. (2014). Diagnostic and prognostic markers for uterine diseases in dogs. *Reprod. Domes. Anim.* 49 (Suppl 2): 16–20.

Hardy, R.M. and Root Kustritz, M.V. (2005). Theriogenology question of the month: hypospadias in a dog. *JAVMA* 227: 887–888.

Hare, W.C.D., McFeely, R.A., and Kelly, D.F. (1974). Familial 78Xx male pseudohermaphroditism in three dogs. *J. Reprod. Fertil.* 36: 207–210.

Hayes, H.M. and Pendergrass, T.W. (1976). Canine testicular tumors: epidemiologic features of 410 dogs. *Int. J. Cancer* 18: 482–487.

Hayes, H.M. and Wilson, G.P. (1986). Hospital incidence of hypospadias in dogs in North America. *Vet. Rec.* 118: 605–606.

Hayes, H.M., Wilson, G.P., Pendergrass, T.W. et al. (1985). Canine cryptorchidism and subsequent testicular neoplasia: case-control study with epidemiologic update. *Teratology* 32: 51–56.

Holt, P.E. and Sayle, B. (1981). Congenital vestibulovaginal stenosis in the bitch. *J. Sm. Anim. Pract.* 22: 67–75.

Howard, P.E. and Bjorling, D.E. (1989). The intersexual animal – associated problems. *Prob. Vet. Med.* 1: 74–84.

Hutchison, J.A. (1973). Persistence of the penile frenulum in dogs. *Can. Vet. J.* 14: 71.

Jacobs, D. and Baughman, G.L. (1977). Preputial defect in a puppy. *Mod. Vet. Pract.* 58: 522–523.

Jurka, P., Galanty, M., Zielinski, P. et al. (2009). Hypospadias in six dogs. *Vet. Rec.* 164: 331–333.

Kawakami, E., Tsutsui, T., Yamada, Y. et al. (1984). Cryptorchidism in the dog: occurrence of cyrptorchidism and semen quality in the cryptorchid dog. *Jap. J. Vet. Sci.* 46: 303–308.

Kieves, N.R., Novo, R.E., and Martin, R.B. (2011). Vaginal resection and anastomosis for treatment of vestibulovaginal stenosis in 4 dogs with recurrent urinary tract infections. *JAVMA* 239: 972–980.

Kipnis, R.M. (1974). Membranous penile urethra and preputial abnormality in a dog. *Vet. Med. Sm. Anim. Clin.* 69: 750–751.

Kitchell, R.L., Kirk, E.J., Johnson, R.D. et al. (1988). Comparative studies of the cutaneous areas of the external genitalia of the dog, tom cat, ram and billy goat. *Anat. Histol. Embryol.* 17: 88–89.

Kyles, A.E., Vaden, S., Hardie, E.M. et al. (1996). Vestibulovaginal stenosis in dogs: 18 cases (1987–1995). *JAVMA* 209: 1889–1893.

Laznicka, A., Jaresova, H., Vitasek, R. et al. (1997). Segmental aplasia of the Mullerian duct in bitches. *Veterinářství* 47: 410–412.

Little, S. (2011). Feline reproduction: problems and clinical challenges. *J. Feline Med. Surg.* 13: 508–515.

Long, S.E., Gruffydd-Jones, T., and David, M. (1981). Male tortoiseshell cats: an examination of testicular histology and chromosome complement. *Res. Vet. Sci.* 30: 274–280.

Loughman, W.D. and Frye, F.L. (1974). XY/XYY bone marrow karyotype in a male Siamese-crossbred cat. *Vet. Med. Sm. Anim. Clin.* 69: 1007–1011.

Loughman, W.D., Frye, F.L., and Condon, T.B. (1970). XX/XXY bone marrow mosaicism in three male tricolor cats. *Am. J. Vet. Res.* 31: 307–314.

Malouf, N., Benirschke, K., and Hoefnagel, D. (1967). XX/XY chimerism in a tricolored male cat. *Cytogenet. Genome Res.* 6: 228–241.

Mantri, M.B. and Vishwasrao, S.V. (1994). Pseudo-hermaphroditism in a German Shepherd dog – a case report. *Ind. Vet. Surg.* 15: 98.

Marcella, K.L., Ramirez, M., and Hammerslag, K.L. (1985). Segmental aplasia of the uterine horn in a cat. *JAVMA* 186: 179–181.

Marino, G., Barna, A., Mannarino, C. et al. (2010). Stromal cysts of the canine ovary: prevalence, diagnosis and clinical implications. *Veterinaria (Cremona)* 24: 9–15.

Mattos, M.R.F., Simoes-Mattos, L., and Domingues, S.F.S. (2000). Cryptorchidism in dog. *Ciência Anim.* 10 (1): 61–70.

McEntee, M. (1990). *The Ovary. Reproductive Pathology of Domestic Mammals*. San Diego, CA: Academic Press.

McGeady, T.A., Quinn, P.J., FitzPatrick, E.S. et al. (2006). Male and female reproductive system. In: *Veterinary Embryology* (eds. T.A. McGeady, P.J. Quinn, E.S. Fitzpatrick, et al.), 244–267. Ames, IA: Wiley Blackwell.

McIntyre, R.L., Levy, J.K., Roberts, J.F. et al. (2010). Developmental uterine anomalies in cats and dogs undergoing elective ovariohysterectomy. *JAVMA* 237: 542–546.

Meij, B.P., Voorhout, G., and VanOosterom, R.A.A. (1990). Agenesis of the vulva in a Maltese dog. *J. Sm. Anim. Pract.* 31: 457–460.

Memon, M.A., Ganjam, V.K., Pavletic, M.M. et al. (1992). Use of human chorionic gonadotropin stimulation test to detect a retained testis in a cat. *JAVMA* 201: 1602.

Meyers-Wallen, V.N. (1991). Clinical approach to infertile male dogs with sperm in the ejaculate. *Vet. Clin. N. Am. Sm. Anim. Pract.* 21: 609–633.

Meyers-Wallen, V.N. (2009). Review and update: genomic and molecular advances in sex determination and differentiation in small animals. *Reprod. Dom. Anim.* 44 (Suppl 2): 40–46.

Meyers-Wallen, V.N. (2012a). Inherited diseases of the reproductive tract in dogs and cats. *Clin. Theriogenol.* 4: 244–250.

Meyers-Wallen, V.N. (2012b). Gonadal and sex differentiation abnormalities of dogs and cats. *Sex. Dev.* 6: 46–60.

Meyers-Wallen, V.N., Wilson, J.D., Griffin, J.E. et al. (1989). Testicular feminization in a cat. *JAVMA* 195: 631–634.

Millis, D.L., Hauptman, J.G., and Johnson, C.A. (1992). Cryptorchidism and monorchism in cats: 25 cases (1980–1989). *JAVMA* 200: 1128–1130.

Nack, R.A. (2000). Theriogenology question of the month. *JAVMA* 217: 182–184.

Nef, S. and Parada, L.F. (2000). Hormones in male sexual development. *Genes Dev.* 14: 3075–3086.

Neilen, A.L.J., Janss, L.L.G., and Knol, B.W. (2001). Heritability estimations for diseases, coat color, body weight, and height in a birth cohort of boxers. *Am. J. Vet. Res.* 62: 1198–1206.

Neilsen, S.W. and Lein, D.H. (1974). International histological classification of tumors of domestic animals. VI. Tumors of the testis. *Bull. World Health Org.* 50: 71–78.

Nelson, R.W. and Couto, C.G. (1994). Distúrbios do pênis, prepúcio e testículos. In: *Fundamentos de medicina interna de pequenos animais*, 2e (eds. R.W. Nelson and C.G. Couto), 513–517. Rio de Janeiro: Koogan.

Nickel, R.F., Ubbink, G., VanDerGaag, I. et al. (1992). Persistent Mullerian duct syndrome in the basset hound. *Tijdschr. Diergeneesk.* 117: 31S.

Nomura, K., Koreeda, T., Kawata, M. et al. (1997). Vaginal atresia with transverse septum in a cat. *J. Vet. Med. Sci.* 59: 1045–1048.

O'Connor, C.L., Schweizer, C., Gradil, C. et al. (2011). Trisomy-X with estrous cycle anomalies in two female dogs. *Theriogenology* 76: 374–380.

Olsen, D. and Salwei, R. (2001). Surgical correction of a congenital preputial and penile deformity in a dog. *J. Am. Anim. Hosp. Assoc.* 37: 187–192.

Papazoglou, L.G. and Kazakos, G.M. (2002). Surgical conditions of the canine penis and prepuce. *Comp. Contin. Educ. Pract. Vet.* 24 (3): 204–218.

Pavletic, M. (2007). Reconstruction of the urethra by use of an inverse tubed bipedicle flap in a dog with hypospadias. *JAVMA* 231: 71–73.

Payan-Carreira, R. (2013). Feline mammary fibroepithelial hyperplasia: a clinical approach. In: *Insights from Veterinary Medicine* (ed. R. Payan-Carreira), Ch. 8. London: IntechOpen https://doi. org/10.5772/55550.

Pendergrass, T.W. and Hayes, H.M. (1975). Cryptorchism and related defects in dogs: epidemiologic comparisons with man. *Teratology* 12: 51–56.

Peter, A.T., Markwelder, D., and Asem, E.K. (1993). Phenotypic feminization in a genetic male dog caused by non-functional androgen receptors. *Theriogenology* 40: 1093–1105.

Pope, E.R. and Swaim, S.F. (1985). Surgical reconstruction of a hypoplastic prepuce. *J. Am. Anim. Hosp. Assoc.* 22: 73–77.

Poth, T., Breuer, W., Walter, B. et al. (2010). Disorders of sex development in the dog – adoption of a new nomenclature and reclassification of reported cases. *Anim. Reprod. Sci.* 121: 197–207.

Prestes, N.C., Bicudo, S.D., Landin Alvarenga, F.C. et al. (1997). Aplasia of one uterine horn associated with pyometra in a female dog. *Vet. Noticias* 3: 133–134.

Priester, W.A., Glass, A.G., and Waggoner, N.S. (1970). Congenital defects in domesticated animals: general considerations. *Am. J. Vet. Res.* 31: 1871–1879.

Proescholdt, T. and DeYoung, D. (1977). Infantile penis in the canine. *ISU Vet.* 2: 59–60.

Pugh, D.G., Caudle, A.B., and Wenzel, J. (1987). A persistent frenulum in a dog. *Canine Pract.* 14: 38–40.

Reif, J.S. and Brodey, R.S. (1969). The relationship between cryptorchidism and canine testicular neoplasia. *JAVMA* 155: 2005–2010.

Reis, R.H. (1966). Unilateral urogenital agenesis with unilateral pregnancy and vascular abnormalities in the cat (Felis domestica). *Wasmann J. Biol.* 24: 209–222.

Richardson, E.F. and Mullen, H. (1993). Cryptorchidism in cats. *Compend. Cont. Educ. Pract.* 15: 1342–1369.

Robinson, G.W. (1965). Uterus unicornis and unilateral renal agenesis in a cat. *JAVMA* 147: 516–518.

Root, M.V., Johnston, S.D., and Johnston, G.R. (1995). Vaginal septa in dogs: 15 cases (1983–1992). *JAVMA* 206: 56–58.

Root, M.V., Johnston, S.D., Johnston, G.R. et al. (1996). The effect of prepuberal and postpuberal gonadectomy on penile extrusion and urethral diameter in the domestic cat. *Vet. Radiol. Ultrasound* 37: 363–366.

Root Kustritz, M.V. (2001). Disorders of the canine penis. *Vet. Clin. N. Am. Sm. Anim. Pract.* 31: 247–258.

Rosset, E., Galet, C., and Buff, S. (2011). A case report of an ectopic fetus in a cat. *J. Feline Med. Surg.* 13: 610–613.

Rousset, N., Abbondati, E., Posch, B. et al. (2011). Unilateral hydronephrosis and hydroureter secondary to ureteric atresia, and uterus unicornis in a young terrier. *J. Sm. Anim. Pract.* 52: 441–444.

Ruble, R.P. and Hird, D.W. (1993). Congenital abnormalities in immature dogs from a pet store: 253 cases (1987–1988). *JAVMA* 202: 633–636.

Ryer, K.A. (1979). Persistent penile frenulum in a cocker spaniel. *Vet. Med. Sm. Anim. Clin.* 74: 688.

Sahay, P.N., Dass, L.L., Mukherjee, R. et al. (1987). Phallocampsis due to persistent frenulum in a dog. *Ind. Vet. J.* 64: 524–525.

Schulman, M.L. and Bolton, L.A. (1997). Uterine horn aplasia with complications in two mixed-breed bitches. *JSAVA* 68: 150–153.

Segura Gil, P., Peris Palau, B., Martínez Martínez, J. et al. (2004). Abdominal pregnancies in farm rabbits. *Theriogenology* 62: 642–651.

Sommer, M.M. and Meyers-Wallen, V.N. (1991). XX true hermaphroditism in a dog. *JAVMA* 198: 435–438.

Stewart, R.W., Menges, R.W., Selby, L.A. et al. (1972). Canine intersexuality in a pug breeding kennel. *Cornell Vet.* 62: 464–472.

Strain, L., Dean, J.C., Hamilton, M.P., and Bonthron, D.T. (1998). A true hermaphrodite chimera resulting from embryo amalgamation after in vitro fertilization. *N. Engl. J. Med.* 338 (3): 166–169.

Sumner, S.M., Grimes, J.A., Wallace, M.L., and Schmiedt, C.W. (2018). *Os clitoris* in dogs: 17 cases (2009–2017). *Can. Vet. J.* 59: 606–610.

Switonski, M., Payan-Carreira, R., Bartz, M. et al. (2012). Hypospadias in a male (78,XY;SRY-positive) dog and sex reversal female (78,XX;SRY-negative) dogs: clinical, histological and genetic studies. *Sex. Dev.* 6: 128–134.

Szczerbal, I., Stachowiak, M., Dzimira, S. et al. (2015). The first case of 38,XX (SRY-positive) disorder of sex development in a cat. *Mol. Cytogen.* 8: 22.

Tangner, C.H., Breider, M.A., and Amoss, M.S. (1982). Lateral hermaphroditism in a dog. *JAVMA* 181: 70–71.

Tivers, M. and Baines, S. (2010). Surgical diseases of the female genital tract. 2. Vagina and external genitalia. *In Pract.* 32: 362–369.

Tsumagari, S., Takagi, K., Takeishi, M. et al. (2001). A case of a bitch with imperforate hymen and hydrocolpos. *J. Vet. Med. Sci.* 63: 475–477.

Turba, E. and Willer, S. (1988). The population genetics of cryptorchidism in German boxers. *Monatsh. Veterinärmed.* 43: 316–319.

Viehoff, F.W. and Sjollema, B.E. (2003). Hydrocolpos in dogs: surgical treatment in two cases. *J. Sm. Anim. Pract.* 44: 404–407.

von Reitzenstein, M., Archbald, L.F., and Newell, S.M. (2000). Theriogenology question of the month. *JAVMA* 216: 1221–1223.

Wu, X., Wan, S., Pujar, S. et al. (2009). A single base pair mutation encoding a premature stop codon in the MIS type II receptor is responsible for canine persistent Mullerian duct syndrome. *J. Androl.* 30: 46–56.

Wykes, P.M. and Soderberg, S.F. (1983). Congenital abnormalities of the canine vagina and vulva. *J. Am. Anim. Hosp. Assoc.* 19: 995–1000.

3

Instrumentation for Spay–Neuter

Amber Burton and Sara White

The purpose of this chapter is to aid the surgeon in the selection of instruments, suture, and needles when performing an ovariohysterectomy (spay) or orchidectomy (neuter) procedure. Instruments and suture are the interface between surgeon and patient, and are integral to every aspect of our surgical performance, including efficiency, precision, patient outcomes, and surgeon comfort.

Instrument Selection

The type and number of surgical instruments vary depending on type of surgery and age and condition of the patient. The surgical instruments used in spay–neuter can be divided into those used for cutting, manipulation of tissue, manipulation of needle and suture, adequate hemostasis, and drape securement.

Cutting Instruments

Instruments used for cutting include scalpel blades, scalpel handles, and scissors (Figure 3.1). The two most commonly used scalpel blades in high-quality high-volume spay–neuter (HQHVSN) are size 10 and size 15. Blade size selection is usually based on the size of the patient (the smaller the patient, the smaller the blade) and on the surgeon's preference. Size 15 blades are particularly useful for achieving small incisions in feline spay procedures.

The scalpel handle used for spay–neuter procedures is the number 3 scalpel handle, which is sized to accommodate size 10 and 15 blades. However, many HQHVSN veterinarians prefer not to use a scalpel handle while cutting with a scalpel blade (White 2018). Although conventional wisdom states that the use of blades on scalpel handles is safer than using unattached blades, other literature suggests that about 10% of scalpel injuries in human healthcare occur during disassembly of the blade from the handle (Perry et al. 2003). At this time, research is not available to determine whether scalpel injuries are more likely in HQHVSN with or without the use of a scalpel handle.

There are advantages and disadvantages to the elimination of the scalpel handle for spay–neuter. Advantages of not using a handle include elimination of the time required to assemble and disassemble the blade and handle, elimination of the risks of injury during assembly and disassembly, and the perceived ability to make smaller and quicker movements with the blade alone than with the blade with handle. The reduction of the number of instruments included in each surgery pack can also be advantageous, by reducing both initial pack purchase price and staff time for instrument cleaning and pack assembly. Disadvantages of using unattached scalpel

High-Quality, High-Volume Spay and Neuter and Other Shelter Surgeries, First Edition. Edited by Sara White.
© 2020 John Wiley & Sons, Inc. Published 2020 by John Wiley & Sons, Inc.

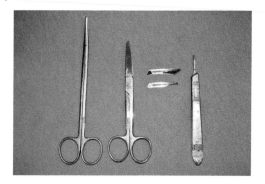

Figure 3.1 Instruments used for cutting. Pictured from left to right: Metzenbaum scissors, Mayo scissors, size 10 blade (top), size 15 blade (bottom), number 3 scalpel handle.

blades include the increased likelihood of losing track of the blade within the surgery field, and potential injury due to lack of visualization of the blade or because of the blade slipping in the fingers.

Scissors are used for cutting tissues, drapes, and suture. The basic types of scissors that may be used in spay or neuter surgeries are general operating scissors, Metzenbaum scissors, and Mayo scissors. Mayo scissors are most often used for cutting heavy tissues, as well as cutting suture and making fenestrations in disposable sterile drapes. Operating scissors may also be used for this purpose, but are less commonly included in HQHVSN surgery packs (White 2018). Curved Metzenbaum scissors are used

for cutting tissue and should not be used for cutting drapes or suture, as this can lead to a significant decrease in sharpness of the scissor blades. Since most HQHVSN surgery packs have only one type of scissors per pack (White 2018), blade sharpness can be preserved by cutting tissues near the point of the blades and sutures near the back of the jaws.

Instruments for Tissue Manipulation

Instruments selected for manipulation of tissue include thumb forceps and the Snook spay hook (Figure 3.2a). Thumb forceps are so named because they are held between the thumb and forefinger. Various types of thumb forceps are used in HQHVSN, and are differentiated by the number and size of teeth at the tip (Figure 3.2b). Adson tissue forceps have delicate rat-tooth (1×2) tips and are suitable for use during suturing of skin and fascia. Brown–Adson forceps have equally delicate, small intermeshing serrated teeth on the end, providing a broader grip on the tissue than Adson forceps and also allowing grasping of the needle (Nieves et al. 1993). Rat-tooth forceps have larger interdigitating teeth and allow a strong grasp on tissues (Brisson 2011). Adson-Brown forceps are the most commonly used thumb forceps in HQHVSN due to their versatility in grasping tissues and needles, although some

(a)

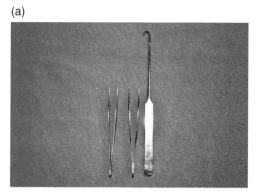

(b)

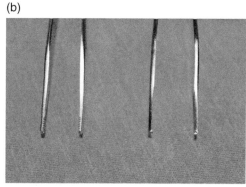

Figure 3.2 (a) Instruments used for manipulation of tissue. Pictured from left to right: Adson-Brown forceps, rat-toothed thumb forceps, and Snook spay hook. (b) Difference in tips of Adson-Brown (left) and rat-toothed forceps (right). Notice the large interlocking teeth of the rat-toothed forceps.

surgeons prefer Adson or larger rat-tooth forceps, or include more than one type of thumb forceps in their surgery packs (White 2018).

The other instrument commonly used for tissue manipulation in HQHVSN is the spay hook, which is used to retrieve the uterine horn during spay surgery. Two styles of spay hook are available, Snook and Covault. Snook hooks have a flat tip and Covault hooks have a ball or button tip (Nieves et al. 1993). Snook hooks are more commonly used and more readily available, and vary considerably in both the width and the curvature of the hook.

Instruments for Needle and Suture Manipulation

The Mayo–Hegar needle holder and the Olsen–Hegar needle holder are two instruments that are commonly used to manipulate suture or to hold needles (Figure 3.3). These instruments differ in that the Olsen–Hegar needle holder has suture scissors incorporated in the jaws, thus eliminating the step of cutting suture with Mayo scissors (Nieves et al. 1993). The Olsen–Hegar needle holder is preferred by most HQHVSN surgeons (White 2018).

While there is some risk with Olsen–Hegar needle holders of inadvertently cutting suture while attempting to grasp the suture or needle, this consequence may be reduced with attention and practice. In addition, since spay–neuter surgeries do not require suturing in deep cavities, it is less likely that suture will be prematurely cut, as this occurs most often when visibility is poor and when suturing in a restricted space.

Instruments for Hemostasis

In order to obtain a clear visualization of surgery, instruments are needed to provide adequate hemostasis. The types of hemostatic forceps used are Halstead mosquito, Kelly, Crile, and Rochester–Carmalt (Figure 3.4). These forceps can be either straight or curved. Mosquito forceps have transverse serrations that extend the full length of the jaws and are used for clamping small vessels to prevent or control hemorrhage. Mosquito forceps are also used for performing instrument ties in the pediatric canine and feline neuter, as well as ovarian pedicle ties in the feline spay. Kelly and Crile hemostatic forceps are used for controlling hemorrhage from small and medium-sized vessels. In addition, they can be used to crush tissue and blood vessels when placing ligatures. These forceps are similar in that they have serrations along the tip of the instrument that are transverse to the jaws. The transverse serrations ensure that the vessel is less likely to slip when the tip of the hemostat is applied to the vessel. The Kelly hemostatic forceps differ from the Crile forceps in that in the Kelly, the

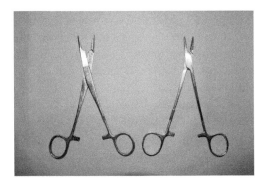

Figure 3.3 Instruments used for manipulation of suture and holding needles. Mayo–Hegar needle holder (left), Olsen–Hegar needle holder (right).

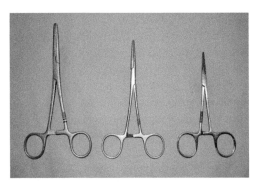

Figure 3.4 Instruments used to provide adequate hemostasis. Pictured from left to right: Rochester–Carmalt forceps, Kelly/Crile hemostatic forceps, Halstead mosquito hemostatic forceps.

transverse serrations only extend half the length of the jaws (Nieves et al. 1993). The Rochester–Carmalt forceps have longitudinal serrations along the jaws, with transverse serrations on the tip of the instrument. These forceps are designed to provide maximum hold of clamped tissue, and are commonly used for clamping the ovarian pedicle of large canine spays.

Instruments for Drape Securement

Some HQHVSN surgeons use towel clamps to secure surgical drapes to the patient's skin. The most commonly used style is the Backhaus towel forceps. Multiple towel forceps may be used to secure each drape to the patient. Towel clamps are most commonly included in dog spay packs, and are more likely to be incorporated in surgery packs that include paper drapes compared to those with cloth drapes (White 2018). This may be due to the differences in the draping qualities of cloth versus paper, or may be related to the desire to avoid damaging reusable cloth drapes and shortening the life of the drape material.

Suture Selection

The primary function of suture is to provide support and apposition of tissue until healing has occurred. The ideal suture should maintain high tensile strength throughout healing, should be easy to handle, and should provide excellent knot security. Suture should also be easy to sterilize and not cause reaction of tissue. Other properties desired in suture include that it be safe, nontoxic, noncarcinogenic, and not facilitate bacterial growth. This section will describe how suture is classified, and will describe the properties of common suture types used in spay–neuter.

Suture Materials and Use

Suture material is generally classified according to three characteristics based on its composition: absorbable or nonabsorbable, natural or synthetic, and monofilament or multifilament. The first major characteristic to consider when selecting a suture is whether the suture is absorbable or nonabsorbable. Absorbable suture loses its tensile strength within 60 days of use and is eventually absorbed by the body by either phagocytosis or hydrolysis (Boothe 1993; Edlich and Long 2008). Absorbable suture is typically utilized for internal ligations and closure of tissues. It is commonly used for closing tissues, including body wall (linea alba), subcutaneous tissues, and skin (buried interrupted or intradermal pattern). Nonabsorbable suture is suture that retains tensile strength for longer than 60 days and is typically not absorbed by natural mechanisms. It is used when suture is desired to be permanently left within the tissues, or to be removed at a later date. Except for the occasional use of stainless steel, nonabsorbable suture material is not typically used in HQHVSN surgeries (White 2018).

The second major characteristic to consider when selecting a suture is whether the suture is natural, synthetic, or metallic. Natural suture is derived from a plant or animal source, and can elicit tissue reactions due to the protein composition of the suture. Tensile strength duration is variable and may range from a couple of days to months, and these materials may have a tendency to fray during knot construction (Edlich and Long 2008). Examples of natural suture include surgical gut (catgut) and silk. Synthetic sutures were introduced in order to reduce risk of tissue reaction, and to have less variability in tensile strength and absorption (Boothe 1993). Synthetic suture is the most common type of suture used in spay–neuter (White 2018).

The third major characteristic to consider when selecting a suture is whether the suture is monofilament or multifilament (braided). Monofilament suture is one single, smooth strand of suture. This type of suture passes easily through tissue, but can be difficult to handle due to a tendency to take the shape that it maintained in the original package, called "memory." Multifilament suture is constructed with several strands of filament braided together. This type of suture allows good knot security and easy handling, but produces "tissue drag" when pulled through tissue. This drag can be traumatic to tissue, as well as create a potential source for bacterial infection in a contaminated environment. In order to avoid this, manufacturers have developed polymer coatings for selected suture types (Edlich and Long 2008). These coatings function to reduce tissue drag and potential for bacterial colonization, but can significantly decrease knot security.

Commonly used sutures in veterinary medicine for spay–neuter procedures include synthetic monofilament absorbable sutures such as poliglecaprone 25 (Monocryl[®]) and polydioxanone (PDS[®] II), synthetic braided absorbable sutures such as polyglactin 910 (Coated Vicryl[®]; all from Ethicon, Inc., Cornelia, GA, USA), and stainless steel. Synthetic monofilament absorbable suture is by far the most commonly used suture type in HQHVSN (White 2018).

Poliglecaprone 25 (Monocryl) is an absorbable monofilament suture that is synthetic in origin. Its properties include moderate tensile strength, low tissue drag, low tissue reactivity, and ease of handling. It has high initial tensile strength with excellent knot security. This suture has rapid loss of tensile strength, with nearly 75% lost by day 14 after implantation. By day 21, almost all suture tensile strength is lost. Undyed Monocryl loses tensile strength about 25% more rapidly than dyed Monocryl (Dunn 2005).

Polydioxanone (PDS II) is an absorbable monofilament suture that is also synthetic in origin. Its properties include excellent tensile strength, low tissue drag, and low tissue reactivity. Polydioxanone maintains the longest tensile strength of nearly all synthetic absorbable sutures, retaining nearly 75% strength after 14 days. By 28 days, nearly half of tensile strength is maintained. Complete absorption does not occur until close to 180 days after suture implantation (Dunn 2005). A disadvantage of polydioxanone is that it retains memory

from packaging, thus decreasing handling ability.

Polyglactin 910 (Coated Vicryl) is a synthetic multifilament suture that is supplied as a coated suture that is easy to handle, with minimal tissue drag and minimal tissue reaction. Coated Vicryl retains 75% of its tensile strength after 14 days and 25% after 28 days, and is completely absorbed between 56 and 70 days (Dunn 2005).

Differences in the amount of tissue reaction between the various types of synthetic absorbable sutures have been studied, and some amount of inflammatory reaction is seen with every absorbable suture type, whether monofilament or braided (Freeman et al. 1987). Any of these suture types are acceptable, and most surgeons will choose their suture based on handling preferences and duration of tensile strength.

The suture material that has the highest tensile strength is stainless steel. Stainless steel has excellent knot security and produces no inflammatory tissue reaction. It is very cost-effective, making it an appropriate choice for situations involving large volumes of daily surgeries, such as animal shelters or spay–neuter clinics (Mackey n.d.). Steel suture may be steam sterilized without loss of tensile strength, but should not be sterilized on a wooden spool, as lignin from the wood may cling to the suture (Dunn 2005). Stainless steel suture can be used on ovarian and uterine pedicles, body wall closure (linea alba), and subcutaneous tissue. Stainless steel is not considered acceptable for external closure of skin. The major disadvantage of stainless steel is the difficulty with handling and the learning curve required for efficient use. Steel suture will also dull the blades on suture scissors or Olsen–Hegar needle holders more quickly than other types of suture (Mackey n.d.). In practice, stainless steel suture is not used in the majority of HQHVSN practices, and those veterinarians who do use it often use monofilament absorbable suture during other portions of the same surgeries in which they use stainless steel (White 2018).

Nylon and polypropylene are synthetic non-absorbable sutures used for external closure of skin. External skin sutures are not recommended for use in HQHVSN practice, and in a survey of 81 spay–neuter veterinarians, none used synthetic nonabsorbable sutures (White 2018). If external closure of skin is desired, it is acceptable to use synthetic absorbable suture in the skin (Sylvestre et al. 2002; Parell and Becker 2003; Rosenzweig et al. 2010) as an alternative to nonabsorbable suture types.

Suture Size

Once the composition type of the suture is selected, another factor that must be considered is the size of the suture. Suture size can range from 11-0 to 7, with 11-0 being the smallest diameter (Dunn 2005). Tensile strength is directly related to the size of the suture, with larger suture having greater tensile strength. Suture size is selected based on how much tensile strength is required by the tissue type, using the smallest diameter suture that will adequately hold the mending tissue (Dunn 2005). The most common suture sizes used in spay–neuter surgery range from 4-0 to 1 (White 2018), with size 0 or 1 utilized in tissue that needs the greatest tensile strength (linea alba of a large dog spay).

It is important to note that stainless steel is sized differently from other suture types. It is sized according to gauge, and ranges from 18 gauge to 41 gauge. The two common sizes used in spay–neuter for stainless steel are 32 gauge and 34 gauge (Mackey n.d.).

Suture Sizes for Canine Spay

The suture selected for a canine spay can be utilized on all tissues, thus only requiring one suture size (or pack) per surgery. However, some surgeons select a smaller suture (such as 3-0) for closure of subcutaneous and subcuticular tissues.

For puppy spays under 10 lb (4.5 kg), most veterinarians select 3-0 suture, and for puppies over 20 lb (9 kg), most select 2-0 suture. For puppies in the 10–20 lb (4.5–9 kg) range, either 3-0 or 2-0 suture is acceptable.

For adult dog spays, suture size preferences vary considerably. Most veterinarians choose 3-0 suture for dogs under 10 lb (4.5 kg), 2-0 for dogs weighing 10–40 lb (4.5–18 kg), 2-0 or 0 for dogs weighing 40–50 lb (18–22 kg), and 0 for dogs over 50 lb (22 kg). Some surgeons select size 1 suture, especially in dogs of 70 lb (30 kg) and over (White 2018).

Suture Sizes for Feline Spay

For kitten spays, 4-0 or 3-0 suture is commonly used and is appropriate. For adult feline spays, most surgeons like to use 3-0 suture (White 2018). Some surgeons prefer to use a larger suture size such as 2-0 on adult cats, especially for the ligation of the uterine body in cats who are pregnant or in estrus.

Suture Sizes for Adult Canine Castration

For dog neuters, most veterinarians choose 3-0 suture for dogs under 20 lb (9 kg) and 2-0 suture for dogs who are 20–50 lb (9–22 kg). For dogs over 50 lb (22 kg), veterinarians may choose 2-0 or 0 suture. In larger dogs, many veterinarians use a large suture (such as 0) for cord ligations, and smaller suture (such as 3-0) for the subcutaneous and/or subcuticular closures and for ligation of subcutaneous bleeders (White 2018).

Suture material is not typically used for pediatric canine castration or for feline castration.

Suture Packaging

Suture material is generally supplied in either single-use packets or multiuse cassettes. Each type of packaging is commonly used in HQHVSN clinics (White 2018).

Suture packets are sterile packages that contain a length of suture, usually between 18 and 36 cm, attached or "swaged on" to a needle. To use a suture packet, the outer layer is peeled open and the entire packet is handed sterilely to the surgeon or dropped sterilely onto the opened surgery pack. Once the suture with its swaged-on needle has been used on one patient, it cannot safely be resterilized for use on a different patient.

Suture cassettes are multiuse suture material dispensers that contain either 25 or 50 m of suture material (Figure 3.5). Cassettes are usually placed within a suture cassette rack, which holds the cassette upright and available for the surgeon's use. The interior of the cassette remains sterile, and the suture material exits the cassette through a small opening. In order to obtain suture, the veterinarian must grasp the exposed suture end with an instrument or gloved fingers and pull upward to dispense the desired amount of suture. The veterinarian then cuts the suture near where it exits the cassette, leaving 1–2 cm of suture exposed. To place sutures using material from a cassette, an eyed needle must be used.

Suture cassettes come with a cover or cap that should be placed over the exposed suture end when not in use. When the cassette is first opened for the day or for the surgical session, the exposed portion of the suture that was in contact with the inside of the cap or cover is no longer sterile. This suture should be "tipped"; that is, the exposed tip of the suture should be removed and discarded prior to obtaining suture for surgery.

Each type of packaging has advantages and disadvantages. The major advantage of suture packets is that they are convenient. The suture

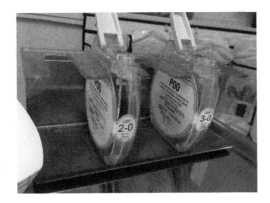

Figure 3.5   Suture cassettes in a cassette rack.

is already attached to the needle, making it unnecessary to thread an eyed needle. Also, since suture packets are supplied sterilely for each surgery, there is less chance that mishandling of the packaging before or between surgeries could lead to contamination of the suture. However, suture packets are more expensive than cassette suture. In addition, the length of suture provided in each packet may be much more than needed for a given surgery, and since leftover suture from packets cannot be reused on a different patient, this excess suture is wasted.

A major advantage of suture cassettes is that they cost less to use than suture packets. This is both because the cost per centimeter of cassette suture is lower, and because fewer centimeters of suture are typically dispensed for each surgery. An additional advantage of using suture cassettes is that they facilitate using different sizes of sutures for different parts of the surgery. It is possible to use a large size of suture for ligations and body wall closure, and a smaller suture for subcuticular and intradermal closure. The disadvantages of cassettes is the learning curve for the use of eyed needles and the care that must be taken to maintain sterility of the contents.

Needle Selection

Suture needles are required in surgery to facilitate the passage of suture through tissues. The appropriate selection of needle type provides easy penetration of tissue with as little trauma as possible. An ideal needle should be strong, stable when held with needle holders, and maintain sharpness of point throughout the procedure.

Basic Needles and Use

Surgical needles are made from stainless steel alloys, and can be categorized based on their structure, shape, size, and point. They have three components: the eye or swage, body, and point. The characteristics and size of the needles can be located on the packaging of the selected needle or suture.

The structure of the needle varies by whether suture comes from the manufacturer already attached at the hub of the needle. When needles are already attached to suture, they are termed "swaged-on" needles; otherwise, they are termed plain needles or eyed needles (Dunn 2005). If a plain needle is used, sterilized suture must be threaded through the eye of the needle in order to suture.

The shape of a needle can either be straight or curved. Straight needles are used when placing sutures in superficial wounds near the skin and are not typically used for spay–neuter surgery. Curved needles can be used for closing all tissue layers, and are appropriate for suturing tissue in spay–neuter. The most commonly used curved needles in spay–neuter are half circle or a three-eighths circle needles.

Measurements of a needle's size include chord length, diameter, and needle length (Figure 3.6; Dunn 2005; Smith and Macsai 2007). The chord length is the straight-line distance measured from the needle point to the swage or eye. The diameter of the needle is the thickness or gauge of the needle. The needle length is the distance measured along the needle itself from point to end (measured in millimeters). Needle length is the most commonly used measurement for needle selection. Increase in needle length should be directly

proportional to an increase in suture size. If a small suture size is selected, such as 3-0, an appropriate needle length would also be small (approximately 26 mm). If a larger suture (2-0) were selected, the appropriate needle length would be larger (approximately 36 mm).

The type of needle point is also important to consider during needle selection. The two primary needle types characterized by the point are cutting and noncutting needles. A cutting needle is designed with three edges that allow the needle to pass easily through dense and thick tissue. The two major types of cutting needles are conventional and reverse-cutting needles. Both have edges that form a triangle, but they differ by which surface of the needle contains the cutting edge. The conventional cutting needle has a cutting edge along the concave (inner) surface, while the reverse-cutting needle has a cutting edge on the convex (outer) surface. Reverse-cutting needles are considered superior to conventional cutting needles due to the reduced risk of cutting out tissue and increased needle strength (Boothe 1993). A noncutting needle is known as a taper or taper-point needle. This needle is rounded in cross-section and does not have any sharp edges. The taper needle passes through tissue by stretching rather than cutting. The sharpness of a taper needle is measured by the taper ratio. A high taper ratio is desired to produce optimum sharpness, thus reducing tissue trauma. In spay–neuter a reverse-cutting needle

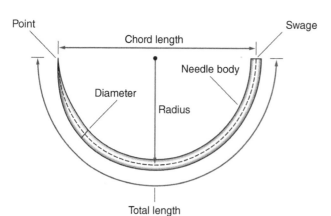

Figure 3.6 Anatomy of a surgical needle. *Source:* Reprinted with permission from Springer Nature: Ophthalmic Microsurgical Suturing Techniques by Jennifer Hasenyager Smith and Marian S. Macsai Smith and Macsai (2007).

is most commonly used, although noncutting (taper) needles are also appropriate.

Surgical Packs

Once instruments are selected, they are placed in surgical packs, wrapped, and sterilized. Surgery pack size and contents vary considerably among HQHVSN clinics. Some HQHVSN clinics assemble different types of surgery pack for different patient categories (based on patient species, sex, age, and size), whereas others assemble a single pack type for use in all surgeries, and wrap and sterilize additional instruments for use as needed.

Adult Canine Spay Pack

The adult canine spay pack is designed for use on any female canine over six months of age (Figure 3.7). The instruments most commonly included are a needle holder (most frequently Olsen–Hegar), a thumb forceps (typically Adson–Brown), one or more scissors (Mayo, Metzenbaum, or both), and a spay hook (White 2018). Various types of hemostats are also included and vary according to surgeon preferences, and may consist of a combination of

Kelly or Crile hemostats, Rochester–Carmalt forceps, and mosquito forceps. If the Rochester–Carmalt forceps are not included in each surgery pack, they should be available as separately wrapped and sterilized instruments. Additional instruments are sometimes incorporated in adult canine spay packs, including a number 3 scalpel handle and towel clamps. Drape material, surgical gauze, and eyed needles (if used) are also either added to each surgery pack or are wrapped separately. A number 10 scalpel blade is most commonly selected for this procedure.

Feline/Pediatric Canine Spay Pack

The feline spay pack is designed for use on any female cat, as well as for most female puppies under six months of age (Figure 3.8). The instruments most often included in the feline spay pack include a needle holder (usually Olsen–Hegar), a thumb forceps (typically Adson–Brown), one or more scissors (Mayo, Metzenbaum, or both), and a spay hook (White 2018). Hemostats are also included and vary according to surgeon preferences, generally consisting of a combination of mosquito forceps and Kelly or Crile hemostats. Additional instruments are sometimes incorporated in

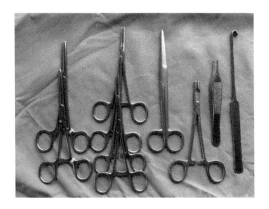

Figure 3.7 An example of a surgery pack for an adult dog spay. This pack contains two Rochester-Carmalt hemostats, four Kelly hemostats, a Mayo scissor, an Olsen-Hegar needle holder, a thumb forceps, and a Snook spay hook.

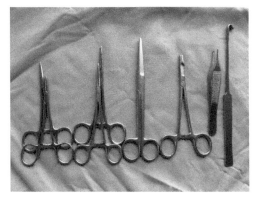

Figure 3.8 An example of a surgery pack for a standard feline spay/pediatric canine spay. This pack contains two mosquito hemostats, two Kelly hemostats, a Mayo scissor, an Olsen-Hegar needle holder, a thumb forcep, and a Snook spay hook.

feline spay packs, including a number 3 scalpel handle, Rochester–Carmalt forceps, and towel clamps. Drape material, surgical gauze, and eyed needles (if used) are also either added to each surgery pack or are wrapped separately. A number 15 scalpel blade is most frequently selected for this procedure, although a number 10 is also commonly used.

Adult Canine Neuter Pack

The adult canine neuter pack is designed for use on any male canine over six months of age, as well as for younger male dogs with testicular development that precludes the use of a pedicle tie (Figure 3.9). The instruments most commonly included in the adult canine spay pack include a needle holder (typically Olsen–Hegar), and a thumb forceps (most often Adson–Brown); most packs also contain scissors (Mayo, Metzenbaum, or both; White 2018). Various types of hemostats are also included and vary according to surgeon preferences, and may consist of a combination of Kelly or Crile hemostats, Rochester–Carmalt forceps, and mosquito forceps. Additional instruments are sometimes added to adult canine spay packs, including a number 3 scalpel handle and towel clamps. Drape material, surgical gauze, and eyed needles (if used) are also either contained in each surgery pack or are wrapped separately. A number 10 scalpel blade is most often selected for this procedure.

It is important to note that if the dog has a cryptorchid testicle(s), the use of a spay hook may be desired, therefore the canine or feline spay pack should be selected instead.

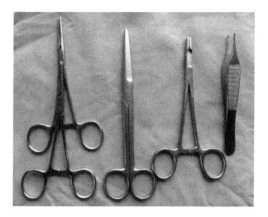

Figure 3.9 An example of a surgery pack for a standard adult canine neuter. This pack contains two Kelly hemostats, a Mayo scissor, an Olsen–Hegar needle holder, and a thumb forceps.

Feline/Pediatric Canine Neuter Pack

The feline/pediatric canine neuter pack is designed for use on male cats of any age who are not cryptorchid, and for male puppies on whom an instrument tie castration technique will be used (see Chapter 14 to learn this technique). Prior to selecting this pack, it is important to palpate and verify that both testicles have descended into the scrotum. The feline/pediatric canine neuter pack generally consists of a single hemostat. Many surgeons prefer a curved hemostat, and mosquito, Kelly, or Crile hemostats are all acceptable for this purpose. In some clinics, several hemostats are packaged together and removed singly by the gloved surgeon for each procedure. The feline/pediatric canine neuter pack may also contain a gauze sponge. A number 15 or number 10 blade is generally selected for this procedure.

References

Boothe, H.W. (1993). Suture materials, tissue adhesives, staplers and ligating clips. In: *Textbook of Small Animal Surgery*, 2e (ed. D. Slatter). Philadelphia, PA: W. B. Saunders.

Brisson, B. (2011). Thumb forceps. Ontario Veterinary College, University of Guelph.

http://www.vetsurgeryonline.com/thumb-forceps (accessed 14 March 2019).

Dunn, D.L. (2005). *Ethicon Wound Closure Manual*. Somerville, NJ: Ethicon.

Edlich, R.F. and Long, W.B. (2008). *Surgical Knot Tying Manual*. Norwalk, CT: Syneture/ Division of US Surgical/Tyco Healthcare.

Freeman, L.J., Pettit, G.D., Robinette, J.D. et al. (1987). Tissue reaction to suture material in the feline linea alba: a retrospective, prospective, and histologic study. *Vet. Surg.* 16: 440–445.

Mackey, W.M. (n.d.). Stainless-steel sutures. QuickSpay. http://quickspay.com/articles.html (accessed 14 March 2019).

Nieves, M.A., Merkley, D.F., and Wagner, S.D. (1993). Surgical instruments. In: *Textbook of Small Animal Surgery*, 2e (ed. D. Slatter). Philadelphia: W. B. Saunders.

Parell, G.J. and Becker, G.D. (2003). Comparison of absorbable with nonabsorbable sutures in closure of facial skin wounds. *Arch. Facial Plast. Surg.* 5: 488–490.

Perry, J., Parker, G., and Jagger, J. (2003). Scalpel blades: reducing injury risk. *Adv. Exposure Prev.* 6: 37–48.

Rosenzweig, L.B., Abdelmalek, M., Ho, J., and Hruza, G.J. (2010). Equal cosmetic outcomes with 5-0 poliglecaprone-25 versus 6-0 polypropylene for superficial closures. *Dermatol. Surg.* 36: 1126–1129.

Smith, J.H. and Macsai, M.S. (2007). Needles, sutures, and instruments. In: *Ophthalmic Microsurgical Suturing Techniques* (ed. M.S. Macsai). Berlin: Springer.

Sylvestre, A., Wilson, J., and Hare, J. (2002). A comparison of 2 different suture patterns for skin closure of canine ovariohysterectomy. *Can. Vet. J.* 43: 699–702.

White, S. (2018). Surgery packs and suture in HQHVSN. *ergovet*. http://ergovet.com/surgery-packs-and-suture-in-hqhvsn (accessed 18 August 2018).

4

Asepsis
Brian A. DiGangi

... it is from the vitality of the atmospheric particles that all the mischief arises ....
—Lord Joseph Lister

Is Asepsis Really a Requirement for Spay–Neuter Surgery?

In 1846, Ignaz Phillip Semmelweiss set out to tackle the 10% mortality rate attributed to sepsis in the First Obstetrical Clinic of the Vienna General Hospital. Over the next year, he correctly surmised the theory of fomite transfer of disease, instituted a handwashing protocol, and dropped the mortality rate to 1.3% seemingly overnight (Longo 1995). Around the same time in Great Britain, Joseph Lister began his successful experimentation with topical antiseptics and the preparation of surgical instruments in the management of contaminated wounds and other afflictions requiring surgical intervention (Lister 1867). With these two medical pioneers leading the way, our understanding of disease transmission was strengthened, countless lives were saved, and the field of infection control along with the concept of aseptic technique was born.

The goals of aseptic technique are to prevent cross-contamination during surgery and to minimize the amount of microorganisms in the surgical environment, thereby preventing their entrance into the surgical wound and the associated morbidity. Maintaining asepsis is considered the standard of care for surgical sterilization and has a direct impact on patient outcome (Association of Operating Room Nurses 2006; Griffin et al. 2016; Hedlund 2007). In addition, the perceived lack of such standards is frequently cited as an argument against shelter animal practice and high-quality high-volume spay–neuter (HQHVSN) clinics (Becker 2011; Tumblin and Hoekstra 2011; Woloshyn 2010). In order to correct these misperceptions, advance the field of shelter medicine, and continue to ensure surgical complication rates lower than those reported by general practitioners and tertiary care institutions, HQHVSN surgeons must be especially strict in their adherence to evidence-based aseptic practices.

In the human medical field, surgical site infections (SSIs) occur in 3% of all surgical procedures and make up 14–22% of all healthcare-associated infections (Barie and Eachempati 2005). As well as contributing a significant economic burden to healthcare systems, such infections result in an estimated 9000–20 000 deaths each year (Emori and Gaynes 1993; Klevens et al. 2007). While two-thirds of human SSIs are limited to incisional infections, the majority of SSI-related deaths were

High-Quality, High-Volume Spay and Neuter and Other Shelter Surgeries, First Edition. Edited by Sara White.
© 2020 John Wiley & Sons, Inc. Published 2020 by John Wiley & Sons, Inc.

attributed to infections of the internal organs or spaces (Mangram et al. 1999).

Comparable data for veterinary medicine is not available; however, nosocomial infections are common and SSIs are the most common type of nosocomial infection reported in small animals, involving up to 24.5% of all surgical procedures (Benedict et al. 2012; Johnson 2002; Vasseur et al. 1988). In one study of 142 adult dogs undergoing elective ovariohysterectomy by senior veterinary students at a teaching hospital, 8.5% of patients showed signs of inflammation consistent with SSIs, making up 41.4% of all complications in this study (Burrow et al. 2005). Other veterinary studies have indicated SSI rates of 4.5–8.5% for clean-contaminated surgical wounds in dogs and cats (Brown et al. 1997; Eugster et al. 2004; Nicholson et al. 2002; Vasseur et al. 1988; Table 4.1). One university-based spay–neuter program reported an overall complication rate of 3%, largely comprising minor SSIs (Isaza and DiGangi 2012). A different study of shelter animal surgeries performed by shelter veterinarians or veterinary students reported an SSI rate under 1% (Kreisler et al. 2018).

Minimum Requirements for Aseptic Surgery

Broad guidelines for surgical care that are attainable in most models of HQHVSN programs have been established (Griffin et al. 2016). In most cases, these represent the minimum requirements necessary to maintain asepsis; however, HQHVSN surgeons should strive to practice above these requirements whenever possible to decrease the chances of wound contamination and surgical complications (Table 4.2). Programs operating below this threshold of care place their professional reputation, that of similar organizations, and, most importantly, the welfare of their patients at unnecessary risk. Should these requirements be impossible to attain, re-analysis of the program mission and resource allocation is warranted.

Operating Environment

The minimum requirements for a functional operating environment include areas designated for animal housing, anesthesia and patient preparation, surgeon preparation,

Table 4.1 Reported rates of surgical site infections (SSIs) in dogs and cats.

References	Species	Procedure type	SSI rate (%)
Vasseur et al. (1988)	Dogs and cats	Clean	2.5
		Clean-contaminated	4.5
		Contaminated	5.8
		Dirty	18.1
Brown et al. (1997)	Dogs and cats	Clean	4.7
		Clean-contaminated	5.0
		Contaminated	12.0
		Dirty	10.1
Nicholson et al. (2002)	Dogs and cats	Clean-contaminated	5.9
Eugster et al. (2004)	Dogs and cats	Clean	6.9
		Clean-contaminated	8.0
		Contaminated	13.7
		Dirty	24.5
Burrow et al. (2005)	Dogs	Clean-contaminated	8.5

Table 4.2 Spectrum of aseptic practices for spay–neuter surgery.

Description	Ideal	Recommended	Minimum
Operating room	Separate working unit isolated from general facility traffic	Single-purpose unit within main facility	Designated area within multipurpose room; identified with physical and visual barriers
Equipment and supplies			
Surgical instruments	Separately wrapped instrument packs for each procedure; steam, gas, or plasma sterilization utilized	Large pack of instruments for multiple surgeries; individual instruments used on a single patient; steam, gas, or plasma sterilization utilized	Liquid chemical sterilization; individual instruments used on a single patient and reprocessed
Suture materials	Individually packaged suture for each patient	Reeled suture, sterilely acquired for each patient	Individually packaged or reeled suture; sterile, unused portions shared between patients
Surgical personnel			
Surgical attire	Dedicated surgical attire worn by all personnel; attire not worn outside operating room; attire changed/laundered daily	Surgical attire worn throughout the day; jacket/lab coat worn outside of operating room	Surgical attire worn throughout the day
	Caps and masks worn at all times within operating room	Caps and masks worn while procedures are in progress	Caps and masks worn for all procedures except for castration of cats and pediatric puppies
	Single-use, sterile, surgical gowns and gloves worn by surgeons for all operating room procedures	Single-use, sterile surgical gowns worn for all abdominal procedures; single-use, sterile gloves worn for all procedures	Sterile gowns not utilized but aseptic technique is maintained; single-use sterile gloves worn for all procedures except cat castrations when single-use examination gloves are worn
Surgeon prep	Surgical scrub or rub performed prior to each procedure and prior to entering operating room	Surgical scrub or rub performed prior to a series of procedures; sterility is maintained between procedures; new single-use sterile gloves are donned prior to each procedure	Surgical scrub or rub performed prior to individual or a series of procedures except for closed castration of cats and pediatric puppies
Patient preparation			
Skin scrub	Hair removal and operative site prepared after anesthetic induction and prior to entering operating room	Hair removal and operative site prepared after anesthetic induction in designated area of operating room	Hair removal and operative site prepared within operating room
Draping	Complete sterile draping performed for all operating room procedures	Complete sterile draping performed for all abdominal procedures and castration of adult dogs; clean barrier draping performed for castration of cats and pediatric puppies	Complete sterile draping performed for all abdominal procedures

surgical procedures, and patient recovery. Additional areas that may enhance efficiency and promote infection control include dressing rooms, supply rooms, an instrument pack preparation room, and a designated area for donning sterile gowns and gloves. Closed doors between clean operating environments and contaminated areas of the facility will aid in infection control and the promotion of aseptic technique (Fossum 2007a).

When designing a surgical facility, careful attention should be paid to traffic flow patterns to ensure maximum efficiency and minimize opportunities for disease transmission. One study of SSI risk in dogs and cats demonstrated a 1.3 times greater risk of SSI for each additional person in the operating room (Eugster et al. 2004). To minimize this risk, only essential personnel should be allowed into the operating room and conversation should be kept to a minimum (Letts and Doermer 1983). Overall traffic flow through the surgical clinic should be thought of as unidirectional and, to promote compliance, the facility should be laid out such that the desired flow pattern is the most direct path for personnel and animals to follow (Figure 4.1).

Although a designated, separate working unit isolated from general facility traffic is the ideal arrangement for an operating room environment (Fossum 2007a), many spay–neuter programs operate under "field" conditions in which this environment must be re-created in a different location on a frequent basis. In such conditions, priority should be given to each of the following points in order to promote

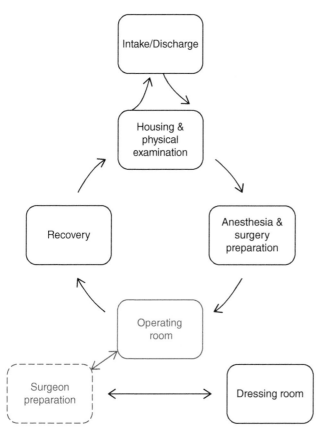

Figure 4.1   Traffic flow through the surgical clinic should be unidirectional to minimize opportunities for contamination of the operating room. Sterile areas are indicated by red lines.

asepsis and minimize the chances of cross-contamination and the occurrence of SSIs (Fossum 2007a; Mangram et al. 1999):

1) Select an area of sufficient size for necessary personnel and equipment.
2) Create physical and/or visual barriers to control and minimize traffic flow (Figure 4.2).
3) Establish a clean, uncluttered environment (e.g. remove wall posters, discard perishable items, cover ceiling fans; place a clean tarpaulin over surfaces that cannot be removed or cleaned prior to use).
4) Select an area with constant humidity and temperature and good air flow.
5) Utilize equipment and surfaces that are amenable to cleaning and disinfection (e.g. smooth, non-porous) or cover surfaces with clean, disposable drape material.

The operating room itself represents a common point for the transfer of infectious disease agents that is often overlooked in clinic sanitation protocols. Environmental character-

istics of the operating room thought to increase the risk of SSI development include contaminated medications, inadequate sanitation practices, and inadequate ventilation (Barie and Eachempati 2005); steps to minimize the risks posed by these factors should be addressed in standard operating protocols. Sanitation practices that should be completed between handling different patients, on a daily basis, and on a weekly basis to maintain a sanitary operating room environment are presented in Table 4.3. Specific disinfectants and their proper usage will be discussed in Chapter 5.

Ancillary Equipment

Countless pieces of equipment and supplies come into contact with spay–neuter patients throughout their clinic experience. Each of these items has the potential to harbor pathogens and transmit disease if not properly sanitized between patients. In fact, biologic contamination and transmission of both bacteria and viruses have been demonstrated

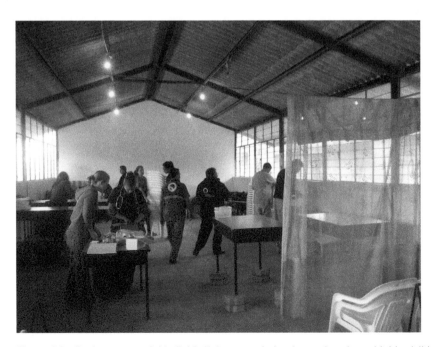

Figure 4.2 During set-up of this field clinic, a curtain has been placed as a highly visible, physical barrier separating the patient receiving area from the operating environment.

Table 4.3 Recommended frequency of sanitation for the operating environment of the spay–neuter clinic.

Between each patient	Daily	Weekly
Patient preparation table	Operating table drip tray	Light fixtures
Operating table surface	Instrument tables	Cabinets and other furniture
Any items contaminated with organic material	Intravenous drip stands	Window sills
	Kick buckets/trash cans	Ventilation grills
	Operating room floor	
	Surgeon scrub sink	
	Door handles and switch plates	

through needles, syringes, intravenous (IV) tubing lines, and laryngoscope blades and handles that have not been thoroughly disinfected between uses (Fleming and Ogilvie 1951; Meier 2002; Morell et al. 1994; Roberts 1973; Shulan et al. 1985; Trepanier et al. 1990). When contaminated items enter the clean operating room environment, they jeopardize the surgeon's ability to maintain surgical asepsis. Common items that are overlooked in spay–neuter clinic sanitation protocols are presented in Box 4.1.

Recommended practices in the human healthcare industry call for complete sterilization of items that come into contact with the vascular system or sterile body tissue (e.g. IV catheters, IV tubing), disinfection of items that contact mucous membranes (e.g. laryngoscope blades, masks), and thorough cleaning of items

that contact intact skin (e.g. electrocardiogram leads, blood pressure cuffs) in between each use. Items such as endotracheal tubes, some breathing circuits, filters, needles, and syringes are considered single-use items to be discarded after use (Association of Operating Room Nurses 2005). Many of these single-use items are commonly reused in veterinary medicine; in these cases following the recommendations for sterilization and disinfection based on level of patient contact already described seems prudent. Maintaining a large stock supply of these items for sanitizing once at the end of each day, utilizing disposable covers or single-use towels to protect equipment surfaces, or limiting shared use of items to groups of patients that are normally exposed to one another (e.g. animals residing in the same household or shelter housing unit) may help promote good sanitary practices without negatively impacting clinic efficiency.

Surgical Instruments

Perhaps the pieces of equipment with the greatest opportunity to impact asepsis are the surgical instruments themselves. Aseptic surgery cannot be achieved unless each surgical instrument that contacts body tissues or blood is sterile at the time of use (Fossum 2007b; Griffin et al. 2016). There are three distinct components to the proper preparation of instruments for use in surgical procedures that warrant discussion: cleaning and decontamination, packaging, and sterilization.

Box 4.1 Commonly Overlooked Surgical and Anesthetic Equipment to Sanitize between Patients

- Pulse oximeters
- Laryngoscopes
- Eye lubricant containers
- Ventilation bags
- Anesthetic circuits
- Clippers
- Stethoscopes
- Thermometers
- Patient positioning devices
- Thermoregulatory devices

Cleaning and Decontamination

Removal of organic contamination (e.g. blood and mucous) through cleaning and decontamination of reusable surgical instruments must be undertaken prior to attempts at sterilization. In fact, the ability to achieve sterilization is dependent upon the number, type, and resistance of microorganisms that are present as well as the presence or absence of biofilms (Association of Operating Room Nurses 2006). Organic contamination of items may inactivate or prevent penetration of chemical germicides as well as increase the bio-burden of the equipment such that sterilization is not possible (Favero and Bond 2001). If allowed to dry on surgical instruments, blood, body fluids, and saline can result in corrosion, rusting, and pitting, which can also impede the sterilization process (Association of Operating Room Nurses 2002b). Cleaning with a detergent and water is likely the most effective as well as cost-efficient means of removing organic material (Dvorak et al. 2008; Quinn and Markey 2001). A pH-neutral, low-foaming, free-rinsing detergent should be safe for most surgical equipment (Association of Operating Room Nurses 2002b). The use of enzymatic cleaners can aid in the removal of proteins from surgical instruments and these are often commercially available in combination products containing detergents. If not removed for decontamination and re-packaging immediately after use, surgical instruments can be immersed in a detergent–water solution (+/− enzymatic cleaner) until processing (Association of Operating Room Nurses 2002b, Association of Surgical Technologists 2009). However, unless indicated by the manufacturer's instructions, instruments should not be immersed in cleaning solutions for extended periods of time (i.e. longer than 20 minutes) in order to preserve integrity and extend useful life (Fossum 2007c). Box 4.2 describes a recommended step-by-step process for manual cleaning and decontamination of surgical instruments.

> **Box 4.2 Manual Cleaning and Decontamination of Surgical Instruments (Association of Operating Room Nurses 2002b; Association of Surgical Technologists 2009)**
>
> - Wipe off visible organic material with a clean, moist sponge
> - Flush instrument lumens with water
> - Immerse in a solution of warm water (80–110 °F) and detergent
> - Scrub instruments with purpose-designed instrument cleaning brush *(Do not use scouring pads or abrasive cleaning agents)*
> - Thoroughly rinse instruments with tap water to remove detergent residue and organic material
> - Rinse instruments with distilled/de-ionized water to prevent staining
> - Place instruments in the unlocked or open position on an absorbent, lint-free towel to dry

Packaging

After appropriate cleaning, decontamination, and drying, surgical instruments must be packaged for processing. The choice of packaging system will depend upon the type of item being sterilized and the method of sterilization being utilized (Association of Operating Room Nurses 2007a). For most stainless-steel surgical instruments utilized in HQHVSN programs, woven cotton muslin (minimum thread count 140), non-woven SMS (spunlace-melt-blown-spunbonded) materials, woven cotton/polyester-blend fabrics, or paper-plastic peel packages will be sufficient (Fossum 2007c). When reusable woven textiles are used, it is important they be laundered between each use, even if no visible contamination is present. In addition to its cleaning effects, laundering serves to rehydrate the material and prevent superheating during the sterilization process, which can inhibit sterilization (Association of Operating Room Nurses

2007a). Although probably unnecessary when non-woven materials are utilized, double-wrapping surgical packs will help prevent bacterial contamination and extend the shelf life of the sterilized pack (Association of Operating Room Nurses 2007a; Fossum 2007c).

Paper-plastic peel pouches can be used for small, lightweight, blunt, low-profile items. The package should be large enough to accommodate the instruments with enough space for steam to circulate around them during the sterilization process (i.e. 3–5 mm), box locks should be opened, and as much air as possible should be removed from the pouch prior to sealing (Association of Operating Room Nurses 2007a; Fossum 2007c). The package should be labeled on indicator tape affixed to the plastic side of the pouch, the plastic side of the self-seal strip, or written directly on the plastic window itself. Caution must be taken not to compromise the permeable, paper side of the pouch, which allows steam penetration, and packages should not be reused unless manufacturers' instructions indicate it is safe to do so (Association of Operating Room Nurses 2007a). Additional tips for successful sterilization with paper-plastic peel pouches are presented in Box 4.3.

Sterilization

While decontamination and packaging are critical to the success of the sterilization process, they do not result in the death or inactivation of bacteria or viruses that are present (Fossum 2007b). A properly performed sterilization process seeks to eliminate all microorganisms, including bacterial spores, from the object of interest, and reduces the probability of organism survival to less than one in one million (Favero and Bond 2001). Sterilization of surgical instruments can be accomplished through steam, ethylene oxide, gas–plasma, liquid chemicals (Box 4.4), ozone, or dry heat (Association of Operating Room Nurses 2006).

Gravity displacement steam sterilization is the most common method of instrument preparation used in HQHVSN programs. The

---

> **Box 4.3   Proper Use of Plastic-Paper Peel Pouches (Association of Operating Room Nurses 2007a, 2007b)**
>
> - Pouches are single use unless otherwise specified by the manufacturer
> - Each pouch can hold 1–2 small, light-weight, low-profile, blunt instruments
> - Use pouches of appropriate size (3–5 mm of space around instrument)
> - Open box locks and disassemble complex instruments prior to placing in pouch
> - Remove air from pouch prior to sealing
> - Seal should be airtight
> - If double pouches are used, do not fold the edges of the inner pouch
> - Place pouches on end on a rack in the sterilizer to allow steam penetration
> - Place paper portion of pouches adjacent to one another in the sterilizer rack
> - Do not place pouches within wrapped instrument packs or other containers
> - Allow pouches to cool within a rack or with paper side up

---

ability of the sterilizer to achieve sterilization is dependent upon its ability to move air through the autoclave and its contents; proper packaging and loose loading of the autoclave are essential to achieve this goal (Fossum 2007b; Reuss-Lamky 2012). Mechanical settings (i.e. time, temperature, and pressure) of the gravity displacement sterilizer must be carefully monitored to ensure sterilization is achieved. The precise settings required for sterilization will vary based on the piece of equipment to be sterilized and the sterilizer itself; however, commonly desired minimum parameters are reported in Table 4.4. After the sterilization cycle is complete, materials should be allowed to dry and cool thoroughly before removal from the sterilizer (i.e. 15–45 minutes). When they are handled prematurely, stacked on top of one another, or placed on a cool surface, residual steam vapor can cause moisture to penetrate the packaging, resulting

Box 4.4	Liquid Chemical Sterilization

Although not specifically addressed in published guidelines for HQHVSN programs (Griffin et al. 2016), liquid chemical or "cold" sterilization is a common technique utilized in veterinary practices and field clinic settings. The active ingredients in commercially available liquid chemical sterilants include glutaraldehyde, peroxyacetic acid, hydrogen peroxide, ortho-phthalaldehyde, and phenol/phenate. It is possible to achieve sterilization with these chemicals; however, specific conditions must be met with each use (Favero and Bond 2001; Fossum 2007b):

1) Items to be sterilized must be clean and dry prior to immersion.
2) Complex instruments must be disassembled prior to immersion.
3) Proper immersion times must be observed; sterilization can be achieved in 6–12 hours depending on formulation.
4) Instruments must be rinsed with sterile water and dried with sterile towels prior to use.
5) Sterilant must be changed after one "cycle" of use; reuse will result in contamination, chemical degradation, and loss of potency.

These requirements, along with the fact that many of the liquid chemical sterilants are known to result in significant toxicities to humans and/or animals (Beauchamp et al. 1992; Block 2001; Favero and Bond 2001; Miller et al. 1973; Morinaga et al. 2010), render liquid chemical sterilization impractical in most spay–neuter practices and its use is not recommended.

Table 4.4 Commonly reported minimum sterilization cycle parameters for surgical equipment in gravity displacement steam sterilizers.

Item	Temperature	Time	Pressure[a]
Instruments	250 °F	30 minutes	15–17 psi
	270 °F	15 minutes	27–30 psi
	275 °F	10 minutes	27–30 psi
Textiles	250 °F	30 minutes	27–30 psi
	270 °F	25 minutes	27–30 psi
	275 °F	10 minutes	27–30 psi
Flash sterilization[b]	270–275 °F	3–10 minutes	27–29 psi

Sources: Rutala and Weber (2008), Fossum (2007b), Association of Operating Room Nurses (2006), Sebben (1984), Young (1993).
[a] For every 1000 ft of altitude, an additional 0.5 psi above 15 psi (normal atmospheric pressure at sea level) is needed.
[b] Item should be unwrapped and placed in a perforated metal tray; observe 10-minute exposure times for porous items or those with lumens.

in the loss of sterilization (Association of Operating Room Nurses 2006; Fossum 2007b).

The sterilizer's mechanical settings should not be relied upon as the sole means of monitoring the effectiveness of sterilization procedures. Additional best practices include the use of both chemical and biological process indicators. Chemical indicators, in the form of tape or paper strips, are available for steam, gas, and plasma sterilization (Fossum 2007b). These devices are commonly placed both inside and outside of each surgical pack and will undergo a color change in response to a threshold temperature (usually between 245 and 270 °F); however, their effectiveness is variable (Association of Operating Room Nurses 2006; Fossum 2007b; Lee et al. 1979). Biologic indicators are perhaps the most accurate means of assessing the sterilization process. A variety of biologic indicators are commercially available; these typically consist of spore-forming bacteria contained in a glass vial that is placed within a "test pack," run through a typical sterilization cycle, and then cultured for bacterial growth. It is recommended that biologic indicators be used a minimum of once per week in veterinary surgical programs (Association of Operating Room Nurses 2006; Fossum 2007b).

In addition to assuring that the sterilization process itself is effective, care should be taken when storing and handling sterilized equipment to prevent contamination. Sterilized packages should be stored in closed cabinets or containers, protected from moisture and aerosolized dust and debris, and should not be stacked on one another (Association of Operating Room Nurses 2006; Fossum 2007c; Renberg 2012). It is also recommended that packs be stored at a constant temperature (<75 °F) and low humidity (<70%); however, the guidance documents making these temperature and humidity recommendations cite no evidence to support such recommendations (McAuley 2009). Handling should be limited to movement from the sterilizer to the storage cabinet/container to the operating room. Excessive handling can lead to seal breakage and package damage (Association of Operating Room Nurses 2006; Fossum 2007c). Events and environmental challenges such as these, rather than time, cause loss of sterilization. However, reported recommended maximum storage times for sterilized packs range from four weeks (for double-wrapped woven packages) to one year (for peel pouches), depending on the specific packaging and storage system utilized (Fossum 2007c).

Surgeon Preparation

Surgeon preparation encompasses the donning of appropriate attire for the procedure – including caps, masks, gowns (if used), and gloves – and surgical hand preparation (Fossum 2007d). Surgical hand preparation has three primary goals: to remove debris and transient microorganisms, to reduce the resident microbial count, and to inhibit rebound growth of microorganisms (Association of Operating Room Nurses 2004; Crabtree et al. 2001). These goals are typically accomplished through the use of commercially available antimicrobial soaps (i.e. an antiseptic–detergent combination) or surgical hand rubs and a standardized surgical scrub procedure (e.g. anatomic timed scrub, counted brush stroke, surgical hand rub; Fossum 2007d).

The ideal antimicrobial product will be rapid acting, broad spectrum, active in the presence of organic matter, non-irritating, have long-acting residual antimicrobial effects, and be economical (Baines 1996; Fossum 2007d). Products containing alcohol, chlorhexidine, iodine/iodophors, phenolic compounds, or some combination of these active ingredients are most common in spay–neuter programs. The pros and cons of each antiseptic along with recommended surgical scrub contact times are presented in Table 4.5. In general, alcohol-based products are considered the most effective agents, followed by chlorhexidine solutions and the iodophors (Hsieh et al. 2006; Noorani et al. 2010; Tanner et al. 2008; Widmer et al. 2010).

Disposable plastic brushes, soap-impregnated sponges, brushless scrub solution, and waterless scrub solutions and rubs are all acceptable and effective methods of applying antiseptic solutions to the hands (Association of Operating Room Nurses 2004; Crabtree et al. 2001; Fossum 2007d; Parienti et al. 2002). However, the use of scrub brushes is thought to be associated with increases in skin damage, skin cell shedding, microbial counts, infection risk, and infection transmission (Kikuchi-Numagami et al. 1999).

Table 4.5   Characteristics of common antiseptics found in surgical scrub solutions.

Antiseptic	Concentration	Pros	Cons	Reported effective contact times
Alcohol	60–95%	Broad-spectrum bactericidal Good fungicide Rapid killing activity Minimal residual activity Inexpensive	Variable efficacy against non-enveloped viruses No residual activity Loss of efficacy in presence of organic debris	1–5 minutes
Chlorhexidine gluconate	0.5–4%	Broad-spectrum bactericidal Strong residual activity Maintains efficacy in presence of organic debris	Poor efficacy against enveloped viruses Ineffective against non-enveloped viruses	2–6 minutes
Para-chloro-meta-xylenol (PCMX)	0.5–4%	Broad-spectrum bactericidal	Variable efficacy against non-enveloped viruses Ineffective against non-enveloped viruses Residual effects unclear	30 seconds –2 minutes
Povidone iodine	0.75–2% (free iodine)	Broad-spectrum bactericidal Moderate fungicide Sporicidal Some residual activity	Variable efficacy against non-enveloped viruses Prolonged time to effect Loss of efficacy in presence of organic debris Staining of skin Tissue toxicity	2–10 minutes

Sources: World Health Organization (2009), Dvorak et al. (2008), Fossum (2007e), Hsieh et al. (2006), Crabtree et al. (2001), Heit and Riviere (2001), Paulson (1994), Larson et al. (1990).

Brushing protocols have not demonstrated enhanced antimicrobial effects compared to brushless methods; in fact, in some cases a greater reduction in microbial counts and lower operating costs were associated with brushless protocols (Barbadoro et al. 2014; Hobson et al. 1998; Howe et al. 2006; Larson et al. 2001; Loeb et al. 1997; Mulberry et al. 2001; Park et al. 2006; Tanner et al. 2008; Tavolacci et al. 2006; Widmer et al. 2010).

It is important to note that not all brushless, waterless, antiseptic rubs or gels have equivalent efficacy and that the contact time required for surgical antisepsis is generally greater than that for purely hygienic purposes. In addition to products intended for surgical antisepsis, manufacturers often have additional waterless products designed for hygienic purposes alone. Program supply coordinators should take care to match the intended use with the labeled indications of the specific product purchased. Surgeons should note that the technique for application of surgical hand rubs (see Figure 4.3) is different than that used for traditional scrub solutions (Kramer et al. 2002; Widmer et al. 2010). In addition, when such products are used, hands should be free from visible contamination and thoroughly dried. In most cases, this will require thorough handwashing with non-medicated soap (WHO 2009).

For the high-volume surgeon, scrubbing prior to each procedure may not be practical or possible. In these cases, it is acceptable to perform a complete surgical scrub at the

Surgical Handrubbing Technique

- Handwash with soap and water on arrival to OR, after having donned theatre clothing (cap/hat/bonnet and mask).
- Use an alcohol-based handrub (ABHR) product for surgical hand preparation, by carefully following the technique illustrated in Images 1 to 17, before every surgical procedure.
- If any residual talc or biological fluids are present when gloves are removed following the operation, handwash with soap and water.

1 Put approximately 5ml (3 doses) of ABHR in the palm of your left hand, using the elbow of your other arm to operate the dispenser.

2 Dip the fingertips of your right hand in the handrub to decontaminate under the nails (5 seconds).

 3   **4**   **5**   **6**   **7**

Images 3-7: Smear the handrub on the right forearm up to the elbow. Ensure that the whole skin area is covered by using circular movements around the forearm until the handrub has fully evaporated (10-15 seconds).

 8   **9**   **10**   **11**   **12**

Images 8-10: Now repeat steps 1-7 for the left hand and forearm.

11 Put approximately 5ml (3 doses) of ABHR in the palm of your left hand as illustrated, to rub both hands at the same time up to the wrists, following all steps in images 12-17 (20-30 seconds).

12 Cover the whole surface of the hands up to the wrist with ABHR, rubbing palm against palm with a rotating movement.

 **13**   **14**   **15**   **16**   **17**

13 Rub the back of the left hand, including the wrist, moving the right palm back and forth, and vice-versa.

14 Rub palm against palm back and forth with fingers interlinked.

15 Rub the back of the fingers by holding them in the palm of the other hand with a sideways back and forth movement.

16 Rub the thumb of the left hand by rotating it in the clasped palm of the right hand and vice versa.

17 When the hands are dry, sterile surgical clothing and gloves can be donned.

Repeat this sequence (average 60 sec) the number of times that adds up to the total duration recommended by the ABHR manufacturer's instructions. This could be two or even three times.

Figure 4.3   World Health Organization surgical handrubbing technique. Reproduced with permission of the World Health Organization: https://www.who.int/infection-prevention/countries/surgical/NewSurgicalA3.pdf.

beginning of the surgical period, with additional scrubs occurring only after breaks in aseptic technique and after procedures lasting longer than 60 minutes. The degree of residual activity and likelihood of skin irritation of the chosen antiseptic agent should be considered when planning the frequency and duration of scrub protocols. However, in most cases, a minimum of five minutes of antiseptic contact time is recommended for the initial scrub, with subsequent scrubs ensuring at least two minutes of contact time (Fossum 2007d). When using surgical hand rubs, contact time generally ranges from one to three minutes depending upon the product formulation (WHO 2009).

Regardless of the scrub technique utilized, it is important to ensure that the hands are fully dried prior to donning surgical gloves. Potentially pathogenic bacteria have been isolated from hospital taps and cultured from the droplets off surgeons' hands after scrubbing, setting up the potential for recontamination of properly scrubbed hands (Heal et al. 2003). This concern may be even greater in developing countries and in field clinic situations where water quality is questionable (Widmer et al. 2010). The permeability of surgical glove wrappers to bacteria in contaminated water has also been demonstrated (Heal et al. 2003). Ensuring that the hands are dry will decrease the chance of inadvertent contamination of the sterile gown and gloves prior to use, may reduce the number of viable bacteria that are present on the hands, and will help ensure that the gloved hands remain an inhospitable environment for bacterial proliferation during the surgical procedure.

The use of sterile surgical gloves is not a substitute for proper hand preparation. The relatively high incidence of glove perforation during surgical procedures is well established and has been directly associated with SSI, particularly when peri-operative antibiotics are not administered (Misteli et al. 2009). One multicenter veterinary study described an overall incidence of glove defects of 23%, with significantly more defects found in gloves worn on the non-dominant hand and those worn during procedures longer than 60 minutes. Surgeon experience was not associated with the incidence of defects (Character et al. 2003). Table 4.2 describes the indications for sterile surgical glove application in spay–neuter programs along with those of additional surgical attire such as caps, masks, and surgical gowns.

Patient Preparation

Patient preparation in veterinary medicine encompasses the removal of hair and scrubbing of the planned surgical site, along with the application of appropriate barrier drapes. The goals of patient preparation are the same as those already described for the surgeon. In addition, the use of surgical drapes serves as both a physical barrier against microbes and a visual establishment of the sterile field (Association of Operating Room Nurses 2006b).

Hair removal in veterinary patients can be performed through the use of electric clippers or depilatory creams. Depilatory creams are less traumatic and result in a smoother skin surface than electric clippers (Fossum 2007e; Weiland et al. 2006); however, a mild, self-limiting inflammatory reaction has been described after using a commercial depilatory cream in rabbits (Foley et al. 2001). Studies comparing the rates of inflammation and risk of SSI between depilatory creams and electric clippers in veterinary patients are not available.

The timing of hair removal can also contribute to the risk of SSI development. One veterinary study utilizing electric clippers for hair removal found that patients clipped ≥4 hours prior to the surgical procedure had significantly greater odds of developing a SSI than those clipped <4 hours prior to surgery (Mayhew et al. 2012); a second found that clipping of the surgical site prior to anesthetic induction resulted in a threefold increase in the likelihood of SSI (Brown et al. 1997). These findings mirror those of human surgical patients, in which lower rates of SSI are seen the closer hair removal is performed to the start of the surgical procedure (Alexander et al. 1983; Seropian and Reynolds 1971). To minimize skin trauma in veterinary patients, hair clipping should be performed with an electric clipper and a sharp number 40 clipper blade in the same direction as the hair growth. In patients with dense hair coats, initially using a coarser blade (e.g. number 10) followed by a number 40 blade may be most effective (Fossum 2007e). The size of the clipped area should be proportional to the size of the patient, the drape fenestration (for prefenestrated drapes), and the anticipated incision, allowing for expansion of the surgical field if necessary. Excess clipping may increase the risk of trauma and infection, promote

hypothermia, and reduce cosmesis, while too small an area may result in contamination of the surgical field (Figure 4.4). Clipped hair should be removed from the environment with a vacuum (Fossum 2007e). For patients with fine hair or in locations without electricity, use of a one-sided adhesive lint roller is also effective.

After thorough hair removal, antiseptic preparation of the surgical site can begin. It is ideal to perform a general cleansing scrub prior to transporting the patient into the operating room where the sterile skin preparation takes place (Fossum 2007e). The purpose of this protocol is to ensure that the surgical site does not become contaminated during transportation

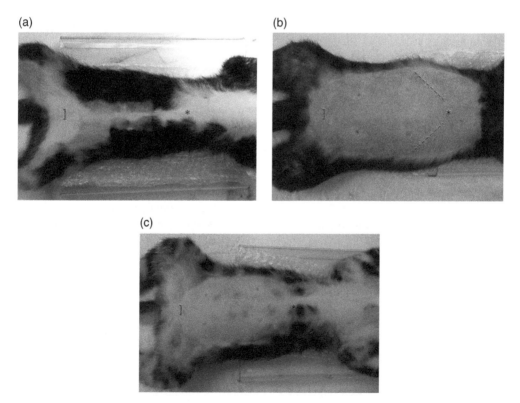

(a)

(b)

(c)

Figure 4.4 Patients being prepared for ovariohysterectomy. (a) The clipped area is too small to maintain aseptic technique. If extension of the incision is necessary, the surgical site will become contaminated. (b) The clipped area is too wide for this patient and will promote hypothermia. In addition, the clipped area extends over the borders of the rib cage – it is unlikely that any complications encountered during ovariohysterectomy will require the surgeon to perform a thoracotomy. (c) This patient is clipped appropriately for its size and the anticipated surgical procedure. The clipped area extends from the xiphoid to the pubis and follows the borders of the rib cage laterally. *, xiphoid;], pubis; - - -, borders of rib cage.

and positioning of the patient on the operating table. Application of an antiseptic-soaked gauze sponge to the anticipated incision site and use of a specific handling technique for small patients may help in protecting the prepared surgical site (Figure 4.5). Should there be any question of contamination after positioning the patient on the operating table, the sterile scrub should be repeated. Alternatively, both hair removal and antiseptic preparation can be performed in one location, as long as precautions are taken not to contaminate the surgical site or operating environment.

Antiseptic agents useful in preparing the surgical site are similar to those described for surgeon preparation (Table 4.5). Phenolic compounds (e.g. hexachlorophene, para-chloro-meta-xylenol or PCMX, triclosan) and quaternary ammonium salts should not be used, as they are associated with significant toxicities in animals and safe, effective alternatives are readily available (Dvorak et al. 2008; Fossum 2007e; Heit and Riviere 2001; Merianos 2001). Many commercially available patient preparation solutions contain one or more additional antiseptics that have been shown to enhance antimicrobial efficacy or persistence (Hibbard

2005; Hibbard et al. 2002). Multiple protocols for the application of antiseptics have proven effective (e.g. alternating antiseptic scrub with alcohol or saline rinse, antiseptic scrub followed by sprays or paints, antiseptic spray alone, wiping skin dry after scrubbing, leaving skin to air dry, etc.; Geelhoed et al. 1983; Kutarski and Grundy 1993; Moen et al. 2002; Osuna et al. 1990; Shirahatti et al. 1993). Perhaps more important than the antiseptic chosen or the application protocol are the provisions that the skin surface is clean prior to beginning the surgical scrub, that the appropriate contact time for the chosen antiseptic is observed, and that application of the agent does not result in recontamination of the surgical site (Association of Operating Room Nurses 2002a). Figure 4.6 describes the appropriate technique for manual application of pre-operative antiseptic solutions.

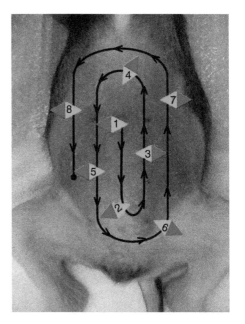

Figure 4.6 Surgical scrubbing pattern. Once the skin surface has been cleaned, application of the antiseptic solution should proceed in gradually expanding circles from the anticipated incision site outward. Care must be taken to rotate the applicator sponge so that the contaminated "tail" end does not contact a previously scrubbed area. Green, "head" of applicator sponge; red, "tail" of applicator sponge.

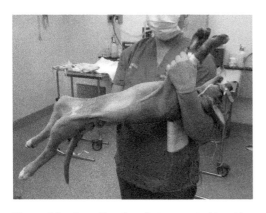

Figure 4.5 A small patient is transported into the operating room without contaminating the prepared surgical site. The technician places the patient's neck against the inside of her elbow to support the head, while holding the front legs with the same hand. The opposite hand is laid flat underneath the patient's pelvis to prevent the hind legs from contacting the surgical site.

Once the scrub of the surgical site is complete, it should be allowed to dry thoroughly prior to draping (Fossum 2007e). Although wet drape material has been shown to enhance bacterial strike-through, the effectiveness of barrier drapes in protecting the patient against SSI is the subject of debate in human surgical care (Belkin 2002; Blom et al. 2002; Hadiati et al. 2012; Mangram et al. 1999). Their role in veterinary surgery, however, seems more obvious given the relatively high risk of hair or fecal contamination of the surgical site (Looney et al. 2008). Patient draping is generally accomplished in two layers: placement of field drapes or towels to cover contaminated areas outside of the prepared surgical field, followed by placement of a fenestrated drape to isolate the anticipated incision site (Fossum 2007e). While a number of human and veterinary studies have demonstrated no reduction in SSI with the use of adhesive incise drapes in combination with barrier drapes, the true impact of the traditional two-layer draping technique in preventing SSI is unknown (Owen et al. 2009; Webster and Alghamdi 2007). It is common in HQHVSN programs to utilize a single fenestrated drape to isolate the incision site. As long as reasonable precautions are taken to keep drape material dry and to remain conscious of the limits of the sterile field, there is no evidence that this technique results in increased risk of SSI. If drapes are not pre-fenestrated, creating a fenestration prior to applying the drape material to the patient may help prevent contamination of sterile surgical scissors by the patient's skin.

How Do you Maintain Asepsis while Increasing Efficiency of HQHVSN Programs?

In healthcare, as in many other industries, ensuring a high-quality outcome goes hand in hand with improvements in efficiency, streamlined operational practices, and the use of individuals with highly specialized skill sets (Ford and Crowther 1922; Gawande 2009; McDonald's 2013). For surgery in particular, the relationship between the performance of a high volume of procedures and low rates of surgical complications has long been scientifically established (Birkmeyer et al. 2013; Donabedian 1984; Flood et al. 1984, 1984b; Luft 1980). Some critical components of reducing SSIs and other surgical complications in both humans and animals include taking steps to reduce both total anesthetic time and surgical procedure time, ensuring adequate host immune defense, maintaining normothermia, ensuring euglycemia, providing supplemental oxygen during and shortly after surgery, and providing adequate analgesia (Brodbelt et al. 2008; Brown et al. 1997; Brunn 1970; Burrow et al. 2005; Cruse and Foord 1973; Eugster et al. 2004; Nicholson et al. 2002; Sessler 2006; Velasco et al. 1996). By its very nature, HQHVSN necessitates the integration of such practices which also promote positive outcomes. Sections Two and Three will discuss specific anesthetic and surgical techniques to help the HQHVSN surgeon achieve these goals.

Frequently Asked Questions

Can Masking Tape Be Used to Secure Paper-Plastic Instrument Pouches?

Masking tape is commonly used as an inexpensive alternative to sealing paper-plastic instrument pouches with sterilization indicator tape. This is not a reliable method of ensuring an airtight seal that will not be compromised throughout the sterilization process. Masking tape adhesive will melt around 150 °F (much lower than the temperatures achieved during steam sterilization), while the adhesive found in indicator tape contains a polyacrylate that maintains its adhesive properties up to 300 °F. Melted adhesive can result in disruption of the seal and/or opening of the package during the sterilization process (Fisher Scientific, personal communication, February 8, 2013).

Are Ultrasonic Instrument Cleaners Effective?

Ultrasonic instrument cleaners can be an effective tool if utilized properly. They should only be used if the following conditions can be met: gross contamination has been mechanically removed, cleaners are regularly "degassed" according to manufacturer's directions, only instruments constructed from the same metal are cleaned together, instruments are fully submerged in the cleaning solution, instruments are rinsed thoroughly after cleaning, and the cleaner is emptied and sanitized when visibly soiled (Association of Operating Room Nurses 2002b). Ultrasonic instrument cleaners do not typically have significant antimicrobial effects of their own, so instruments must be properly packaged and sterilized prior to reuse (Jatzwauk et al. 2001; Muqbil et al. 2005).

Can a Pressure Cooker Be Used to Sterilize Surgical Instruments?

In some field clinic situations where use of an autoclave is not feasible or possible (i.e. there is no electricity), it may be desirable to utilize a pressure cooker to sterilize surgical instruments (Mulcahy 2003). The ability of a pressure cooker to inactivate bacterial spores has been established (Expanded Program on Immunization in the Americas 1984). In order to ensure effectiveness and operator safety, the same procedures for preparing and packaging instruments as already discussed must be followed, instruments must not contact the water in the bottom of the cooker, and time and pressure measurements should not begin until the entire cooking chamber has filled with steam (i.e. steam rushes out of the open air vent, which is subsequently closed to start the sterilization process; Expanded Program on Immunization in the Americas 1984; Frobisher 1939). See Table 4.4 for desired time, temperature, and pressure settings. As proper sterilization relies on a human operator to monitor cycle parameters, the use of sterilization

indicators is especially important to ensure sterilization has been achieved.

Should Shoe Covers Be Worn in the Operating Room?

Shoe covers have not been shown to impact bacterial counts on operating room floors or decrease the risk of SSI (Humphreys et al. 1991; Mangram et al. 1999). Similarly, tacky mats and foot baths are fraught with logistical problems, poor efficacy, and evidence that they may even promote the spread of infectious organisms (Amass et al. 2000; Ayliffe et al. 1967; Stockton et al. 2006). As the appropriate use of these items comes at the expense of significant resources, it may be more effective to require surgical staff members to wear clean shoes designated for use only within the surgical suite (Weightman and Banfield 1994).

How Many Times Can Reusable Surgical Gowns and Drapes Be Laundered?

Textile manufacturers provide recommended usage guidelines for specific products – in some cases this is indicated by a "usage grid" on the item itself which is marked each time it is used; when all the grids are full the item should be discarded (Association of Operating Room Nurses 2007a; Reuss-Lamky 2012). Maintenance of a thread count greater than 270 and limiting woven fabrics to 75 reuses have also been suggested as means of ensuring textile integrity (Association of Surgical Technologists 2008). In the absence of such information, reusable materials should be inspected after each use for holes, punctures, and tears which may compromise their ability to provide an antimicrobial barrier. The material should be easy to handle, flexible, and free of residues. Small holes or areas of worn fabric can be patched with the same type of drape material which must be heat sealed in place (stitching the patch in place is not acceptable, as this compromises the integrity of the material; Association of Surgical Technologists 2008).

Is There a Benefit to Using Antibiotic-Coated Suture?

Antibiotic-coated suture material is marketed by a variety of veterinary supply distributors as a means of reducing rates of SSI in certain types of surgical wounds. A number of in-vitro and in-vivo studies have demonstrated the ability of these products to inhibit bacterial colonization under experimental conditions, but comparisons of clinical efficacy in veterinary patients are limited (Edmiston et al. 2006; Marco et al. 2007; Ming et al. 2007; Storch et al. 2004). A recent retrospective study in dogs undergoing tibial plateau-leveling osteotomy and a prospective, randomized study of horses undergoing exploratory celiotomy both found no difference in SSI rates between patients that were sutured with antibiotic-impregnated suture and those with non-impregnated suture (Bischofberger et al. 2010; Etter et al. 2013). However, in human surgical patients, the use of antibiotic-coated suture has resulted in fewer SSIs, particularly in adults, patients undergoing abdominal surgery, and in clean or clean-contaminated procedures (Justinger et al. 2009; Nakamura et al. 2013; Wang et al. 2013). Pediatric patients reported less pain one day post-operatively when antibiotic-coated suture was used compared to other suture types (Ford et al. 2005). Additional veterinary studies may elucidate a clearer role for this material in HQHVSN programs.

Can I Use a Tattoo Gun to Identify Neutered Patients?

Application of tattoo ink is a common method of identifying neutered animals. A variety of methods can be employed to apply the ink, including the use of a tattoo gun (Griffin et al. 2016). Since the tattoo gun's needle comes into contact with sterile body tissue, it should be sterile at the time of use (Association of Operating Room Nurses 2005; Griffin et al. 2016). Indeed, transmission of a variety of serious infectious diseases has been reported in people when aseptic technique is not followed during tattoo application (Centers for Disease Control and Prevention 2010; Nishioka and Gyorkos 2001; Sun et al. 1996). With the constant discovery of new infectious organisms in veterinary medicine, it is naïve to assume that we are not transmitting infectious organisms in our veterinary patients simply because we have not diagnosed an as yet undiscovered infectious disease (Belák et al. 2013). In most spay–neuter programs it is safer and more cost-effective to utilize another method of tattoo application. See Chapter 16 for more information.

References

Alexander, J.W., Fischer, J.E., Boyajian, M. et al. (1983). The influence of hair-removal methods on wound infections. *Arch. Surg.* 118 (3): 347–352.

Amass, S.F., Vyverberg, B.D., Ragland, D. et al. (2000). Evaluating the efficacy of boot baths in biosecurity protocols. *J. Swine Health Prod.* 8 (4): 169–173.

Association of Operating Room Nurses (2002a). Recommended practices for skin preparation of patients. *AORN J.* 75 (1): 184–187.

Association of Operating Room Nurses (2002b). Recommended practices for cleaning and caring for surgical instruments and powered equipment. *AORN J.* 75 (3): 627–638.

Association of Operating Room Nurses (2004). Recommended practices for surgical hand: antisepsis/hand scrubs. *AORN J.* 79 (2): 416–431.

Association of Operating Room Nurses (2005). Recommended practices for cleaning, handling, and processing anesthesia equipment. *AORN J.* 81 (4): 856–870.

Association of Operating Room Nurses (2006). Recommended practices for sterilization in the perioperative practice setting. *AORN J.* 83 (3): 700–722.

Association of Operating Room Nurses (2006b). Recommended practices for maintaining a sterile field. *AORN J.* 83 (2): 402–416.

Association of Operating Room Nurses (2007a). Recommended practices for selection and use of packaging systems for sterilization. *AORN J.* 85 (4): 801–812.

Association of Operating Room Nurses (2007b). Using peel packages inside containers or wrapped instrument trays. *AORN J.* 86 (3): 461–462.

Association of Surgical Technologists (2008). AST recommended standards of practice for surgical drapes. http://www.ast.org/pdf/Standards_of_Practice/RSOP_Surgical_Drapes.pdf (accessed 17 February 2013).

Association of Surgical Technologists (2009). Recommended standards of practice for the decontamination of surgical instruments. http://www.ast.org/pdf/Standards_of_Practice/RSOP_Decontamination_%20 Surgical%20Instruments_.pdf (accessed 8 February 2013).

Ayliffe, G.A., Collins, B.J., Lowbury, E.J. et al. (1967). Ward floors and other surfaces as reservoirs of hospital infection. *J. Hyg.* 65 (4): 515–536.

Baines, S. (1996). Surgical asepsis: principles and protocols. *In Pract* 18: 23–33.

Barbadoro, P., Martini, E., Savini, S. et al. (2014). *In vivo* comparative efficacy of three surgical hand preparation agents in reducing bacterial count. *J. Hosp. Disinfect.* 86: 64–67.

Barie, P.S. and Eachempati, S.R. (2005). Surgical site infections. *Surg. Clin. N. Am.* 85 (6): 1115–1135.

Beauchamp, R.O., St. Clair, M.B., Fennell, T.R. et al. (1992). A critical review of the toxicology of glutaraldehyde. *Crit. Rev. Toxicol.* 22 (3–4): 143–174.

Becker, M. (2011). Should veterinarians offer spays below cost? http://www.vetstreet.com/dr-marty-becker/should-veterinarians-offer-spays-below-cost?WT.mc_id=mbfacebook%3 Bcostofspaying (accessed 8 February 2013).

Belák, S., Karlsson, O.E., Blomström, A.L. et al. (2013). New viruses in veterinary medicine, detected by metagenomic approaches. *Vet. Microbiol.* 165 (1–2): 95–101.

Belkin, N.L. (2002). Barrier surgical gowns and drapes: just how necessary are they? *Text. Rent.* 1: 66–73.

Benedict, K.M., Morley, P.S., and Van Metre, D.C. (2012). Characteristics of biosecurity and infection control programs at veterinary teaching hospitals. *JAVMA* 233 (5): 767–773.

Birkmeyer, J.D., Finks, J.F., O'Reilly, A. et al. (2013). Surgical skill and complication rates after bariatric surgery. *N. Eng. J. Med.* 369: 1434–1442.

Bischofberger, A.S., Brauer, T., Gugelchuk, G. et al. (2010). Difference in incisional complications following exploratory celiotomies using antibacterial-coated suture material for subcutaneous closure: prospective randomised study in 100 horses. *Equine Vet. J.* 42 (4): 304–309.

Block, S.S. (2001). Peroxygen compounds. In: *Disinfection, Sterilization, and Preservation*, 5e (ed. S.S. Block), 185–204. Philadelphia, PA: Lippincott Williams & Wilkins.

Blom, A.W., Gozzard, C., Heal, J. et al. (2002). Bacterial strike-through of re-usable surgical drapes: the effect of different wetting agents. *J. Hosp. Infect.* 52 (1): 52–55.

Brodbelt, D.C., Pfeiffer, D.U., Young, L.E. et al. (2008). Results of the confidential enquiry into perioperative small animal fatalities regarding risk factors for anesthetic-related death in dogs. *JAVMA* 233 (7): 1096–1104.

Brown, D.C., Conzemius, M.G., Shofer, F. et al. (1997). Epidemiologic evaluation of postoperative wound infections in dogs and cats. *JAVMA* 210 (9): 1302–1306.

Brunn, J. (1970). Post-operative wound infection. Predisposing factors and the effect of a reduction in the dissemination of staphylococci. *Acta Medica Scandinavica* S514: 1–89.

Burrow, R., Batchelor, D., and Cripps, P. (2005). Complications observed during and after ovariohysterectomy of 142 bitches at a veterinary teaching hospital. *Vet. Rec.* 157: 829–833.

Centers for Disease Control and Prevention (2010). HIV transmission. http://www.cdc.gov/hiv/resources/qa/transmission.htm (accessed 17 February 2013).

Character, B.J., McLaughlin, R.M., Hedlund, C.S. et al. (2003). Postoperative integrity of veterinary surgical gloves. *J. Am. Anim. Hosp. Assoc.* 39 (3): 311–320.

Crabtree, T.D., Pelletier, S.J., and Pruett, T.L. (2001). Surgical antisepsis. In: *Disinfection, Sterilization, and Preservation*, 5e (ed. S.S. Block), 919–934. Philadelphia, PA: Lippincott Williams & Wilkins.

Cruse, P.J. and Foord, R. (1973). A five-year prospective study of 23,649 surgical wounds. *Arch. Surg.* 107 (2): 206–210.

Donabedian, A. (1984). Volume, quality, and the regionalization of health care services. *Med. Care* 22 (2): 95–97.

Dvorak, G., Petersen, C.A., Rovid Spickler, A. et al. (2008). Disinfection 101. In: *Maddie's Infection Control Manual for Animal Shelters* (eds. C.A. Petersen, G. Dvorak and A. Rovid Spickler), 42–65. Ames, IA: Center for Food Security and Public Health, Iowa State University, College of Veterinary Medicine.

Edmiston, C.E., Seabrook, G.R., Goheen, M.P. et al. (2006). Bacterial adherence to surgical sutures: can antibacterial-coated sutures reduce the risk of microbial contamination? *J. Am. Coll. Surg.* 203 (4): 481–489.

Emori, T.G. and Gaynes, R.P. (1993). An overview of nosocomial infections. *Clin. Microbiol. Rev.* 6 (4): 428–442.

Etter, S.W., Ragetly, G.R., Bennett, R.A. et al. (2013). Effect of using triclosan-impregnated suture for incisional closure on surgical site infection and inflammation following tibial plateau leveling osteotomy in dogs. *JAVMA* 242 (3): 355–358.

Eugster, S., Schawalder, P., Gaschen, F. et al. (2004). A prospective study of postoperative surgical site infections in dogs and cats. *Vet. Surg.* 33: 542–550.

Expanded Program on Immunization in the Americas (1984). Using a pressure cooker as an autoclave. *Expanded Program on Immunization in the Americas Newsletter* 6 (6): 5–8.

Favero, M.S. and Bond, W.W. (2001). Chemical disinfection of medical and surgical materials. In: *Disinfection, Sterilization, and Preservation*, 5e (ed. S.S. Block), 881–917. Philadelphia, PA: Lippincott Williams & Wilkins.

Fleming, A. and Ogilvie, A.C. (1951). Syringe needles and mass inoculation technique. *BMJ* 1 (4706): 543–546.

Flood, A.B., Scott, W.R., and Ewy, W. (1984). Does practice make perfect? Part I: the relation between hospital volume and outcomes for selected diagnostic categories. *Med. Care* 22 (2): 98–114.

Flood, A.B., Scott, W.R., and Ewy, W. (1984b). Does practice make perfect? Part II: the relation between volume and outcomes and other hospital characteristics. *Med. Care* 22 (2): 115–125.

Foley, P.L., Henderson, A.L., Bissonette, E.A. et al. (2001). Evaluation of fentanyl transdermal patches in rabbits: blood concentrations and physiologic response. *Comparative Med.* 51 (3): 239–244.

Ford, H. and Crowther, S. (1922). *My Life and Work*. Garden City, NY: Garden City Publishing.

Ford, H.R., Jones, P., Gaines, V. et al. (2005). Intraoperative handling and wound healing: controlled clinical trial comparing coated VICRYL plus antibacterial suture (coated polyglactin 910 suture with triclosan) with coated VICRYL suture (coated polyglactin 910 suture). *Surg. Infect.* 6 (3): 313–321.

Fossum, T.W. (2007a). Surgical facilities, equipment, and personnel. In: *Small Animal Surgery*, 3e (ed. T.W. Fossum), 15–18. St. Louis, MO: Mosby Elsevier.

Fossum, T.W. (2007b). Sterilization and disinfection. In: *Small Animal Surgery*, 3e (ed. T.W. Fossum), 9–14. St. Louis, MO: Mosby Elsevier.

Fossum, T.W. (2007c). Principles of surgical asepsis. In: *Small Animal Surgery*, 3e (ed. T.W. Fossum), 1–8. St. Louis, MO: Mosby Elsevier.

Fossum, T.W. (2007d). Preparation of the surgical team. In: *Small Animal Surgery*,

3e (ed. T.W. Fossum), 38–45. St. Louis, MO: Mosby Elsevier.

Fossum, T.W. (2007e). Preparation of the operative site. In: *Small Animal Surgery*, 3e (ed. T.W. Fossum), 32–37. St. Louis, MO: Mosby Elsevier.

Frobisher, M. (1939). Disinfection in the home. *Am. J. Nurs.* 39 (1): 833–839.

Gawande, A. (2009). *The Checklist Manifesto*. New York: Metropolitan Books.

Geelhoed, G.W., Sharpe, K., and Simon, G.L. (1983). A comparative study of surgical skin preparation methods. *Surg. Gynecol. Obstet.* 157 (3): 265–268.

Griffin, B., Bushby, P.A., McCobb, E. et al. (2016). The Association of Shelter Veterinarians' 2016 veterinary medical care guidelines for spay-neuter programs. *JAVMA* 249 (2): 165–188.

Hadiati, D.R., Hakimi, M., and Nurdiati, D.S. (2012). Skin preparation for preventing infection following caesarean section. *Cochrane Database Syst. Rev.*, Sep 12 (9): CD007462. https://doi.org/10.1002/14651858. CD007462.pub2.

Heal, J.S., Blom, A.W., Titcomb, D. et al. (2003). Bacterial contamination of surgical gloves by water droplets spilt after scrubbing. *J. Hosp. Infect.* 53 (2): 136–139.

Hedlund, C.S. (2007). Surgery of the reproductive and genital systems. In: *Small Animal Surgery*, 3e (ed. T.W. Fossum), 702–774. St. Louis, MO: Mosby Elsevier.

Heit, M.C. and Riviere, J.E. (2001). Chemotherapy of microbial diseases. In: *Veterinary Pharmacology and Therapeutics*, 8e (eds. J.E. Riviere and M.G. Papich), 783–795. Hoboken, NJ: Wiley-Blackwell.

Hibbard, J.S. (2005). Analyses comparing the antimicrobial activity and safety of current antiseptic agents: a review. *J. Infus. Nurs.* 28 (3): 194–207.

Hibbard, J.S., Mulberry, G.K., and Brady, A.R. (2002). A clinical study comparing the skin antisepsis and safety of ChloraPrep, 70% isopropyl alcohol, and 2% aqueous chlorhexidine. *J. Infus. Nurs.* 25 (4): 244–249.

Hobson, D.W., Woller, W., Anderson, L. et al. (1998). Development and evaluation of a new alcohol-based surgical hand scrub formulation with persistent antimicrobial characteristics and brushless application. *Am. J. Infect. Cont.* 26 (5): 507–512.

Howe, L.M., Halvorson, K.T., Simpson, R.B. et al. (2006). Waterless, scrubless, alcohol-based surgical scrub agent compared to traditional surgical scrub using chlorhexidine. *Am. J. Infect. Cont.* 34 (5): 112–113.

Hsieh, H., Chiu, H., and Lee, F. (2006). Surgical hand scrubs in relation to microbial counts: systematic literature review. *J. Adv. Nurs.* 55 (1): 68–78.

Humphreys, H., Marshall, R.J., Ricketts, V.E. et al. (1991). Theatre over-shoes do not reduce operating theatre floor bacterial counts. *J. Hosp. Infect.* 17 (2): 117–123.

Isaza, N. and DiGangi, B.A. (2012). Cultivating compassion: University of Florida Merial shelter animal medicine clerkship. 2012 Maddie's Shelter Medicine Conference, University of Florida, Gainesville.

Jatzwauk, L., Schone, H., and Pietsch, H. (2001). How to improve instrument disinfection by ultrasound. *J. Hosp. Infect.* 48: S80–S83.

Johnson, J.A. (2002). Nosocomial infections. *Vet. Clin. N. Am. Small* 32: 1101–1126.

Justinger, C., Moussavian, M.R., Schlueter, C. et al. (2009). Antibacterial [corrected] coating of abdominal closure sutures and wound infection. *Surgery* 145 (3): 330–334.

Kikuchi-Numagami, K., Saishu, T., Fukaya, M. et al. (1999). Irritancy of scrubbing up for surgery with or without a brush. *Acta Derm. Venereol.* 79 (3): 230–232.

Klevens, R., Edwards, J., Richards, C.L. et al. (2007). Estimating health care-associated infections and deaths in U.S. hospitals, 2002. *Public Health Rep.* 122 (2): 160–166.

Kramer, A., Rudolph, P., Kampf, G. et al. (2002). Limited efficacy of alcohol-based hand gels. *Lancet* 359 (9316): 1489–1490.

Kreisler, R.E., Shaver, S.L., and Holmes, J.H. (2018). Outcomes of elective gonadectomy procedures performed on dogs and cats by veterinary students and shelter veterinarians in a shelter environment. *JAVMA* 253: 1294–1299.

Kutarski, P.W. and Grundy, H.C. (1993). To dry or not to dry? An assessment of the possible degradation in efficiency of preoperative skin preparation caused by wiping skin dry. *Ann. R. Coll. Surg. Engl.* 75 (3): 181–185.

Larson, E.L., Aiello, A.E., Heilman, J.M. et al. (2001). Comparison of different regimens for surgical hand preparation. *AORN J.* 73 (2): 412–420.

Larson, E.L., Butz, A.M., Gullette, D.L. et al. (1990). Alcohol for surgical scrubbing? *Infect. Contr. Hosp. Epidemiol.* 11 (3): 139–143.

Lee, C.H., Montville, T.J., and Sinskey, A.J. (1979). Comparison of the efficacy of steam sterilization indicators. *Appl. Environ. Microbiol.* 37 (6): 1113–1137.

Letts, R.M. and Doermer, E. (1983). Conversation in the operating theatre as a cause of airborne bacterial contamination. *J. Bone Joint Surg. Am.* 65 (3): 357–362.

Lister, J. (1867). On the antiseptic principle in the practice of surgery. *BMJ* 8: 246–248.

Loeb, M.B., Wilcox, L., Smaill, F. et al. (1997). A randomized trial of surgical scrubbing with a brush compared to antiseptic soap alone. *Am. J. Infect. Cont.* 25 (1): 11–15.

Longo, L.D. (1995). Classic pages in obstetrics and gynecology. *Am. J. Obstet. Gynecol.* 172 (1): 236–237.

Looney, A., Bohling, M., Bushby, P. et al. (2008). The Association of Shelter Veterinarians veterinary medical care guidelines for spay-neuter programs. *JAVMA* 233 (1): 74–86.

Luft, H.S. (1980). The relation between surgical volume and mortality: an exploration of causal factors and alternative models. *Med. Care* 18 (9): 940–959.

Mangram, A.J., Horan, T.C., Pearson, M.L. et al. (1999). Guideline for prevention of surgical site infection, 1999. *Infect. Cont. Hosp. Epidemiol.* 20 (4): 250–280.

Marco, F., Vallez, R., Gonzalez, P. et al. (2007). Study of the efficacy of coated Vicryl plus antibacterial suture in an animal model of orthopedic surgery. *Surg. Infect.* 8 (3): 359–365.

Mayhew, P.D., Freeman, L., Kwan, T. et al. (2012). Comparison of surgical site infection rates in clean and clean-contaminated wound in dogs and cats after minimally invasive versus open surgery: 179 cases (2007–2008). *JAVMA* 240 (2): 193–198.

McAuley, T. (2009). Specifications for temperature and humidity in sterile storage environments – Where's the evidence? *Healthcare Infect.* 14: 131–137.

McDonald's (2013). The Ray Kroc story. http://www.mcdonalds.com/us/en/our_story/our_history/the_ray_kroc_story.html (accessed 16 February 2013).

Meier, B. (2002). Reuse of needle at hospital infects 50 with hepatitis C. *New York Times* (10 October), p. 22. http://www.nytimes.com/2002/10/10/us/reuse-of-needle-at-hospital-infects-50-with-hepatitis-c.html (accessed 8 February 2013).

Merianos, J.J. (2001). Surface-active agents. In: *Disinfection, Sterilization, and Preservation*, 5e (ed. S.S. Block), 283–320. Philadelphia, PA: Lippincott Williams & Wilkins.

Miller, J.J., Powell, G.M., Olavesen, A.H. et al. (1973). The metabolism and toxicity of phenols in cats. 540th Meeting of the Biochemical Society University of Oxford 10 and 11, pp. 1163–165.

Ming, X., Nichols, M., and Rothenburger, S. (2007). In vivo antibacterial efficacy of MONOCRYL plus antibacterial suture (Poliglecaprone 25 with triclosan). *Surg. Infect.* 8 (2): 209–214.

Misteli, H., Weber, W.P., Reck, S. et al. (2009). Surgical glove perforation and the risk of surgical site infection. *Arch. Surg.* 144 (6): 553–558.

Moen, M.D., Noone, M.B., and Kirson, I. (2002). Povidone-iodine spray technique versus traditional scrub-paint technique for preoperative abdominal wall preparation. *Am. J. Obstet. Gynecol.* 187 (6): 1436–1437.

Morell, R.C., Ririe, D., James, R.L. et al. (1994). A survey of laryngoscope contamination at a university and a community hospital. *Anesthesiology* 80 (94): 960.

Morinaga, T., Hasegawa, G., Koyama, S. et al. (2010). Acute inflammation and immunoresponses induced by ortho-phthalaldehyde in mice. *Arch. Toxicol.* 84 (5): 397–404.

Mulberry, G., Snyder, A.T., Heilman, J. et al. (2001). Evaluation of a waterless, scrubless chlorhexidine gluconate/ethanol surgical scrub for antimicrobial efficacy. *Am. J. Infect. Cont.* 29 (6): 277–382.

Mulcahy, D.M. (2003). Surgical implantation of transmitters into fish. *Inst. Lab. Anim. Res. J.* 44 (4): 295–306.

Muqbil, I., Burke, F.J., Miller, C.H. et al. (2005). Antimicrobial activity of ultrasonic cleaners. *J. Hosp. Infect.* 60 (3): 249–255.

Nakamura, T., Kashimura, N., Noji, T. et al. (2013). Triclosan-coated sutures reduce the incidence of wound infections and the costs after colorectal surgery: a randomized controlled trial. *Surgery* 153 (4): 576–583.

Nicholson, M., Beal, M., Shofer, F. et al. (2002). Epidemiologic evaluation of postoperative wound infection in clean-contaminated wounds: a retrospective study of 239 dogs and cats. *Vet. Surg.* 31: 577–581.

Nishioka, S. and Gyorkos, T.W. (2001). Tattoos as risk factors for transfusion-transmitted diseases. *Int. J. Infect. Dis.* 5 (1): 27–34.

Noorani, A., Rabey, N., Walsh, S.R. et al. (2010). Systematic review and meta-analysis of preoperative antisepsis with chlorhexidine versus povidone-iodine in clean-contaminated surgery. *Brit. J. Surg.* 97 (11): 1614–1620.

Osuna, D.J., DeYoung, D.J., and Walker, R.L. (1990). Comparison of three skin preparation techniques. Part 2: clinical trial in 100 dogs. *Vet. Surg.* 19 (1): 20–23.

Owen, L.J., Gines, J.A., Knowles, T.G. et al. (2009). Efficacy of adhesive incise drapes in preventing bacterial contamination of clean canine surgical wounds. *Vet. Surg.* 38 (6): 732–737.

Parienti, J.J., Thibon, P., Heller, R. et al. (2002). Hand-rubbing with an aqueous alcoholic solution vs traditional surgical hand-scrubbing and 30-day surgical site infection rates: a randomized equivalence study. *JAMA* 288 (6): 722–727.

Park, E.S., Jang, S.Y., and Kim, J.M. (2006). Comparison of a waterless, scrubless CHG/ethanol surgical scrub to povidone-iodine surgical scrubs. *Am. J. Infect. Cont.* 34 (5): 30–31.

Paulson, D. (1994). Comparative evaluation of five surgical hand scrub preparations. *AORN J.* 60 (2): 249–256.

Quinn, P.J. and Markey, B.K. (2001). Disinfection and disease prevention in veterinary medicine. In: *Disinfection, Sterilization, and Preservation*, 5e (ed. S.S. Block), 1069–1103. Philadelphia, PA: Lippincott Williams & Wilkins.

Renberg, W.C. (2012). Sterilization. In: *Veterinary Surgery Small Animal* (eds. K.M. Tobias and S.A. Johnston), 147–151. St. Louis, MO: Elsevier Saunders.

Reuss-Lamky, H. (2012). Beating the bugs: sterilization is instrumental. AAHA Denver 2012 Yearly Conference Proceedings.

Roberts, R.B. (1973). Cleaning the laryngoscope blade. *Can. J. Anaesth.* 20 (2): 241–244.

Rutala, W.A., Weber, D.J., and Healthcare Infection Control Practices Advisory Committee (2008). Guideline for disinfection and sterilization in healthcare facilities. http://www.cdc.gov/hicpac/pdf/guidelines/disinfection_nov_2008.pdf (accessed 8 February 2013).

Sebben, J.E. (1984). Sterilization and care of surgical instruments and supplies. *J. Am. Acad. Dermatol.* 11 (3): 381–392.

Seropian, R. and Reynolds, B.M. (1971). Wound infections after preoperative depilatory versus razor preparation. *Am. J. Surg.* 121 (3): 251–254.

Sessler, D.L. (2006). Non-pharmacologic prevention of surgical wound infection. *Anesthesiol. Clin.* 24 (2): 279–297.

Shirahatti, R.G., Hoshi, R.M., Vishwanath, Y.K. et al. (1993). Effect of pre-operative skin preparation on post-operative wound infection. *J. Postgrad. Med.* 39 (3): 134–136.

Shulan, D.J., Weiler, J.M., Koontz, F. et al. (1985). Contamination of intradermal skin test syringes. *J. Allergy Clin. Immunol.* 76 (2): 226–227.

Stockton, K.A., Morley, P.S., Hyatt, D.R. et al. (2006). Evaluation of the effects of footwear hygiene protocols on nonspecific bacterial contamination of floor surfaces in an equine hospital. *JAVMA* 228 (7): 1068–1073.

Storch, M.L., Rothenburger, S.J., and Jacinto, G. (2004). Experimental efficacy study of coated VICRYL plus antibacterial suture in guinea pigs challenged with *Staphylococcus aureus*. *Surg. Infect.* 5 (3): 281–288.

Sun, D.X., Zhang, F.G., Geng, Y.Q. et al. (1996). Hepatitis C transmission by cosmetic tattooing in women. *Lancet* 347 (9000): 541.

Tanner, J., Swarbrook, S., Stuart, J. et al. (2008). Surgical hand antisepsis to reduce surgical site infection. *Cochrane Database Syst. Rev.* 1: 1, CD004288–49. https://doi.org/10.1002/14651858.

Tavolacci, M.P., Pitrou, I., Merle, V. et al. (2006). Surgical hand rubbing compared with surgical hand scrubbing: comparison of efficacy and costs. *J. Hosp. Infect.* 63 (1): 55–59.

Trepanier, C.A., Lessard, M.R., Brochu, J.G. et al. (1990). Risk of cross-infection related to the multiple use of disposable syringes. *Can. J. Anaesth.* 37 (2): 156–159.

Tumblin, D. and Hoekstra, H. (2011). How to compete with spay-neuter clinics. *dvm360*, Jan. 1. http://veterinarybusiness.dvm360.com/how-compete-with-spay-neuter-clinics (accessed 21 August 2019).

Vasseur, P.B., Levy, J.K., Dowd, E. et al. (1988). Surgical wound infection rates in dogs and cats. Data from a teaching hospital. *Vet. Surg.* 17 (2): 60–64.

Velasco, E., Thuler, L.C., Martins, C.A. et al. (1996). Risk factors for infectious complications after abdominal surgery for malignant disease. *Am. J. Infect. Cont.* 24 (1): 1–6.

Wang, Z.X., Jiang, C.P., Cao, Y. et al. (2013). Systematic review and meta-analysis of triclosan-coated sutures for the prevention of surgical site infection. *Brit. J. Surg.* 100 (4): 465–473.

Webster, J. and Alghamdi, A.A. (2007). Use of plastic adhesive drapes during surgery for preventing surgical site infection. *Cochrane Database Syst. Rev.*, Oct 17 (4): CD006353.

Weightman, N.C. and Banfield, K.R. (1994). Protective over-shoes are unnecessary in a day surgery unit. *J. Hosp. Infect.* 28 (1): 1–3.

Weiland, L., Croubels, S., Baert, K. et al. (2006). Pharmacokinetics of a lidocaine patch 5% in dogs. *J. Vet. Med.* 53 (1): 34–39.

Widmer, A.F., Rotter, M., Voss, A. et al. (2010). Surgical hand preparation: state-of-the-art. *J. Hosp. Infect.* 74: 112–122.

Woloshyn, C. (2010). Cheap spays, neuters won't fix the animal overpopulation. *Veterinary Economics* (15 November). http://veterinarybusiness.dvm360.com/vetec/Veterinary+business/Cheap-spays-neuters-wont-fix-the-animal-overpopula/ArticleStandard/Article/detail/693827 (accessed 8 February 2013).

World Health Organization (2009). *WHO Guidelines on Hand Hygiene in Healthcare*. Geneva: World Health Organization.

Young, J.H. (1993). Sterilization with steam under pressure. In: *Sterilization Technology* (eds. R.F. Morrissey and G. Briggs Phillips), 120–151. New York: Van Nostrand Reinhold.

5

Infectious Disease Control in Spay–Neuter Facilities
Sara White and Natalie Isaza

The importance of adequate infection control in veterinary hospitals cannot be overstated, and it may be even more important in spay–neuter facilities where there are a high number of animals belonging to different owners, shelters, or rescue groups admitted to the facility daily. Animals may come from different geographic regions; may have received little or no veterinary care, including vaccinations, prior to presenting to the clinic; and may be juvenile or with an altered immune status that may make them more susceptible to disease. Some of the animals will have owners, while others will come from animal shelters or rescue groups. Some of the animals may be clinically ill, while others may be sub-clinically infected with an infectious disease and also be contagious to other animals in the facility. It is especially important in this setting that strict sanitation guidelines are in place, and, if possible, requirements for vaccination prior to elective surgery. Many diseases can be prevented by vaccination, and young puppies and kittens are particularly vulnerable in these settings due to their immature immune systems and probable maternal antibody interference to vaccination.

There are many ways to decrease the risk of exposure to diseases in animal hospitals and shelters. Infectious disease control and prevention depend on interrupting the transmission of pathogens from the infected animal to new hosts and locations. Infectious disease transmission can occur via direct contact, fomites, aerosols, and oral and vector-borne routes (Stull et al. 2018). Sanitation protocols, hygiene while handling animals, and traffic flow through the facility are all important factors in preventing disease transmission, as is the isolation of all sick animals from apparently healthy ones and separation of animals by source, age, and vaccination status (Peterson et al. 2008; Newbury et al. 2010; Miller and Zawistowski 2013).

This chapter will provide an overview of best practices regarding sanitation, hygiene in animal handling, vaccination, and prevention of infectious disease outbreaks in a spay–neuter clinic setting. In addition, the routine use of antibiotics for animals undergoing elective spay–neuter procedures will be discussed.

Hygiene

Animal housing protocols, animal handling, and employee hygiene are of particular concern in the prevention of infectious disease in high-quality high-volume spay–neuter (HQHVSN) clinic settings. With the potential to have many unrelated animals from differing geographic areas in a relatively small space, there is an increased risk of disease spread if strict animal handling protocols are not in

High-Quality, High-Volume Spay and Neuter and Other Shelter Surgeries, First Edition. Edited by Sara White.
© 2020 John Wiley & Sons, Inc. Published 2020 by John Wiley & Sons, Inc.

place. In addition, areas with animal contact including housing, surgical prep, surgery, and recovery areas must be adequately sanitized at the end of each day or when the animals leave, to ensure that animals arriving the next day for surgery are not at risk.

Animal Housing

Housing in the HQHVSN clinic will vary with clinic size and delivery model, and may consist of individual cages or runs, or portable crates or pet carriers (Griffin et al. 2016). In addition, the animal housing area of the clinic may be limited to a single room or vehicle (as in a mobile clinic), or may include multiple housing spaces that allow for physical separation between groups or categories of animals. Regardless of this variability, clinics should develop strategies to limit cross-contamination among patients from multiple sources and in differing states of health. In facilities that have space for physical divisions among housing areas, clinics should consider housing and handling animals in cohorts by source, age, health, and vaccination status; in facilities with limited space or physical barriers, cohort housing may be accomplished by grouping cohort animals near each other and by handling in order from most to least vulnerable. An alternative for reducing exposure and cross-contamination between cohorts might be to schedule patients from different sources on different days (Griffin et al. 2016).

Pediatric patients pose a significant challenge to spay–neuter facilities. Due to their immature immune systems, presence of maternal antibodies, and probable lack of vaccination, they are particularly susceptible to infection. To prevent the spread of infectious diseases to vulnerable animals, puppies, kittens, and any unvaccinated animals should be housed separately from other dogs and cats (Newbury et al. 2010). Adult animals, especially those that have no known vaccine history, should never be housed with unrelated pediatric patients. Ideally, litters of puppies or

kittens will be housed together or with their mother, or at least in pairs if kennel space does not allow the entire litter to be housed in one cage or run. The stress of being separated from littermates can lead to fear imprinting and a higher susceptibility to disease caused by exposure to infectious organisms.

As described in the section on sanitation later in this chapter, in clinics whose housing areas are not "all in/all out," the order of sanitation should proceed from most vulnerable to least vulnerable patients in order to reduce the likelihood of infectious disease spread.

Animal Handling and Clinic Flow

Animal handling is an important component in infection control, especially in settings where there is a high daily turnover of patients.

Potentially Infectious Patients

Patients should be watched for signs of infectious disease from arrival until discharge. If potential signs of infectious disease are noted, the affected animal(s) and any littermates or animals from the same household or source should be segregated from other patients for the duration of their clinic stay. If the sick or exposed animals are determined to be appropriate surgical candidates, they should be scheduled for surgery after surgeries on all apparently healthy animals have been completed (Griffin et al. 2016).

Infectious Disease Control through the Clinic Day

All staff should be aware of the potential for the spread of infectious microorganisms as the animal moves through the clinic throughout the surgery day. Animal contact surfaces should be cleaned and disinfected between patients, including areas and equipment used during examinations, surgical preparation, surgery, and recovery (Stull et al. 2018). Direct contact between unrelated animals should be avoided during the animals' stay at the clinic; this may be most challenging on the recovery

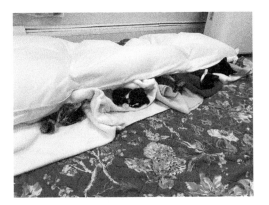

Figure 5.1 Individual towels separate cats recovering on the "beach" from each other and from the underlying bedding. *Source:* Photo courtesy of Pamela Krausz.

"beach" where multiple animals may be placed in close proximity. Many HQHVSN clinics use a towel or other bedding under each patient that travels through the clinic with them, isolating that patient from the surface that they are placed upon, as well as isolating them from other animals on the recovery beach (see Figure 5.1).

Items contacting mucous membranes such as laryngoscopes and pulse-oximeter probes used on the tongue require particular attention for disinfection between each patient with agents known to destroy common veterinary pathogens, including unenveloped viruses (Rutala and Weber 2008; Griffin et al. 2016).

Employee Hygiene

Hand Hygiene

In addition to ensuring animal holding areas are properly disinfected, it is equally important that employees adhere to hand hygiene protocols that should be in place in any veterinary facility. Ensuring that staff are trained to be keenly aware of the necessity of personal hygiene following animal handling will help to prevent the spread of nosocomial infections, as many animals may carry infective organisms on their skin and hair coats (Weese 2004).

Hand hygiene may be accomplished via hand washing or the use of alcohol-based hand sanitizers (AHS). In cases where hands are not visibly soiled, AHS may be better than hand washing because of their superior ability to kill many microorganisms on the skin, their quick application, minimal skin irritation, and the ease and convenience of providing dispensers throughout the workspace (Stull et al. 2018).

Veterinarians, veterinary technicians, and kennel staff are often targeted for increased hand washing between handling animal patients, but all employees in a facility should make a practice of regular and thorough hand hygiene. Receptionists and office personnel may have contact with animals in the lobby or waiting area of the facility, so it is important that these employees are also vigilant about personal hygiene.

Hand-washing stations or AHS dispensers should be readily available to all personnel, and diagrams depicting proper hand washing and hand sanitizer use techniques should be posted for all visitors and employees. Hand hygiene is only effective at preventing the spread of disease if it is done properly, so care must be taken to ensure that all staff know the proper steps in effective hand hygiene (Larson 1995; Weese 2004).

Other Fomites

Infectious organisms can be transported into the clinic via contaminated leashes, collars, and crates, so it is important that all personnel handling animals take appropriate precautions to prevent disease spread.

Employee clothing can also serve as a fomite. Cats and kittens in particular have been shown to harbor infectious organisms in their hair and dander, so ensuring that animals are not contaminating clothing is essential. Many respiratory diseases of cats, as well as fungal spores of *Microsporum canis*, can easily transfer to clothing and be spread to other animals in the facility via fomite transmission. The use of personal protective equipment (PPE) such as an exam coat and exam gloves when handling potentially infectious animals is recommended (Stull et al. 2018).

Sanitation

Sanitation is an important tool for prevention of the spread of infectious diseases in veterinary hospitals. The goal of sanitation is to lower the numbers of infectious organisms to a non-infective dose in the environment by using physical cleaning and chemical or physical disinfection to destroy susceptible pathogens (Peterson et al. 2008). Sanitation is especially important in clinics with a high turnover of patients daily, and proper sanitation is imperative when animals with unknown vaccination histories or disease exposures are housed in close proximity to one another.

Order of Sanitation

In clinics that operate on an "all in/all out" basis, the order in which cages and kennels are cleaned may not be important. However, in veterinary clinics and animal shelters that house animals before and after their scheduled surgery, the order of cleaning becomes more important. In general, the most vulnerable animals should be cared for first; this includes pediatric patients regardless of vaccination status. These patients' immune systems may not be fully developed, and because of possible maternal antibody interference with vaccination, they may be more susceptible to infection. Pathogenic organisms from other animals may infect these animals via fomite transmission by staff if other areas are cleaned first. The next to be sanitized is the housing area of any unvaccinated adult animals, or adult animals with an unknown vaccine history. While many adult dogs in households have immunity to parvovirus infection by one year of age, over 60% of adult dogs entering a southern animal shelter had insufficient immunity to canine distemper virus (CDV) and canine parvovirus (CPV) (Lechner et al. 2010). These animals

would be particularly vulnerable in a clinic where there may be sub-clinical shedding of virus occurring from neighboring animals.

Physical Cleaning

A proper sanitation protocol begins with the basics. Physical cleaning is an important yet often overlooked step in the sanitation process. Physical cleaning includes the removal of all organic material (feces, urine, vomitus, blood, and dirt) prior to application of an appropriate detergent. Fecal material should be removed manually and not hosed down the kennel drain, a practice that can contaminate neighboring areas by aerosolizing pathogens. In addition, kennel drains are often overlooked in the sanitation process, so that residual infective feces could pose an infection risk for future patients.

Following physical removal of feces, all surfaces of the cage or kennel should be cleaned with a detergent to remove residual organic material from the enclosure. Any commercial dishwashing detergent will suffice, and there is no need to purchase specialty detergents from chemical companies for this purpose. Remember that each cage has six surfaces, including the doors, and all should be thoroughly cleaned prior to application of the disinfectant. Cage and kennel doors are often overlooked in the cleaning process, and it may be especially difficult to remove dried organic material from the cage or kennel bars prior to applying disinfectants. Many cage doors can be removed and placed in trays to soak before scrubbing. Cleaning may also require "elbow grease" to scrub stubborn stains and dried-on material from surfaces. Periodically, and depending on traffic through the facility, surfaces should be cleaned with special degreaser detergents to remove accumulated biofilm.

Following physical cleaning, any residual detergent should be rinsed or wiped away with a clean, damp cloth before applying the disinfectant product. This is especially important because many disinfectants are deactivated by detergents. In addition, excess water used for rinsing should be squeegeed or wiped away prior to applying the disinfectant to prevent further dilution of the disinfectant product.

Disinfection

Disinfection refers to the application of a chemical or the use of a physical force (heat or steam) to kill pathogens in the environment. Disinfectants are applied to inanimate objects in order to kill microorganisms, whereas antiseptics are applied directly to the animal for the same purpose (Peterson et al. 2008). While chemical disinfectants are essential to the development of sanitation protocols, there are safety concerns for both the animals and the personnel using the products.

There are many classes of disinfectants with different efficacies for certain pathogens. It is important to know which type of disinfectant destroys what type of microorganism, as that will inform infection control protocols. It is also important that the manufacturer's guidelines for dilution be followed, as too dilute or too concentrated disinfectants may not result in the desired effect. Too much dilution will result in loss of efficacy, whereas a concentrated product may result in injury to the animals (Figure 5.2). Disinfectants applied to very

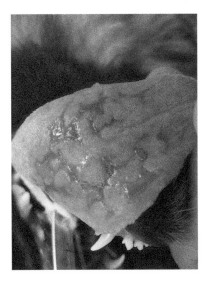

Figure 5.2 Lingual burns on a puppy from licking chemical disinfectant.

wet surfaces further dilute the product, so removing excess water prior to disinfectant application is also important.

Adequate contact time should be allowed to ensure the efficacy of the disinfectant product. Most products require a minimum of 10 minutes of contact time prior to rinsing, but as with mixing, the manufacturer's guidelines should always be followed. Some newer disinfectants require only two to three minutes of contact time with surfaces prior to rinsing (Omidbakash and Satter 2006).

Another important consideration when mixing disinfectants from a stock solution of concentrated product is adequate labeling of the mixed product. The container should be labeled with the name of the product, the date it was mixed, the name of the person preparing the mixture, as well as an expiration date. Disinfectants may have very different ranges of efficacy after the product is mixed. For example, when sodium hypochlorite is diluted with water at appropriate concentrations to destroy microorganisms, it is only efficacious for 24 hours (Miller and Zawistowski 2013).

Broad-spectrum disinfectants destroy a wide range of infectious organisms, but may not cover a particular pathogen the clinic is concerned about. Therefore, some knowledge about some of the more common disinfectants used in veterinary practice is imperative for developing effective disease control strategies (Figure 5.3).

Quaternary Ammonium Compounds

Quaternary ammonium compounds (QUATS) are broad-spectrum disinfectants that are used routinely in veterinary practice. Some of the familiar names of QUATS are Broadcide®, Roccal-D®, and Parvosol®. They have excellent efficacy against Gram-positive bacteria, and good efficacy against Gram-negative bacteria, some fungi, and enveloped viruses. For most QUATS, 10 minutes of contact time with contaminated surfaces prior to rinsing is required to reduce the infectious load of susceptible organisms in the environment. There are a

Characteristics of Selected Disinfectants

This table provides general information for each disinfectant chemical classes. Antimicrobial activity may vary with formulation and concentration. Always read and follow the product label for proper preparation and application directions.

Disinfectant Category	Alcohols	Alkalis	Aldehydes	Oxidizing Agents				Phenols	Quaternary Ammonium Compounds
				Halogens: Chlorine	Halogens: Iodine	Peroxygen Compounds			
Common Active Ingredients	ethanol, isopropanol	calcium hydroxide, sodium carbonate, calcium oxide	formaldehyde, glutaraldehyde, ortho-phthalaldehyde,	sodium hypochlorite (bleach), calcium hypochlorite, chlorine dioxide	povidone-iodine	hydrogen peroxide/ accelerated HP, peracetic acid, potassium peroxymonosulfate		ortho-phenylphenol, orthobenzylpara-chlorophenol	benzalkonium chloride, alkyldimethyl ammonium chloride
Sample Trade Names*			Synergize®	Clorox®, Wysiwash®		Rescue®, Oxy-Sept 333®, Virkon-S®		One-Stroke Environ®, Pheno-Tek II®, Tek-Trol®, Lysol®	Roccal-D®, DiQuat®, D-256®
Mechanism of Action	Precipitates proteins; denatures lipids	Alters pH through hydroxyl ions; fat saponification	Denatures proteins; alkylates nucleic acids	Denatures proteins	Denatures proteins	Denature proteins and lipids		Denatures proteins; disrupts cell wall	Denatures proteins; binds phospholipids of cell membrane
Characteristics	• Fast acting • Rapid evaporation • Leaves no residue • Can swell or harden rubber and plastics	• Slow acting • Affected by pH • Best at high temps • Corrosive to metals • Severe skin burns; mucous membrane irritation • Environmental hazard	• Slow acting • Affected by pH and temperature • Irritation of skin/mucous membrane • Only use in well ventilated areas • Pungent odor • Noncorrosive	• Fast acting • Affected by pH • Frequent application • Inactivated by UV radiation • Corrodes metals, rubber, fabrics, • Corrosive • Stains clothes and treated surfaces	• Stable in storage • Affected by pH • Requires frequent application • Corrosive • Stains clothes and treated surfaces • Mucous membrane irritation	• Fast acting • May damage some metals (e.g., lead, copper, brass, zinc) • Powdered form may cause mucous membrane irritation • Low toxicity at lower concentrations • Environmentally friendly		• Can leave residual film on surfaces • Can damage rubber, plastic; • non-corrosive • Stable in storage • Irritation to skin and eyes	• Stable in storage • Best at neutral or alkaline pH • Effective at high temps • High concentrations corrosive to metals • Irritation to skin, eyes, and respiratory tract

Figure 5.3   Characteristics of different disinfectants.

Disinfectant Category	Alcohols	Alkalis	Aldehydes	Oxidizing Agents Halogens: Chlorine	Oxidizing Agents Halogens: Iodine	Oxidizing Agents Peroxygen Compounds	Phenols	Quaternary Ammonium Compounds
Precautions	Flammable	Very caustic	Carcinogenic	Toxic gas released if mixed with strong acids or ammonia			May be toxic to animals, especially cats and pigs	
Bactericidal	+	+	+	+	+	+	+	+
Virucidal	±[a]	+	±	+	+	+	+	+ Enveloped
Fungicidal	+	+	+	+	+	±	+	+
Tuberculocidal	+	±	+	+	+	±	+	−
Sporicidal	−	+	+	+	±	+	−	+
Factors Affecting Effectiveness	Inactivated by organic matter	Variable	Inactivated by organic matter, hard water, soaps and detergents	Rapidly inactivated by organic matter	Rapidly inactivated by organic matter	Effective in presence of organic matter, hard water, soaps, and detergents	Effective in presence of organic matter, hard water, soaps, and detergents	Inactivated by organic matter, hard water, soaps and anionic detergents

+ = effective; ± = variable or limited activity; − = not effective   a - slow acting against nonenveloped viruses (e.g., norovirus)

DISCLAIMER: The use of trade names serves only as examples and does not in any way signify endorsement of a particular product.

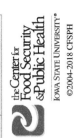

the Center for Food Security & Public Health
IOWA STATE UNIVERSITY®
©2004-2018 CFSPH

REFERENCES: Fraise AP, Lambert PA et al. (eds).Russell, Hugo & Ayliffe's Principles and Practice of Disinfection, Preservation and Sterilization. 5th ed. 2013. Ames, IA: Wiley-Blackwell; McDonnell GE. Antisepsis, Disinfection, and Sterilization: Types, Action, and Resistance. 2007. ASM Press, Washington DC. Rutala WA, Weber DJ, Healthcare Infection Control Practices Advisory Committee (HICPAC). 2008. Guideline for disinfection and sterilization in healthcare facilities. Available at: http://www.cdc.gov/hicpac/Disinfection_Sterilization/toc.html; Quinn PJ, Markey FC et al. (eds). Veterinary Microbiology and Microbial Disease. 2nd ed. 2011. West Sussex, UK: Wiley-Blackwell, pp 851-889.

Figure 5.3   (Continued)

wide variety of products to choose from, and in addition to their disinfection properties, QUATS also have some detergent action, which decreases with successive newer generations of these compounds. QUATS destroy microorganisms by denaturing proteins and binding the phospholipids of cell membranes.

In general, QUATS are efficacious against many important viral and bacterial pathogens of dogs and cats. Enveloped viruses such as CDV, feline herpesvirus (FHV), and canine influenza virus (CIV), and bacterial pathogens like *Bordetella* and *Streptococcus zooepidemicus*, are destroyed by QUATS when applied appropriately and with adequate contact time necessary to ensure efficacy. However, QUATS do not provide reliable disinfection against some of the deadliest pathogens in veterinary medicine, namely CPV and feline panleukopenia virus (FPV) (Eterpi et al. 2009). These viruses, together with other non-enveloped viruses like feline calicivirus (FCV) and canine adenovirus-1, are not destroyed by the routine use of these disinfectants. In addition, these compounds do not destroy fungal spores of *Microsporum canis*, which can survive for months to years on untreated surfaces and are of particular concern in animal shelters (Miller and Hurley 2009; Newbury et al. 2010).

Increasing the concentration of QUATS in solution does not result in improved efficacy against non-enveloped viruses like parvovirus and calicivirus, and in fact can be harmful, as exposure to a concentrated QUAT product can result in tissue damage (Figures 5.2 and 5.4). Additionally, many veterinary patients are enticed by the smell of these products and may lick any residual disinfectant left on cage or kennel surfaces. QUATS are irritating to tissues and can cause oral and skin ulcerations, secondary bacterial infections, and signs of systemic illness. The animal may be unable to eat or drink due to severe mouth pain. This is especially important in pediatric patients, where an inability to eat or drink can result in dehydration and hypoglycemia, rapid decline, and even death.

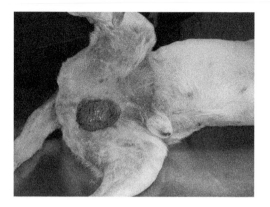

Figure 5.4 Scrotal burns on an adult dog from lying on surfaces not properly rinsed following chemical disinfection.

Oxidizing Agents

Oxidizing agents destroy pathogens by denaturing the proteins and lipids of the microorganism and disrupting cell permeability (Rutala and Weber 2008). Disinfectant agents like Virkon* and Trifectant*, both potassium peroxymonosulfate compounds, and accelerated hydrogen peroxide compounds like Rescue* (formerly marketed as Accel), are oxidizing agents and have excellent efficacy against many pathogens, and are also effectively reliable against non-enveloped viruses like CPV and FPV. A recent study has shown that when applied for 10 minutes, both accelerated hydrogen peroxide and 2% potassium peroxymonosulfate are effective against spores of ringworm fungi *Microsporum canis* and *Trichophyton* sp. (Moriello 2015).

In addition to their disinfectant qualities, oxidizing agents have limited detergent action, and are not corrosive to metal as are halogen (bleach) compounds. They are also less toxic to tissues than QUATS when diluted properly, and retain some activity in the presence of organic material like blood, urine, and feces. The potassium peroxymonosulfate compounds may leave a powdery residue on metal surfaces if not properly rinsed following application. Another negative is the relative expense of these products when compared to the cost of QUATS and halogen compounds like bleach.

The use of accelerated hydrogen peroxide compounds (Rescue) has become more common in animal shelters and veterinary hospitals due to the relative safety of these products and their efficacy against major veterinary pathogens like the non-enveloped viruses and ringworm pathogens. These products require shorter contact time with contaminated surfaces to destroy most pathogens (1–5 minutes of contact time); however, 10 minutes of contact time is necessary to destroy parvoviruses and ringworm spores. In addition, the byproducts of these compounds are water and oxygen, so there are no toxic residues left on hard surfaces following application (Omidbakash and Satter 2006).

Halogen Compounds

Halogen compounds are generally inexpensive disinfectants that have low toxicity when diluted properly. They include chlorine compounds like bleach (sodium hypochlorite) and Wysiwash® (calcium hypochlorite), and iodine and iodophor compounds (iodine complexes) like povidone-iodine. Their effect on microorganisms is determined by their negatively charged ions (chlorine or iodine) which denature the proteins of the pathogen, resulting in their destruction (Peterson et al. 2008). The iodophors are used mainly as antiseptics in patient preparation for surgery and not for routine surface disinfection. However, bleach is commonly used in animal hospitals and shelters because it is inexpensive, readily available, and is efficacious against important veterinary pathogens when diluted appropriately. For example, a 1 : 32 dilution (1/2 cup per gallon of water) of household bleach (0.16% NaOCl) destroys non-enveloped viruses like parvovirus and spores of *Microsporum canis* and *Trichophyton* sp. (Moriello 2015), as well as more labile respiratory pathogens like canine distemper and *Bordetella*. It should be noted that Wysiwash (calcium hypochlorite) was shown in one study not to have efficacy against spores of *Microsporum canis* and *Trichophyton* sp. (Moriello 2015).

Because sodium hypochlorite is corrosive to metal surfaces and chain-link fencing material, many facilities may be reluctant to use it for routine disinfection. Bleach also has very limited efficacy in the presence of organic material, and has no detergent action. Bleach is inactivated by sunlight and diluted product should be made daily for the best efficacy of the product. Wysiwash may be a reliable alternative to standard bleach compounds, since it is composed of calcium hypochlorite and is therefore less corrosive to metal.

Phenols and Aldehydes

Phenolic compounds like Lysol®, and aldehyde compounds including glutaraldehyde, are extremely toxic to companion animals, especially cats. Their routine use for disinfection of animal holding areas is not recommended (Peterson et al. 2008).

Alcohols

Alcohol compounds are generally used as antiseptics in veterinary medicine and not as surface disinfectants. Most hand sanitizers contain alcohol as the active ingredient. Isopropyl alcohol (70%) will destroy many pathogens important in veterinary medicine, including FCV (Gehrke et al. 2004). Although not particularly important in small animal medicine, alcohols are more efficacious against *Mycobacteria* than are phenols (Peterson et al. 2008).

Biguanides

Chlorhexidine (the active ingredient in Nolvasan®) is a familiar example of a biguanide, and works by reacting with the negatively charged groups on cell membranes to alter the permeability. Like alcohols, biguanides are used in veterinary medicine as antiseptics, but these compounds are not suitable as surface disinfectants due to their limited spectrum. Biguanides' broad antibacterial spectrum makes them effective for skin antisepsis prior to surgery, but they are limited in their effectiveness against enveloped viruses, are not effective against non-enveloped viruses, and are not sporicidal, mycobacteriocidal, or fungicidal (Dvorak 2008).

Vaccination

It is highly recommended that animals entering HQHVSN clinics be vaccinated with modified live (MLV) vaccines at least one week *prior* to admission whenever possible (Miller and Hurley 2009; Newbury et al. 2010). While perioperative vaccination is safe and acceptable when necessary and can effectively confer immunity (Griffin et al. 2016), it is in most cases ineffective at protecting animals during their clinic stay. The use of MLV vaccines is recommended over the use of killed vaccine because killed products require booster vaccination after three weeks to provide adequate protection, whereas MLV and recombinant vaccines begin to provide protection within hours to days (Abdelmagid et al. 2004; Larson and Schultz 2006; Miller and Hurley 2009). In addition, when used in pediatric patients, MLV vaccine products are better able to overcome maternal antibody interference than killed vaccines. Pediatric patients are particularly vulnerable to contracting infectious diseases due to a number of factors, including maternal antibody interference with vaccination, inability to mount an effective immune response due to an immature immune system, and increased stress due to separation from littermates or being in unfamiliar surroundings (Buonavoglia et al. 1992; Jas et al. 2009; DeCramer et al. 2011). This increase risk to pediatric animals is present even in private veterinary hospitals, even though a lower volume of animals is presented for surgery in these settings.

Despite the recommendation for vaccination prior to admission, it is unrealistic to assume that all animals will have received timely vaccination with core vaccines prior to presentation to the spay–neuter facility. Many clients may not have the financial resources to provide routine veterinary care for their animals, and in many cases their arrival at the HQHVSN clinic is the first time their pet has visited a veterinarian (White et al. 2018). Other owners may not have continued their pets' veterinary visits to complete the recommended vaccination schedule. In addition, many pet owners may be concerned with what they consider the overvaccination of their pet and refuse vaccination. Nevertheless, HQHVSN facilities should follow the recommended standard of care for vaccination, inform owners of the importance of vaccination prior to admission for surgery, and discuss the risks to animals that have not received adequate vaccination prior to admission.

Core Vaccinations

Vaccination guidelines for companion animals have been established by the American Animal Hospital Association (AAHA; Ford et al. 2017) and the American Association of Feline Practitioners (AAFP; Scherk et al. 2013). Dogs and cats should be vaccinated with core vaccines beginning at six to eight weeks of age, or as early as four weeks for puppies and kittens housed in animal shelters or high-density environments. Vaccination should continue every three to four weeks (or every two weeks in an animal shelter) until the animal is at least sixteen weeks of age. Animals over six months of age with an unknown vaccination history should be vaccinated prior to admission whenever possible. Subsequent vaccinations for adult animals should be repeated once in three to four weeks, or two weeks from initial vaccination if in a shelter environment (Richards et al. 2006; Welborn et al. 2011).

Core vaccines for dogs include a combination MLV or recombinant vaccine for CDV, canine parainfluenza virus (CPiV), CPV, and canine adenovirus-2 (CAV-2). *Bordetella bronchiseptica* vaccine is not a core vaccine for dogs living in the community, but it is considered a core vaccine for shelter dogs (Ford et al. 2017). Core vaccines for cats include feline herpesvirus-1 (FHV), FCV, and FPV

(Scherk et al. 2013). It is important to remember that vaccination for some diseases provides incomplete or inadequate protection against infection in most animals, although clinical signs may be less pronounced. For example, vaccination with FHV-1 provided protection in ≤75% of vaccinated cats. Conversely, vaccination for FPV can provide excellent immunity (≥99%) even after only one vaccine (Schultz 2006).

It is recommended that veterinarians follow the AAFP vaccination site guidelines for cats and kittens, with FVRCP vaccine administered below the elbow in the right forelimb, rabies vaccine below the knee in the right hindlimb, and any vaccine containing killed feline leukemia virus (FeLV) below the knee in the left hindlimb (Richards et al. 2006).

For more information on infectious diseases and vaccination of animals in the shelter setting, the reader is referred to the books *Infectious Disease Management in Animal Shelters* (Miller and Hurley 2009) and *Shelter Medicine for Veterinarians and Staff*, 2nd edn (Miller and Zawistowski 2013).

Rabies Vaccine

Rabies vaccination, though not generally considered a core vaccine, should be required of all dogs and cats old enough to receive it prior to or at the time of elective surgery. Because rabies infection in humans is an almost uniformly fatal zoonotic disease, most municipalities require rabies vaccination in companion animals. If an animal has not been vaccinated against rabies prior to admission for surgery, many clinics will vaccinate at the time of spay–neuter surgery to fulfill the legal requirements for rabies vaccination. The required age for rabies vaccination is determined by the county or municipality where the animal resides. Most commercially available rabies vaccines are labeled for use in dogs and cats 12 weeks of age and older, are killed virus vaccines, and require the addition of an adjuvant to stimulate the immune system to elicit an immune response. The exception to this is the feline rabies Purevax® vaccine, which uses a canary pox vector and is labeled for use in kittens as young as 8 weeks of age; however, most municipalities throughout the United States will not recognize a vaccine given before 12 weeks of age, regardless of the label.

Use of Antibiotics in Elective Surgical Procedures

The use of prophylactic antibiotics to prevent infection during routine spay–neuter procedures is not recommended. In general, the risk of infection at the surgical site is directly related to the length of the surgical procedure and whether there are breaks in asepsis (Brown et al. 1997). Antibiotics should be reserved for those patients in whom a known break in asepsis has occurred, the surgical procedure is prolonged, the animal has significant skin disease or other infection that may result in contamination during surgery, or the animal has a traumatic infected wound or other condition such as pyometra that could benefit from a prescribed course of antibiotics. Unless indicated for other current active infection, prolonged use of antibiotics after surgery should be avoided in animals with clean wounds (Griffin et al. 2016).

References

Abdelmagid, O., Larson, L., Payne, L. et al. (2004). Evaluation of the efficacy and duration of immunity of a canine combination vaccine against virulent parvovirus, infectious canine hepatitis, and distemper virus challenges. *Vet. Ther.* 5 (3): 173–186.

Brown, D.C., Conzemius, M.G., Shofer, F. et al. (1997). Epidemiologic evaluation of postoperative wound infection in dogs and cats. *JAVMA* 10 (9): 1302–1306.

Buonavoglia, C., Tollis, M., Buonavoglia, D. et al. (1992). Response of pups with maternal derived antibody to modified-live canine parvovirus vaccine. *Comp. Immunol., Microbiol. Infect. Dis.* 15 (4): 281–283.

DeCramer, K.G.M., Stylanides, E., and van Vuuren, M. (2011). Efficacy of vaccination at 4 and 6 weeks in the control of canine parvovirus. *Vet. Microbiol.* 149 (1–2): 126–132.

Dvorak, G.D. (2008). *Disinfection 101*. Ames, IA: Center for Food Security and Public Health.

Eterpi, M., McDonnell, G., and Thomas, V. (2009). Disinfection efficacy against parvoviruses compared with reference viruses. *J. Hosp. Infect.* 73: 64–70.

Ford, R.B., Larson, L.J., McClure, K.D. et al. (2017). 2017 AAHA canine vaccination guidelines. *J. Am. Anim. Hosp. Assoc.* 53: 243–251.

Fraise, A.P., Maillard, J.-Y., Sattar, S. et al. (eds.) (2013). *Russell, Hugo & Ayliffe's Principles and Practice of Disinfection, Preservation and Sterilization*, 5e. Ames, IA: Wiley-Blackwell.

Gehrke, C., Steinmann, J., and Goroncy-Bermes, P. (2004). Inactivation of feline calicivirus, a surrogate of norovirus (formerly Norwalk-like viruses), by different types of alcohol *in vitro* and *in vivo*. *J. Hosp. Infect.* 56 (1): 49–55.

Griffin, B., Bushby, P.A., McCobb, E. et al. (2016). The Association of Shelter Veterinarians' 2016 veterinary medical care guidelines for spay-neuter programs. *JAVMA* 249: 165–188.

Jas, D., Aeberle, C., Lacombe, V. et al. (2009). Onset of immunity in kittens after vaccination with a non-adjuvanted vaccine against feline panleukopenia, feline calicivirus, and feline herpesvirus. *Vet. J.* 182 (1): 86–93.

Larson, E.L. (1995). APIC guidelines for handwashing and hand antisepsis in health care settings. *Am. J. Infect. Cont.* 23 (4): 251–269.

Larson, L.J. and Schultz, R.D. (2006). Effect of vaccination with recombinant canine distemper virus vaccine immediately before

exposure under shelter-like conditions. *Vet. Ther.* 7 (2): 113–118.

Lechner, E.S., Crawford, P.C., and Levy, J.K. (2010). Prevalence of protective antibody titers for canine distemper virus and canine parvovirus in dogs entering a Florida animal shelter. *JAVMA* 236 (12): 1317–1321.

McDonnell, G.E. (2007). *Antisepsis, Disinfection, and Sterilization: Types, Action, and Resistance*. Washington, DC: ASM Press.

Miller, L. and Hurley, K. (2009). *Infectious Disease Management in Animal Shelters*. Ames, IA: Wiley-Blackwell.

Miller, L. and Zawistowski, S. (2013). *Shelter Medicine for Veterinarians and Staff*, 2e. Ames, IA: Wiley-Blackwell.

Moriello, K.A. (2015). Kennel disinfectants for *Microsporum canis* and *Trichophyton sp. Vet. Med. Int.* 2015: 853937.

Newbury, S., Blinn, M.K., Bushby, P.A. et al. (2010). *Guidelines for Standards of Care in Animal Shelters*. Apex, NC: Association of Shelter Veterinarians.

Omidbakash, N. and Satter, S.A. (2006). Broad-spectrum microbial activity, toxicologic assessment, and materials compatibility of a new generation of accelerated hydrogen peroxide-based environmental surface disinfectant. *Am. J. Infect. Cont.* 34 (5): 251–257.

Peterson, C.A., Dvorak, G., and Spickler, A.R. (2008). *Maddie's® Infection Control Manual for Animal Shelters*. Ames, IA: Center for Food Safety and Public Health, Iowa State University.

Quinn, P.J., Markey, B.K., Leonard, F.C. et al. (eds.) (2011). *Veterinary Microbiology and Microbial Disease*, 2e. Chichester: Wiley-Blackwell.

Richards, J.R., Elston, T.H., Ford, R.B. et al. (2006). The 2006 American Association of Feline Practitioners Feline Vaccine Advisory Panel report. *JAVMA* 229 (9): 1405–1441.

Rutala, W. and Weber, D. (2008). *Guideline for Disinfection and Sterilization in Healthcare Facilities, 2008*. Atlanta, GA: Centers for Disease Control and Prevention.

Rutala, W.A., Weber, D.J., and Healthcare Infection Control Practices Advisory Committee (HICPAC) (2008). Guideline for disinfection and sterilization in healthcare facilities. http://www.cdc.gov/hicpac/ Disinfection_Sterilization/toc.html (accessed 16 August 2019).

Scherk, M.A., Ford, R.B., Gaskell, R.M. et al. (2013). 2013 AAFP feline vaccination advisory panel report. *J. Feline Med. Surg.* 15: 785–808.

Schultz, R.D. (2006). Duration of immunity for canine and feline vaccines: a review. *Vet. Microbiol.* 117 (1): 75–79.

Stull, J.W., Bjorvik, E., Bub, J. et al. (2018). 2018 AAHA infection control, prevention, and biosecurity guidelines. *JAAHA* 54: 297–326.

Weese, J.S. (2004). Barrier precautions, isolation protocols, and personal hygiene in veterinary hospitals. *Vet. Clin. N. Am. Equine Pract.* 20 (3): 543–559.

Welborn, L.V., DeVries, J.G., Ford, R. et al. (2011). American Animal Hospital Association canine vaccination guidelines. http://www.aahanet.org/PublicDocuments/ CanineVaccineGuidelines.pdf (accessed 7 March 2013).

White, S.C., Scarlett, J.M., and Levy, J.K. (2018). Characteristics of clients and animals served by high-volume, stationary, nonprofit spay-neuter clinics. *JAVMA* 253: 737–745.

6

Strategies to Reduce Stress and Enhance Patient Comfort during the Spay–Neuter Process
Brenda Griffin

The Association of Shelter Veterinarians' Veterinary Medical Care Guidelines for Spay–Neuter Programs state: "Proactive strategies to decrease patient stress and fear while promoting patient comfort are essential components of patient care in all clinical settings. Among these strategies, safe, low-stress handling is a key requirement for animal health and well-being" (Griffin et al. 2016). In addition to being "good medicine," this approach will enhance not only the quality of patient care but also efficiency, further improving the overall quality of care in a high-volume setting. In turn, reduced patient stress levels will result in lower levels of staff stress, creating a safer and more pleasant work environment for animals and people alike. This approach may also enhance a spay–neuter program's community reputation and relations.

Triggers for Stress and Fear in the Spay–Neuter Clinic

From start to finish, the process of spaying and neutering animals presents enormous opportunities for introducing stressors and inducing stress and fear in patients. Commonly encountered stressors include transport, housing in a new environment, slippery floors, separation from familiar caregivers or animals, strange smells, noises, the presence of unfamiliar animals or caregivers, unpredictable events, handling, examination, restraint, and administration of injections. Furthermore, anything unfamiliar to a cat or dog can activate the stress response and induce fear. For many animals, coping with such stress is difficult. This is true even during short-term confinement, especially if they are unable to engage in activities that would otherwise comfort them. For example, many dogs are motivated to seek human companionship when they are stressed or fearful, but may be unable to do so because they are confined or because they are simply too emotionally upset or fearful to do so. Fear often motivates cats to retreat to a quiet spot to hide, but they may have no option for doing so and/or may be unable to escape the sounds of barking dogs.

Impact on Health and Behavior

Both acute stress and fear are accompanied by catecholamine (also known as adrenalin) release, which prepares the body for "fight" or "flight." Even temporary activation of the stress response can have deleterious effects on patient health. Catecholamine release increases heart and respiratory rate, as well as blood pressure, and can impact an animal's response to anesthetic agents. For example,

High-Quality, High-Volume Spay and Neuter and Other Shelter Surgeries, First Edition. Edited by Sara White.
© 2020 John Wiley & Sons, Inc. Published 2020 by John Wiley & Sons, Inc.

fear-induced tachycardia increases the risk of serious cardiac arrhythmias during anesthetic induction (Trim 1999). Furthermore, ongoing stress can impede patient recovery by inhibiting normal maintenance behaviors such as eating, eliminating, and restful sleeping. It can also impact immunity. In cats, the role of acute stress in the development of respiratory infection, particularly feline viral rhinotracheitis (feline herpesvirus), has been well documented (Sparkes et al. 2016).

Proactively managing patient stress and fear improves patient wellbeing by positively impacting both physical health and behavior. In terms of behavior, animals that remain calm are generally much easier to handle, while animals that are stressed or fearful frequently resist handling. If a more forceful approach is used to handle a fearful or resistant subject, the individual's fear will increase and displays of aggressive behavior will be more likely, increasing the odds of injury to the animal and staff. For some animals, fear imprinting may occur – in this case, a single traumatic event such as forceful handling can result in the patient learning a lasting negative association, which could make handling and care much more difficult in the future. In contrast, if patient stress and fear are minimized, animals are calmer and more tractable, facilitating the delivery of efficient, quality care.

Signs of Patient Stress and Fear

Individual animals display a wide variety of emotional reactions in the spay–neuter clinic depending on their species, genetic makeup, personality, prior socialization, and past experiences. In other words, what one animal finds distressful, versus positively stimulating or even relaxing, will be different from one to the next. With training and experience, staff can ascertain a great deal about an animal's emotional state by observing their behavior. Indeed, behavior is a reflection of the animal's emotional state. Dogs and cats actively communicate how they are feeling through a constant stream of

signals, the most obvious of which involve changes in their body postures and vocalizations. When animals experience stress and fear, they generally become tense – their bodies stiffen, and tension can also be seen in their faces (Figure 6.1). They are often wide-eyed, and their ears tend to shift back or sideways. Some individuals remain silent, while others may hiss, growl, bark, whine, or even scream.

In addition to active communication, animals also communicate passively. Passive communication includes both "lack of behavior" (such as refusing to eat a tasty treat, freezing in place, or avoiding contact) and physiologic changes that one might discover through very careful observation or physical examination. For example, one might notice rapid breathing and dilated pupils in a fearful animal. Excessive shedding is also common when animals are nervous or otherwise stressed. A careful observer can deduce what an individual animal is experiencing emotionally by accurately interpreting body language and vocalizations, as well as by understanding these more passive forms of communication.

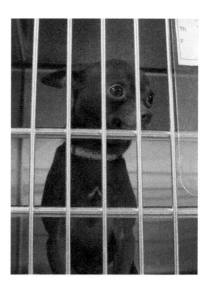

Figure 6.1 Admission to a spay–neuter clinic is stressful and potentially fear evoking for animals. This little dog is communicating his discomfort and apprehension with his body language. Both his body and face appear slightly tense, his pupils are dilated, and his ears are held low and are rotated backward.

It is important to recognize that there are many ways in which dogs and cats communicate that they are experiencing stress and fear – behavioral responses vary greatly among individuals. The "four Fs" are often used to describe common types of behaviors associated with fear and stress: these are fight, flight, fret/fidget, and freeze behaviors. Some animals display "fight" behaviors, including struggling, growling, snarling, hissing, biting, or lunging. Such aggressive behavior is the animal's attempt to drive away a perceived threat. Other animals display "flight behaviors." In this case, they may cower, look away, and move away as they attempt to escape, hide, or otherwise avoid or evade contact. They often tuck their tails and try to retreat or roll over to resist handling. Still other animals display "fret or fidget" behaviors – they might move restlessly, pacing, shifting, or nervously jumping about. A careful observer might notice that they nervously lick their lips, lift a paw, yawn, or scratch themselves. Finally, some animals display "freeze" behaviors. These animals should not be mistaken as relaxed; instead they are tense and frozen in a helpless sort of state. Many stressed and fearful animals display a mixture of fight, flight, fret/fidget, and freeze behaviors. The presence of these behaviors tells us that the animal is stressed and fearful, and not that they are mean, nasty, or unsocialized. When one sees these behaviors, one should respond with compassion, adjusting interactions with the animal to reduce their perception of a threat. In addition, an attempt should be made to ascertain additional triggers that may be contributing to the patient's stress and fear, so that steps can be taken to reduce or eliminate them as soon as possible.

Reducing Patient Stress and Fear

Reducing patients' fear and stress begins with understanding the potential impact of the clinic environment. While it is true that each individual animal will respond a little differently, staff can learn to prevent and minimize negative emotional responses during the spay–neuter process by carefully considering how animals are likely to perceive the environment and making adjustments to avoid or mitigate potential stressors and fear-inducing stimuli. When staff are observant and in tune with how the environment, as well as their own actions, can impact patient stress, they can take simple, practical steps to mitigate it. The response of an individual animal will depend not only on their unique genetic makeup, level of socialization, personality, and prior experience, but also on the severity and number of given stressors and their duration of exposure to them. Obviously, the more severe the stress and the longer it lasts, the more difficult it is for an animal to cope and the more likely they will be to suffer harmful effects from it. When stress is perceived as unescapable, uncontrollable, or unpredictable, it is especially severe.

When individual animals experience stress and fear, their emotional reactions can affect the responses of others in the clinic. Stress and fear are literally "contagious" among groups of animals: the process of "emotional contagion" is a simple and widespread form of emotional transfer that occurs among animals whereby animals shift their own emotional state, upon perceiving the emotions of other animals, in the same direction (Spinka 2012). This process can multiply both negative and positive emotions in animal groups. This has important implications in the clinic setting and should be carefully considered when determining the timing of caring for those patients that are considered to potentially be the most reactive.

Regardless of the precise nature of a particular spay–neuter program or the physical facilities in which it operates, there are many simple things that staff can do to mitigate environmental stressors and promote a positive emotional environment for animals and people alike. A healthy emotional environment provides positive, compassionate caregiving by well-trained staff members and actively reduces potential stressors and fear-inducing stimuli such as loud noises, other intense or overwhelming stimuli, haphazard interactions, and frequent interruptions. Animals can cope with new and unknown stimuli provided that fear responses are not overwhelming or sensitizing. It is especially helpful for staff to critically consider the environment from the animals' perspective.

Animals' Senses, Perceptions, and Environmental Management

Dogs and cats have astonishing and unique sensory capabilities, and the ways in which they perceive the environment around them are greatly influenced by these senses. Possessing some knowledge and understanding of how animals' senses contribute to their unique perceptions can go a long way toward helping staff to create an environment that is less intimidating and more relaxing for patients. Thinking in terms of what the animals are experiencing – what they are hearing, smelling, seeing, and feeling – is a key to environmental management for stress reduction.

Sense of Hearing

Dogs and cats possess very acute hearing, and can detect many sounds that go unnoticed by caregivers. They are highly sensitive to sounds and loud noises, especially in an unfamiliar environment. Vocal signals from other animals such as howling, crying, yowling, or hissing can invoke apprehension and fear for those in audible range. In particular, the sounds of barking dogs are especially stressful and fear invoking for cats. For all of these reasons, minimizing loud and sudden noises, including barking, is a crucial component of environmental management to reduce patient stress and promote comfort.

Sense of Smell

Dogs and cats also possess incredibly keen senses of smell. As such, avoiding strong and noxious odors (such as the smell of isopropyl alcohol) has the potential to reduce stress and fear.

The ability of animals to detect even very small amounts of scent in the environment makes it particularly important to remove potentially stressful scents to the extent possible. In contrast, pleasant, soothing odors such as lavender may be useful additions to the environment, because they may be calming for animals and people alike.

Sense of Sight

Compared to human beings, dogs and cats possess a considerably wider visual field, while their visual acuity, depth perception, and color vision remain less well developed. They are highly sensitive to movement, and can see and function in very dim light. Because of their greater peripheral vision, dogs and cats often see things beyond the field of view of their human caregivers. Rapid movements frequently startle them, particularly when they are in a novel environment, and may invoke abrupt, impulsive, and/or exaggerated responses. Furthermore, sudden or rapid movement toward an animal is likely to induce fear because it is generally interpreted as a threat. Similarly, animals are likely to view certain postures, such as leaning over them or reaching toward them, as threatening. With all of this in mind, caregivers can avoid triggering stress and fear responses simply by moving slowly, calmly, and deliberately, and by avoiding threatening postures while working with patients. Blocking visual stimuli in the environment is often a very effective means of reducing patient stress and fear. For example, doors can be shut to block outside activity; towels can be used to cover an animal's head, blocking their vision during a procedure; a towel can be draped over a carrier; or a visual barrier can be hung on the front of a cage or run.

Sense of Touch

Dogs and cats can be very sensitive to touch – and remembering this is a key to reducing stress during handling. The way in which they are touched greatly influences their response to it. Using slow, steady contact while avoiding rapid stroking, sudden manipulations, or overly restrictive restraint helps animals to remain calmer and more relaxed. Stress can also be reduced by avoiding contact with areas of the body that tend to be most sensitive, such as the feet and ventral abdomen.

Practice Tips for Stress Reduction in the Spay–Neuter Clinic

There are numerous practical and cost-effective means of mitigating patient stress and fear during the spay–neuter process, beginning before admission and continuing until, or even after, the time that an animal is discharged. Staff should be trained to be proactive and encouraged to always think ahead to minimize stress. Even small changes in a clinic's practices and its environment have the potential to dramatically impact patient care. Spay–neuter programs should have policies and protocols in place for environmental management of patient stress and fear, including low-stress handling of animals. Of course, there will always be some patients for which reducing stress and fear is more difficult. In addition to general protocols, special protocols should also be established for those animals displaying signs of severe stress and fear, including feral-behaving animals. It is clearly understood that each spay–neuter program is unique in terms of the types of patients it serves and the physical location in which services are provided. Nonetheless, in all cases it is possible for staff to create a lower-stress, positive emotional environment by unitedly embracing and implementing such protocols. By applying the tips and concepts in Box 6.1 to the extent possible in the context of a given program, staff can successfully reduce patient fear and stress and improve the quality and efficiency of patient care.

Train Staff in Low-Stress Handling Techniques

In the context of spay–neuter programs, handling and restraint of animals of varying ages,

---

Box 6.1   Practice Tips for Stress and Fear Reduction in the Spay–Neuter Clinic

- Train staff in low-stress handling techniques
- Provide information to caregivers in advance
- Maintain a calm reception area
- Separate species
- Control noise
- Control odors and consider use of aromatherapy and/or pheromones
- Reduce visual stimuli
- Provide consistent housing
- Keep littermates together
- Provide creature comforts
- Ensure warmth
- Ensure secure footing
- Use tasty treats
- Minimize stress during injections
- Facilitate elimination
- Ensure proper analgesia
- Develop protocols for animals with high levels of fear and stress
- Use trazodone and gabapentin

---

personality types, social experiences, and stress/fear levels requires skill, knowledge of normal canine and feline behavior and signaling, finesse, and proper equipment. Staff members should be well trained to recognize signs of stress and fear in patients and to mitigate them through environmental management and positive, calming interactions. Minimal, gentle restraint should be used to handle tractable patients, since research indicates that gentle human contact can attenuate the adverse effects of unpleasant stimuli, eliminate fear responses, and alleviate signs of pain in animals (McMillan 2002). Providing even a short period of time for animals to acclimate to new surroundings prior to handling is often a helpful means of facilitating the delivery of care in a low-stress manner, because it may reduce the amount of restraint required. For some animals, appraisal of their behavior may indicate that selection of a more private and quiet environment will be the key to providing a low-stress handling experience. As such, animal care protocols should be flexible enough to allow staff to meet the needs of individual patients whenever possible. Avoiding escapes and the need to recapture is also crucial, because these will greatly increase stress, as well as the risk of animal and staff injury. Simply ensuring that doors and windows are closed prior to opening animal enclosures is an imperative part of low-stress handling.

Most animals respond best to gentle restraint and react negatively when "over-restrained." In many instances, skillful, patient, and/or creative management and handling will avoid the need for additional physical restraint, improving animal and staff safety while reducing stress. When physical restraint is necessary to avoid human injury or injury to an animal, it should be of the least intensity and duration necessary. Proper equipment in good working order and adequate staff should be readily available in the event that either is needed to ensure safe and successful handling. The way in which equipment is used is crucial to ensure that it mitigates and limits stress versus increasing the risk of physical or emotional harm. Techniques or equipment suitable for one animal or situation may be inappropriate for another, thus a "one size fits all" approach is best avoided. Instead, several tools should be available and selected based on the appraisal of the individual animal and situation. Towel wraps are often useful aids for handling cats and small dogs. Well-fitted basket muzzles are useful for preventing dog bites and are generally better tolerated and safer for patients that traditional cone or tie muzzles. Likewise, Elizabethan collars can be useful and humane tools for protecting the handler from bites from both dogs and cats. In some cases, chemical restraint should be administered with the use of humane restraint equipment such as nets or squeeze devices. The use of control poles should be avoided and they should never be used to restrain cats. In all cases, calm handling is essential. Box 6.2 contains a list of resources for low-stress handling.

Provide Information to Caregivers in Advance

Providing key information to caregivers in advance can reduce patient stress during transport and admission. In particular, caregivers will benefit from instruction regarding selection of transport carriers, acclimating pets to carriers and securing them in place, and ensuring comfortable temperatures during transport, as

---

Box 6.2   Resources for Low-Stress Handling and Veterinary Care

(2011). American Association of Feline Practitioners and International Society of Feline Medicine feline-friendly handling guidelines. *J. Feline Med. Surg.* 13 (5): 364–375. https://icatcare.org/sites/default/files/PDF/ffhg-english.pdf.

(2012). American Association of Feline Practitioners and International Society of Feline Medicine feline-friendly nursing care guidelines. *J. Feline Med. Sur.* 14: 337–349. https://www.catvets.com/public/PDFs/PracticeGuidelines/NursingCareGLS.pdf.

(2015). AAHA canine and feline behavior management guidelines. *JAAHA* 51 (4): 205–221. https://www.aaha.org/graphics/original/professional/resources/guidelines/2015_aaha_canine_and_feline_behavior_management_guidelines_final.pdf.

Fear Free, LLC. https://fearfreepets.com.

International Society of Feline Medicine (2016). Guide to feline stress and health. https://icatcare.org/shop/publications/isfm-guide-feline-stress-and-health.

Yin S. (2009). *Low Stress Handling, Restraint and Behavior Modification of Dogs and Cats.* Davis, CA: Cattle Dog Publishing. https://lowstresshandling.com.

well as knowing what to expect when they arrive at the clinic. In many instances, information can be made readily available through the program's website or via volunteers. For cats, using plastic carriers from which the top half can be easily removed is recommended to facilitate getting a reluctant cat out in a low-stress manner. Most plastic carriers also have the advantage of affording cats some privacy, since they typically have solid, partially slatted sides. Caregivers should be instructed to loosely cover wire carriers with a towel or sheet to shield cats from visual stimuli. Whenever possible, staff should ask in advance if patients have a history of being highly reactive during veterinary visits or are feral, so that staff can plan ahead accordingly.

Maintain a Calm Reception Area

Reception areas can be busy, crowded, and stressful during the time of patient admission and discharge. Scheduling should strive to alleviate bottlenecks and minimize wait times. Staff should always take care to maintain a calm demeanor during admission and release processes by working in a quiet, steady manner and talking in calm and soothing tones. Simply taking care to minimize noise and rapid movements will go a long way to making animals feel comfortable during these processes. Weather permitting, leaving animals in cars until such time that someone is available to transport them directly to housing areas will minimize congestion and stress in reception areas. Likewise, leaving them in housing areas until discharge procedures are complete will minimize the time spent in reception areas during release.

Separate Species

Dogs and cats should always be kept separate to the greatest extent possible (Griffin et al. 2016). Naturally possessing heightened fight-or-flight responses, feline patients are particularly prone to experiencing acute stress and fear in novel environments, and the presence and sounds of unfamiliar dogs are extremely distressing and fear invoking to them. As such, from the time they arrive at the clinic and continuing throughout their stay, care should be taken not to place cats within spatial, visual, or auditory range of dogs whenever possible. For this reason, some programs rotate surgery days for dogs and cats, admitting only one species on a given day to avoid exposing cats to the sights, sounds, and smells of canine patients. If canine and feline patients are admitted on the same day, they should be kept as separate as possible in waiting, housing, surgery, and recovery areas. The order and timing of the day's surgery schedule can facilitate such separation.

Providing elevated surfaces, such as counter tops or shelving, on which to rest carriers containing cats is a simple but powerful means of reducing patient stress, because cats instinctively feel more secure when they can perch at a high vantage point, "out of a predator's reach." In addition, the use of visual barriers can also provide separation and privacy for animals. Towels or sheets can be provided in the waiting room for covering carriers containing cats immediately upon entry, shielding them visually from stress-invoking stimuli.

Control Noise

Minimizing loud and sudden noises, including barking, is a crucial component of environmental management to reduce patient stress and promote comfort at all time points during the spay–neuter process. Housing design and soundproofing systems can help. Noise can be also be blunted by using background sounds such as soothing music, water fountains, or white noise machines. In particular, a radio playing soft music at a low volume will provide a welcome distraction and may prevent animals from being startled by loud noises. Importantly, most caregivers enjoy listening to the radio, and happy caregivers positively contribute to a low-stress, relaxed environment. Staff and volunteers should refrain from loud talking and always take care to minimize noise during the course of their duties.

Administration of anesthetic pre-medications to dogs at the time of entry is a very effective means of reducing patient stress and promoting calm and quiet dog housing areas before surgery. Their anxiolytic and sedative effects can greatly reduce patient barking. This practice benefits not only the dogs, but also cats within auditory range. To quiet barking dogs at other times, an examination of the motivation behind the barking will help to solve the problem, alleviating the individual's distress as well as its impact on other animals. Anxiety or pain medication, being walked outside to eliminate, providing visual shielding, or movement to a different housing area may be all that is necessary.

Taking care to mitigate noise during cleaning and feeding time is also important. For example, staff should avoid clanging metal gates, cage doors, and food bowls. Many spay–neuter programs utilize inexpensive paper trays for feeding, which can aid in noise reduction and save time. When possible, cats should be allowed to retreat to a hiding spot if they choose while their cage is quietly tidied and replenished around them as needed. Commercially available "cat dens" are ideal for this purpose (Figure 6.2). Whenever possible, dogs should be removed from their enclosures during cleaning procedures or, as a minimum, moved from side to side of a double-sided enclosure to prevent undue stress.

Control Odors and Consider Use of Aromatherapy and/or Pheromones

Good air ventilation and routine sanitation protocols are important means of reducing stress-triggering odors from the environment. Using enzymatic cleaners and other products that help to eliminate odors as part of the clinic's routine sanitation protocols will help ensure a more pleasant environment for animals and people alike. Noxious odors, such as the smell of isopropyl alcohol or strong fumes from cleaning and disinfectant products, should be avoided around animals. In addition, staff and volunteers should refrain from

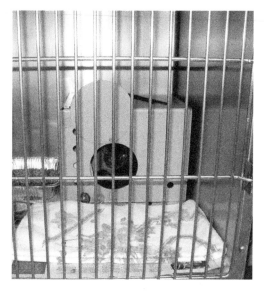

Figure 6.2 A commercially available "cat den" (Animal Care and Equipment Services [ACES], Boulder, CO) serves as a secure hiding place for a cat. The den's circular portal door can be closed from a safe and non-threatening distance while the cage is spot cleaned as needed. The cat can also be securely transported in the den.

wearing strong-smelling perfumes or lotions during work hours. In some instances, soothing lavender aromatherapy may enhance the clinic environment. Animals may also respond positively to the potentially calming effects of commercially available diffusers containing synthetic analogues of naturally occurring feline facial pheromones or dog-appeasing pheromones (Siracusa et al. 2010; Pereira et al. 2016). These products can be sprayed onto bedding or preferentially used in wards designated for housing animals displaying marked signs of stress and fear.

Reduce Visual Stimuli

Blocking visual stimuli in the environment can be a very effective means of reducing patient stress and fear. Closing doors to block outside activities, covering carriers containing patients, and draping a towel over an animal's head to block their vision during a procedure are all examples (Figure 6.3). When possible, and in a manner that does not interfere with peri-anesthetic monitoring, the use

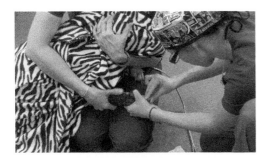

Figure 6.3   A soft blanket is used to block a dog's vision, helping to keep him calm and lowering stress and fear, during anesthetic induction via an intravenous injection. The blanket will be removed straight after the dog responds to the anesthetic (immediately upon induction).

of visual barriers or hiding places is also very useful for animals in their enclosures. For dogs that are fearful or otherwise reactive in their runs, attaching a barrier such as a sheet or shower curtain to the bottom of the run will afford them a much-needed refuge and a bit of privacy, which can help them adjust to the environment because they will be able to shield themselves from the things that they find stressful. For cats and small dogs, the provision of a hiding box or towel to cover the cage can substantially reduce stress and fear. Indeed, the ability to control aversive stimuli through hiding profoundly decreases the stress response (Carlstead et al. 1993).

Provide Consistent Housing
Procedures for temporary housing before and after surgery should enhance patient comfort and safety. Tractable adults should be housed in individual enclosures that allow for good visibility of the animals so they may be readily monitored as needed, and adequate space for them to stand and turn around (Griffin et al. 2016). Whenever possible, animals should be housed in the same enclosure before and after surgery, and only spot cleaning as needed should be performed in between in order to preserve their scent, which is necessary for stress reduction. Cats instinctively feel more secure when they can perch at a high point, and studies indicate that feline stress responses

are significantly reduced when cats are housed in elevated cages compared to floor-level cages (McCobb et al. 2005). For these reasons, placing carriers containing cats on the floor should be avoided if possible and cats should be preferentially transferred to the highest available holding cage when practical. Stress reduction will also be aided by minimizing foot traffic in housing areas by limiting entry only to essential personnel. Finally, whenever possible dimming lights and keeping doors closed in housing areas will contribute substantially to stress control.

Keep Littermates Together
From the time of admission, pediatric littermates or housemates often benefit greatly from being housed together to prevent stress induced by separation. This practice also helps to support a quiet environment, since puppies and kittens often cry loudly when experiencing separation stress. Following surgery, pediatric patients may benefit from co-housing. According to the Association of Shelter Veterinarians' Veterinary Medical Care Guidelines for Spay–Neuter Programs, "For pediatric patients, recovery with littermates is recommended when possible to provide warmth and reduce anxiety associated with separation. However, given that littermates normally pile one on top of another to sleep, inadvertent respiratory compromise may occur when littermates in various stages of recovery are housed together. When littermates are housed together during recovery, direct continuous observation is required until each animal is oriented and strongly ambulatory" (Griffin et al. 2016).

Provide Creature Comforts
Animal housing should include basic creature comforts, including bedding (Figure 6.4). Soft bedding should be available not only for comfort, but so that animals may establish a familiar scent which aides in acclimation to a new environment. Animals will also benefit from being cared for by consistent, familiar people whenever possible.

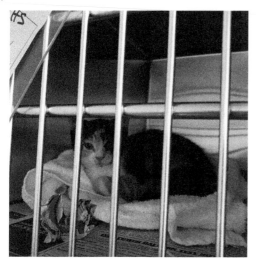

Figure 6.4 A kitten awaiting spay surgery rests on a soft towel. Bedding is an important creature comfort that also reduces stress by aiding scent familiarization and helping to keep patients warm and dry.

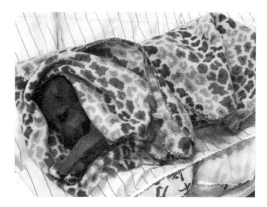

Figure 6.5 A puppy is swaddled in a cozy blanket during initial anesthetic recovery. Providing each patient with individual bedding that will stay with him/her throughout the spay–neuter process not only supports patient comfort and warmth, but also improves biosecurity and infectious disease control by providing a physical barrier that reduces cross-contamination among patients.

Ensure Warmth

Patient comfort relies on ensuring appropriate ambient temperatures and adequate patient warmth throughout the clinic, before, during, and after surgery. Hypothermia may lead to anesthetic complications and prolonged recoveries, and being chilled contributes substantially to patient stress and discomfort. For all of these reasons, ambient temperature and humidity should be well controlled in the clinic, avoiding drafts. Bedding materials, such as papers, towels, or blankets, should be used to help keep animals warm and dry. By providing each individual animal with a cozy towel or blanket, staff can improve body warmth and patient comfort as well as improving general biosecurity by reducing cross-contamination among patients (Figure 6.5). The Association of Shelter Veterinarians' Veterinary Medical Care Guidelines for Spay–Neuter Programs include numerous recommendations for preserving body temperature and actively warming patients (Griffin et al. 2016).

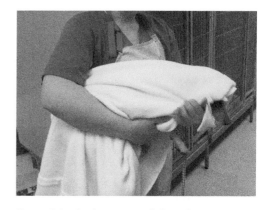

Figure 6.6 A reluctant small dog who was uncomfortable walking on a leash is carried through a ward in the arms of a caregiver. Note the use of a soft blanket to visually shield her from the environment.

Ensure Secure Footing

Many dogs are uncomfortable walking on tile floors and older animals may have difficulty standing or walking on traditional flooring. If a dog refuses to walk, placing a non-slip mat in front of him may help him to get started. This will be enough for many dogs to gain confidence walking in the building. Dogs should never be dragged by the scruff or on a leash. If they are too uncomfortable to walk, they should be lifted and carried (Griffin et al. 2016; Figure 6.6). Ensuring secure footing for both dogs and cats will ease stress and fear, while facilitating animal movement, handling, and examination. Other examples include placing a non-slip mat on a scale, or a towel or sheet of newspaper on a slick exam surface.

Use Tasty Treats

Tasty treats are powerful tools for putting pets at ease in new situations. They can aid in distraction, redirection, and counterconditioning of both dogs and cats, though dogs are more likely to partake of treats than many cats. Even in a surgical clinic, treats can be safely used to facilitate administration of both oral and injectable medications. Depending on the program's surgery schedule, the use of solid treats may or may not be feasible given the need for withholding food for a few hours prior to surgery. However, a tiny amount of soft cheese spread, such as canned cheese or cream cheese products, can be used to facilitate administration of oral medications, such as trazodone or gabapentin, when given a couple of hours or more prior to anesthesia. Freezing clear broth in a small paper cup and allowing an animal to lick it briefly is a safe option prior to anesthesia and can be used to facilitate low-stress handling during examination and anesthetic injection. Following postoperative recovery, many patients will benefit both physically and emotionally from a small, palatable meal. Canned foods or soft cheese spreads can also simplify administration of oral analgesics in the post-operative period.

Minimize Stress during Injections

"Total intramuscular anesthesia" is an efficient and safe technique utilized by many spay–neuter programs. The Association of Shelter Veterinarians' Veterinary Medical Care Guidelines for Spay-Neuter Programs state: "Administering a single injection that includes sedative, analgesic, and anesthetic induction agents may reduce patient pain and stress, compared with administering multiple injections ... Recommended combinations for single injections include α2-adrenoreceptor agonists, opioids, and dissociative drugs because such combinations provide patients with multimodal analgesia and balanced anesthesia when administered in appropriate doses" (Griffin et al. 2016). Stress and pain during injections are also mitigated by using low-stress handling techniques and small-gauge needles, and by changing needles prior to injection to ensure they are as sharp and smooth as possible.

Facilitate Elimination

For dogs that are house trained, regular opportunities to go outside to eliminate are very important, because eliminating inside can be extremely stressful for them. If cats are to be held for more than 12 hours, a litter box should be provided once the patient is ambulatory. According to the Association of Shelter Veterinarians' Veterinary Medical Care Guidelines for Spay-Neuter Programs, "Prolonged confinement without opportunities for urination and defecation away from the enclosure can increase patient stress and discomfort. This problem may be exacerbated by perioperative administration of fluids and certain anesthetic agents such as α2-adrenoceptor agonists, which can increase urine output. In addition, confinement inhibits elimination behavior in some patients. For all of these reasons, expression of the patient's bladder, including both male and female patients, during anesthesia may improve comfort in the immediate post-operative period. For overnight stays, an absorbent substrate, such as paper, litter, or bedding, should be provided for cats. Dogs should be walked, provided that doing so does not pose a safety risk to staff; housed in an enclosure such as a run that allows for elimination away from the resting area; or provided with an absorbent substrate in their enclosures. Traps housing community cats should be covered to decrease patient stress and should be elevated to allow urine and feces to fall through the wire bottoms away from the patient or lined with absorbent material that can be safely changed if soiled" (Griffin et al. 2016; Figure 6.7).

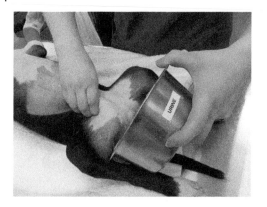

Figure 6.7 Expressing the bladder of both male and female patients while they are anesthetized will enhance patient comfort post-operatively. This is because a full bladder can be very uncomfortable and distressing for patients, especially those that are house trained.

Ensure Proper Analgesia

Pain is a huge physiologic stressor and ensuring proper analgesia is of paramount importance during the spay–neuter process. Pre-emptive and multimodal analgesia techniques are recommended (see Chapters 7 and 8 for specific recommendations regarding pain management before, during, and after surgery).

Develop Protocols for Animals with High Levels of Stress and Fear

Plan ahead whenever possible for how the clinic will handle particular patients that are highly stressed, fearful, and/or reactive. Such patients may do best as either the first or last case of the day. Because of the power of emotional contagion, it is very important to limit exposure of other animals to the negative emotional reactions of highly reactive animals. Whenever possible, individual animals that are exhibiting marked stress and fear at the time of entry should be housed in specially designated quiet areas away from other animals and foot traffic within the clinic. When an animal does not need urgent intervention, delaying a procedure to allow that animal time to relax in a quiet environment before handling is often the best option. The precise means by which the animal is handled will

depend on the individual. Handling methods must be approached and tailored according to the individual animal's needs and responses. In all instances, the use of forceful handling should be minimized and "chemical restraint" should be utilized to limit patient stress and ensure patient and staff safety. Whenever possible, use of a hands-off approach for delivery of care is best. For feral cats, this approach is discussed in additional detail in a subsequent section of this chapter.

Protocols for animals with high levels of stress and fear must be flexible and should afford a variety of options. Staff training should include working with animal models to practice using handling tools and techniques before attempting to use them on patients. Improper or forceful use of any of tool or technique can escalate a high-stress situation rather than diffusing it, compromising animal welfare and creating an unsafe situation for both animals and people. Successful low-stress handling requires patience, practice, good timing, finesse, and the ability to continuously apprise and assess the animal's signals and situation and adjust your response accordingly.

Administration of "pre-visit" oral doses of trazodone or gabapentin is ideal whenever possible (see next section). Likewise, administration of injectable pre-medications upon arrival should also be strongly considered whenever possible. Many fearful dogs can be walked into the clinic and weighed, but may be difficult to later remove from a cage or other enclosure due to defensive behavior. By weighing, briefly examining (as possible), and pre-medicating such patients prior to putting them into their enclosures, staff can avoid the difficult situation of removing a reluctant or reactive dog from an enclosure. In dogs, combining a tranquilizer, such as acepromazine, with a narcotic analgesic, such as hydromorphone, will provide sedation, anxiolysis, and pre-emptive analgesia, as well as greatly facilitating handling. For small dogs, a rolled towel wrap can be used to facilitate examination and injection (Figure 6.8). With this technique, a rolled-up

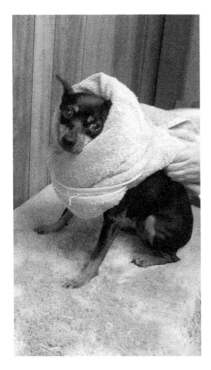

Figure 6.8 A rolled towel was placed around the neck of a nervous dog by the handler, who is standing behind her. The towel can be held in place to steady the dog and prevent her from turning to bite so that she can be gently examined.

towel is used to encircle the dog's neck. Standing behind the dog facilitates placement of the towel, because the handler will appear less threatening since he/she will not be facing or leaning over the dog during placement. The towel is then held snugly in place with one hand in order to keep the dog steady and secure, preventing their head from turning to bite.

At times, situations will arise in which staff must remove reluctant animals from their enclosures. There is no single recipe for accomplishing this task. For some dogs, if a slip leash can be maneuvered over their head, they may choose to walk out on their own or be readily coaxed to do so. In this case, the handler should gently swing the door to the enclosure open wide, and step aside while holding the end of the leash, allowing the dog to exit. Once out of their enclosure, many dogs will feel less threatened or vulnerable and will accept handling.

In other cases, ensuring a smooth exit from the enclosure will be considerably more challenging. Some dogs will refuse to walk out and instead will freeze once the leash is over their head. Still others will resist, or even panic and try to escape. A slip lead should never be used to drag out a resistant animal. In some instances, a Snappy Snare (Campbell Pet Company, Vancouver, WA) can be used to facilitate removal of a reluctant subject from a cage. This tool provides a loop on the end of a rigid pole that facilitates placement over the animal's head from a greater distance – creating less of a threat from the handler during placement. For animals that will not willingly walk out once leashed, a thick towel or blanket can be thrown over them and they can be lifted out and carried, while the leash is used only as necessary to protect the handler during placement of the towel/blanket and lifting. For fractious large dogs that are unsafe to handle, a pole syringe or blow pipe can be safely used as a hands-off means of administering a small volume of anesthetic agent for heavy sedation, such as tiletamine/zolazepam for injection.

For reluctant cats that remain in carriers, removing the lid and using a towel to cover the cat as needed may be all that is necessary for successful and humane handling. If the cat is in a cage, a commercially available feral cat den can be used to facilitate low-stress handling. Cat dens are designed as secure boxes and are equipped with both a guillotine-style door and a side portal door which can easily be closed from a distance (Figure 6.9). In addition to their use as hiding boxes for cats, cat dens can be used to transport cats as well as to facilitate safe transfer of cats to other enclosures with guillotine-style doors, including commercially available squeeze cages, which can be used to facilitate administration of anesthetic injections (Figure 6.10). Alternatively, a commercially available "hand shield" can be used to facilitate injection of a cat in a den (Figure 6.11). Transferring a cat from a carrier or other container with a swinging door rather than a guillotine-style door is not recommended because of the risk of escape.

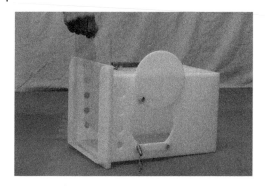

Figure 6.9 A commercially available cat den (Tomahawk Live Trap, Hazelhurst, WI). Note the guillotine-style door on the front in addition to the side portal door.

A net is another potentially useful tool for handling highly stressed cats. Several commercially available cat nets are available. In some cases, the design allows the user to close the opening of the net using a special sliding mechanism on the handle (Figure 6.12). This type of net (often called a cage net) is designed for use when a cat is enclosed in a cage or other confined space. Once a cat is securely netted, chemical restraint may be administered through the netting. Covering the cat with a thick towel or blanket will aid in safe and humane restraint while an injectable anesthetic is administered. As soon as the cat is

(a)

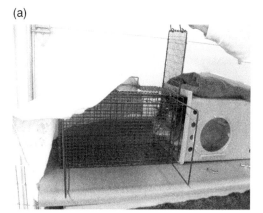

(b)

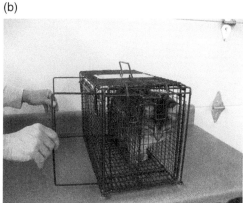

Figure 6.10 (a) By raising and lowering the guillotine doors, a cat is safely and humanely transferred from a cat den to a squeeze cage for restraint. Note the use of a cage cover. (b) The design of the squeeze cage allows the cat to be gently pushed over to one side to facilitate injection through the bars of the cage. Following injection, the cat can be covered to reduce stress.

(a)

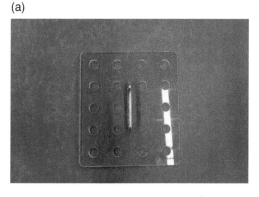

(b)

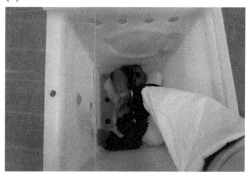

Figure 6.11 (a) Commercially available "hand shield" for use with a cat den (Tomahawk Live Trap, Hazelhurst, WI). (b) An injection can be administered through one of the circular holes in the durable transparent plastic shield while the handler uses it to gently confine the cat in the back of the den. Note that the cat den is positioned on its end and that the handler is wearing protective gloves for added safety.

(a)

(b)

(c)

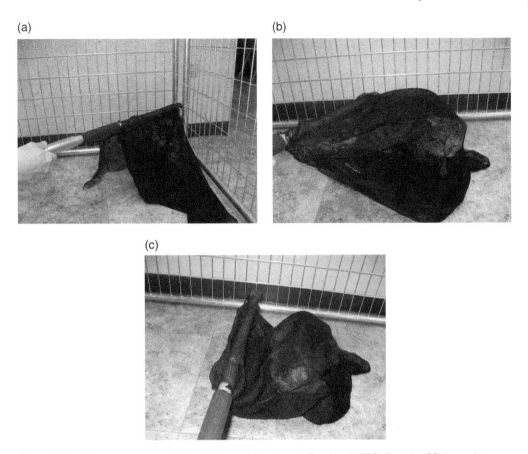

Figure 6.12 Freeman cage net (Animal Care and Equipment Services [ACES], Boulder, CO) is used to humanely handle a cat in an enclosure. The design of the net allows the user to close the opening to the net using a special sliding mechanism on the handle of the pole. (a) The net is placed over the cat. (b) As the handler moves closer, the cat moves farther into the net and the net is closed. (c) The handler calmly and gently rolls the net onto the pole to confine the cat securely, preventing thrashing. A towel can then be used to cover the cat while an anesthetic injection is administered.

relaxed and immobilized, he/she should be removed from the net. When used properly, nets minimize stress, prevent injury of the animal, and ensure staff safety. In contrast, commercially available cat tongs should never be used for routine movement or handling of cats (Griffin 2011).

A variety of other useful tools and techniques are available. Continuing education and training are highly recommended in order to continually refine and improve protocols and skills for safe and humane handling. As previously mentioned, Box 6.2 contains a list of resources for low-stress handling.

Use Trazodone and Gabapentin

Administration of oral pre-anesthetic medications, such as trazodone or gabapentin, to aid in anxiolysis and sedation immediately upon or prior to arrival can be very helpful for patients. In fact, several recent studies have evaluated the use of trazodone in dogs and cats for stress reduction (Gruen and Sherman 2008; Gruen et al. 2014; Gilbert-Gregory et al. 2016; Stevens et al. 2016), as well as the use of gabapentin in cats for the same (Pankratz et al. 2018; van Haaften et al. 2017). Drug therapy is often used to reduce patient stress and when stress is mitigated in this way, dogs and cats are more likely to respond to good environmental management and behavioral care. Even for individuals who are not highly stressed, medications such as trazodone and gabapentin may lessen stress, facilitate smooth delivery of care, and improve the patient's overall emotional experience during the process of spay–neuter. Both of these drugs are widely available, highly cost-effective, and have a wide margin of safety. Neither is a controlled substance. They can be safely administered at home by caregivers one to two hours prior to arrival at the clinic or by program personnel immediately upon a patient's arrival at the clinic. For all of these reasons, the routine use of these drugs for all spay–neuter patients is an attractive option. Of note is that their use does not preclude the use of additional (injectable) pre-medications if needed.

The drug trazodone is a safe and effective sedative and anxiolytic medication in both dogs and cats. Trazodone is classified as a serotonin antagonist and reuptake inhibitor. It has a rapid onset of action: one to two hours following oral dosing. It has a wide safety margin and can be used concurrently with many other drugs, including selective serotonin reuptake inhibitors (SSRIs). However, concurrent use of monoamine oxidase inhibitors (MAOIs) must be avoided, including amitraz-containing products, because of the risk of serotonin syndrome. Trazodone dosage for dogs ranges from 4 to 12 mg/kg every 8–12 hours. A typical starting dosage is 4–7 mg/kg and this can be increased as needed. For cats, the typical dosage is 50 mg/cat once or twice daily. Trazodone may take up to two hours to exert its full effects. In general, adverse side effects are uncommon; however, patients should be monitored for the following potential side effects: excessive sedation, vomiting and/or diarrhea, tremors, and increased anxiety (Gruen and Sherman 2008; Gruen et al. 2014; Gilbert-Gregory et al. 2016; Stevens et al. 2016).

The drug gabapentin is structurally related to gamma aminobutyric acid (GABA), but its actions are not fully understood. It apparently binds to voltage-sensitive calcium channels in the brain, decreasing calcium influx, which in turn inhibits the release of excitatory neurotransmitters. Its use for behavioral calming has been studied in cats, but not in dogs (Pankratz et al. 2018; van Haaften et al. 2017). In cats, the recommended dosage is 50–100 mg/cat. Its use visibly reduces signs of feline stress. In dogs, it is used as an adjunctive treatment for seizures and for pain control. Although its use for behavioral calming has not been specifically evaluated, sedation is a common side effect and it has anecdotally been reported to produce behavioral calming in some dogs. In dogs, the dosage ranges from 5 to 20 mg/kg orally every 6–12 hours, with starting doses of 5–10 mg/kg being typical. In both species, the drug reaches its peak action 1–2 hours following oral administration. Gabapentin is supplied in both capsule and liquid forms. The commercially available liquid suspension contains xylitol, which is toxic to both dogs and cats and must be avoided. The capsule form lends itself to administration for all but the smallest dogs. Administration of a gabapentin suspension to community cats is discussed in a later section of this chapter.

Special Considerations for Community Cats

It is crucial to provide the least stressful environment possible when working with community cats. Feral and poorly socialized cats, as well as tame cats that have been through the traumatic experience of being captured in a live trap, should all be assumed to be highly stressed and fearful. Regardless of their socialization level, these cats may be overtly aggressive or may be "teetering on the edge" of defensive aggression. The entire process of capture, transport, and admission to a spay-neuter program can induce severe fear and terror in these animals, and truly feral cats will not be able to adapt. They simply will not be able to learn to accept handling, and will not acclimate to their captive environment.

Although it is impossible to eliminate fear responses in feral cats, caregivers can help these cats to cope during the time they must be confined to undergo these procedures by actively working to create the least stressful environment possible, and by limiting their exposure to people and other stimuli as much as possible (Griffin et al. 2010; Griffin 2011).

For more information on feral cat natural history and feral cat clinics, see Chapters 25 and 35.

Environmental Management Considerations for Community Cats

Environmental management should include previously described practices to minimize and mitigate cat stress and fear. A calm and quiet environment is essential, and cats should be left undisturbed to the extent possible. Only when necessary for proper care and monitoring should caregivers disturb cats in any way. Caregivers should always move slowly and deliberately around cats to avoid startling or overwhelming them. Caregivers should work to actively reduce potential stressors and fear-inducing stimuli such as loud noises, other intense or overwhelming stimuli, and interruptions. Cats should always be visually shielded from stimuli – covering traps or other enclosures containing cats is crucial to reduce the impact of threatening stimuli. Cats must always be protected from the sight and sounds of dogs. Creature comforts, such as bedding, should be provided to the extent possible. The way in which the environment is managed will have a profound influence on the emotional responses and wellbeing of cats undergoing these procedures (Griffin et al. 2010; Griffin 2011).

Using a Hands-Off Approach

Because of their lack of socialization, capture and handling are extremely stressful for feral cats. In addition to environmental management, proper education of caregivers and veterinary staff on the use of equipment to facilitate a "hands-off" approach is key to minimizing feline stress and fear, while keeping caregivers and cats safe. In most instances, cats should be humanely trapped using commercially available live traps (Figure 6.13). For those cats that are elusive, a drop trap is a humane alternative, but generally requires substantial time and patience (Figure 6.14). Once captured, cats may be held securely in their covered traps while awaiting surgery. Transferring them to larger enclosures increases the risk of human injury as well as

(a)

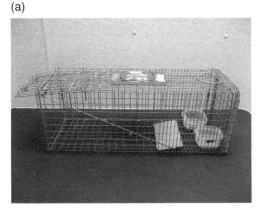

(b)

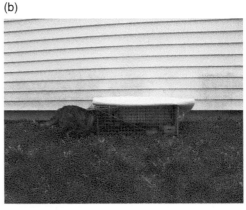

Figure 6.13   (a) A commercially available box trap (Tomahawk Live Trap, Tomahawk, WI). When a cat steps on the spring-loaded foot plate to reach the food bait, the trap door will close and lock. (b) A cat enters a box trap. Covering the trap serves to make it more inviting. In addition, it will help to reduce stress and fear by providing cover and security, helping to calm the cat once captured.

cat escape. Indeed, if provided an opportunity, most cats will successfully escape, and serious injury can occur if individuals have to recapture them. In addition, escaped cats can be destructive as they attempt to hide and resist recapture.

Caregivers should be required to present cats for surgery in individual covered traps. Some

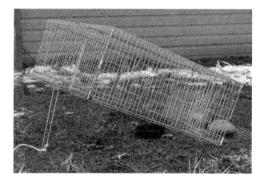

Figure 6.14 Commercially available drop trap, which is fully collapsible for ease of transport (Tomahawk Live Trap, Hazelhurst, WI). A drop trap can be used to humanely capture cats that will not enter a box trap. Strong-smelling food is placed on the ground beneath the trap, and the caregiver waits covertly nearby until the cat takes the bait. From the remote location, the caregiver pulls a string to remove the prop stick, causing the trap to drop, capturing the cat. A guillotine-style transfer door is used to safely transfer the cat from the drop trap into a regular box trap or transfer cage for transport.

spay–neuter programs provide services exclusively to community cats or do so only on particular days; others integrate their care into the clinic's daily routine while caring for a variety of both canine and feline patients. In the latter case, arranging for cats to be admitted during a "quiet" time, or through a separate entrance, is highly recommended. Clinic personnel should have sheets or towels readily available to cover cats at the time of entry in case they arrive uncovered. Staff should immediately transfer cats in their covered traps to dedicated holding wards, which are quiet, dimly lit, and free of non-essential foot traffic (Figure 6.15). Exit doors should always remain securely closed to reduce stress as well as to prevent escapes in the event that a cat is somehow released from a trap.

Keeping cats confined in traps not only reduces stress and the risk of escapes, it facilitates administration of anesthetics. With the cat confined in a trap, this can be done without extensive handling, minimizing stress and enhancing safety for both cats and personnel. This is accomplished by quietly but quickly standing the trap on end and using a commercially available "trap divider" to more tightly confine the cat. This allows an intramuscular injection to be administered to the cat between the trap's wire bars (Figure 6.16). In this way,

(a)

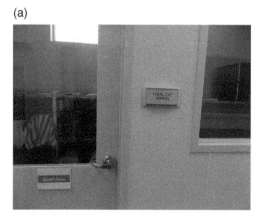

(b)

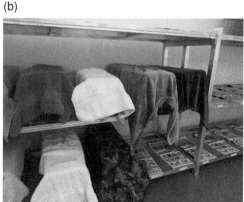

Figure 6.15 Proper holding procedures for feral cats. (a) A dedicated ward is provided for holding community cats that arrive in traps. (b) To reduce stress, traps remain covered and the ward is kept quiet and dimly lit. For safety and security, cats remain in their covered traps before and after surgery.

(a)

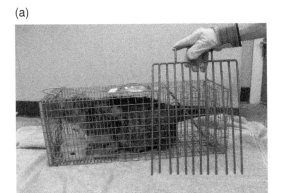

(b)

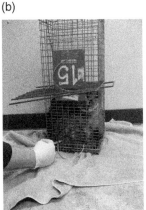

Figure 6.16 (a) A commercially available "trap divider" (Animal Care and Equipment Services [ACES], Boulder, CO) is used to humanely restrain a cat in a box trap to facilitate intramuscular injection of an anesthetic agent. (b) The trap is gently and swiftly turned on one end, and the device is inserted, confining the cat for the injection.

cats are kept in their traps and only removed once they have been heavily sedated or anesthetized. Then, at the completion of surgery and before awakening, they can be returned to their traps for recovery. With this system, cats are never handled while conscious, and there are no opportunities for escape or injury. And, importantly, they do not sustain any additional stress from unnecessary handling (Griffin 2011).

Use of Oral Gabapentin for Community Cats

In addition to environmental management and hands-off handling techniques, administration of oral gabapentin may further attenuate cat fear responses during the process of trap–neuter–return (TNR). A recent study demonstrated that the drug can be safely and humanely administered to confined cats using a tomcat catheter and that dosages of 50–100 mg/cat were safe and not associated with increased sedation (Pankratz et al. 2018). An added benefit of this protocol is that it is inexpensive.

Because commercially available gabapentin solutions often contain xylitol, which is toxic to cats, the use of such solutions must be strictly avoided. Oral solutions of gabapentin may be prepared by mixing the contents of capsules with xylitol-free flavored syrup vehicles or

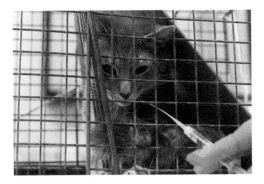

Figure 6.17 An oral suspension of gabapentin is administered to a community cat in a trap using an open tomcat catheter attached to a dosing syringe. Note the use of a trap divider to confine the cat to one end of the trap, facilitating administration. *Source:* Photo courtesy of John Joyner, North Carolina State University.

other palatable liquids (e.g. tuna juice, milk). To administer an oral suspension, a trap divider should be used to temporarily restrict the cat to one end of the trap. Immediately following restriction of the cat, the end of an open tomcat catheter, which is attached to a dosing syringe, is slowly and deliberately inserted into the corner of the cat's mouth to deliver the suspension (Figure 6.17). Alternatively, capsule contents can be mixed directly into highly palatable food at the time of trapping and with subsequent feedings. For community cats, a starting oral dosage of 50 mg/cat can be used and repeated as needed up to every six hours.

Conclusion

With training, experience, and a willingness to work together, spay–neuter program staff can create low-stress, positive emotional environments in the workplace, which will result in calmer patients that pose fewer risks to themselves and their caregivers. Calmer patients facilitate high-quality, efficient, and humane care. Simply stated, reducing patient stress and fear translates into better medicine. By using a holistic approach to reducing patient stress and fear, staff will ultimately create a more pleasant work environment for everyone, animals and humans alike.

References

Carlstead, K., Brown, J.L., and Strawn, W. (1993). Behavioral and physiological correlates of stress in laboratory cats. *Appl. Anim. Behav. Sci.* 38: 143.

Gilbert-Gregory, S.E., Stull, J.W., Rice, M.R., and Herron, M.E. (2016). Effects of trazodone on behavioral signs of stress in hospitalized dogs. *JAVMA* 249 (11): 1281–1291.

Griffin, B. (2011). Care and control of community cats. In: *The Cat: Clinical Medicine and Management* (ed. S.E. Little), 1290–1309. St. Louis, MO: Elsevier.

Griffin, B., Bushby, P.A., McCobb, E. et al. (2016). The Association of Shelter Veterinarians' 2016 veterinary medical care guidelines for spay-neuter programs. *JAVMA* 249 (2): 165–188.

Griffin, B., DiGangi, B., and Bohling, M.A. (2010). Review of neutering cats. In: *Consultations in Feline Internal Medicine VI* (ed. J.R. August), 776–790. St. Louis, MO: Elsevier/Saunders.

Gruen, M.E. and Sherman, B.L. (2008). Use of trazodone as an adjunctive agent in the treatment of canine anxiety disorders: 56 cases (1995–2007). *JAVMA* 233 (12): 1902–1907.

Gruen, M.E., Roe, S.C., Griffith, E. et al. (2014). Use of trazodone to facilitate postsurgical confinement in dogs. *JAVMA* 245 (3): 296–301.

McCobb, E.C., Patronek, G.J., Marder, A. et al. (2005). Assessment of stress levels among cats in four shelters. *JAVMA* 226: 548.

McMillan, F.D. (2002). Development of a mental wellness program for animals. *JAVMA* 220: 965.

Pankratz, K.E., Ferris, K.K., Griffith, E.H. et al. (2018). Use of single-dose oral gabapentin to attenuate fear responses in cage-trap confined community cats: a double-blind, placebo-controlled field trial. *J. Feline Med. Surg.* 20 (6): 535–543.

Pereira, J.S., Fragoso, S., Beck, A. et al. (2016). Improving the feline veterinary consultation: the usefulness of Feliway spray in reducing cats' stress. *J. Feline Med. Surg.* 18 (12): 959–964.

Siracusa, C., Manteca, X., Cuenca, R. et al. (2010). Effect of a synthetic appeasing pheromone on behavioral, neuroendocrine, immune, and acute-phase perioperative stress responses in dogs. *JAVMA* 237 (6): 673–681.

Sparkes, A., Bond, R., Buffington, T. et al. (2016). Impact of stress and distress on physiology and clinical disease in cats. In: *International Society of Feline Medicine Guide to Feline Stress and Health: Managing Negative Emotions to Improve Feline Health and Wellbeing*, 39–52. Tisbury: International Cat Care www.icatcare.org.

Spinka, M. (2012). Social dimension of emotions and its implication for animal welfare. *Appl. Anim. Behav. Sci.* 138: 170–181.

Stevens, B.J., Frantz, E.M., Orlando, J.M. et al. (2016). Efficacy of a single dose of trazodone hydrochloride given to cats prior to veterinary visits to reduce signs of transport- and examination-related anxiety. *JAVMA* 249 (2): 202–207.

Trim, C.M. (1999). Anesthetic emergencies and complications. In: *Manual of Small Animal Anesthesia* (ed. R.R. Paddleford), 147–195. Philadelphia, PA: W.B. Saunders.

van Haaften, K.A., Eichstadt, L.R., Stelow, E.A. et al. (2017). Effects of a single pre-appointment dose of gabapentin on signs of stress in cats during transportation and veterinary examination. *JAVMA* 251 (10): 1175–1181.

Section Two

Anesthesia for Spay–Neuter Surgery

7

Principles of Anesthesia, Analgesia, Safety, and Monitoring
Sheilah Robertson

Anesthesia comprises several steps, which include pre-anesthetic evaluation and pre-medication; the induction, maintenance, and recovery phases of anesthesia; and post-anesthetic care. The essential components of general anesthesia include reversible unconsciousness, muscle relaxation, amnesia, and blockade of autonomic reflexes. Pain is a conscious perception, so by definition an animal under general anesthesia cannot be aware of pain; however, provision of pre- and intraoperative analgesia is an important component of anesthesia to minimize transduction and transmission of noxious stimuli and for modulation of pain-related signals – the processes involved in nociception. By using preventive (formerly referred to as pre-emptive) analgesia, pain is minimized when the patient regains consciousness. Many animals in a sheltering setting are vulnerable: they may be very young and one negative experience such as pain or rough handling may precipitate behavioral problems relating to interactions with humans or other animals. It is clear that we must strive to ensure that during the peri-operative period we maximize comfort and minimize stress in our patients.

In a shelter or high-quality high-volume spay–neuter (HQHVSN) clinic environment, large numbers of animals may undergo anesthesia and surgery in a short period of time, usually for the purposes of neutering. This is the high-volume (HV) component of the HQHVSN acronym. However, it must be emphasized that these clinics are also obligated to provide high-quality veterinary care, and for this reason the Association of Shelter Veterinarians (ASV) has published anesthesia and surgery guidelines (Griffin et al. 2016).

Anesthetic Mortality

"What are the risks of anesthesia in dogs and cats today?" The data generated by the Confidential Enquiry into Perioperative Small Animal Fatalities (CEPSAF) supplied comprehensive information on this topic based on data collected between 2002 and 2004. Data was prospectively collected for approximately 98 000 dogs and 79 000 cats with an American Society of Anesthesiologists (ASA) physical status of 1–5, undergoing a wide variety of both elective and emergency procedures (http://www.asahq.org/standards-and-guidelines/asa-physical-status-classification-system). A total of 117 clinics representing small animal, mixed animal, and referral institutions participated. This study recorded patient outcome (alive, dead, or euthanized) from the time of pre-medication through to 48 hours after the end of the procedure and calculated species-specific risks of anesthetic-related death. An anesthesia-or sedation-related death was defined as "death where surgical or

High-Quality, High-Volume Spay and Neuter and Other Shelter Surgeries, First Edition. Edited by Sara White.
© 2020 John Wiley & Sons, Inc. Published 2020 by John Wiley & Sons, Inc.

pre-existing medical causes did not solely cause death." This study generated risk factors for different species and paved the way for improving anesthetic management in small animals (Brodbelt et al. 2007, 2008a, b; Brodbelt 2009).

Animals were assigned a health status; animals with an ASA status of 1 or 2 were considered "healthy" and those with an ASA status of 3–5 "sick." Assignment of ASA status is shown in Table 7.1. The *overall* risk of death was 0.17% in dogs and 0.24% in cats. In *healthy* dogs and cats the risks were 0.05 and 0.11%, respectively. In *sick* dogs and cats the risks were 1.33 and 1.40%, respectively.

Peri-operative mortality statistics are now available for dogs and cats undergoing spay or castration in a high-volume setting. Medical records and mortality logs for 42 349 dogs and 71 557 cats that were neutered between 2010 and 2016 at a single high-volume clinic were analyzed (Levy et al. 2017). In this study perioperative mortality was defined as a death that occurred in the 24-hour period beginning with the first administration of sedation or anesthesia drugs. The results are summarized in Table 7.2.

In the Levy et al. study, the mortality rate was almost 10-fold lower than in animals classified as "healthy" in the CEPSAF study, but as in the CEPSAF study, mortality in cats was higher than in dogs. The overall low mortality rate in the spay and castration study may be explained by the patient population being healthy, surgery being elective, short procedure times, and surgeons who are specialized in these surgical procedures. In both dogs and cats, mortality in males was less than in females, which may reflect the longer anesthesia times and more invasive surgery of the latter. Community cats represented 76% (26/34) of the feline deaths and for all feline deaths (34), a likely reason or contributing factor was found in 13: upper respiratory tract disease (n = 5), suspected diaphragmatic hernia (n = 2), and pregnancy (n = 6).

Table 7.1 The American Society of Anesthesiologists (ASA) physical status classification system with examples.

ASA physical status	Criteria Example
1	A normal healthy patient A healthy cat for ovariohysterectomy
2	A patient with mild systemic disease A dog with an infected skin mass, a dog with compensated cardiac disease
3	A patient with severe systemic disease A severely dehydrated and anemic patient
4	A patient with severe systemic disease that is a constant threat to life A dog with a large splenic tumor, a cat with advanced chronic kidney disease
5	A moribund patient that is not expected to survive without surgery or intervention A patient with septic shock secondary to a gastrointestinal perforation
E	"E" can be added to any ASA status to denote it is an emergency procedure

Table 7.2 Perioperative mortality data for dogs and cats undergoing spay or castration at a single high-volume facility (Levy et al. 2017).

	Number of surgeries	Deaths	Mortality (%)
CATS			
Male	33 531	10	0.030
Female	38 026	24	0.063
DOGS			
Male	20 800	0	0
Female	21 549	4	0.019
SEX			
All males	54 331	10	0.018
All females	59 575	28	0.047
SPECIES			
Dogs (all)	42 349	4	0.009
Cats (all)	71 557	34	0.048

When Do Most Deaths Occur?

The CEPSAF results reveal that most deaths occur *post-operatively*: in dogs, 47% of deaths occurred during this time and in cats the figure is 61%. Based on this study the most critical time appears to be the *first three hours* after the end of anesthesia. Despite the lower overall mortality rate in the Levy et al. (2017) study, the timing of death was similar to that reported by Brodbelt and colleagues: 21 of the 34 cat deaths (61%) occurred post-operatively, with 20 occurring prior to discharge and 1 after discharge, and all 4 of the canine deaths occurred post-operatively, with 2 (50%) before discharge and 2 after discharge. Of note was that 10 cats scheduled for surgery died pre-operatively; this was during preparation, when patients may not have been as closely monitored as during surgery in the operating room (Levy et al. 2017). This underscores the recommendation that staff must be vigilant at all times; close observation and monitoring increase the likelihood of recognizing problems and initiating rapid intervention.

What Are the Causes of Death?

In the CEPSAF study, an independent panel reviewed details of each anesthetic death and tried to ascertain a cause. Cardiovascular or respiratory causes accounted for 74 and 72% of deaths in dogs and cats, respectively. Likely contributing factors in cats in the spay and castration study were upper respiratory tract disease, suspected ruptured diaphragm, and pregnancy. As in human anesthetic-related deaths, human error plays a role. For example, in the CEPSAF study, two dogs died after the adjustable pressure-limiting (APL or "pop-off") valve of the anesthetic machine was left closed (Brodbelt et al. 2008a). Safety equipment for preventing this accident will be discussed later in this chapter.

Risk Factors

Dogs

Dogs with lower bodyweights (<5 kg) may be at increased risk of anesthetic-related death (Brodbelt et al. 2008b). Due to their greater surface area to bodyweight ratio, smaller patients lose more body heat; the complications of hypothermia are discussed later in the chapter.

Mask induction of anesthesia was found to significantly increase mortality (a 5.9-fold increase in risk compared to induction with an injectable agent followed by maintenance with an inhalant agent; Brodbelt et al. 2008b). For this reason, either the use of pre-medication followed by induction of anesthesia with injectable drugs, or an "all-in-one" injectable induction technique is recommended. Inhalant agents are potent cardiovascular and respiratory depressant drugs and techniques to decrease their use are encouraged; this includes pre-medication with analgesics, sedatives, and tranquilizers, and the use of local analgesics.

In the CEPSAF study increasing age was a risk factor in dogs, with dogs over 12 years of age having an odds ratio of 7 if dogs 6 months to ≤8 years of age were used as a reference point (Brodbelt et al. 2008b). However, breed and weight were not accounted for, therefore it is difficult to interpret these results given the differences in life expectancy related to size. In the study by Levy and others, patient age was only available in the final year of the study (approximately 12% of dogs), but there was no difference in mortality between juveniles (<6 months of age) and adults in this sub-set of dogs, suggesting that anesthesia at a young age is not a risk factor.

Cats

Overall the risk associated with anesthesia in cats is significantly higher than for dogs (Brodbelt et al. 2008a; Levy et al. 2017). Of particular interest is the data showing that the risk in "healthy cats" is greater than in "healthy dogs," but mortality is similar in both species when they are classified as "sick" (Brodbelt et al. 2007). This may be a result of some cats being more difficult than dogs to examine leading to incorrect health classification, or may be due to the presence of difficult to detect or "silent" diseases.

One such reason for the higher risk in "healthy" cats may be the presence of subclinical cardiac disease. In "overtly" or "apparently" healthy cats, the incidence of hypertrophic cardiomyopathy (HCM) may be as high as 15% (Cote et al. 2004; Paige et al. 2009), thus cats may be misclassified. However, since cats with cardiac disease can appear clinically healthy and do not all have murmurs, it is difficult to detect or even suspect these patients without echocardiography or N-terminal pro-brain natriuretic peptide (NT-proBNP) testing (Oyama 2016), neither of which is easily accessible in a HVHQSN or shelter setting.

The number of deaths from all respiratory causes were similar in dogs and cats (20 and 16%, respectively), but respiratory obstruction was reported more frequently in cats (Brodbelt et al. 2008a). There are increased odds of death associated with endotracheal intubation in cats that initially seem counterintuitive (Clarke and Hall 1990; Brodbelt et al. 2007). However, the cat's larynx is small and laryngospasm can make intubation challenging, and it has been suggested that trauma and resultant swelling may contribute to post-anesthetic obstruction. Airway management is discussed later in this chapter.

Body weights at either end of the spectrum (<2 kg or >6 kg) increased the risk of death in cats (Brodbelt et al. 2007). Small cats may be susceptible to hypothermia and its associated complications and may pose more challenges related to intubation and monitoring. Heavy cats may be at increased risk of respiratory compromise (e.g. reduced diaphragmatic excursions due to abdominal and thoracic fat, especially when placed in dorsal recumbency) and excess tissue mass around the neck may result in post-operative obstruction.

Cats older than 12 years are twice as likely to die compared to cats aged 6 months to 5 years. This increased risk was independent of their ASA status, and may be a result of decreased respiratory and cardiovascular reserve, or because older patients have decreased anesthetic requirements, leading to relative overdosing (Brodbelt et al. 2007). However, mortality in juvenile cats (<6 months of age) is no different to that of adult cats (Nutt et al. 2016).

A surprising finding was that the use of intravenous (IV) fluids increased the risks of death in both healthy and sick cats (Brodbelt et al. 2007). One reason may be inaccurate and inappropriate fluid volume delivery. The blood volume in cats is smaller in cats than in dogs – approximately 40–60 ml/kg compared to 80–90 ml/kg in dogs – yet historically intraoperative fluid rates of 10 ml/kg/hour have been recommended for both species (Raskin 2009; Davis et al. 2013). If an apparently healthy cat has underlying cardiac disease, it is likely they cannot tolerate fluid loads. The 2013 American Animal Hospital Association (AAHA) and American Association of Feline Practitioners (AAFP) fluid therapy guidelines suggest lower fluid rates than in the past (Davis et al. 2013).

Pre-anesthetic Evaluation

Ideally, pre-anesthetic assessment includes obtaining a history from the owner, a full physical examination and in some cases biochemical and hematologic analyses of blood, or other screening tests such as a urinalysis. In some cases a history and/or physical examination is not obtainable (e.g. stray and feral animals). The animal's temperament should be assessed and recorded, as this will influence the choice of anesthetic protocol; for example, unsocialized animals will require an "all-in-one" technique whereby a single injection of a mix of drugs will render them unconscious, whereas a calm and friendly adult dog may receive acepromazine and an opioid followed by induction of anesthesia with an IV agent.

An accurate bodyweight is desirable, especially in very small animals, to ensure accurate dosing of drugs, but in some cases the bodyweight will only be estimated. When dealing with community cats that will be trapped, one can weigh each trap in advance and write the weight of the trap clearly with a permanent marker on the top of the trap; at intake, the trap with the cat can be weighed and the weight of the cat calculated.

Assigning Health Status

Assigning a patient's health status is important for assessing peri-operative risks, for determining which pre-operative tests to perform, and for choosing anesthetic drugs. Using a standardized assessment system also assists in retrospective and prospective studies of peri-operative morbidity and mortality. The recommended system is based on the ASA physical status classification which has six categories; in veterinary medicine we use statuses 1 through 5 because status 6 (anesthesia to remove organs for donor purposes) is not applicable; see http://www.asahq.org/standards-and-guidelines/asa-physical-status-classification-system and Table 7.1.

Pre-anesthetic Blood Work

There is little disagreement that prior blood chemistry and hematologic analyses are valuable in some patient groups, but it is debated whether this can be justified for every patient, especially healthy animals undergoing elective procedures. In many situations pre-operative blood work cannot be obtained, for example from non-socialized cats. In other cases there are economic constraints to performing screening tests or limited access to equipment for analyses. Several studies in human anesthesiology question the need for pre-anesthetic laboratory testing in healthy patients and most conclude that pre-operative testing is overused. When no abnormalities surface during history taking and clinical examination, there appears to be little value in conducting pre-anesthetic blood tests (Chung et al. 2009; Benarroch-Gampel et al. 2012). Reference ranges established by laboratories usually incorporate 80% of the population, therefore 20% of healthy

animals may have a result that is outside this range, which can delay the procedure or lead to further, sometimes unnecessary testing. A study of 1500 dogs stated that when no potential issues were noted in the history or physical examination, any abnormalities in the preoperative blood work were usually of little clinical significance and did not lead to any major changes in the anesthetic protocol (Alef et al. 2008). The same study revealed that based on pre-anesthetic screening blood work, approximately 8% of dogs were assigned a higher ASA status, surgery was delayed in 0.8%, additional pre-anesthetic treatment was undertaken in 1.5%, and in 0.2% the anesthetic protocol was changed. Hematologic and biochemical analyses of 101 dogs aged over 7 years resulted in 30 new diagnoses (e.g. neoplasia, hyperadrenocorticism) and cancelation of surgery in 13 of these patients (Joubert 2007). When analyzing risk factors for anesthetic death in sick dogs (ASA 3–5), having a pre-operative blood test was associated with reduced odds of death, particularly in ASA category 4–5 dogs (Brodbelt 2006). In a UK veterinary practice where preanesthesia blood tests in dogs and cats are optional (owner decision), it was clear that clients opted in when their pet was older, with the mean age of dogs and cats undergoing screening being 9.6 and 11.6 years, respectively (Davies and Kawaguchi 2014). This study found that at least one blood test fell outside the reference range established for the clinic in 95 and 97% of dogs and cats, but was not necessarily clinically significant. Clinicians voiced concern over blood results in approximately 8% of dogs and changed the anesthetic protocol in 4% of cases. In cats, concern was expressed about the results in 15% of patients and in 9% decisions about the anesthetic protocol were changed. In 1% of all cases, a problem that was not suspected from the pet's history or physical examination was uncovered and the authors concluded that pre-anesthetic screening can be valuable for the management of dogs and cats undergoing anesthesia (Davies and Kawaguchi 2014).

Based on evidence from human anesthesia and from a smaller number of veterinary studies, there appears to be negligible benefit to biochemical or hematologic screening in apparently healthy animals (ASA 1–2). In animals assigned a higher ASA status and in geriatric patients it is more clear-cut, with the published veterinary studies providing justification that pre-anesthetic screening is of value in terms of anesthetic management and outcome. However, there is still no substitute for a thorough clinical examination by trained personnel, and if pre-anesthetic blood screening and other tests are conducted they should be regarded as adjuncts, not alternatives to the patient's physical assessment.

Components of Anesthesia

Pre-medication

The goals of pre-medication include sedation of the patient to facilitate handling and reduce stress, provision of preventive analgesia, and reduction of the dose of anesthetic agents. Attainment of these goals is associated with a decrease in the risk of anesthetic-related death (Brodbelt 2009), and may be accomplished with sedatives, tranquilizers, and opioids, administered either alone or in combination. In most cases pre-medicant drugs are given intramuscularly (IM), but some are suitable for administration by the subcutaneous (SC; e.g. acepromazine) or oral transmucosal route (e.g. dexmedetomidine in cats; Slingsby et al. 2009). If IV access is easy to achieve or an IV catheter is in place, most pre-medicant drugs can be given by this route at reduced doses.

Stress Reduction

Stress, fear, and anxiety should be minimized as much as possible in the peri-operative period, as this may alleviate negative physiologic changes, including tachycardia, hypertension, ileus, and increased circulating catecholamines, and enhance the overall emotional experience of the patient. This can be achieved with a combination of carefully selected drugs, pheromones, and implementation of low-stress and fear-free handling. See Chapter 6 for more information about stress reduction in the spay–neuter clinic.

Pheromones

Synthetic analogues of feline facial pheromone (FFP; Feliway®, Ceva Animal Health Care, Libourne, France) are widely used to reduce stress and stress-related problems in cats (Mills et al. 2011). Handling and the process of anesthesia may be stressful for cats due to the novel interventions they encounter, a strange environment, and exposure to unknown animals and personnel. Kronen and colleagues looked at the benefits of FFP (sprayed on cage paper before placing the cat in the cage) in the pre-anesthetic period and reported that it had additional calming effects in cats that received acepromazine and helped calm cats that had not received acepromazine (Kronen et al. 2006). FFP has also been reported to increase food consumption and grooming behavior in cats (Griffith et al. 2000). Pheromone therapy, including dog-appeasing pheromone (Adaptil®, Ceva Animal Health) may have a role to play in a shelter or HVHQSN environment.

Gabapentin and Trazodone

Gabapentin (50 or 100 mg per cat) administered in a suspension (Ora-Plus suspending vehicle and Ora-Sweet flavored syrup vehicle, Perrigo®, Dublin, Ireland, in a 50:50 ratio) to community cats after trapping decreased their fear responses when compared to placebo treatment (Pankratz et al. 2018). After weighing the cats, the dose used ranged from 9.2 to 47.6 mg/kg. Peak effect occurred two hours after administration, but there were no differences in sedation scores between gabapentin- and placebo-treated cats.

Trazodone is a serotonin (5-HT) antagonist/reuptake inhibitor and is classified as an "atypical" antidepressant. Favorable results have been published on its use for decreasing behavioral signs of stress in hospitalized dogs and for enhancing behavioral calmness when dogs are confined during recovery form surgery (Gruen et al. 2014; Gilbert-Gregory et al. 2016). Recommended doses range from 4 to 12 mg/kg.

Induction

This phase of anesthesia renders the patient unconscious. This state is commonly achieved by administering IV induction drugs (e.g. alfaxalone, propofol, ketamine). Although inhalant agents delivered via a face mask continue to be used for induction, this practice should be discouraged. In dogs, mask induction is associated with a higher mortality rate (Brodbelt et al. 2008b); reasons for this may include the stress of the technique, which requires physical restraint for several minutes during which patients may resist and struggle, resulting in catecholamine release and arrhythmias. In addition, with mask induction there is no option for rapid airway control if respiratory obstruction occurs, and the risks of regurgitation and aspiration are increased. The technique exposes the patient to a large dose of inhalant agent; both isoflurane and sevoflurane are potent cardiac and respiratory depressants. This technique also exposes personnel to waste anesthetic gases (see Chapter 31 for more information on waste gas exposure risks and prevention).

Pre-oxygenation
Pre-oxygenation is recommended in compromised patients, brachycephalic breeds, obese patients, and pregnant animals, as these situations involve animals with limited respiratory reserves or an anticipated difficult intubation. If a healthy dog breathing room air prior to induction becomes apneic, the dog will desaturate – peripheral capillary oxygen saturation (SpO_2) ≤90%, partial pressure of oxygen (PaO_2) ≤60 mmHg – within 69.6 ± 10.6 seconds, and in some cases within 30 seconds. For the same animal breathing oxygen via a face mask for 3 minutes prior to induction, this time is extended to 297.8 ± 42 seconds, a difference of almost 4 minutes (McNally et al. 2009).

"One-Step" Induction
In several situations there is no separation between pre-medication and induction: induction of anesthesia is achieved by a single injection, usually of several different drugs, for example dexmedetomidine, ketamine, and buprenorphine, usually given IM. Protocols that combine pre-medication and induction drugs are widely used, particularly in pediatric patients (see Chapter 9), in feral or non-socialized animals, and in HVHQSN clinics (see Chapter 8). These techniques reduce the number of times the animal is restrained and are time saving without compromising safety.

Maintenance

Maintenance of anesthesia may be by inhalant anesthetic agents, repeated boluses ("top-ups"), or continuous infusions of IV agents. In some cases the initial induction technique may be of sufficient duration to last for the intended procedure. The duration of action of a "one-step" induction technique described above is often sufficient to perform a feline spay. In many cases a canine castration can be completed after pre-medication and a single bolus of propofol – and if more time is needed a "top-up" dose can be given.

Recovery

As highlighted by the results of the CEPSAF study and the data from a high-volume spay and castration clinic, the recovery period is when most anesthetic mortalities occur (Brodbelt 2009; Levy et al. 2017). It is highly recommended that patients recovering from anesthesia are closely observed for at least three hours. If sufficient staff are available, a dedicated recovery area should be set up where staff are always present. If this is not possible, a recovery area can be set up in an area of the clinic where people are always present who may be performing several tasks, including observing recovering patients – this is not

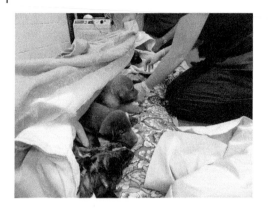

Figure 7.1 Puppies at different stages of recovery. They have been placed under a forced warm air blanket and are being closely observed.

ideal, but is better than leaving animals alone and unattended. During recovery animals should be kept warm, and supplemental heat (e.g. forced warm air devices) may be required until they become normothermic (Figure 7.1). At this time patients are also assessed for comfort and additional analgesics given if needed; peri-operative analgesia, pain assessment, and thermoregulation are discussed in the next part of the chapter.

Peri-operative Pain Assessment and Analgesia

Assessing Pain in Dogs and Cats

One of the main reasons for inadequately treating pain in dogs and cats is the difficulty of recognizing and "measuring" their pain. To treat pain, we must first look for it, recognize it, and quantify it in some way so we can assess the efficacy of our interventions. Pain is a complex, multidimensional experience with both sensory and emotional components. The sensory component includes the type of pain, its location, duration, and intensity. Pain is a conscious emotion and is always unpleasant. Pain is a subjective experience and even after the same surgical procedure, humans who can self-report do not experience the same sensory

and emotional consequences, so how can animal caregivers determine with any degree of certainty what an animal feels? Put simply, in humans that can communicate, pain is what the patient says it is, and in animals, it is what *we* say it is. People involved in the care of patients in the peri-operative period must make "proxy" assessments on behalf of the animal, so it is important that we use validated assessment tools to ensure their comfort.

There is currently no gold standard for assessing acute pain in animals. Many different scoring methods that include physiologic and behavioral variables have been published, but only a few are validated. The correlations between pain and easily measured physiologic (objective) variables such as heart rate, respiratory rate, and blood pressure have been disappointing (Smith et al. 1996; Cambridge et al. 2000; Brondani et al. 2011). This is not surprising, since these variables can be affected by many other factors, including fear, anxiety, drugs, fluid status, and the stress of the clinic environment (Quimby et al. 2011).

Scoring systems that depend on human observers are subjective to some degree and prone to errors of either over- or underestimation of the animal's pain; significant inter-observer disagreement occurs with some assessment methods and this makes them unsuitable when multiple people are involved in pain assessment. Any system that is used must be validated as being reliable (repeatable), sensitive, and specific (accurate). By using trained observers to apply carefully defined criteria, pain scoring systems can achieve acceptable levels of repeatability and accuracy.

The most basic pain scales are simple descriptive scales (SDS), numeric rating scales (NRS), and visual analogue scales (VAS). Holton and others (Holton et al. 1998) compared the use of simple descriptive, numeric rating, and visual analogue scales for assessing pain in dogs following surgery and reported significant inter-observer variability – as high as 36% – with all three scales. An extension of the classic VAS system is the dynamic and interactive visual analogue scale (DIVAS). With this system, animals are first observed undisturbed and from a distance. The reason for this is that some animals do not display overt pain behaviors in the presence of a caregiver, but may do so when they think they are unobserved; this is likely a protective mechanism against potential "predators." Following the initial observation, the assessor approaches, handles the patient, and encourages it to move around; the surgical incision (or injured area) and surrounding area is palpated, and a final overall assessment of pain is made. This approach overcomes some of the deficiencies of purely observational systems; for example, an animal in pain may remain very still and quiet because they are in pain and would be overlooked and untreated without an interaction.

It is now accepted that quantitative measurements of behavior are the most reliable methods for assessing pain in animals, and that if the methodology used to develop and validate these systems is rigorous, they can be objective, with minimal observer bias (Holton et al. 2001). Multidimensional systems are particularly important when self-reporting is not possible. They must incorporate components that have been proven to be sensitive and specific indicators of pain in the species being studied. Knowledge of the normal behavior of a species and the individual being evaluated is important, as deviations from normal behavior may suggest pain, anxiety, fear, or other stressors. Normal behaviors should be maintained postoperatively if an animal is comfortable. Grooming is a normal behavior, but licking excessively at a wound or incision can be an indicator of pain, so the two should be differentiated. The occurrence of new behaviors such as a previously friendly animal becoming aggressive, or a playful and friendly animal becoming reclusive, should raise our suspicion that pain may not have been adequately addressed.

Dogs

In dogs, the Glasgow Composite Measure Pain Scale (GCMPS) is a reliable and widely used tool (Holton et al. 2001). The original tool has been shortened to give it utility in a busy clinical setting (Reid et al. 2007; Murrell et al. 2008). This tool is available for download from http://www.newmetrica.com/acute-pain-measurement. The categories for assessment include vocalization, attention to the wound, mobility on rising, response to palpation of the wound or painful area, posture, and overall demeanor.

Cats

Brondani and colleagues (Brondani et al. 2011, 2013) created a multidimensional composite scale by observing cats undergoing ovariohysterectomy. Brondani and colleagues have created a website with videos that demonstrate the behaviors in their tool, as well as cases to test yourself and a download link (http://www.animalpain.com.br/en-us). This is an excellent resource for staff training.

Another tool is the Glasgow Composite Measures Pain Scale-Feline (rCMPS-Feline), which includes facial expressions (Calvo et al. 2014; Holden et al. 2014; Reid et al. 2017). This tool was developed using cats undergoing different types of surgery or with medically related pain. English and Spanish versions are available for download from http://www.newmetrica.com/acute-pain-measurement.

There are seven assessments (questions) in the Glasgow acute pain scale:

1) Vocalization
2) Posture
3) Attention to the wound
4) Interaction with people
5) Response to palpation of the wound or painful area
6) Facial expressions
7) Overall demeanor

The maximum score a cat can achieve is 20, and intervention is suggested with a score of ≥5.

A feline grimace scale is currently being developed and shows promise for ease of use, validity, reliability, and inter- and intraobserver agreement (Evangelista et al. 2018).

Pathophysiology of Pain

Understanding the mechanisms of pain is the key to its successful treatment. If the pathophysiology of pain is understood, logical choices regarding analgesic protocols can be made. The "pain experience" can be considered under two headings:

1) *Nociception*, which includes transduction, transmission, and modulation
2) *Perception*, which is the unpleasant experience that we call pain

Transduction is the process that involves translation of noxious stimuli (e.g. surgical incisions) into electrical activity at sensory nerve endings. Nociceptors respond to thermal, mechanical, and chemical stimulation. *Transmission* is the process of transmitting or sending the impulses throughout the sensory nervous system. Afferent signals from the periphery are relayed through the dorsal root ganglia to the dorsal horn of the spinal cord. These signals travel up the spinal cord, finally reaching the brain. *Modulation* is the modification of nociceptive transmission. The body can regulate and modify incoming impulses at the dorsal horn; this involves release of enkephalins and endorphins, and activation of serotonergic and noradrenergic pathways. Transmission can also be modified pharmacologically by the administration of analgesic drugs. The perception of pain can only occur in a conscious animal and is a result of the interaction of transduction, transmission, and modulation.

The concepts of peripheral and central sensitization explain much of an animal's response to an injury, and why analgesia may succeed or fail. The inflammatory response to a wound produces a change in sensitivity to noxious stimuli. As the local area of tissue injury becomes more sensitive, the threshold for subsequent stimuli decreases; this is termed *primary hyperalgesia*. Clinically this is observed when an animal demonstrates sensitivity to touch in the immediate area of a surgical wound. Peripheral sensitization is a result of inflammatory mediators and the severity is directly related to the degree of trauma, for example a small incision versus a large incision. This post-injury hypersensitivity is not confined to the original site of injury; rather, it spreads to other parts of the body, creating what is termed *secondary hyperalgesia*. For example, following ovariohysterectomy, there is a decrease in the mechanical nociceptive threshold not only at the incision site, but also at remote sites (Lascelles et al. 1998).

When neurons in the dorsal horn are repeatedly stimulated, their rate of discharge dramatically increases over time; this is termed *central hypersensitization* (Woolf 2011). The barrage of signals that arrive in the spinal cord cause changes in the dorsal horn neurons and as a result of these changes, the response to subsequent incoming signals is dramatically changed. The neurons remain hypersensitive for a time, even after the noxious stimulus stops. Activation and modulation of N-methyl-D-aspartate (NMDA) receptors by the excitatory neurotransmitter glutamate are thought to be the primary mechanism in the development of *central sensitization* and *secondary hyperalgesia*.

How Long Do We Need to Treat?

There are two phases associated with tissue injury: the first is the sensory input arising directly from the surgical wound; and the second is from the resultant, more prolonged inflammatory response. It is now understood that unless effective and appropriate analgesics are provided during the inflammatory period, "re-initiation" of pain is possible (Kissin et al. 1998; Kelly et al. 2001). The term "preventive" is preferred to "pre-emptive" analgesia because the latter suggests that all that is required for effective analgesia is the administration of pre-operative analgesics. Although it is true that pre-operative use of analgesic agents, especially opioids, is more effective than administration after surgery, continued dosing in the post-operative period is often required to prevent post-operative pain. To prevent prolonged or persistent post-operative pain, analgesic therapy should be started prior to surgery, maintained during surgery, be robust in the immediate post-operative period, and be continued until the inflammatory response has subsided. Different analgesic drugs may be used during each of these phases; for example, opioids and non-steroidal anti-inflammatory drugs (NSAIDs) may be given pre-operatively along with sedative agents. Opioids may be continued in the immediate post-operative period, then stopped. If there are no contraindications to their use, NSAIDs are used throughout the entire perioperative period and are often the only drug required in the later stages of healing. Duration of treatment will depend on the degree of surgical trauma and resultant inflammatory response. Ovariohysterectomy in cats can be associated with changes in behavior suggestive of pain for up to three days (Vaisanen et al. 2007).

Multimodal or Balanced Analgesia

Nociception and pain involve many steps and pathways, so it seems unlikely that one analgesic agent could completely prevent or alleviate pain. Multimodal analgesia, also termed balanced analgesia, describes the combined use of drugs that have different modes of action, working at different receptors and at different sites along the "pain pathway." The assumption is that this will provide superior analgesia and/or allow lower doses of each drug to be used, thereby reducing the risk of adverse side effects. The most commonly used combinations of drugs are opioids, NSAIDs, and local anesthetics. In cats and dogs, a combination of buprenorphine and carprofen was superior to either drug used alone (Shih et al. 2008; Steagall et al. 2009).

Airway Management and Oxygen Administration

During anesthesia dogs and cats may breathe room air or receive oxygen and/or inhalant agents via a face mask or following intubation.

Oxygen supplementation is recommended in anesthetized animals. In some settings, providing oxygen to every anesthetized patient is not possible; for example, in high-volume clinics where total injectable protocols are often used, multiple patients are anesthetized at the same time and there is limited equipment for inhalant anesthetic or oxygen delivery. Although low SpO_2 readings indicative of desaturation have been reported in anesthetized cats breathing room air, the long-term effects are unknown (Williams et al. 2002; Harrison et al. 2011).

There is little controversy over the use of endotracheal tubes (ETTs) in dogs where placement is easy to perform and few complications are reported; however, there is more concern regarding airway management in cats. The CEPSAF study (Brodbelt et al. 2007) reported a link between mortality and intubation for short procedures (<30 minutes) in cats. Respiratory obstruction as a cause of death has been reported more frequently in cats than in dogs, suggesting that intubation is not a benign procedure in cats. It is important to take steps to prevent trauma and swelling of delicate mucosa (Clarke and Hall 1990; Dyson et al. 1998; Brodbelt et al. 2007; Robertson et al. 2018).

Endotracheal intubation should be performed with care, under the correct plane of anesthesia (not too light) and with direct visualization (using a laryngoscope). Because of the propensity of laryngospasm in cats, local anesthetics (e.g. lidocaine) may need to be applied to the arytenoids and vocal cords (see also Chapter 10, Figure 10.1). The ETT should only be advanced when the vocal cords are open. Tracheal tears within the thorax are associated with a poor outcome (Hardie et al. 1999), therefore the length of the ETT should be measured against the cat prior to insertion and the tip of the tube should not extend beyond the point of the shoulder (Figure 7.2). However, when this procedure is followed, in dogs or cats, many ETTs are too long – the portion of the tube that extends beyond the incisor teeth may create excessive dead space and

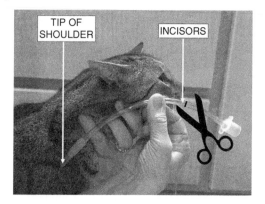

Figure 7.2 The endotracheal tube should reach form the incisors to the point of the shoulder. If it is too long, cut at the appropriate site (black mark on the tube).

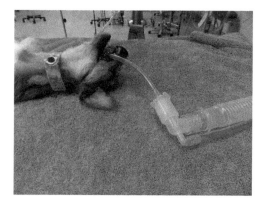

Figure 7.3 In this image, there is excessive dead space because the endotracheal tube is excessively long.

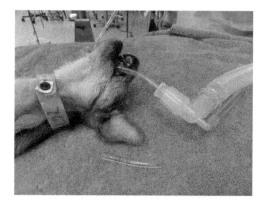

Figure 7.4 Dead space has been decreased by shortening the endotracheal tube.

result in rebreathing. After measuring the ETT, it should be cut to the correct length (Figure 7.2). Figure 7.3 shows placement of an ETT that was excessively long in a puppy and Figure 7.4 shows the tube after it was cut.

Tracheal injury related to intubation is well documented in cats (Hardie et al. 1999; Mitchell et al. 2000; Bhandal and Kuzma 2008; Bauer et al. 2009), as is damage to the larynx (Hofmeister et al. 2007). Approximately 70–75% of tracheal ruptures reported are in cats that have undergone dental procedures. Presenting signs include subcutaneous emphysema, coughing, gagging, and varying severity of dyspnea occurring any time from 4 hours to 12 days post-anesthesia.

In a cadaveric model, Hardie and others (Hardie et al. 1999) documented that overinflation of the cuff is the cause of tears in cats and that they occur directly over the cuff. One theory is that cuffs are overinflated due to a fear of aspiration, especially when performing dental and other oral procedures. Larger tears are more difficult to repair or medically manage; therefore, the choice of ETT should be made with care. Two different types of cuffs are available on ETTs: one is a low-volume, high-pressure cuff and the other is a high-volume, low-pressure cuff. High-volume, low-pressure cuffs have a larger contact area with the tracheal wall and, because tears occur directly over the cuff, they will be longer than with low-volume, high-pressure cuffs. The cuff should only be inflated if necessary; this is contrary to the common technique of routinely inflating every cuff immediately after intubation. The seal can be tested by occluding the APL valve (the "pop-off") and squeezing the reservoir bag – air is added in small increments to the cuff until there is no leak at 15 cmH$_2$O. As an added safety measure, a small (1 ml or 3 ml) syringe should be used to restrict the volume of air that can be added to the cuff. The use of water-soluble gel on the cuff improves the airway seal, even at low cuff inflation pressures (Blunt et al. 2001). Oxygen masks and supraglottic airway devices (SGADs) are alternatives to cuffed ETTs in cats; their use will depend on the conformation of the cat (e.g. brachycephalic), and the type and duration of the procedure.

One SGAD (Cat v-gel[*], Docsinnovent Ltd., London, UK; Figure 7.5) has been designed to conform to the shape of the feline larynx and pharynx and has undergone clinical assessment (Crotaz 2013; van Oostrom et al. 2013; Barletta et al. 2015; Prasse et al. 2016). This device rests over the laryngeal inlet and the tip lodges in the esophageal opening. There was less stridor and greater food consumption in the immediate recovery period after use of an SGAD compared to an ETT (van Oostrom et al. 2013; Barletta et al. 2015). In spontaneously breathing cats there was no difference in the measured isoflurane concentration at the mouth when ETTs and SGADs were compared (van Oostrom et al. 2013). During mechanical ventilation up to an airway pressure of 16 cmH_2O, there was less leakage with an SGAD than an ETT (Prasse et al. 2016). Inexperienced veterinary students were able to secure an airway more quickly and with fewer attempts when they used an SGAD instead of an ETT and less propofol was required with the former device (Barletta et al. 2015).

If intubation is not routinely performed, equipment for emergency intubation and ventilation must always be available for emergency use; this includes a range of ETT sizes, a laryngoscope, Ambu bag, or anesthesia machine, and a source of oxygen. See Chapter 11 for details on emergency procedures and cardiopulmonary resuscitation.

Fluid Therapy

A cost– and time–benefit analysis of IV fluid administration sets and IV catheter use should be made based on the procedure being performed. Healthy adult and pediatric patients do not necessarily require fluids during short, elective surgical procedures that are associated with minimal blood loss; one study reported no differences in blood pressure in healthy dogs undergoing elective surgical procedures with or without IV fluids (Gaynor et al. 1996). However, clinics should have the ability to administer fluids in specific cases on an as-needed basis, for example pregnant animals undergoing ovariohysterectomy or cesarean section, dehydrated or compromised animals, and in cases where significant blood loss may be anticipated (e.g. limb amputation or enucleation surgery). When intraoperative IV fluids are used, the appropriate dose should be administered. The 2013 AAHA and AAFP fluid therapy guidelines suggest lower doses than in the past, for example 5 ml/kg/hour in healthy dogs, with a 25% reduction in rate every hour (Davis et al. 2013).

As previously discussed, the use of IV fluids was associated with an increased risk of mortality in healthy and sick cats (Brodbelt et al. 2007). Although confounding factors should be considered (i.e. those cats receiving IV fluids may have been at greater anesthetic risk to begin with), these findings warrant reassessment of fluid therapy protocols in anesthetized cats. As previously discussed, the blood volume of cats is approximately 60 ml/kg compared to 80–90 ml/kg in dogs (Raskin 2009). The 2013 AAHA and AAFP Fluid Therapy Guidelines for Dogs and Cats suggest 3 ml/kg/hr

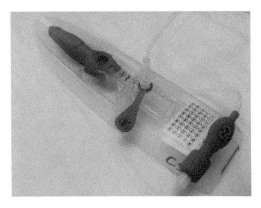

Figure 7.5   A supraglottic airway device specifically designed for cats. The side port is attached to a side-stream capnograph.

as a starting rate for crystalloid fluids in cats (Davis et al. 2013).

Even at lower rates of intraoperative fluid administration, accurate dosing and administration are required if inadvertent fluid overload is to be avoided. The use of correctly programmed infusion or syringe pumps or a buretrol is advised in cats to ensure accurate volume delivery; the latter prevents free flow of fluids from the fluid bag after the volume in the chamber is delivered. Most buretrols hold 100–150 ml of fluid, but should never be filled to capacity; no more than 60 minutes' worth of fluids should be put in the chamber at a time, so that administration is limited even if the drip rate is set incorrectly or the roller clamp left wide open.

Equipment

A complete review of anesthetic and monitoring equipment is outside the scope of this chapter and can be found elsewhere (Shelby and McKune 2014; Robertson et al. 2018), but specific and pertinent points related to anesthetic principles will be addressed.

Oxygen Supply

Traditionally, most veterinary clinics have used oxygen cylinders or bulk tanks of liquid oxygen as their source of oxygen for anesthesia machines. A feasible alternative are oxygen concentrators, which are commercially available as small portable units. An oxygen concentrator uses room air (21% oxygen) to produce a gas that contains 95% oxygen, which is comparable to medical-grade oxygen supplied in cylinders (Barrand 2011). Oxygen concentrators require a power source, but can be run off a power inverter (Barrand 2011). The advantages include cost savings after the initial outlay, minimal maintenance, and an "on demand" source of oxygen. Investing in this equipment will result in long-term cost savings and may be ideal for mobile or MASH (mobile animal sterilization hospital) clinics.

Breathing Circuits

Two types of breathing circuits should be available to accommodate the wide range of patient sizes and weights encountered in shelter medicine and HQHVSN. Non-rebreathing circuits (e.g. Bain or Ayre's T-piece) are recommended for patients ≤3 kg. To prevent rebreathing, the flow rate in these systems must be 200–300 ml/kg/min. Rebreathing systems (e.g. a circle system) can be used in patients ≥3 kg; at lower weight ranges (3–10 kg) pediatric, rather than adult, breathing hoses should be used. Because rebreathing systems incorporate a carbon dioxide absorbent (e.g. soda lime or baralyme), oxygen flow rates are much lower (10–20 ml/kg/min) compared to non-rebreathing systems.

Safety Equipment

A patient safety incident is one that causes injury or is potentially harmful to the patient. Many of these events are caused by human error and are preventable (Hofmeister et al. 2014).

All anesthesia machines should be fitted with an in-circuit manometer and a device to prevent high airway pressures occurring, which can cause barotrauma (Robertson et al. 2018). A manometer is essential for safely delivering manual breaths or if a mechanical ventilator is used; the pressure should never exceed 20 cmH$_2$O and a range of 12–16 cmH$_2$O is usually adequate for delivering a normal tidal volume (10–15 ml/kg) to a patient. The manometer is also required when checking for leaks around an ETT (Figure 7.6).

One potentially lethal accident is leaving the APL valve ("pop-off") closed, which results in a rapid rise in airway pressure and risk of barotrauma and cardiac arrest – this occurs very quickly (<30 seconds) in small patients on a non-rebreathing system. In a university teaching hospital, patient safety incidents were recorded over a 11.5-month period; approximately 26% of incidents were due to closed APL valves. After this finding, a checklist was

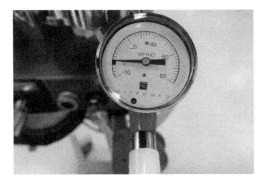

Figure 7.6 An in-circuit manometer to measure pressure within the anesthetic circuit and therefore applied to the patient's lungs.

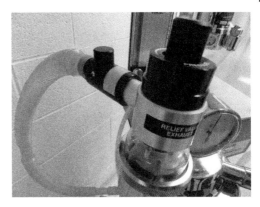

Figure 7.8 A pop-off occlusion valve; this allows the adjustable pressure-limiting (pop-off) valve to be left open at all times; when a manual breath is to be delivered the button is depressed by the operator using their thumb. A breath is given, then the operator's thumb is removed, and the valve reopens.

Devices may vent into room air or the scavenger system. Another technique is to use a pop-off occlusion valve (Figure 7.8). This device allows the APL valve to be left open at all times. When a breath is manually delivered, the operator presses the button during delivery of the breath, and as soon as they remove their finger, the occlusion valve reopens.

Body Temperature

Maintaining normothermia is important for cardiac function, metabolism, normal enzyme activity, nerve conduction, hemostasis, preventing post-operative wound infections, and improving post-operative comfort, and is an important goal of anesthetic management.

Hypothermia occurs commonly in dogs and cats that undergo anesthesia and the consequences are greatly underestimated (Evans et al. 1973; Waterman 1975; Pottie et al. 2007; Redondo et al. 2012a, b). In humans, peri-anesthetic hypothermia is linked to increased mortality. In veterinary medicine, studies show that cats weighing less than 2 kg, dogs under 5 kg, senior patients, and those undergoing long procedures have a greater peri-operative

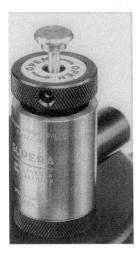

Figure 7.7 A pop-off safety relief valve; this opens at a preset pressure to relieve patient circuit pressure and prevent barotrauma.

implemented to include checking that the APL valve was open before attaching a patient to the anesthesia machine. After this intervention, problems were logged again and the incidence of closed APL valves dropped to 16% (Hofmeister et al. 2014). By adding a pop-off safety relief valve or a pop-off occlusion valve to every anesthesia machine, the occurrence of this accident should be minimal, but it requires that the safety devices themselves are checked, as they can malfunction. A pop-off safety relief valve is shown in Figure 7.7; these automatically relieve patient circuit pressure by opening at a preset pressure (e.g. 20 cmH$_2$O).

mortality risk (Brodbelt et al. 2007, 2008b); hypothermia is likely in these patient populations. It is important to identify at-risk patients and understand why animals become cold, the adverse effects of low body temperatures, and current options for the prevention and treatment of peri-operative hypothermia.

Thermoregulation

The body is divided into two compartments: the core, containing the most metabolically active organs; and the periphery, which acts as a buffer between the external environment and the core. Thermoreceptors in the skin, the hypothalamus, and other areas of the body provide feedback to the posterior hypothalamus, which regulates body temperature. In a conscious animal, temperature is tightly controlled to within an inter-threshold range of ±0.2 °C (Clark-Price 2015). This is accomplished via behavioral responses, changes in body metabolism and blood flow to the skin, and shivering or panting.

Heat loss occurs by four main mechanisms:

Conductive heat loss is the transfer of heat from a warmer object to a cooler one when they are in direct contact with each other. An example is an animal lying directly on a cold stainless-steel table.

Convective heat loss occurs when warm air next to the body is displaced by cool air ("wind chill"). An example is placing the animal near an air vent or in a draft.

Radiative heat losses occur due to infrared emission from an object to cooler surroundings. One example is housing an animal in a cold room.

Evaporative heat losses occur when liquids change to vapors, taking heat with them. Examples include evaporation of moisture from exposed serosal surfaces and the respiratory tract, and evaporation of alcohol or other liquids used to prepare surgical sites.

Homeothermy, the balance between heat loss and heat gain, involves complex sensing processes that drive the mechanisms controlling heat loss or gain in the correct direction. Temperature sensors exist centrally (hypothalamus, spinal cord, brain stem, abdominal organs, and skeletal muscles) and peripherally (warm and cold receptors in the skin). The hypothalamus acts by integrating thermal input and controlling effector organs, in many ways acting as a thermostat. Heat gains can be obligatory or facultative. Obligatory gains occur independently of thermoregulation and include heat from basal metabolism, eating, and exercise. Facultative gains act to restore thermal balance; the most important source is from shivering. In animals, over 75% of heat losses occur from the body surface, with the remainder coming from the respiratory tract.

When an animal is anesthetized, many factors interrupt normal thermoregulation. Anesthesia abolishes behavioral responses – for example, the animal cannot no longer seek out a warm environment. Anesthesia also reduces the metabolic rate, alters hypothalamic function, and reduces muscle tone and effector responses (shivering). In addition, operating room environments and surgical procedures (exposure of body cavities) impose large thermal losses on patients. In anesthetized patients, the inter-threshold range increases to ±2.5 °C and mechanisms to stem heat loss do not come into play until there is a significant drop in body temperature.

Anesthesia-induced hypothermia (AIH) can be divided into three phases. In phase 1 there is redistribution of heat from the core to the periphery. This phase begins as soon as animals are pre-medicated, due to direct effects on central (hypothalamic) thermoregulation by sedatives, tranquilizers, and opioids; in addition, peripheral vasodilation associated with the use of acepromazine increases heat loss from the body surface. After induction of anesthesia there is loss of autonomic control and anesthetic agents such as propofol and inhalant anesthetics cause vasodilation. Heat loss in phase 1 is primarily via conduction and convection, which account for up to 80% of total heat loss. Body temperature can drop quickly, with the greatest rate of heat loss occurring in the first 20 minutes following induction; in one study, cats' temperatures fell on average by 1.2 °C during the first hour of anesthesia (Redondo et al. 2012a). The second phase of AIH is a continued but slower loss of heat to the cooler surrounding environment. Additional losses occur by evaporation from exposed serosal surfaces and via the respiratory tract; respiratory losses are increased when the animal is breathing cold, dry oxygen and/or inhalant agents. Heat production is also reduced due to a decrease in metabolic rate caused by anesthesia. The third phase of AIH is termed the plateau phase and typically occurs after three hours of anesthesia. The plateau occurs due to two mechanisms: first, although reduced from normal, the animal's heat production begins to exceed heat losses; and second, the lower end of the inter-threshold range is reached, triggering autonomic responses to preserve heat such as vasoconstriction.

Which Patients Are at Risk?

Every patient undergoing general anesthesia is at risk for developing hypothermia. In the CEPSAF study, overall mortality rates in dogs and cats were 0.17 and 0.24%, respectively, but cats weighing less than 2 kg, dogs under 5 kg, and older animals were at increased risk (Brodbelt et al. 2008b). Duration of anesthesia increases the risk of mortality; Brodbelt and colleagues (Brodbelt et al. 2008b) showed an increased risk when duration of anesthesia exceeded 1.5 hours and this may be related to hypothermia. In a review of 275 feline anesthesia cases, Redondo and colleagues (Redondo et al. 2012a) reported that at the end of the procedure mild hypothermia was present in 26.5% of cats, moderate hypothermia in 60.4%, and severe hypothermia in 10.5%. No mortalities occurred in normothermic cats (38.5–39.5 °C), whereas the mortality index (%) was 6.89 in severely hypothermic cats (<34.0 °C). In this study the greatest drops in temperature were associated with longer anesthesia, major versus minor procedures, and increasing ASA status (Redondo et al. 2012a). Other studies in cats showed a correlation between duration of anesthesia and severity of heat loss (Kelly et al. 2012). In a review of 1525 canine anesthesia records, the prevalence of hypothermia at the end of the procedure was mild 51.5%, moderate 29.3%, and severe 2.8% (Redondo et al. 2012b). Factors that were related to a greater drop in temperature included the time from pre-medication to induction of anesthesia, duration of anesthesia, physical status, type of procedure, and body surface area.

Physiologic Effects of Hypothermia

Hypothermia causes changes in metabolism, coagulation, and cardiovascular function (heart rate and rhythm), increases the likelihood of wound infection, and contributes to patient discomfort during recovery. Recovery is delayed in hypothermic patients due to decreased metabolism and elimination of injectable anesthetic agents (Pottie et al. 2007). Inhalant agents are more soluble in blood at lower than normal temperature, and this, combined with a decrease in anesthetic requirements in these patients, can lead to a relative anesthetic overdose and prolonged recovery times. Return of spontaneous respiration is delayed by hypothermia. In dogs anesthetized for neutering, the esophageal temperature at the end of the procedure had a significant impact on recovery times (Pottie et al. 2007). Normothermic dogs (>38.0 °C) assumed sternal recumbency in a mean of 7.7 ± 3.8 minutes (time from turning off the vaporizer to extubation), whereas those that were between 35.0 and 35.4 °C took 23.4 ± 22.1 minutes (Pottie et al. 2007).

Blood loss increases in hypothermic patients, and this effect is well documented in humans. Blood viscosity is increased and coagulopathies occur due to inhibition of platelet function, platelet sequestration, and diminished enzymatic activity in the clotting cascade. In dogs, clot formation takes longer in hypothermic blood, but the clots formed are equivalent in strength to clots formed in normothermic blood (Taggart et al. 2012).

The correlation between wound infection and hypothermia is well documented in humans. Several factors contribute to this, including impairment of the immune response, cutaneous vasoconstriction, and local tissue hypoxia. Leukocyte phagocytosis, antibody production, and cytokine production also decrease as body temperature drops. In dogs and cats, wound infection has been linked to the duration of anesthesia, and again hypothermia may play a contributing role (Beal et al. 2000; Eugster et al. 2004).

Severe hypothermia causes bradycardia, decreased cardiac output, and hypotension. Catecholamine levels are increased in hypothermia, as is cardiac irritability. Bradyarrhythmias such as atrioventricular block are common and ventricular fibrillation and asystole can occur. The usual intervention to treat bradycardia is to administer atropine or glycopyrrolate, but in hypothermic patients the heart is less responsive to these drugs (Cookson and DiPalma 1955).

During recovery, shivering increases metabolic oxygen consumption and can lead to hypoxemia and metabolic acidosis. Intraocular and intracranial pressures are increased and discomfort results from muscle rigidity and movement around surgical incisions. Humans describe feeling cold and shivering as extremely unpleasant in the immediate recovery period. In newborn babies, warmth is an effective non-pharmacologic analgesic technique during painful procedures such as vaccination (Gray et al. 2012).

Temperature Monitoring

Body temperature is not always closely monitored or recorded in anesthetized patients; therefore, hypothermia often goes undetected. In one study, temperature was recorded in only 1–2% of cats during surgery and in 11–15% of cats post-operatively (Brodbelt et al. 2007). Sites for temperature monitoring include the rectum, ear, and esophagus. Rectal or auricular readings are affected by perfusion at the site of monitoring, local inflammation, and fecal material. Although auricular readings are quick to obtain, one study in cats reported poor correlation between auricular and rectal temperature when readings were taken with a veterinary-specific infrared thermometer (Kunkle et al. 2004). Another investigator observed good agreement when an auricular thermometer designed for humans was used in cats (Sousa et al. 2013); however, in an earlier paper, the authors reported discordance between the two sites when similar equipment was used in dogs (Sousa et al. 2011). Esophageal temperature probes can be used in anesthetized patients to provide an estimate of core temperature and should be placed in the distal third of the esophagus. In order to track trends, it is best to choose one site and one device and use these consistently.

Because rectal and auricular measurements are invasive, time consuming, and stressful to many animals and may result in cross-contamination, non-contact infrared thermometry is attractive in a shelter setting. However, in cats, different devices and recording sites failed to provide reliable results (Nutt et al. 2016).

Prevention and Treatment

Because of the many negative effects of hypothermia, steps should be taken to recognize, prevent, and treat it. In humans, pre-warming with forced air warming of skin for 10–20 minutes before general anesthesia is documented to significantly reduce the incidence of hypothermia and post-operative shivering (Horn et al. 2012). The goal of this technique is to increase the peripheral temperature, thereby minimizing redistribution hypothermia (phase 1), which occurs after pre-medication and induction of anesthesia. Although a similar study has not been published in small dogs or cats, placing dogs weighing ≤10 kg in an incubator before induction of anesthesia had no positive effect on peri-operative hypothermia or post-operative shivering (Rigotti et al. 2015; Aarnes et al. 2017).

Warming techniques can be divided into two types: passive and active. Passive warming methods include the use of blankets, bubble wrap, reflective blankets, and placing socks over limbs to minimize heat loss to the environment. Warmer ambient temperatures in the patient preparation areas, operating rooms, and recovery areas also decrease patient–environment temperature gradients. Active warming methods include circulating warm water blankets, forced air warmers, or heating mats made from conductive fabric. Circulating warm water blankets are often placed under animals during surgery. These blankets have been employed in various ways: in one study warm water blankets were placed over, under, or around the feet of dogs, and the latter position was most effective at reducing heat loss (Cabell et al. 1997). These blankets are less popular in the recovery areas as they are often punctured by claws and nails. Forced warm air devices (e.g. 3M™ Bair Hugger™ Therapy, 3M, St Paul, MN; WarmTouch™, Covidien, Boulder, CO; Thermacare® Warming System, Stryker, Portage, MI) can minimize heat loss in anesthetized cats (Machon et al. 1999) and are widely used in veterinary medicine. These work best if they are used continuously from the time of pre-medication until animals are returned to their cages or kennels. However, when resources are limited, a single unit can be used to rewarm multiple animals at once during recovery (Figure 7.1). In dogs, a forced warm air device was superior to a circulating warm water blanket in minimizing AIH (Clark-Price et al. 2013).

Heating blankets made from semi-conductive polymeric fabric are available (HotDog®, Augustine Temperature Management, Eden Prairie, MN). These blankets come in different sizes, are flexible, reusable, and durable. In dogs, this device was compared to a forced warm air system in dogs of similar weight and undergoing similar procedures and duration of anesthesia. The dogs placed on the heated mat had a higher nadir and end-of-procedure temperature (Kibanda and Gurney 2012). A patient simulation study using the HotDog system showed that heating is not uniform across the entire blanket: 95% of the time test sites did not reach the set temperature on the control unit, and in 2.3% of readings exceeded it (McCarthy et al. 2018). These authors warn that hyperthermic injury may be possible with this technology along with inefficient and uneven warming. It is common for fluid (e.g. lavage solutions, urine) to accumulate between the patient and blanket in clinical scenarios; when saline was used in the simulator model to mimic this, blanket temperatures became significantly lower, therefore the anesthetist should ensure good patient–blanket contact and remove accumulated fluid.

Warmed rice bags, heated fluid-filled bags, and hot water bottles are popular, but must be used with caution as they can cause thermal burns. In addition, these devices cool quickly to room temperature and will then draw heat from the patient, defeating their purpose. Thermal burns can also occur with the use of electric blankets, infrared lamps, and a forced warm air device hose without attaching it to a diffusion blankets.

Additional areas where small changes in protocol can help mitigate heat losses include the use of warm preparation solutions for cleansing the surgical site, and removing any excess solution from the animal.

The use of warm IV fluids has been advocated, but at the administration rates used and the duration of most elective procedures, this intervention will not have a significant influence on body temperature. There was no difference in body temperatures in cats undergoing ovariohysterectomy when a non-rebreathing circuit and a pediatric circle system were compared (Kelly et al. 2012). Proprietary data shows that a heated breathing circuit specially designed to attach to all standard anesthesia machines reduces heat loss from the respiratory tract (DarvallVet, Gladesville, NSW, Australia). These two pieces of equipment are unlikely to be a good investment for a shelter or HVHQSN clinic.

Peri-operative hypothermia is a common complication of general anesthesia in small animal patients. By keeping procedure times to a minimum and using simple measures to prevent and treat hypothermia, patient comfort will be improved and morbidity and mortality decreased.

Monitoring

A monitor can be described as an instrument or device used for observing, checking, or keeping a continuous record. The verb "to monitor" means to observe and check the progress or quality of something over a period of time. Monitors extend the human senses, but do not replace them. As such, a monitor can only warn the user of an adverse event; it cannot intervene. Initiating a response remains a vital function of the person in charge of a patient's anesthetic event. It is imperative that practitioners understand the data the monitors display and what to do when an abnormality arises. Much of the reduction in anesthetic patient mortality in humans is a result of better anesthetic drugs, equipment, and monitoring devices, yet an intraoperative incident still occurs in 1 out of 10 of patients (Haller et al. 2011) and these events are primarily due to human error, underscoring the importance of the anesthesia team members in delivery of safe anesthesia to patients.

The American College of Veterinary Anesthesia and Analgesia has developed small animal monitoring guidelines (http://www.acvaa.org/docs/Small_Animal_Monitoring_2009.doc). The ASV also includes suggestions for monitoring anesthetized patients in its guidelines for spay and neuter programs (Griffin et al. 2016). Monitoring of the depth of anesthesia (by assessing jaw tone, eye position, and reflexes), adequacy of

circulatory function (by palpating and assessing pulse rate, rhythm, and quality, or using a blood pressure monitor), oxygenation (by assessing mucus membrane color or using a pulse oximeter), ventilation (by observation of the patient's respiratory rate and pattern or use of a capnograph), and body temperature is vital to patient safety.

Dyson and colleagues showed the value of trained personnel in veterinary medicine: the presence of a technician whose primary focus was anesthetic management of the patient significantly reduced the odds of a complication occurring (Dyson et al. 1998); the value of trained personnel is also emphasized in the ASV 2016 Veterinary Medical Care Guidelines for Spay–Neuter Programs (Griffin et al. 2016). The Academy of Veterinary Technicians in Anesthesia and Analgesia is the organization that oversees specialization in this discipline, with a rigorous application and examination process (www.avtaa-vts.org). Many veterinary conferences have lectures and laboratory sessions dedicated to improving the skills of veterinary technicians that are charged with overseeing a patients' anesthesia care. The AAHA anesthesia guidelines for dogs and cats toolkit is an excellent resource and includes anesthesia staff training questionnaires (http://www.aaha.org/professional/resources/anesthesia.aspx).

The study spearheaded by Brodbelt (Brodbelt et al. 2007) is the first time that the value of monitoring has been shown to save lives in veterinary medicine: monitoring the pulse and using a pulse oximeter significantly reduced mortality in cats, although the same advantages could not be statistically demonstrated in dogs. It is well worth investing time in learning how best to utilize a pulse oximeter; one study indicated that the best site for probe placement in cats is the rear paw (Matthews et al. 2003). This is an ideal site when performing oral procedures or if a cat is not intubated but receiving oxygen via face mask. Fluorescent and operating room lights can interfere with the light-emitting diode of the probe and sensor; therefore, it is recommended to place a barrier (e.g. a gauze sponge) over the probe after it is placed on the patient to prevent this.

When selecting a monitor, it is important to choose one which has a good audible signal, for example a pulse oximeter or Doppler ultrasonic flow detector, because personnel respond more rapidly to a change in sound than to a visual display. In addition, in a busy setting where multitasking is common, it is not possible to observe a visual display at all times. Another inexpensive monitoring device is an esophageal stethoscope, which allows heart rate and respiratory rate to be auscultated; this can be checked frequently by personnel or attached to an audible amplification and visual (flashing red light) output device for continuous assessment (APM Audible Patient Monitor, A.M. Bickford, Inc., New York, www.ambickford.com).

Record Keeping

Anesthesia records must be kept for legal purposes and to help advance our understanding of risks associated with anesthesia, as was done with the valuable CEPSAF study. The legal requirements vary between countries and within the United States from state to state. Veterinarians are responsible for knowing what the requirements for record keeping in their locale are and adhering to or ideally exceeding these. The AAHA has a comprehensive yet user-friendly sedation and anesthesia form for purchase. The Association of Veterinary Anaesthetists (AVA) based in Europe has various anesthesia and monitoring forms and checklists available for download at no cost (https://ava.eu.com).

Use of Standard Operating Procedures and Checklists

Standard operating procedures (SOPs) should be embraced in clinical practice: they improve safety, compliance, and accountability and ensure things are done in a consistent manner despite turnover of staff. For example, anesthesia machines should be checked prior to each use; excellent downloadable check lists are available (http://www.abbottanimalhealth.com/veterinary-professionals/education/anesthesia/tools.html) and these can be laminated and attached to the machine.

Perhaps one of the biggest mistakes we can make in clinical medicine is not to learn from our previous mistakes. Based on how the aviation industry has dealt with "critical incidents," the medical profession is also seeing the benefits of SOPs, checklists, clinical guidelines, improved specialty training, teamwork, and communication (Haller et al. 2011; Arriaga et al. 2013). When surgical-crisis checklists were available, only 6% of life-saving steps were missed during a crisis such as a cardiac arrest, compared to 23% when checklists were unavailable (Arriaga et al. 2013). Each clinic should develop specific SOPs and checklists that are relevant to its practice. Ready-to-use checklists that span the time from pre-induction to recovery are available from the AVA (https://ava.eu.com).

Incident reporting is also important for improving patient safety (Mahajan 2010). When an adverse event occurs in a clinic there are lessons to be learned; the incident should be documented in detail and carefully analyzed during a debrief so that protocols can be adjusted to prevent the same incident in the future.

Conclusions

Anesthesia and analgesia are key components to the success of a shelter's spay and neuter program. Anesthesia must be time and cost efficient and associated with a low morbidity and mortality rate. When appropriate anesthetic protocols are used that include multimodal analgesia, along with close monitoring by trained personnel and attention to detail, these goals can be achieved.

References

Aarnes, T.K., Bednarski, R.M., Lerche, P., and Hubbell, J.A. (2017). Effect of pre-warming on perioperative hypothermia and anesthetic recovery in small breed dogs undergoing ovariohysterectomy. *Can. Vet. J.* 58: 175–179.

Alef, M., von Praun, F., and Oechtering, G. (2008). Is routine pre-anaesthetic haematological and biochemical screening justified in dogs? *Vet. Anaesth. Analg.* 35: 132–140.

Arriaga, A.F., Bader, A.M., Wong, J.M. et al. (2013). Simulation-based trial of surgical-crisis checklists. *N. Engl. J. Med.* 368: 246–253.

Barletta, M., Kleine, S.A., and Quandt, J.E. (2015). Assessment of v-gel supraglottic airway device placement in cats performed by inexperienced veterinary students. *Vet. Rec.* 177: 523.

Barrand, K. (2011). Oxygen supply – a possible alternative. *In Pract.* 33: 42–45.

Bauer, M.D., Clark-Price, S.C., and McFadden, M.S. (2009). Anesthesia case of the month. *JAVMA* 234: 1539–1541.

Beal, M.W., Brown, D.C., and Shofer, F.S. (2000). The effects of perioperative hypothermia and the duration of anesthesia on postoperative wound infection rate in clean wounds: a retrospective study. *Vet. Surg.* 29: 123–127.

Benarroch-Gampel, J., Sheffield, K.M., Duncan, C.B. et al. (2012). Preoperative laboratory testing in patients undergoing elective, low-risk ambulatory surgery. *Ann. Surg.* 256: 518–528.

Bhandal, J. and Kuzma, A. (2008). Tracheal rupture in a cat: diagnosis by computed tomography. *Can. Vet. J.* 49: 595–597.

Blunt, M.C., Young, P.J., Patil, A., and Haddock, A. (2001). Gel lubrication of the tracheal tube cuff reduces pulmonary aspiration. *Anesthesiology* 95: 377–381.

Brodbelt, D.C. (2006). The confidential enquiry into perioperative small animal fatalities. PhD thesis. London University.

Brodbelt, D. (2009). Perioperative mortality in small animal anaesthesia. *Vet. J.* 182: 152–161.

Brodbelt, D.C., Pfeiffer, D.U., Young, L.E., and Wood, J.L. (2007). Risk factors for anaesthetic-related death in cats: results from the confidential enquiry into perioperative small animal fatalities (CEPSAF). *Br. J. Anaesth.* 99: 617–623.

Brodbelt, D.C., Blissitt, K.J., Hammond, R.A. et al. (2008a). The risk of death: the confidential enquiry into perioperative small animal fatalities. *Vet. Anaesth. Analg.* 35: 365–373.

Brodbelt, D.C., Pfeiffer, D.U., Young, L.E., and Wood, J.L. (2008b). Results of the confidential enquiry into perioperative small animal fatalities regarding risk factors for anesthetic-related death in dogs. *JAVMA* 233: 1096–1104.

Brondani, J.T., Luna, S.P., and Padovani, C.R. (2011). Refinement and initial validation of a multidimensional composite scale for use in assessing acute postoperative pain in cats. *Am. J. Vet. Res.* 72: 174–183.

Brondani, J.T., Mama, K.R., Luna, S.P. et al. (2013). Validation of the English version of the UNESP-Botucatu multidimensional composite pain scale for assessing postoperative pain in cats. *BMC Vet. Res.* 9: 143.

Cabell, L.W., Perkowski, S.Z., Gregor, T., and Smith, G.K. (1997). The effects of active peripheral skin warming on perioperative hypothermia in dogs. *Vet. Surg.* 26: 79–85.

Calvo, G., Holden, E., Reid, J. et al. (2014). Development of a behaviour-based measurement tool with defined intervention level for assessing acute pain in cats. *J. Small Anim. Pract.* 55: 622–629.

Cambridge, A.J., Tobias, K.M., Newberry, R.C., and Sarkar, D.K. (2000). Subjective and objective measurements of postoperative pain in cats. *JAVMA* 217: 685–690.

Chung, F., Yuan, H., Yin, L. et al. (2009). Elimination of preoperative testing in

when it was used as a tranquilizer during their hospital stay. In the same report, 10 dogs that were actively seizing were given acepromazine; in 6 seizures ceased for between 1.5 and 8 hours and in 2 dogs seizures did not recur (Tobias et al. 2006).

Alpha₂-Adrenergic Agonists

The three most commonly used alpha$_2$-adrenergic agonist drugs in small animal anesthesia are xylazine, medetomidine, and dexmedetomidine. All three drugs provide sedation, analgesia, and muscle relaxation, but they differ in their selectivity for the alpha$_2$-receptor compared to the alpha$_1$-receptor; selectivity for alpha$_2$-receptors is greatest for dexmedetomidine, followed by medetomidine, then xylazine (Murrell and Hellebrekers 2005).

In historical mortality studies (Clarke and Hall 1990; Dyson et al. 1998), the alpha$_2$-adrenergic agonist xylazine was associated with an increased risk of death in dogs; however, in the Confidential Enquiry into Perioperative Small Animal Fatality (CEPSAF) study, medetomidine was not associated with an increased risk (Brodbelt et al. 2008) and it is assumed that this would hold true for dexmedetomidine. One explanation for the risk associated with xylazine is that it can sensitize the heart to ventricular arrhythmias (Tranquilli et al. 1986), whereas the more specific alpha$_2$-adrenergic agonist drug dexmedetomidine does not (Hayashi et al. 1991). The contribution of xylazine to perianesthetic mortality in cats is less clear. One study showed an increased risk when xylazine was used with ketamine (Clarke and Hall 1990); in contrast, a different study found that xylazine combined with ketamine did not increase the risk of cardiac arrest in cats (Dyson et al. 1998). It is difficult to say what the risks of xylazine use are in cats because of different study designs, drug combinations, and health status of the cats in the reports.

Medetomidine and dexmedetomidine provide reliable dose-related sedation, muscle relaxation, and analgesia (Slingsby and Waterman-Pearson 2000b; Kuusela et al. 2001;

Pypendop and Ilkiw 2014). It may be difficult to differentiate sedation from analgesia after administration of these drugs, but it should be remembered that the dose required for analgesia is much higher than that required for sedation (Slingsby and Taylor 2008).

Although dogs and cats may appear deeply sedated, it is important to be aware that animals are arousable; this can happen if there is a sudden loud noise or a painful procedure is attempted, for example suturing a wound without using additional analgesia such as a local anesthetic. Arousal can be extremely sudden, and animals may bite or scratch clinic personnel; such unexpected arousal is anecdotally reported most frequently when alpha$_2$-adrenergic agents have been given. To avoid injury, never let your guard down around a dog or cat that is sedated.

Medetomidine is a racemic mixture of two optical stereoisomers: dexmedetomidine (the active enantiomer) and levomedetomidine, with the latter thought to be pharmacologically inactive (Murrell and Hellebrekers 2005). In some countries both are available, but in the United States dexmedetomidine has replaced medetomidine and is labeled for use in dogs and cats. Medetomidine can be compounded to reduce drug costs. Dexmedetomidine is available in two concentrations: 500 µg (0.5 mg)/ml and 100 µg (0.1 mg)/ml; the latter is appropriate for accurate administration in dogs under 10 kg and in cats. It can be given IV or IM in dogs, but only the IM route is recommended in cats. The recommended doses, based on body surface area (BSA), route of administration, and purpose (pre-anesthetic medication or sedation and analgesia) are available in an easy-to-read chart format which is available for download at the manufacturer's website (http://www.zoetisus.com/products/cats/dexdomitor/index.aspx). It may be especially important to dose based on BSA to account for metabolic scaling in very small puppies and kittens. Inadequate depth of anesthesia in kittens under 1.5 kg given injectable combinations was thought to be a result of them having a higher BSA to body mass ratio; therefore some clinicians have created protocols that take this into account, so smaller patients receive a larger dose on a mg/kg basis (Joyce and Yates 2011).

Dexmedetomidine and medetomidine are extremely reliable, useful, and effective agents in a wide variety of settings and are especially useful in patients that are not well socialized or difficult to handle due to fear, stress, or behavioral issues. The differences between the two drugs are difficult to summarize despite multiple studies, because of the range of doses used and physiologic and clinical effects that are dose dependent (Murrell and Hellebrekers 2005). An injectable anesthetic protocol using a combination of ketamine, buprenorphine, midazolam, and either dexmedetomidine or medetomidine was evaluated in kittens and adult cats undergoing castration (Bruniges et al. 2016). All cats were given atipamezole at the same dose 40 minutes after induction and the investigators stated that the choice of alpha$_2$-adrenergic drug had little effect.

The alpha$_2$-adrenergic drugs may be used alone for sedation or combined with an opioid to provide additional analgesia and sedation. They are common components of a total injectable induction protocol, for example when combined with ketamine or tiletamine/zolazepam and an opioid.

In fractious, aggressive, or extremely fearful animals, oral transmucosal (OTM) administration can be extremely effective and is a safe technique for veterinary staff. In cats, buccal or OTM administration of dexmedetomidine at 40 μg/kg provided similar sedation to the same dose given IM (Slingsby et al. 2009). A case series in dogs (n = 4) using a mean dose of 32.6 μg/kg provided satisfactory sedation and safe handling of the dogs. It was possible to deliver the drug by spraying into a dog's mouth from a distance of 0.6 m, using a 3 ml syringe and 22-gauge needle; onset time to suitable sedation was approximately 20 minutes (Cohen and Bennett 2015). Note that these studies use the injectable formulation of dexmedetomidine

and not the OTM gel marketed for canine noise aversion (Sileo® Orion Pharma Animal Health, Zoetis, Parsippany, NJ).

All alpha$_2$-adrenergic agonist drugs have profound effects on the cardiovascular system. These include bradycardia, bradyarrhythmias, decreased cardiac output, increased systemic vascular resistance, and increased blood pressure (Murrell and Hellebrekers 2005). Dexmedetomidine and medetomidine significantly reduce the requirements for injectable and inhalant anesthetic drugs, in some cases by up to 80%. The decrease in anesthetic requirements, cardiac output, and bradycardia have clinical significance: when administering IV anesthetic induction drugs, the injection site (e.g. cephalic vein) to brain circulation time is prolonged, therefore injectable anesthetic drugs should be given initially at low doses and time allowed for the drug to have an effect before deciding to give more. If mask inductions are performed, loss of consciousness may occur very rapidly. It is easy to overdose animals with injectable or inhalant agents if the effects of an alpha$_2$-adrenergic agonist are not taken into consideration. Other consequences resulting from the cardiovascular changes include paler mucus membranes, difficulty in obtaining pulse oximeter readings, and finding it more challenging to place an intravenous catheter.

The use of dexmedetomidine and medetomidine in the face of cardiac disease is controversial. In cats with hypertrophic cardiomyopathy, in particular those with left ventricular outflow obstruction, no detrimental effects were seen after administration of medetomidine (20 μg/kg IM). In dogs with poor ventricular function, the increase in afterload caused by alpha$_2$-adrenergic agonist drugs is not well tolerated.

The alpha$_2$-adrenergic agonists are emetogenic; however, specific drug and species differences are reported. Vomiting increases intraocular and intracranial pressure; contraindications would include patients with a penetrating corneal foreign body or deep corneal ulcer, and if there is any suspicion or history of head trauma. Aspiration is a possible sequela because sedation occurs rapidly with this class of drug, therefore all patients should be observed closely following administration.

The alpha$_2$ drugs are used to induce vomiting in cats after toxin ingestion, so this side effect should be expected when they are used as sedatives. When used alone in cats, one study reported vomiting with xylazine and dexmedetomidine in 51.1% and 58% of cats, respectively, which was not statistically different (Willey et al. 2016). After xylazine was given at approximately 0.5 mg/kg IM, 60% of cats vomited (Thies et al. 2017). When dexmedetomidine was used as a pre-medicant prior to general anesthesia in cats (McSweeney et al. 2012), 31% of cats vomited compared to 6% of placebo-treated cats. Administering ondansetron (0.22 mg/kg IM) with dexmedetomidine (40 µg/kg) at the same time (mixed in the same syringe) reduced the incidence of vomiting from 78% (placebo group) to 33%; pre-treatment with ondansetron 30 minutes before dexmedetomidine was not effective, with 67% of cats vomiting (Santos et al. 2011). The alpha$_2$-agonists are frequently used in combination with an opioid and dissociative agent as a total intramuscular anesthetic (TIMA) technique in cats, and when used as such vomiting is less likely but is not eliminated. When medetomidine, buprenorphine, and ketamine were combined and used in community cats undergoing sterilization, 8% vomited (Harrison et al. 2011).

Vomiting is also reported in dogs following administration of alpha$_2$-adrenergic agonists. Review articles state that 20–50% of dogs vomit following xylazine and 8–20% after medetomidine (Sinclair 2003; Lemke 2004).

In the author's experience, all three alpha$_2$-adrenergic agonist drugs are extremely valuable components of shelter medicine anesthesia protocols. The reports of xylazine use and increased mortality in dogs (Clarke and Hall 1990; Dyson et al. 1998) should be carefully critiqued (Sinclair 2003). The safety of sedative and anesthetic drugs depends on how they are used, combined with a robust understanding of their pharmacologic properties. When xylazine was launched in the early 1970s its potency, anesthetic-sparing effects, and side effects were underestimated; it was used in a cavalier manner and in patients we would not use it on today based on our experience and knowledge of drugs in this class (Sinclair 2003). The safety outcomes of these drugs have improved in parallel with our increased knowledge and experience of them.

Alpha$_2$-adrenergic agonist drugs are reversible. Atipamezole (5 mg/ml) is a specific reversal agent for dexmedetomidine and medetomidine. Reversal is not always required, and some anesthetists prefer to allow patients to remain sedated and wake up slowly. Atipamezole is used when a rapid recovery is beneficial; for example, in pediatric patients when it is desirable for them to eat soon after a procedure. Although used widely in both dogs and cats, it is only labeled for IM use in dogs. After administration of atipamezole, it must be remembered that any residual analgesia as well as sedation is reversed, therefore other analgesics should already be on board. In a report of applying "fast-track surgery principles" in a clinical feline neutering setting, pain scores were not different between cats that did or did not receive atipamezole; all cats were anesthetized with a combination of dexmedetomidine, ketamine, and hydromorphone and received meloxicam immediately after surgery (Hasiuk et al. 2015). Atipamezole reliably shortened recovery time in adult cats and kittens given ketamine, buprenorphine, midazolam, and either dexmedetomidine or medetomidine for castration, with kittens recovering faster than adults (Bruniges et al. 2016).

In dogs, the recommended dose of atipamezole is a volume equal to the volume of dexmedetomidine (based on the 500 µg/ml concentration) given. It is not labeled for use in cats but when used, the volume of atipamezole usually given is half (if the 500 µg/ml of dexmedetomidine is used) or one-tenth (if the 100 µg/ml concentration is used) of the initial dexmedetomidine volume. Joyce and

Yates (2011) suggest a dose of atipamezole of between 10 and 50% of the original volume of medetomidine in their "quad" protocol for cats (discussed later in this chapter). Some authors have reported that giving atipamezole subcutaneously (SC) results in calmer albeit slower recoveries in cats compared to IM administration (Harrison et al. 2011). Atipamezole (25–50 µg/kg IM) can be used to reverse xylazine in dogs and cats.

Yohimbine (0.1 mg/kg IM, SC, or slow IV) has historically been used to reverse the effects of xylazine, but is difficult to source commercially and has largely been replaced by atipamezole. Yohimbine can be compounded, but users are reminded that compounded drugs do not undergo efficacy testing.

Reversal of alpha₂-drugs is not recommended until at least 20 minutes after the original injection unless emergency reversal is required (Joyce and Yates 2011).

Benzodiazepines

Benzodiazepines (midazolam and diazepam) are not recommended as pre-medicant agents in healthy dogs and cats because their effects are unpredictable; animals may become disinhibited, resulting in a patient that is agitated, excited, and difficult to restrain. The beneficial effects of benzodiazepines (sedation) are more predictable in senior or debilitated animals; midazolam is more versatile as it can be given IV or IM, whereas diazepam can only be given IV. Benzodiazepines are beneficial as co-induction agents; when given after a small dose of propofol or alfaxalone, the total dose of the latter drugs required to intubate dogs is significantly reduced, quality of induction is improved, and it can be cost saving (Sanchez et al. 2013; Liao et al. 2017). Benzodiazepines should be available in the event a patient has a seizure and should be readily available or given pre-emptively to cases with a known history of seizures. Another advantage of benzodiazepines is the additional muscle relaxation they provide, which is beneficial during abdominal surgery in obese patients.

Induction of Anesthesia

For recommended doses of induction agents, see Table 8.2.

Table 8.2 Drugs and doses for intravenous induction of anesthesia. After pre-medication (Table 8.1) lower doses may be sufficient.

Drug	Dose mg/kg Dogs	Dose mg/kg Cats	Comments
Alfaxalone	2.0–4.0	3.0–5.0	Always give to effect (e.g. to permit intubation). Give initial dose over 60 seconds. Apnea is common after rapid administration. Can be given intramuscularly (IM) in cats (see text for details).
Propofol	2.0–6.0	4.0–8.0	Give initial dose over 60 seconds. Apnea is common after rapid administration.
Ketamine	5.0	5.0	Give after an alpha₂-adrenergic agonist and/or with midazolam or diazepam to decrease muscle rigidity.
Tiletamine/ zolazepam	2.0–4.0	2.0–4.0	Intravenous use is off-label in cats in the United States. May be given intramuscularly at 2–3 times the intravenous dose. Note: IM injection may not induce general anesthesia, but can provide deep sedation. Additional doses or other drugs (e.g. inhalant agent) can be given to produce anesthesia. Local anesthetic techniques can be used for some procedures (e.g. skin laceration repair).

Injectable anesthetic agents are preferred over inhalant agents for the induction of anesthesia. Many factors will influence the choice of agent, including availability, safety, versatility (suitable for dogs and cats; route of administration, i.e. IV only, IV and IM; single injection only, "top-ups," infusions), shelf life, cost, and personal experience and preference. It is advisable to be familiar with more than one protocol due to the increasing occurrence of drug shortages and "back orders" in veterinary medicine. Cost is becoming increasingly difficult to predict because prices change rapidly as a result of drug shortages.

Injectable agents and protocols include propofol, ketamine plus a benzodiazepine (diazepam or midazolam), tiletamine/zolazepam, and alfaxalone.

Propofol

Propofol (2,6 diisopropylphenol) is available as a 1% (10 mg/ml) solution for intravenous induction and short-term maintenance of anesthesia in dogs and cats. In some geographic locations propofol is a controlled substance and scheduling oversight is likely to increase. There are two formulations. The original product is a single-use oil-in-water emulsion containing no preservative which, if not used within six hours after the vial or bottle is breached, must be discarded due to the risk of contamination. The second formulation is similar to the original product but contains the preservative 2% benzyl alcohol, which is effective against Gram-positive bacteria, molds, and fungi. This latter product is only approved for use in dogs. It has a shelf life of 28 days and performs similarly to the original product (Mama et al. 2013). Although not approved for use in cats, preservative-containing propofol has been used in this species and no adverse effects were reported when normal to high clinical doses were used (Taylor et al. 2012). Using the preservative-containing solution may offer some cost benefits due to reduced waste. Neither formulation is irritating to tissues in the event of a peri-vascular injection and, compared to humans, pain on injection appears to be rare in animals.

The major side effects of propofol are related to respiratory and cardiovascular function. Respiratory depression, including apnea, is related to the dose of propofol and the rate of administration. Hypotension, which can be severe in hypovolemic animals, occurs as a result of vasodilation and lack of a reflex increase in heart rate. Induction doses are significantly reduced in pre-medicated dogs and cats, resulting in fewer adverse effects (Glowaski and Wetmore 1999; Shih et al. 2008). The induction dose required to reach a set end point (endotracheal intubation) in dogs is influenced by body condition score. Overweight dogs require less propofol on a mg/kg basis than normal weight dogs (Boveri et al. 2013). To prevent apnea, it is recommended that the induction dose is given over 60–90 seconds or at 1–2 mg/kg/minute. The induction dose should be "given to effect"; the end result the anesthetist is aiming for will be variable, with more drug required to achieve a sufficient depth of anesthesia for intubation than for placing a face mask.

Using a benzodiazepine and propofol for induction can significantly reduce the dose of propofol and decrease the incidence of apnea. In dogs pre-medicated IM with acepromazine (0.02 mg/kg) and morphine (0.4 mg/kg), three IV techniques were compared: (1) midazolam (0.25 mg/kg) then propofol (1 mg/kg); (2) propofol then midazolam; and (3) saline then propofol; additional boluses of propofol (0.5 mg/kg) were given until conditions were suitable for orotracheal intubation (Sanchez et al. 2013). The dose of propofol (mg/kg) used in group 1, 2, and 3 were 1.7 ± 0.6, 1.1 ± 0.2, and 3.2 ± 0.6, respectively; the propofol requirements in group 2 were significantly lower than with the other two protocols, and this protocol was associated with less apnea (Sanchez et al. 2013).

Onset of action will take longer in animals that have received an alpha$_2$-adrenergic agonist due to an increase in the injection site to brain circulation time. A single dose of propofol is expected to last 5–10 minutes and anesthesia can be continued with additional "top-ups" (1–2 mg/kg when needed) or a continuous-rate infusion (3–4 μg/kg/minute), or by an inhalant agent. Recoveries are usually smooth, rapid, and complete following propofol.

Ketamine plus Benzodiazepines

Ketamine is a dissociative agent that is widely used in multiple species. Due to its abuse potential it is a scheduled drug. When used as an anesthetic it has a high therapeutic index (wide margin of safety). It is a sympathetic nervous system stimulant and supports cardiovascular function even in hypovolemic animals (Haskins and Patz 1990). The cardiovascular effects are well tolerated in most animals, but in those with cardiac disease the tachycardia and decreased systolic filling time, which may result in decreased stroke volume and cardiac output combined with increased oxygen demands, can be detrimental.

Ketamine causes minimal respiratory depression (Haskins and Patz 1990), but may produce a change in respiratory pattern; apneustic breathing (the animal holds its breath at the end of inspiration before exhaling) is commonly observed.

One unique feature of ketamine that makes it stand out from other injectable anesthetic agents is its action at the N-methyl-D-aspartate (NMDA) receptors in the dorsal horn of the spinal cord, which are involved in central sensitization and plasticity (Pozzi et al. 2006). Its role in pain management is discussed later in this chapter.

Ketamine used alone causes rigidity, so it must be used in combination with drugs that produce muscle relaxation, such as the $alpha_2$-adrenergic agonists or benzodiazepines. A very popular technique is to combine ketamine with either diazepam or midazolam in the same syringe and administer IV "to effect." If 5 mg/kg of ketamine (100 mg/ml) and 0.25 mg/kg of diazepam or midazolam (5 mg/ml) are used, this results in equal volumes of each drug. Ketamine at anesthetic doses should be used with caution in animals with head trauma and eye injuries or glaucoma, as ketamine can increase intracranial and intraocular pressure. Sub-anesthetic doses used to supplement anesthesia or analgesia (see later) are unlikely to cause problems.

Tiletamine and Zolazepam

A tiletamine (a dissociative agent) and zolazepam (a benzodiazepine) mixture is available as a sterile powder which is reconstituted with sterile water before use, resulting in 50 mg tiletamine base and 50 mg zolazepam base per milliliter (100 mg/ml combined). It is labeled for IV and IM use in dogs and IM use only in cats. Very little specific information is known about each drug, as they are only available in this combination. Recovery is significantly faster after IV administration compared to IM administration. In cats the half-life of zolazepam is longer than that of tiletamine and recoveries are usually smooth, but sometimes prolonged after IM use. In dogs, tiletamine outlasts zolazepam and dogs may be agitated during recovery.

Tiletamine/zolazepam can be recommended for induction of anesthesia in healthy dogs and cats, but additional analgesics – opioids, nonsteroidal anti-inflammatory drugs (NSAIDs)± local anesthetic agents – must be administered in patients undergoing surgery. IM administration (5 mg/kg) is a useful technique in aggressive dogs and usually results in lateral recumbency within 5–10 minutes. Tiletamine/zolazepam can also be incorporated into total injectable protocols for feline anesthesia (see later in this chapter).

In cats, tiletamine–zolazepam is absorbed through the oral mucus membranes, which offers an alternative route of administration in cats that are difficult to inject. When 10 mg/kg and 15 mg/kg of the reconstituted solution (100 mg/ml) were evaluated in a cross-over study, both doses produced lateral recumbency within 15 minutes, with no response to clippers or physical restraint (Nejamkin et al. 2019).

Sedation lasted for approximately 120 minutes. Neither dose resulted in pulse oximeter readings (SpO$_2$) falling below 95% when cats breathed room air, there was no dose-related effect on heart rate, and although systolic arterial pressure (SAP) and respiratory rate were higher in the low-dose group, values were within clinically acceptable ranges (SAP ≥100 mmHg). Retching and vomiting did not occur at either dose, but hypersalivation was seen in cats given the higher dose; based on these results, 5 mg of tiletamine and 5 mg of zolazepam per kg administered onto the mucosal surface is recommended (Nejamkin et al. 2019). In the study described here, the drug was placed in the buccal pouch with a syringe; this author has had success when tiletamine and zolazepam have been sprayed into the mouths of cats, which was achieved using a Luer Lock syringe and needle or IV catheter with the stylet removed.

Alfaxalone

Alfaxalone (Alfaxan®, Jurox, Rutherford, NSW, Australia; Alfaxan multidose, 10 mg/ml) is a synthetic neurosteroid that is solubilized in 2-hydroxypropyl-beta-cyclodextrin and used in a wide range of species, but labeled for use in dogs and cats, to produce general anesthesia and muscle relaxation. In the United States alfaxalone is a Schedule IV drug and appropriate records must be kept. When it was first launched, a big disadvantage was the lack of preservative, which dictated discard of unused drug six hours after the bottle was broached. The newer formulation (Alfaxan multidose) contains a mixture of preservatives and has a 28-day shelf life after the first dose is withdrawn. Alfaxalone has a high therapeutic index (significantly greater than propofol), but should be given slowly and "to effect" for induction of anesthesia; the manufacturer recommends that the induction dose is given over 60 seconds. Cats require a higher induction dose than dogs (see Table 8.2). Duration of anesthesia can be extended by giving additional "top-up" doses and constant-rate infusions can also be used – these methods are approved and "on label."

Adequate pre-medication is recommended in dogs and cats to ensure a smooth recovery (Jimenez et al. 2012). Alfaxalone has been evaluated for induction of anesthesia in puppies and kittens under 12 weeks of age after pre-medication with acepromazine (0.03 mg/kg), morphine (0.3 mg/kg), and atropine (0.04 mg/kg; O'Hagan et al. 2012a, b). The mean induction dose in kittens was 4.7 ± 0.5 mg/kg and 1.7 ± 0.3 mg/kg in puppies. In kittens, anesthesia was maintained with isoflurane or supplemental doses of alfaxalone, and puppies were maintained on isoflurane. In both studies the quality of induction and recovery was acceptable and cardiovascular and respiratory parameters were well maintained.

Alfaxalone is an appropriate induction agent for healthy or compromised patients and, based on the vitality scores of newborn puppies, is a good choice for cesarean section (Doebeli et al. 2013; Metcalfe et al. 2014).

In some countries, but not the United States, IM administration of alfaxalone is approved in cats. Recent data suggests a dose of 5 mg/kg (0.5 ml/kg) to produce deep sedation but not general anesthesia (Deutsch et al. 2017; Rodrigo-Mocholi et al. 2018). Butorphanol is often combined with alfaxalone to provide analgesia and additional sedation (Ribas et al. 2015; Deutsch et al. 2017). A combination of alfaxalone (3 mg/kg), butorphanol (0.2 mg/kg), and dexmedetomidine (10 µg/kg) was sufficient to perform castration, and produced a better-quality albeit longer recovery compared to cats that were given ketamine (5 mg/kg) as a substitute for alfaxalone (Khenissi et al. 2017). Reports on the quality of recovery after IM alfaxalone range from good to poor, with the most commonly reported side effects being opisthotonos, exaggerated responses to touch and noise, and twitching (Deutsch et al. 2017; Rodrigo-Mocholi et al. 2018). To decrease these side effects cats should be recovered in a quiet area with subdued lighting. Partial pressure of oxygen (PaO$_2$) values should be monitored and supplemental oxygen is often required (Deutsch et al. 2017).

Inhalant Anesthetic Agents

Mask inductions are discouraged as they are stressful for patients, expose personnel to waste anesthetic gas, and in dogs increase the risk of anesthetic death (Brodbelt et al. 2008). If they are performed, this should be an exception, not the rule, and prior sedation is preferable. Face masks made of clear plastic and fitted with a rubber gasket should be used so that the color of the tongue or lips can be observed, and a seal achieved. To prevent breath holding and struggling, a "stepwise" induction technique is advised. The circuit should be filled with oxygen and the face mask placed over the animal's muzzle for 30–60 seconds, then the vaporizer turned on and the setting on the dial increased every 30 seconds. There may be a short-lived excitement phase and if this happens increasing the vaporizer setting more rapidly helps overcome this. For mask inductions sevoflurane may offer some advantages. When induction of anesthesia in a stepwise fashion was compared using isoflurane or sevoflurane in non-pre-medicated dogs, the latter was smoother and faster (Johnson et al. 1998); in this study both agents resulted in a rapid and smooth recovery. In another study there was no difference in induction time between sevoflurane and isoflurane, nor in pre-medicated versus non-pre-medicated dogs, although sedation did result in a better quality of induction (Pottie et al. 2008). Regardless of the inhalant agent used or if dogs are sedated or not, induction time (defined as the time to reach a plane of anesthesia sufficient for endotracheal intubation) can be over three minutes (Pottie et al. 2008); in a high-volume spay–neuter setting routine mask inductions are unacceptable (Association of Shelter Veterinarians' Veterinary Task Force to Advance et al. 2016).

In cats pre-medicated with acepromazine (0.05 mg/kg IM), sevoflurane and isoflurane had similar induction qualities, but time to intubation was faster with sevoflurane (210 ± 57 seconds versus 236 ± 60 seconds respectively; Lerche et al. 2002). Chamber or "tank" inductions may be necessary in some cats, but IM injection of drug combinations (see later in this chapter) is recommended. Use of feline facial pheromones sprayed on the inside of the chamber or on a towel which is then placed in the chamber is recommended. A similar stepwise process as described for mask inductions should be followed: after the cat is placed in the chamber and the lid secured, oxygen should be given first, then the vaporizer turned on and turned up every 30 seconds. Before removing the lid, the cat's righting reflex should be checked by turning the box from side to side.

Maintenance of Anesthesia

Following induction of anesthesia with an injectable agent, anesthesia may be continued, if needed, with repeated boluses of some induction agents (propofol or alfaxalone) or with an inhalant anesthetic agent delivered via endotracheal tube, supraglottic airway device (cats), or face mask. Even if inhalant agents are not used, SpO$_2$ should be monitored and equipment for oxygen supplementation be readily available.

Isoflurane and sevoflurane are the most commonly available agents and there is no data to support that one is "safer" than the other; therefore, choice of agent may be based on cost, with isoflurane being considerably less expensive when compared in an equipotent manner. Both agents produce significant dose-related cardiovascular and respiratory depression. Vasodilation causes hypotension and also enhances heat loss from the periphery. Although sevoflurane is less soluble and should result in more rapid changes of anesthetic depth and recovery, the clinical differences are minimal. One of the goals of pre-medication and use of injectable induction drugs is to decrease the animal's requirements for these agents; the alpha$_2$-adrenergic agents may reduce inhalant requirements by up to 90% (Reed and Doherty 2018). During the procedure the patient's depth of anesthesia should be checked frequently and the vaporizer setting adjusted accordingly; the vaporizer should never be set on a fixed setting for the entire procedure.

Total Injectable Anesthetic Protocols

Total injectable protocols use a combination of drugs given IM to provide the key components of anesthesia: unconsciousness, analgesia, and muscle relaxation. Although these TIMA techniques were first trialed with feline trap–neuter–return (TNR) programs, they have evolved over the years and are suitable for a wide range of patients because of their simplicity and efficiency.

Tiletamine/Zolazepam/Ketamine/ Xylazine (TKX)

One well documented protocol for use in large community cat programs is commonly referred to as "TKX" and is a mixture of tiletamine and zolazepam, ketamine, and xylazine (Box 8.1) that is given IM. It should be noted that although the individual components of this mixture are approved for use in cats in many countries, the mixture is "off-label" and in some jurisdictions would be considered compounding, therefore all local regulations should be consulted and followed. Tiletamine/ zolazepam and ketamine are scheduled drugs and all regulations related to purchasing, storing, recording, and disposal of these drugs must be strictly adhered to. Williams et al. (2002) reviewed the use of this injectable anesthetic in 5766 cats. A single (0.24 ± 0.04 ml/cat) dose of the mixture was sufficient 79.5% of the time and the total mean dose for all cats was 0.27 ± 0.09 ml. Additional doses required were as follows (number of additional doses followed by percentage of cats): 1 (16.8%),

---

Box 8.1   Instructions for Formulating the Combination of Tiletamine, Zolazepam, Ketamine, and Xylazine (TKX)

Drugs:

1) Tiletamine–zolazepam powder (250 mg tiletamine, 250 mg zolazepam)
2) Ketamine 100 mg/ml
3) Xylazine (10%) 100 mg/ml

Reconstitute the tiletamine–zolazepam with 4 ml of ketamine and 1 ml of xylazine. Each milliliter of the mixture contains:

50 mg of tiletamine
50 mg of zolazepam
80 mg of ketamine
20 mg of xylazine

The recommended dose for an adult cat (6.6 lb, 3.0 kg) is 0.25 ml of the mixture given IM. If required, additional doses of 0.05 ml can be given until sufficient anesthetic depth is reached.

Source: Based on Williams et al. (2002).

---

2 (3.1%), 3 (0.5%), and 4 (0.1%). Onset of effect after IM administration is approximately 4 ± 1 minutes (Cistola et al. 2004). After drug administration cats should be observed but left undisturbed. Approximately 5 minutes after injection the cat should be recumbent, but should not be removed from the trap until its righting reflex and response to a noxious stimulus have been lost. This can be tested by turning the trap 90° left then right: if the cat is unresponsive and does not "right" itself, next a toe should be squeezed from outside the trap; if the cat does not respond, the trap door can be opened and the cat removed. The depth of anesthesia should be monitored frequently as the cat progresses through the different stations in the clinic and caution always exercised when handling or moving the cat. If the cat is still responsive after the first injection, a "top-up" is given based on how reactive it is, but usually additional doses range from 0.1 to

0.2 ml. After a further 5 minutes, repeat these steps before removing the cat from the trap or administering further doses. Follow-up studies with this drug combination recommend a dose of 0.25 ml in most adult cats (Cistola et al. 2004), but slightly larger volumes (0.27–0.30 ml) are often given to large cats and pregnant females. Recorded weights from one study were 1.9–3.9 kg for females and 2.2–4.6 kg for males (Cistola et al. 2004).

Over a four-year period, 7502 cats were sterilized using this protocol with a total of 26 deaths, 17 of which were deemed to be solely attributed to anesthesia (Williams et al. 2002). This anesthesia mortality rate of 0.23% is similar to that reported by Brodbelt et al. (2007) (0.24%) for owned cats undergoing anesthesia at primary care and referral clinics.

The TKX protocol provides sufficient depth and duration of anesthesia to permit ear tipping, pre-operative clipping and preparation, surgery, vaccination, and administration of various other medications (e.g. parasiticides and antibiotics) in most cats. Based on other published studies, the expected duration of action of TKX is approximately 40 minutes (Ko et al. 1993). Cistola et al. (2004) reported that a single dose of TKX was sufficient to complete all procedures in 92% of cats; in the remaining 8% an additional 0.15 ml of TKX was required at the start of surgery.

In the studies reported by Williams et al. (2002) and Cistola et al. (2004), cats were not intubated and breathed room air. Recent studies suggest that not intubating cats for short procedures (<30 minutes) may reduce peri-operative deaths, most of which occur in the first three hours after surgery and are frequently related to airway dysfunction or obstruction that may be a result of trauma and swelling caused by intubation (Brodbelt et al. 2007). However, the equipment required for intubation and ventilation should always be available for use in specific cases and in the event of an emergency. Intubation is advised in pregnant cats due to their increased risk of aspiration and in brachycephalic cats due to their increased risk of airway obstruction. Intubation also allows assisted ventilation, which is more likely in overweight and pregnant animals; anesthesia for pregnant animals is discussed later in this chapter. Based on pulse oximeter readings (recorded from the tongue), oxygen saturation of hemoglobin (SpO_2) was $92 \pm 3\%$ in males and $90 \pm 4\%$ in females during anesthesia, but an SpO_2 of less than 90% was recorded at least once in most cats following administration of TKX (Cistola et al. 2004). The consequences of low SpO_2 readings are unknown in this population of cats. Other physiologic parameters reported by Cistola and colleagues include indirectly measured mean blood pressures (average $\pm$ standard deviation [SD]) of 136 ± 30 mmHg in males and 113 ± 29 mmHg in females, heart rates of 156 ± 19 beats per minute, and respiratory rates of 18 ± 8 breaths per minute.

After all procedures were completed, adult cats and kittens received 0.5 mg or 0.3 mg of the alpha$_2$-adrenergic antagonist yohimbine IV, respectively, and were placed back in their original trap to recover. As discussed earlier, atipamezole (IM or SC) can be used for reversal of xylazine. Recovery from anesthesia following TKX is reported to be smooth but prolonged; the time from administration of yohimbine to the time cats regained sternal recumbency was 72 ± 42 minutes (Cistola et al. 2004). A slow recovery can be problematic, as it delays return to normal function including eating, and community cats should not be released until fully recovered; this requires them to remain in traps, which may be stressful. Reasons for these prolonged recovery times include the fact that yohimbine is a non-selective reversal agent and only serves to reverse or partially reverse the effects of xylazine, and there are no clinically available reversal agents for tiletamine or ketamine.

Hypothermia delays recovery from anesthesia and has negative consequences. Cistola et al. (2004) reported rectal temperatures of $38.0 \pm 0.8\,^\circ C$ (mean of $100.4\,^\circ F$) in male cats and $36.6 \pm 0.8\,^\circ C$ (mean of $97.8\,^\circ F$) in females at the time of reversal. Although TKX meets many of the unique requirements for trap, neuter, vaccinate, and return (TNVR) clinics, there have been concerns about sufficient analgesia and prolonged recovery times. To rectify the analgesia concerns, an opioid, usually buprenorphine, and/or an injectable NSAID (meloxicam or robenacoxib) can be given before returning the cat to the trap for recovery. Based on the limitations of TKX, other protocols have and continue to be developed.

Medetomidine/Ketamine/ Buprenorphine (MKB 1)

Medetomidine is no longer commercially available in the United States, but it is sold in other countries. Medetomidine can be compounded and many clinics do this because of the significant cost savings. A combination of medetomidine, ketamine, and buprenorphine has been evaluated in a TNVR clinic (Harrison et al. 2011). The hypotheses were that this combination would result in shorter recovery times because medetomidine is a more specific alpha$_2$-adrenergic agonist than xylazine and a specific antagonist (atipamezole) is available, and that buprenorphine would provide good peri-operative analgesia. Following preliminary trials, a combination of medetomidine (100 μg/kg), ketamine (10 mg/kg), and buprenorphine (10 μg/kg) was chosen for the study, which included 101 cats (53 males and 48 females), and administered IM; for a 3 kg cat the total volume injected was 0.7 ml. Atipamezole (125 μg/kg) was given SC at the end of surgery. In this study the dose of atipamezole was lower than usually recommended and was given SC rather than IM. These clinicians noted that when the suggested dose (half the volume of medetomidine) and route (IM) were used, a significant number of cats awoke very quickly and became hyperexcitable; the lower dose given SC resulted in a better quality of recovery.

Cats were not intubated and breathed room air. Time to lateral recumbency was similar to that reported for TKX (four to five minutes). Eleven cats required additional doses of medetomidine and/or ketamine before they could be removed from their trap. Eleven cats received supplemental anesthesia with isoflurane administered via a face mask to complete the surgical procedure; in all of these cats the depth of anesthesia did not become inadequate until ≥45 minutes after administration of MKB. Although SpO$_2$ values were higher than those reported for TKX, a value of less than 95% was recorded at least once in all cats. The time from injection of atipamezole to sternal recumbency was 33 ± 31 minutes and was not different between males and females. These recovery times were faster than those reported for TKX, despite rectal temperatures at the time of reversal being similar with both injectable protocols. In some countries medetomidine is no longer available but dexmedetomidine can be used instead, at half of the medetomidine dose based on micrograms per kilogram. MKB can be used in dogs and is especially useful in puppies.

Medetomidine/Ketamine/ Butorphanol (MKB 2)

MKB, with B representing butorphanol, is widely used in both dogs and cats and results in a highly versatile TIMA. Butorphanol provides more sedation than buprenorphine and has a faster onset of action, which has likely led to the popularity and success of this technique. To provide longer analgesia, an NSAID can be given after the procedure; some veterinarians also give buprenorphine at this time. Reversal of medetomidine with atipamezole results in a fast recovery.

Dexmedetomidine/Ketamine/ Butorphanol (DKB)

Clinically there is no obvious difference when medetomidine is substituted with dexmedetomidine. If the concentration of medetomidine used is 1 mg/ml and the dexmedetomidine 0.5 mg/ml, the preparation of the mixture on a volume basis is identical (see Box 8.2). Butorphanol can be replaced with buprenorphine, and again, when

Box 8.2 Instructions for Formulating the Combination of Dexmedetomidine, Ketamine, and Butorphanol (DKB)

Drugs

1) Dexmedetomidine 0.5 mg/ml (500 μg/ml)
2) Ketamine 100 mg/ml
3) Butorphanol 10 mg/ml

Draw up equal volumes (1:1:1) of each drug and add them to a sterile vial using aseptic technique (wipe all rubber stoppers with alcohol and allow it to evaporate before inserting the needle into each vial). Each milliliter of the mixture contains:

0.167 mg (167 μg) of dexmedetomidine
33.3 mg of ketamine
3.3 mg of butorphanol

Source: Based on Bushby and Griffin (2011).

butorphanol is 10 mg/ml and buprenorphine 0.3 mg/ml, a direct substitution by volume can be done.

Dosing charts of the DKB combination for dogs and cats (doses are different) can be downloaded from an open access site (Bushby and Griffin 2011; also see kitten and puppy dosing charts available in Chapter 9). These can be printed off and laminated for easy access in the induction area. In this author's experience DKB alone is sufficient for feline ovariohysterectomies or ovariectomies and castrations and for canine castrations; female dogs may require additional anesthesia, and this can easily be provided with an inhalant agent or incremental doses of propofol to effect. Reversal is at the discretion of the clinician, but should not be performed until 20 minutes after injection. An NSAID is recommended to provide follow-up analgesia.

Tiletamine/Zolazepam/ Butorphanol/Dexmedetomidine

This mixture is widely known as TTD based on the original drug names: T = Telazol (tiletamine/zolazepam), T = Torbugesic (butorphanol), and D = Dexdomitor (dexmedetomidine). All three components are now available as generics, but the name TTD has stuck. To minimize the volume for IM injection, the powdered tiletamine/zolazepam is reconstituted with 2.5 ml of butorphanol (10 mg/ml) and 2.5 ml of dexmedetomidine (0.5 mg/ml; Ko and Berman 2010). This results in a total volume of 0.12 ml for surgical anesthesia in a 3 kg patient. This drug combination is equally useful in dogs and cats, and at the same dose, simplifying clinic flow when dogs and cats are being anesthetized at the same time. Another attractive feature is that by varying the dose, one can achieve mild, moderate, or deep sedation, or surgical anesthesia (Ko and Berman 2010). As with other injectable protocols already described, reversal with atipamezole and additional analgesics can be given as deemed necessary.

Printable dosage charts (dogs and cats) are available (Ko and Berman 2010) and a detailed feline chart giving dosage volumes in small weight increments from 1.0 to 6.4 kg is available for download from the ASPCAPro website (http://www.aspcapro.org/resource/spayneuter-clinic-drug-charts-logs).

The Cat and Kitten "Quad" Protocol

This protocol combines medetomidine, ketamine, midazolam, and buprenorphine and is widely used in the UK (Joyce and Yates 2011). Doses are based on BSA to account for metabolic scaling and differences in BSA to mass ratios between very small kittens and adult cats. The addition of midazolam, which is an excellent muscle relaxant, allows a lower dose of medetomidine to be used, which may decrease cardiovascular side effects and also shortens the duration of action. The authors suggest that midazolam promotes early return to feeding. More details about this protocol including a dosing chart are discussed later in this chapter in the section on anesthesia for the young and old and in Chapter 9.

Perioperative Analgesia

Analgesic agents should always be administered to animals undergoing surgery. The major categories of analgesic agents are:

- Opioids
- NSAIDs
- Local anesthetics
- Ketamine

The World Small Animal Veterinary Association (WSAVA), Global Pain Council Guidelines for the Recognition, Assessment and Treatment of Pain are an excellent resource and available for download at no cost. These guidelines take into account availability of drugs in different parts of the world (Mathews et al. 2014).

Opioids

Since 2017 there has been a tremendous change in the landscape of opioid use in human medicine in the United States which has greatly impacted veterinary medicine. In response to the human opioid abuse and addiction crisis, the US Food and Drug Administration (FDA) decreased the production of opioids and plans to continue on this path, urging physicians to use alternative analgesics. The decreased availability of fentanyl, hydromorphone, and morphine led manufacturers that had provided these drugs to veterinarians to restrict their supplies only for use in humans. Implementation of these changes has led to many opioids being unavailable or in short supply, and unpredictable price swings have negatively impacted their use in veterinary patients. Because of these changes there has been a renewed focus on multimodal analgesia, utilizing more local anesthetics and ketamine, and in some cases using the one available non-scheduled opioid nalbuphine (Kreisler et al. 2019).

The only veterinary-approved opioids in the United States are butorphanol (a Schedule IV drug) and Simbadol™ (Zoetis; injectable buprenorphine for cats, CIII).

Opioids are highly effective analgesic agents in dogs and cats and are the cornerstone of acute pain management protocols. Nearly all opioids are scheduled (controlled) drugs, therefore a license to purchase and prescribe is needed and all state and federal regulations for record keeping and storage must be followed.

Ideally opioids should be given prior to surgery for greatest benefit. Opioids are routinely administered along with a sedative agent as part of a "pre-med" protocol. Opioids rarely cause excitement in cats and euphoria (rubbing, purring, and kneading) is commonly noted after administration. IV administration is ideal but not always possible. IM administration is more effective and associated with fewer side effects than the SC route (Robertson et al. 2009; Steagall et al. 2013, 2014). The buccal or OTM route may be used, especially in cats, for the administration of some opioids. The opioid most commonly administered by this route is buprenorphine and although the effects are reported to be variable (Robertson et al. 2005; Giordano et al. 2010; Hedges et al. 2014; Steagall et al. 2014), it is a viable option for treating cats when physical restraint and IM injections are not easy to perform. Although bioavailability was reduced in cats with gingivostomatitis, 6 out of 6 cats ate 30 minutes after buccal administration of buprenorphine compared to only 2 out of 6 of the same cats when given saline (Stathopoulou et al. 2018). Two formulations of buprenorphine (preservative free and a multidose with preservative) given by the OTM route were compared in a randomized cross-over study using glucose as a control (Bortolami et al. 2012). Adverse events such as salivation or vomiting were not seen after any treatment and cats appeared to prefer the preservative-free formulation, but it was still simple to give.

The bioavailability of mu-opioid agonist opioids including morphine, methadone, hydromorphone, and oxymorphone has been reported in cats, with methadone having the greatest uptake (Ferreira et al. 2011; Pypendop et al. 2014).

The most commonly used perioperative opioids include butorphanol, buprenorphine, hydromorphone, methadone, and morphine. Recommended doses are shown in Table 8.3.

Butorphanol

Butorphanol is one of only two opioids licensed for veterinary use in the United States and is unlikely to be affected by the FDA's decision to decrease opioid production. Butorphanol is classified as an agonist–antagonist opioid and therefore reaches a ceiling effect where increasing doses (e.g. from 0.1 to 0.8 mg/kg) do not provide any further analgesia (Lascelles and Robertson 2004). In addition, it is a short-acting agent – in a thermal threshold model it provided antinociception for ≤90 minutes (Lascelles and Robertson 2004) – and repeated dosing is time consuming and costly. Despite its popularity, butorphanol's analgesic properties have been questioned for a long time (Wagner 1999). Clinical studies have shown that when butorphanol is the primary analgesic it does not provide adequate pain relief for surgical procedures such as ovariohysterectomy in cats (Taylor et al. 2010; Warne et al. 2014).

However, a dismissal of butorphanol as a component of anesthetic and analgesic protocols is unwarranted after careful scrutiny of several studies that compare it to other opioids. When studies were designed to compare butorphanol to buprenorphine (Taylor et al. 2010; Warne et al. 2014) or methadone (Warne et al. 2013) in cats undergoing surgery (predominantly ovariohysterectomy), no other analgesics were given. Rarely is an opioid the only analgesic used in animals undergoing surgery; a multimodal approach using ketamine, NSAIDs, alpha$_2$-adrenergic agonist drugs, and local anesthetic agents is commonly used and provides good intra- and post-operative analgesia.

Nalbuphine

Pre-mixed combinations of an opioid, dissociative, and alpha$_2$-adreneric agonist (also known as "kitty magic") are often used for IM induction in cats in a variety of settings. Nalbuphine is not a controlled substance and is an agonist–antagonist opioid similar to butorphanol. A randomized clinical trial in cats presented to a mobile TNR clinic demonstrated non-inferiority of nalbuphine compared to butorphanol (Kreisler et al. 2019). The protocol used was a combination of tiletamine–zolazepam (3 mg/kg), dexmedetomidine (7.5 µg/kg) and either butorphanol or nalbuphine at 0.15 mg/kg given IM. The authors concluded that "nalbuphine is an effective substitute for butorphanol" (Kreisler et al. 2019). Record keeping and safe storage of opioids are essential and the use of nalbuphine can reduce this burden.

Buprenorphine

Buprenorphine is a partial mu agonist which can be used in cats and dogs, but is more widely used in cats.

There are three different formulations of buprenorphine currently available:

1) The "traditional" injectable product – in the United States the human formulation (brand name Buprenex®, generic formulations) is often used off-label. In several countries there are veterinary-approved multidose products containing preservatives. These formulations have a concentration of 0.3 mg/ml. Recommended dose rates are 0.02–0.04 mg/kg (IV and IM) in dogs and cats. The OTM route has been discussed earlier and is an option, but when possible the IV and IM routes should be used. The SC route is not as efficacious for this formulation of buprenorphine due to erratic absorption, which may be worse when animals are cold or have received an alpha$_2$-adrenergic drug that causes peripheral vasoconstriction (Steagall et al. 2014).

The time to onset of action, peak effect, and duration of buprenorphine have been investigated, but are often misunderstood. Based on research models and clinical studies, onset of analgesia occurs

Table 8.3 Opioid drugs recommended for alleviation of acute pain in dogs and cats. The suggested frequency of administration is for guidance; patients may require more or less frequent treatment and this is based on assessing their pain. Availability of opioids and market authorization for dogs and cats varies widely in different countries.

Drug Class Drug	Dose, mg/kg Dog	Dose, mg/kg Cat	Route	Frequency hours	Comments
Agonist-antagonists					
Butorphanol	0.2–0.4	0.2–0.4	IM, IV	q 1–2	Drugs in this class have a ceiling effect and used alone are only sufficient for minor procedures. They are best used in a multimodal plan or as part of a TIMA protocol where other analgesics are used (e.g. NSAIDs, alpha₂-adrenergic agonists, ketamine, tiletamine–zolazepam).
Nalbuphine	0.2–0.4	0.2–0.4	IM, IV	q 1–2	Butorphanol provides better sedation than other opioids. Nalbuphine is a non-scheduled drug in the United States.
Partial agonists					
Buprenorphine 0.3 mg/ml	0.02–0.04	0.02–0.04	IM, IV, OTM	q 4–8	OTM uptake may be less in dogs than cats; use the higher end of the dose range if using this route.
Buprenorphine 1.8 mg/ml (Simbadol®)	Not labeled for dogs	0.24	SC	q 24	Buprenorphine 1.8 mg/ml (Simbadol) is currently FDA approved only for use in cats. There are no generic formulations.
Buprenorphine SR (sustained release)	0.03–0.06	0.12	SC	q 72	Appropriate for use when handling of the patient after recovery is not possible.
Agonists					
Morphine	0.5–1.0	0.2–0.5	IM, IV*	q 4–6	*IV administration may cause histamine releases; give over 1–3 minutes. Likely to cause nausea and vomiting.
Methadone	0.5–1.0	0.3–0.5	IM, IV, OTM**	q 4	**Cats only. Vomiting is rare. Has N-methyl-D-aspartate (NMDA) receptor antagonist properties. Sporadically available.
Oxymorphone	0.05–0.1	0.025–0.10	IM, IV		Likely to cause nausea and vomiting.
Hydromorphone	0.1–0.2	0.05–0.10	IM, IV		May cause hyperthermia in cats.

FDA, Food and Drug Administration; IM, intramuscular; IV, intravenous; NSAIDs, non-steroidal anti-inflammatory drugs; OTM, oral transmucosal; q, every; SC, subcutaneous; TIMA, total intramuscular anesthetic.

between 15 and 30 minutes and peak effect at 60–90 minutes, with a duration of 4–6 hours (Steagall et al. 2014).

2) Buprenorphine SR™ (sustained release) formulation (SR Veterinary Technologies; supplied by ZooPharm, Windsor, CO). This is formulated in a sustained-release biodegradable matrix and is not FDA approved. It is available at a concentration of 10 mg/ml and 3 mg/ml for use in dogs and cats, and a 1 mg/ml formulation is available for use in laboratory rats and mice. This biodegradable liquid polymer matrix can be given SC in cats and dogs and plasma levels are consistent with those required for analgesia; one dose may provide analgesia for up to 72 hours. Recommended buprenorphine SR dose rates are 0.12 mg/kg for cats and 0.03–0.06 mg/kg for dogs. A clinical study compared sustained-release buprenorphine with OTM buprenorphine in cats undergoing ovariohysterectomy. Cats were given a single dose of sustained-release buprenorphine SC once, or OTM buprenorphine every 12 hours, and evaluated over 72 hours; no cats required rescue analgesia and there were no significant differences in pain scores between the two treatment groups. There are no peer-reviewed studies of sustained release buprenorphine in dogs, but anecdotal reports are positive.

3) Simbadol (buprenorphine injection for cats). The concentration of this product is 1.8 mg/ml. It is intended for SC administration and may provide analgesia for up to 24 hours. The label dose is 0.24 mg/kg administered SC once daily, for up to three days. It is only labeled for use in cats and should not be dispensed for use outside the clinic.

Hydromorphone

Hydromorphone is a potent mu agonist opioid that is widely used in veterinary medicine, particularly in North America (Pettifer and Dyson 2000). It causes vomiting in approximately 50% of dogs when used as a pre-medicant for elective surgery, the incidence of which can be decreased by prior (15 minutes) or co-administration of acepromazine (Valverde et al. 2004). Vomiting occurs much less frequently when opioids are given to dogs in pain. Vomiting is rarely detrimental in healthy dogs, but is contraindicated in brachycephalic breeds, dogs with laryngeal paralysis, cervical injuries, or megaesophagus due to the danger of aspiration, in dogs with glaucoma or a deep corneal laceration due to the danger of further increases in intraocular pressure or globe rupture, and in dogs with head trauma or an intracranial mass due to the risks of increased intracranial pressure.

It is an excellent antinociceptive agent in cats (Wegner and Robertson 2007), but can result in significant hyperthermia for several hours (Niedfeldt and Robertson 2006; Posner et al. 2007); this is discussed later in the chapter along with the effect of other opioids on body temperature in cats.

Methadone

Methadone is a mu-opioid agonist, but is unique in this class as it also has activity at the NMDA receptor, providing an additional mode of action. The NMDA receptors in the dorsal horn of the spinal cord are important in the phenomenon of central plasticity and "wind up" pain; this is the same site that ketamine exerts its antihyperalgesic effects. Methadone is licensed for use in dogs and cats in some countries, but not in the United States, where currently it is not widely used due to cost and limited availability. Methadone rarely causes vomiting or excitement when used alone and is a versatile opioid as it can be given IV or IM, and data in cats supports OTM administration (Ferreira et al. 2011; Murrell 2011; Pypendop et al. 2014). Dosed at 0.6 mg/kg by the OTM route in cats, antinociceptive effects were detected at 10 minutes after administration for approximately four hours (Ferreira et al. 2011). In cats that were anesthetized with ketamine, midazolam, medetomidine, and either buprenorphine or methadone, the latter provided superior post-operative analgesia after neutering; however, cats were not given post-operative NSAIDs (Shah et al. 2018). When IM medetomidine plus either buprenorphine or methadone was compared to SC meloxicam followed by IM alfaxalone (for anesthesia induction) and maintenance with isoflurane in cats undergoing ovariohysterectomy, no significant differences in the anesthetic conditions or post-operative pain scores were detected; no cats required rescue analgesia (Mahdmina et al. 2019). This emphasizes once again the value of multimodal analgesia and the efficacy of NSAIDs for acute post-operative pain.

Morphine

Morphine has been used successfully for many years in dogs and cats. As with hydromorphone, vomiting is often seen in healthy dogs, but the incidence is decreased with the use of acepromazine or maropitant. Morphine can cause histamine release, so if given IV it should be injected slowly (over two to five minutes) and avoided in animals with mast cell tumors.

Historically people have avoided morphine in cats due to reports of "morphine mania." If these studies are looked at closely, cats received 20 mg/kg, which is at least 40 times a clinically relevant dose (Fertziger et al. 1974). Because of the fear of manic reactions which are now unfounded, low doses of morphine (e.g. 0.2 mg/kg) were used in cats, with a lack of efficacy. Unlike most dogs and humans, cats produce very little morphine-6-glucuronide which is an active metabolite, therefore they depend on the parent compound for analgesia. This means that doses greater than 0.2 mg/kg are recommended, and this author uses 0.5 mg/kg IM (Taylor et al. 2001; Robertson and Taylor 2004). Although opioid-related vomiting is less common in cats than dogs, it still occurs, and cats should be carefully observed after administration of any potential emetogenic drug.

Opioid-Related Hyperthermia in Cats

Published studies and anecdotal reports indicate that hyperthermia may occur with opioid administration in cats (Niedfeldt and Robertson

2006; Posner et al. 2007, 2010). Hydromorphone is the drug most often implicated, with one cat reaching a rectal temperature of 42.5 °C (108.5 °F; Niedfeldt and Robertson 2006); the increased temperatures with hydromorphone were seen with doses of 0.05, 0.1, and 0.2 mg/kg (Posner et al. 2010). Posner et al. (2010) reported that morphine, butorphanol, buprenorphine, and hydromorphone alone or in combination with ketamine or isoflurane can result in elevated core body temperatures for four to five hours after administration; in that study temperatures did not exceed 40.3 °C (104.5 °F) and resolved without intervention. Removing heating devices, using a fan, and/or applying cool water to the paws are recommended when temperatures reach 40 °C (104 °F). Many clinicians administer acepromazine to promote vasodilation and heat loss. In the one cat that reached 42.5 °C (108.5 °F) reversal with naloxone was successful; this patient had not undergone a painful procedure (Niedfeldt and Robertson 2006). Opioid-related hyperthermia does not seem to be NSAID responsive. If a painful procedure has been performed and reversal is deemed necessary, butorphanol (e.g. 0.1 mg/kg) can be given if the causative opioid is a mu agonist. If naloxone is used, another analgesic should be administered and the patient assessed for pain. Opioid-related hyperthermia is also discussed in Chapter 10.

Tramadol

Tramadol has opioid (mu agonist) effects and inhibits the reuptake of norepinephrine and serotonin. Some of its analgesic effects depend on active metabolites, the primary one being O-desmethyltramadol, also known as M1, which is produced in cats but produced only minimally in dogs (Pypendop and Ilkiw 2008; Schutter et al. 2017). In the past, tramadol was widely used in dogs for alleviation of acute and chronic pain, despite limited evidence of its efficacy. Well-designed clinical and experimental studies indicate that in dogs, tramadol used alone does not provide sufficient antinociception or analgesia and cannot be recommended for peri-operative use (Davila et al. 2013; Schutter et al. 2017). Cats do produce active tramadol metabolites and experimental studies demonstrate its antinociceptive properties, with 4.0 mg/kg orally (PO) having approximately a six-hour duration (Pypendop et al. 2009). After administration cats exhibit opioid-related behavior, including sedation, pupil dilation, and euphoria. In cats undergoing ovariohysterectomy, tramadol (2 mg/kg SC) combined with the NSAID vedaprofen (0.5 mg/kg PO) provided superior post-operative analgesia than either drug alone (Brondani et al. 2009).

In the United States, tramadol is a Schedule IV drug and is only available in an oral (tablet) formulation; it is on the Drug Enforcement Administration (DEA) list of drugs that are of concern for diversion. The oral tablets are rarely found to be palatable in cats, even after compounding with cat-specific flavors. The product with the tradename Ultracet® should never be used in cats because it contains acetaminophen (paracetamol). In some countries an injectable product is available and is popular in combination with an NSAID to provide analgesia for feline soft tissue procedures.

Non-steroidal Anti-Inflammatory Drugs

NSAIDs are non-scheduled drugs that, depending on dosing, can provide up to 24 hours of pain relief. Used alone they are appropriate for mild to moderate pain (Lascelles et al. 1998; Slingsby and Waterman-Pearson 2000b), but are often combined with an opioid to provide multimodal or balanced analgesia (Shih et al. 2008; Steagall et al. 2009). Injectable and oral formulations are available for treatment of both acute and long-term pain in dogs and cats, but labeling varies considerably around the world. In the peri-operative setting a drug that is available as an injectable and oral formulation is ideal; the injectable agent can be administered after induction or during recovery, and further post-operative treatment can

be with the oral formulation (caplets, tablets, or liquid).

This class of drugs should be used with caution in animals of unknown health status, when renal or hepatic function is unknown, and in the face of dehydration, hypovolemia, and hypotension. In the face of low perfusion pressure, renal prostaglandins are released to preserve renal perfusion, a response that is inhibited by the use of NSAIDs.

Several NSAIDs are labeled for peri-operative use, including prior to surgery, but these drugs are not anesthetic sparing so should be combined with sedatives, tranquilizers, opioids, and local anesthetics. Pre-operative administration has some advantages over post-operative use (Lascelles et al. 1998). The pre-emptive effects of NSAIDs are less than those of the opioids, so if an opioid is on board prior to surgery, many practitioners choose to give NSAIDs in recovery when the patient is waking up and only if surgery was uneventful. Ketoprofen is not recommended for pre-surgical use based on reports of it causing increased bleeding times in dogs (Grisneaux et al. 1999). For recommended doses of NSAIDs, see Tables 8.4 and 8.5.

Acetaminophen (Paracetamol)

Acetaminophen (paracetamol) is available as a sole agent and combined with codeine; with the addition of codeine it is a controlled substance. The mode of action of paracetamol is not fully understood, but involves peripheral and central activity at cyclo-oxygenase pathways. It has analgesic and antipyretic effects, but minimal anti-inflammatory action. For acute pain in dogs, the suggested dose of acetaminophen is 10–15 mg PO, every 8–12 hours. Because acetaminophen plus codeine is a controlled drug with a high risk of diversion, it is less commonly used in the peri-operative period in a shelter setting. Acetaminophen is toxic to cats and should not be used in this species.

Table 8.4 Non-steroidal anti-inflammatory drugs (NSAIDs) recommended for alleviation of acute pain in dogs. Availability of NSAIDs and market authorization for dogs and cats vary widely in different countries.

Drug	Route	Dose, mg/kg	Comments
Carprofen	IV, SC	2	Twice a day.
		4	Once a day.
	PO	2	Twice a day.
		4	Once a day. Can give for 4 days.
Cimicoxib	PO	2	Once a day for 4–8 days.
Deracoxib	PO	3–4	Once daily for up to 7 days.
Firocoxib	PO	5	Once daily for up to 3 days.
Ketoprofen	IV, SC	2	Not recommended pre-operatively due to reports of increased bleeding. Can be given for 3 days post-operatively.
	PO	1	
Meloxicam	IV, SC	0.1–0.2*	Injectable and oral liquid formulations are available.
	PO	0.1–0.2*	*First dose is 0.2 mg/kg, successive doses are 0.1 mg/kg for up to 4 days.
Robenacoxib	SC, IV	1–2	Injectable formulation and oral tablets are available. Can be used for up to 6 days. Can interchange injectable and oral formulations.
	PO	1–2	
Tolfenamic acid	SC	4	Not recommended for pre-operative use. Once daily for 3–5 days.
	PO	4	

IV, intravenously; PO, orally; SC, subcutaneously.

Local Anesthetics

Local anesthetics are extremely effective, inexpensive, and non-scheduled analgesic agents with a wide safety margin. Local anesthetics are unique among analgesic drugs because they can provide *complete* analgesia (loss of sensation). Local anesthetic drugs are associated with very few adverse events. The two most commonly used local anesthetic agents in veterinary practice are lidocaine and bupivacaine, but ropivacaine is gaining popularity, and these can be incorporated into the analgesic plan for many procedures. The peri-operative use in ovariohysterectomy and castration surgeries in dogs and cats is discussed here.

Incisional and Intra-peritoneal Use

Intra-peritoneal (IP) administration of local anesthetics is beneficial in humans and is recommended by the WSAVA's Global Pain Council in veterinary patients (Mathews et al. 2014).

Canine Studies In a clinical setting (student surgeons), dogs that received butorphanol (IM) plus bupivacaine 0.75% both IP (4.4 mg/kg) and at the incision (splash of 2 ml over the incision site) required less rescue analgesia and had lower pain scores than control dogs (butorphanol only); the administration of IP and incisional lidocaine 2% with epinephrine did not show these benefits (Carpenter et al. 2004). Autonomic responses to surgery were

Table 8.5 Non-steroidal anti-inflammatory drugs (NSAIDs) recommended for alleviation of acute pain in cats. Injectable formulations can be given in the peri-operative period; ketoprofen and tolfenamic acid are not recommended for pre-operative use. A few select oral formulations can be given post-operatively. When repeated, the dosing interval for listed NSAIDs is 24 hours.

Drug	Route	Dose, mg/kg	Comments
Carprofen	SC	2–4	Once only.
Ketoprofen	IV, SC	2	Not recommended pre-operatively. Can be given for 3 days post-operatively.
	PO	1	
Meloxicam	SC	0.2	Injectable and oral liquid formulations are available. Can be given PO for 1–4 days after an initial dose of 0.2 mg/kg.
	PO	0.02–0.05	
Robenacoxib	SC	1–2	Injectable formulation and oral tablets (6 mg) are available. Can interchange injectable and oral formulations Can be given for up to 6 days.
	PO	1–2	
Tolfenamic acid	SC	4	Not recommended for pre-operative use. Once daily for 3–5 days.

IV, intravenously; PO, orally; SC, subcutaneously.

not inhibited by incisional infiltration of the linea alba with lidocaine 1% (2 mg/kg) and anesthesia of the mesovarium (0.5 ml of lidocaine 2%; Bubalo et al. 2008). Therefore, longer-acting local anesthetics such as bupivacaine or ropivacaine should be used for these techniques.

Published reports on the use of incisional anesthesia alone are conflicting. SC and IM infiltration of bupivacaine (0.25% 2 mg/kg) at the incision site before surgery was associated with significantly lower pain scores and less need for post-operative opioids compared to post-operative administration of incisional bupivacaine (splash block) or placebo in dogs undergoing celiotomy, suggesting that timing (pre-emptive use) is important (Savvas et al. 2008). In contrast, benefits of incisional anesthesia in dogs undergoing ovariohysterectomy were not apparent in two other studies, and the reasons put forth were that when robust multimodal analgesia is used, additional benefits are difficult to discern, and that recognizing pain in the clinical setting is challenging (Fitzpatrick et al. 2010; McKune et al. 2014).

A recent study showed no benefits in dogs undergoing ovariohysterectomy of using IP

(3 mg/kg) and incisional bupivacaine ("splash" application; 1 mg/kg after ovariohysterectomy and before complete closure) over the IP technique alone; all dogs received morphine and carprofen (Kalchofner Guerrero et al. 2016). IP administration of ropivacaine 0.75% (3 mg/kg) or bupivacaine 0.5% (3 mg/kg) provided similar post-operative analgesia when administered in combination with morphine and carprofen (Lambertini et al. 2018).

In summary, when performing abdominal surgery in dogs, use bupivacaine or ropivacaine, and if only one technique is to be used, choose intraperitoneal administration. This technique should be considered for any intraabdominal procedure, including foreign body removal and splenectomy. The WSAVA's Global Pain Council site provides links to videos of several local anesthetic techniques, including incisional and intraperitoneal anesthesia (http://www.wsava.org/Committees/Global-Pain-Council).

Feline Studies The pharmacokinetics, safety, and efficacy of IP bupivacaine have been reported in cats (Benito et al. 2016a, b, 2018). When bupivacaine 0.25% (2 mg/kg) was placed in the intraperitoneal cavity, it was detectable in plasma, but at significantly lower concentrations than those reported to cause toxic effects (Benito et al. 2016a). Efficacy was confirmed in a prospective, randomized clinical trial. When IP bupivacaine (0.25%, 2 mg/kg) was used in cats pre-medicated with buprenorphine, their post-operative pain scores and need for rescue analgesia were similar to cats that received meloxicam and buprenorphine (no IP treatment), and superior to cats that only received buprenorphine for the first eight hours post-operatively (Benito et al. 2016a). In this study bupivacaine was splashed on the ovarian ligaments and on the cervix of the uterus before their removal, using a catheter attached to a syringe. A good question to ask is whether these techniques, performed on relatively small numbers of clinical research animals, are transferable to cats in a high-volume surgery setting. A recent prospective, randomized, double-blinded, placebo-controlled study that included over 200 cats shows that they are (Fudge et al. 2019). Cats were anesthetized with an IM combination of buprenorphine, ketamine, and dexmedetomidine and maintained with isoflurane. Cats were divided into three groups: one was administered bupivacaine (2 mg/kg); a second, saline; and a third group were "sham" controls in which infiltration sites were observed only. Infiltration was performed at four places (total volume divided equally): both ovarian suspensory ligaments and vessels, the uterine body just caudal to the bifurcation, and incisional subcutaneous tissues. A 25-gauge needle was used. The time taken to perform the block was approximately one minute. An additional few drops were also applied to the cut ends of tissues. At one hour into recovery and at the time of discharge, pain scores were lower in the bupivacaine group, and reached statistical significance in larger cats (>2.7 kg; Fudge et al. 2019).

Vasoconstrictors are often added to local anesthetic agents to prevent systemic uptake and prolong their duration of action. Intraperitoneal bupivacaine with epinephrine (2.0 µg/kg) or dexmedetomidine (1.0 µg/kg) produced plasma concentrations below toxic levels and prolonged the terminal half-life compared to bupivacaine alone; due to low study numbers, it is too soon to know if these drug combinations improve efficacy (Benito et al. 2018).

Cats anesthetized with an injectable anesthetic protocol (medetomidine and ketamine) undergoing ovariohysterectomy benefited from the addition of pre-incisional local anesthesia as measured by the reduced need for supplemental ketamine during surgery (Zilberstein et al. 2008). These clinicians used a total of 6 mg/kg of a 2% lidocaine solution as follows: 1 mg/kg infiltrated SC at the incision site prior to surgery, 2 mg/kg "splashed" on each ovary, and a further 1 mg/kg dripped on the muscle layers of the abdominal wound prior to closure. Post-operative analgesia was not assessed in this study (Zilberstein et al. 2008).

Use of Local Anesthetics for Orchiectomy
Dogs Intratesticular injection of lidocaine has been used for many years during castration of stallions and the technique has been widely adapted to other species. Autoradiographs taken of the surgically removed testicles and spermatic cords of two horses after intratesticular injection of radiolabeled lidocaine showed diffuse distribution of lidocaine within the well-innervated spermatic cord (Haga et al. 2006), and explains why there is no need to inject the cord itself.

Intratesticular injection of local anesthetic agents has been evaluated in dogs (McMillan et al. 2012; Huuskonen et al. 2013; Perez et al. 2013; Stevens et al. 2013) and cats (Moldal et al. 2012). In these studies, local anesthetic without epinephrine was used, because uptake from the vascular testes is possible and would result in cardiovascular effects such as tachycardia and hypertension.

McMillan et al. (2012) studied the effect of 1 mg/kg of a 2% lidocaine solution (1 ml/20 kg) injected into the body of each testicle, or no treatment, on isoflurane requirements during surgery and post-operative pain scores; all dogs received pre-operative buprenorphine and carprofen. The isoflurane requirements were significantly lower, as were pain scores at the time of discharge (five to six hours post-operatively) in the lidocaine group. In another study all dogs received pre-operative morphine and meloxicam and either an intratesticular injection of 2 mg/kg of lidocaine or an equal volume of saline; dogs in the lidocaine group had significantly lower heart rates and mean arterial blood pressure during surgery, indicating an antinociceptive effect (Huuskonen et al. 2013). Although fewer dogs in the lidocaine group required post-operative rescue analgesia, this was not statistically significant (Huuskonen et al. 2013). Perez et al. (2013) compared three protocols for dogs undergoing castration: hydromorphone and carprofen alone; hydromorphone and carprofen plus intratesticular bupivacaine (0.5 mg/kg per testis); and hydromorphone and carprofen plus epidural morphine (0.1 mg/kg). Dogs that received intratesticular bupivacaine or epidural morphine required fewer intraoperative doses of fentanyl to obtund responses to surgery (changes in heart rate, mean arterial pressure, and respiratory rate), required less hydromorphone post-operatively, and had lower post-operative pain scores; there were no differences between the intratesticular bupivacaine group and the epidural morphine group for these parameters. Serum cortisol values were also measured and were lowest in the intratesticular group. Another study compared intratesticular lidocaine (1 mg/kg) plus bupivacaine (1 mg/kg) to placebo (saline) in dogs that also received morphine and carprofen for castration (Stevens et al. 2013). All dogs in this study had low post-operative pain scores, with no difference between placebo and local anesthetic groups. Dogs in the local anesthetic group were less likely to produce a cremaster muscle twitch during ligation than the placebo-treated dogs.

Overall, there is good evidence to support the use of intratesticular local anesthetics in dogs undergoing castration. None of the studies discussed reported unacceptable adverse effects related to the procedure. This block should be part of a multimodal approach to pain management and should be in addition to opioids and/or NSAIDs, not a substitute for these drugs. This author recommends the use of lidocaine at a dose of 1–2 mg/kg (2% solution), as it is readily available worldwide, inexpensive, and has a greater margin of safety than bupivacaine (Neal et al. 2010). The recommended technique is as follows and performed under sterile conditions: use a 22-gauge 25 mm (1 in.) needle and appropriate-sized syringe to draw up the lidocaine; if the drug is drawn up through a rubber stopper, use a separate needle for the intratesticular injection, since the rubber stopper blunts and deforms the tip of the needle. With the dog in dorsal recumbency, hold the testicle and insert the needle at the caudal pole of the testicle and direct it toward the spermatic cord, aspirate the syringe to check for the absence of blood, then inject the calculated volume of lidocaine; the testicle may become turgid, but the injection is stopped prematurely only if there is marked resistance to injection; repeat the procedure on the other side. Occasionally some blood oozes from the needle site, suggesting that a hematoma may have formed or a small vessel has been damaged. After injection, surgery can begin within one minute. The WSAVA's Global Pain Council site provides links to videos of several local anesthetic techniques, including intratesticular blocks (http://www.wsava.org/Committees/Global-Pain-Council).

Cats Intratesticular injections of lidocaine can be used in adult male cats and are documented to reduce the nociceptive response to castration under anesthesia, as measured by pulse rate, heart rate variability, and mean arterial blood pressure (Moldal et al. 2012). The dose of lidocaine is 2 mg/kg, therefore 0.1 ml/kg of 2% (20 mg/ml) lidocaine is drawn up; the technique described by Moldal and colleagues is as follows. One-third of this is injected (using a 25- or 27-gauge needle) into each testicle; with the cat in dorsal recumbency the injection is made in a craniodorsal location, directing the needle caudoventrally; and the remaining one-third is injected SC where the incision will be made.

Ketamine

Ketamine has traditionally been considered a dissociative anesthetic, but its role as a potential analgesic, or antihyperalgesic agent, has evolved over the years in human and veterinary medicine (Kohrs and Durieux 1998; Pozzi et al. 2006). Ketamine is a non-competitive NMDA receptor antagonist. Activation and modulation of NMDA receptors by the excitatory neurotransmitter glutamate are thought to be the primary mechanism in the development of central sensitization and secondary hyperalgesia.

In a study of female dogs undergoing ovariohysterectomy, dogs received a sub-anesthetic dose of ketamine (2.5 mg/kg IM) pre-operatively or post-operatively (at extubation), or saline (Slingsby and Waterman-Pearson 2000a). Other analgesic agents were not given, and pre-medication was with acepromazine and anesthesia induced with thiopental. Mechanical nociceptive thresholds were measured, and pain scores recorded before pre-medication and post-operatively for up to 18 hours after extubation. Dogs in the control (saline) group required more rescue analgesics, showed more wound sensitivity, and had higher pain scores throughout the post-operative period than those in the two ketamine groups. Administration of ketamine before surgery was more effective than administration after surgery (Slingsby and Waterman-Pearson 2000a). Ketamine should not be the sole agent used to alleviate acute pain, but can be used as part of a multimodal peri-operative anesthesia and analgesia plan. Ketamine can also be a valuable addition to an anesthetic or analgesic plan when used at sub-anesthetic doses as an infusion (Wagner et al. 2002). It decreases the requirements for inhalant agents (Muir et al. 2003) and provides protection against central sensitization; this can be an effective technique for major surgeries such as amputations or following severe trauma (e.g. fractures, burns, extensive wounds) and is extremely economical. Ketamine has been shown to reduce C-reactive proteins in dogs with pyometra and may have immunomodulating effects in the face of endotoxemia (DeClue et al. 2008; Liao et al. 2014).

Other Strategies for Preventing or Alleviating Pain

The surgical technique itself can impact on post-operative pain. In cats, ovariohysterectomy performed via the flank was more painful than when performed via a midline abdominal approach (Grint et al. 2006); however, no differences in post-operative pain scores were noted in cats undergoing ovariectomy via the flank or midline, with all cats receiving the same anesthetic and analgesic protocol (Swaffield et al. 2019). Kittens were less painful than adult cats following ovariohysterectomy (Polson et al. 2013) and this could be related to the smaller incisions required in pediatric patients, which in turn produce less inflammation.

The effects of providing good patient nursing care and reducing stress should never be underestimated as adjuncts to pain management strategies.

Cryotherapy

Cryotherapy or cold therapy is one of the most underutilized analgesic techniques, yet it is inexpensive and simple to provide. Cold reduces swelling and inflammation, slows local metabolism, and decreases vascular permeability. Cold also activates specific transient receptor potential (TRP) ion channels in sensory neurons that reduce pain after injury (Liu et al. 2013). Incisions can be iced with commercially available cold packs or crushed ice in zip-lock bags wrapped in a thin towel. Use for 10–20 minutes at a time and repeat every 4–6 hours. To save on personal time, ice packs can be held in place with wraps, such as 3M™ Vetrap™ (3M, St. Paul, MN), elasticated bandages, and T-shirts.

Anesthesia for Other Procedures

In addition to surgical sterilization, many other procedures may be required in a shelter setting; these include but are not limited to limb and tail amputations, surgery involving the eye such as enucleation, rectal and vaginal prolapse, and dental extractions. Although the principles of anesthesia, pain management, and monitoring apply to these cases, they present special challenges and are covered in more detail in Chapters 19–22.

Anesthesia for Special Populations

Anesthesia in Pregnant and Lactating Animals

The WSAVA Global Pain Council provides open access summaries on the analgesic care of pregnant and lactating animals (http://www.wsava.org/Guidelines/Global-Pain-Council-Guidelines).

Pregnant Animals

Pregnant bitches and queens may undergo cesarean section where the intent is to deliver live offspring, or ovariohysterectomy during any stage of gestation where the uterus and fetuses are removed and the pregnancy terminated. In addition, a pregnant animal may require anesthesia for a procedure other than ovariohysterectomy, for example a laceration or fracture repair. There is very little information on how pregnancy alters the pharmacokinetics or actions of drugs in dogs and cats, nor on the potential for drugs to disrupt organogenesis at different stages of fetal development. Increased uterine activity and decreased uterine blood flow are undesirable because this could lead to premature labor or fetal ischemia, respectively. As a class, the alpha$_2$-adrenergic agonist drugs (xylazine, medetomidine, and dexmedetomi-dine) increase uterine tone, but the effect is variable between drugs and species. However, they do cause vasoconstriction and decreased blood flow to vital organs, including the uterus, and should not be used during pregnancy when survival of fetuses is intended. Extrapolating the extensive data in rodents, rabbits, and humans to our patients seems prudent. The placental barrier is a lipoprotein which is highly permeable to lipid-soluble drugs, namely most analgesics (especially opioids) and anesthetics. Ionized, protein-bound, or polar drugs will remain in the maternal circulation; these include glycopyrrolate and neuromuscular blocking agents, both of which are adjunctive anesthetic drugs. Although NSAIDs are protein bound and poorly lipid soluble, there are concerns that they are teratogenic, especially affecting renal organogenesis, and it is not advised to administer this class of drug during pregnancy. Details on anesthetic and surgical procedures for cesarean section can be found in Chapter 13.

Physiologic Changes Related to Pregnancy and Their Impact on Anesthetic Management

All major body systems undergo adaptation during pregnancy and many of these changes have a significant impact on anesthetic management. As the gestational age of the neonates progresses, the greater are the physiologic changes and demands on the dam. Some data is extrapolated from humans (Tan and Tan 2013) and some data has been published based on dog studies, but much less is known about cats.

Cardiovascular System Significant cardiovascular changes have been documented as early as mid-pregnancy in dogs and continue to progress until term. There is a decrease in blood pressure and an increase in heart rate and cardiac output (Pascoe and Moon 2001). Total blood volume increases, but red blood cells do not keep pace with plasma expansion, resulting in a decreased packed cell volume, the magnitude of which is correlated with the number of puppies (Kaneko et al. 1993). Changes in the mother's cardiovascular system directly impact the fetus, because fetal blood flow is not autoregulated. Uterine blood flow is directly proportional to the arterial–venous blood pressure difference and inversely proportional to systemic vascular resistance. Anesthetic drugs, dehydration, and intraoperative fluid losses will result in maternal hypotension. Fear, stress, excitement, and pain increase sympathetic nervous system activity, resulting in vasoconstriction and increased systemic vascular resistance; these changes adversely affect the fetus. Pregnant animals have blunted cardiovascular responses and are less able to tolerate hypovolemia (Brooks and Keil 1994). Hypotension occurs more rapidly after hemorrhage in pregnant compared with non-pregnant animals, and resuscitative efforts are often less effective. Moon et al. (1998) reported that intraoperative fluids were only administered to 53% of dogs undergoing cesarean section, suggesting that cardiovascular support for these patients is an area that can be improved.

Respiratory System Due to a reduced functional residual capacity and increased oxygen demands, pregnant patients are at risk for hypoxemia. Maternal hypoventilation can lead to fetal hypoxia and acidosis and either manual or mechanical intermittent positive pressure ventilation may be required. However, overventilation causing hypocapnia ($PaCO_2 < 32\,mmHg$) is detrimental because alkalosis increases uterine vascular resistance and reduces fetal unloading of oxygen. When available, pulse oximeters should be used to evaluate oxygen saturation and capnometers to indicate the adequacy of ventilation. Positioning in a head-up (reverse Trendelenburg) position may improve respiratory parameters and can easily be done by tipping the table 30° head up, with foam wedges placed under the head and thorax, or, as shown in Figure 8.1, raising the spay tray.

Gastrointestinal System Gastric reflux is more likely because of an increase in intraabdominal pressure and relaxation of the gastroesophageal

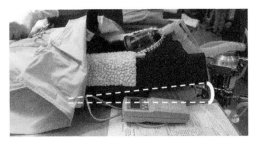

Figure 8.1 Positioning pregnant patients in a head-up (reverse Trendelenburg) position may improve respiratory parameters and decrease the work of breathing.

junction. Gastric emptying is delayed and the stomach contents are more acidic, and aspiration is a possible consequence if rapid intubation is not achieved. Moon et al. (1998) reported that five out of nine bitches whose death was associated with cesarean section had pneumonia. This information justifies the recommendation for rapid airway control with an endotracheal tube after anesthetic induction.

Inhalant Anesthetic Requirements The minimum alveolar concentration (MAC) of inhalant agents is significantly reduced in women during pregnancy and is correlated with serum progesterone levels and beta-endorphins. Decreases of up to 30% are reported as early as 8–12 weeks of gestation (Gin and Chan 1994; Chan et al. 1996). There are no published MAC studies in bitches and queens during pregnancy or at term. Depending on the stage of pregnancy and progesterone levels, the MAC may be significantly reduced, therefore careful assessment of anesthetic depth in the dam is essential.

Ovariohysterectomy of Pregnant Animals

The concerns for the dam are the same as when a cesarean section is performed, but because delivering live offspring is not a goal, neonatal depression is not an issue. Thus, the primary concerns are regurgitation and aspiration and hypoxemia. Pre-oxygenation and intravenous induction of anesthesia followed by rapid airway control are warranted. Based on information from other species, placing heavily pregnant or obese animals in a reverse Trendelenburg position (head elevated by 15–30°) may enhance respiratory function. This is likely due to decreased pressure on the diaphragm by the gravid uterus, and increased thoracic excursions and lung volumes (De Jong et al. 2014; Figure 8.1).

The welfare of the in-utero fetuses removed from the dam must be considered and the most appropriate way to ensure their humane death has been a concern for veterinarians performing these procedures (White 2012). Until recently there was a paucity of information on whether or not fetuses could suffer, leading to diverse opinions on what to do with pregnant animals presented for ovariohysterectomy, ranging from injecting each fetus with a euthanasia solution to refusing to perform the procedure (White 2012).

The prerequisites for suffering are sentience and consciousness (Mellor and Diesch 2006). To perceive sensations animals must have a sufficiently developed neural system that can receive and process incoming information and be conscious. If these sensations are painful or aversive, suffering may result (Mellor and Diesch 2006). Scientific research indicates that mammalian embryos and fetuses are unconscious during gestation and the birth process. The moderately immature neurologic function of dogs and cats at this life stage is thought to contribute to this unconscious state. In these species, sentience is not achieved until several days after parturition. Other factors including chemical inhibitors such as adenosine, prostaglandins, and allopregnalone contribute to unconsciousness or a neuro-inhibited state while in utero (Mellor and Diesch 2006; Mellor 2010; Aleman et al. 2017). Based on this data, the 2013 AVMA Guidelines for the Euthanasia of Animals state that "embryos and fetuses cannot consciously experience feelings such as pain or breathlessness" and Mellor and Diesch (2006) also conclude that embryos and fetuses cannot suffer before birth. An additional factor that protects unborn kittens and puppies

during ovariohysterectomy is the transfer of anesthetic drugs from the maternal circulation across the placenta to the fetuses (White 2012). Based on the AVMA euthanasia guidelines and a commentary on this topic (White 2012), it is recommended that when pregnant dogs and cats undergo ovariohysterectomy, the uterine blood vessels be ligated and the fetuses left undisturbed and in situ to ensure fetal death without suffering. If for some reason the uterus is to be opened to remove the fetuses, this should not be done for at least one hour (White 2012).

Lactating Animals

Secretion into milk would be enhanced if a drug was highly lipid soluble, non-ionized, and had a low molecular weight. Little is known about excretion of drugs into dog or cat milk, but extrapolation from species where milk withholding is mandatory after the animal is treated suggests that approximately 1–2% of the maternal dose reaches the neonate. Opioid drugs are lipid soluble and more likely to reach milk when compared to NSAIDs, which are highly protein bound and poorly lipid soluble. If opioids are given to the dam, the neonates should be observed for side effects such as somnolence. Short-term (one to two days') treatment of lactating animals with NSAIDs appears to be safe for offspring.

Anesthesia for the Young and Old

Anesthesia for dogs and cats at either end of the age spectrum deserves special consideration. The unique needs of dogs and cats at different life stages have led to the publication of several excellent resources: American Association of Feline Practitioners (AAFP)-American Animal Hospital Association (AAHA) Feline Life Stages Guidelines (https://catvets.com/guidelines/practice-guidelines/life-stage-guidelines); AAFP Senior Care Guidelines (https://catvets.com/guidelines/practice-guidelines/senior-care-guidelines);

AAHA Senior Care Guidelines for Dogs and Cats (https://www.aaha.org/globalassets/02-guidelines/senior-care/senior-care-guidelines). Anesthesia and analgesia for pediatric patients are covered in Chapter 9; however, it is worth reiterating that with many anesthetic and analgesic drugs in very young and therefore small animals, they may require relatively larger doses of drugs because of their grater BSA to body mass ratio (Bushby and Griffin 2011; Joyce and Yates 2011; Tables 8.6 and 8.7).

Dogs age at different rates, depending on their breed and size; dogs may be considered "senior" when they have reached 75% of their expected life span. Cats tend to age more uniformly and could be considered senior between 11 and 14 years of age and geriatric between 15 and 25 years of age. In human medicine, senior is a term reserved for a specific age in a spectrum, but geriatric is more than just aging. Frailty is considered a distinct syndrome when three or more of the following are present: weakness, slowness, poor physical endurance, and unintended weight loss; this can be applied to our veterinary patients, too (Chen et al. 2014). It must be remembered that regardless of age, a dog or cat's physical status is important to consider when planning for anesthesia and surgery.

Anesthetic Mortality Related to Advancing Age

Older cats were reported to have a higher anesthetic risk – cats older than 12 years were twice as likely to die compared to cats aged 6 months to 5 years, independent from the American Society of Anesthesiologists (ASA) status (Brodbelt et al. 2007; see Chapter 7). No meaningful data is available for dogs because their longevity depends on weight and breed. A 10-year-old dog could be at the very far end of its expected life span or somewhere in the middle. However, aging results in a decrease in reserve capacity of all vital organs and a change in body composition which affects drug distribution and metabolism.

Age-Related Changes and Their Influence on Anesthesia

The most important age-related changes in cardiac function in older animals are decreased ventricular compliance and cardiac reserve. This renders older animals less tolerant of acute changes in intravascular volume – both fluid loss and fluid overload.

Older patients have a decreased respiratory reserve. Vital capacity is reduced, the chest wall and lungs become less compliant, and anatomic dead space increases, making them more susceptible to hypoxia and hypercapnia.

Table 8.6 The Kitten Quad protocol. Body surface area (BSA) is calculated using the formula BSA = $(10.4 \times$ bodyweight in $kg^{0.67})/100$. 10.4 is a calculated constant (K) for cats. Dosing of drugs based on BSA: medetomidine ($600\,microg/m^2$), ketamine ($60\,mg/m^2$), midazolam ($3\,mg/m^2$), and buprenorphine ($180\,microg/m^2$) in very small (0.5 – 2.0 kg) kittens (Joyce and Yates 2011). For clinical use, the volumes of each drug are also given in milliliters.

Bodyweight (BW), kg	BW, lb	BSA (m^2)	Volume of each drug (ml)	Total volume (ml)
0.5	1.1	0.07	0.04	0.16
1.0	2.2	0.1	0.06	0.24
1.5	3.3	0.14	0.08	0.32
2.0	4.4	0.17	0.1	0.40

Notes: Drug concentrations medetomidine 1.0 mg/ml, ketamine 100 mg/ml, midazolam 5 mg/ml, buprenorphine 0.3 mg/ml. The concentration of dexmedetomidine is 0.5 mg/ml and can be substituted in equal volume for medetomidine. Ketamine, midazolam, and buprenorphine are controlled drugs and must be correctly logged.

Table 8.7 Suggested doses of dexmedetomidine, ketamine, and butorphanol for kittens less than 2 kg (Bushby and Griffin 2011). Note the metabolic scaling used: the smaller the kitten, the more drug it receives on a mg/kg basis.

Bodyweight (BW) kg	BW lb	Volume of each drug (ml)	Total volume (ml) rounded up
0.5	1.1	0.044	0.13
0.6	1.3	0.053	0.16
0.7	1.5	0.062	0.18
0.8	1.8	0.070	0.21
0.9	2.0	0.075	0.23
1.0	2.2	0.770	0.23
1.1	2.4	0.790	0.24
1.2	2.6	0.079	0.24
1.3	2.9	0.068	0.26
1.4	3.1	0.092	0.28
1.5	3.3	0.099	0.30
1.6	3.5	0.106	0.32
1.7	3.7	0.112	0.34
1.8	4.0	0.119	0.36
1.9	4.2	0.125	0.38
2.0	4.4	0.132	0.40

Notes: Drug concentrations dexmedetomidine 0.5 mg/ml, ketamine 100 mg/ml, butorphanol 10 mg/ml. See Box 8.2 for details on preparing this "premix."
Ketamine and butorphanol are controlled drugs and must be correctly logged.

With a decrease in respiratory reserve, older animals may rapidly become hypoxic in the immediate post-induction period and for this reason, pre-oxygenation is recommended in older patients (McNally et al. 2009).

As animals age, renal blood flow decreases, as does glomerular filtration rate and the number of functional glomeruli. Older animals may have underlying renal pathology which is well compensated for until they are stressed in the peri-operative period (fasting, fluid deprivation, and hypotension), therefore overt post-anesthetic renal failure is a real concern. These patients may be administered NSAIDs for chronic pain or be given them for the acute pain associated with surgical procedures. These drugs block prostaglandin production, which is important for maintaining renal blood flow during periods of hypotension. If an NSAID is used in the peri-anesthetic period, great care must be taken to prevent, recognize,

and treat hypotension and to maintain normal fluid balance and organ perfusion.

Brain mass decreases with age as a result of neuronal loss, cerebral blood flow declines, and the quantity of neurotransmitters is reduced. Specific age-related changes indicative of neurodegeneration similar to those seen in aged people have been identified in the brain, brain stem, and spinal cord of cats (Zhang et al. 2005; Gunn-Moore et al. 2006). In humans the requirements for inhalant agents decrease with advancing age (Nickalls and Mapleson 2003) and this has also been demonstrated in dogs (Magnusson et al. 2000; Yamashita et al. 2009). Because of the documented decrease in anesthetic requirements in older patients, the depth of anesthesia must be closely monitored.

Age can cause changes in drug concentration at the site of action and also alter drug action per se. Some of these changes are related to altered body composition, blood flow, and organ perfusion, and some are a result of altered metabolism and excretion and changes in the number and density of receptors in target organs. In essence, advanced age can result in unpredictable drug effects, therefore careful choice and administration are the key to a good outcome. It is prudent to choose drugs that are reversible, can be given "to effect," and have a short duration of action.

As with all patients, a complete history (to the extent that can be obtained) and physical examination are mandatory. Clinical findings will dictate which pre-anesthetic blood work and tests are undertaken; however, hematologic and biochemical analyses of 101 dogs aged over seven years resulted in 30 new diagnoses and cancelation of surgery in 13 patients (Joubert 2007). Therefore if the resources are available, pre-anesthetic blood work is recommended in older patients.

One of the most commonly made mistakes when anesthetizing older patients is to depend primarily on inhalant agents and avoid pre-medicant agents, in the misunderstanding that inhalant agents are somehow "safer." Sedation is recommended to decrease anxiety and fear that lead to increased catecholamine release, which predisposes to cardiac arrhythmias, peripheral vasoconstriction, increased cardiac work, and decreased tissue perfusion. Acepromazine is not contraindicated in geriatric patients, although dose requirements (on an mg/kg basis) may be decreased. Acepromazine is an antiemetic and antiarrhythmic, but one of its most important properties is its anesthetic-sparing effect (Heard et al. 1986). Two studies have examined the effects of acepromazine on systemic blood pressure and glomerular filtration rate (Newell et al. 1997; Bostrom et al. 2003); acepromazine appears to protect renal function, at least in normal dogs, despite a decrease in blood pressure. Preserving renal blood flow and glomerular filtration rate is especially important in older patients, who may have decreased renal reserve or are receiving NSAIDs.

Benzodiazepines such as midazolam and diazepam produce more reliable sedation in older patients than in younger ones. For pre-medication, midazolam has an advantage over diazepam because it can be given IM. These drugs are also reversible with flumazenil should an adverse event occur or if recovery is prolonged. Opioids produce sedation and provide analgesia and should be a part of the anesthetic protocols. Ketamine may cause a significant increase in heart rate and blood pressure, which may be detrimental to some older patients. Propofol can be titrated slowly "to effect" without causing excitement, and when used after pre-medication the dose required for induction is significantly reduced. When preceded by intravenous diazepam or midazolam, induction is smooth and the dose can be significantly reduced (Sanchez et al. 2013). Alfaxalone can also be used as described previously and has a higher therapeutic index than propofol.

Although our older patients may be "more delicate" and challenging to anesthetize, with careful assessment and choice of anesthetic protocols a good outcome should be the rule and not the exception. The key points are that they have less reserve capacity, and when possible anesthesia should be induced with injectable agents (IV) to effect, as they usually require lower drug doses on a mg/kg basis.

Anesthesia of Non-socialized Cats

The term "feral" as applied to cats is not well defined, is used to mean different things within and between countries, and is sometimes interchanged with the terms "free-roaming," "street," or "community cat" (Gosling et al. 2013). See Chapter 25 in this text for more information on these cats and their life histories, and Chapter 35 for information on organizing feral cat clinics. It is important to understand the behavior of these cats when working with them to safeguard both personnel and the welfare of the cats themselves. One proposed definition is "a feral cat is one that is unapproachable in its free-roaming environment and is capable of surviving with or without direct human intervention, and may additionally show fearful or defensive behavior on human contact" (Gosling et al. 2013). One approach to population management is TNVR. This may be done on a small or large scale and the anesthetic protocol is essential to a successful outcome (Williams et al. 2002). Humane traps are used to secure these cats and the cat remains in the trap during transport, for anesthesia, and during recovery; at no time is the cat outside the trap while conscious. Because these cats cannot be handled while awake, no pre-operative evaluation other than a visual assessment of the cat within the trap can be made. Anesthesia must be achieved via IM injection with the cat safely restrained in its trap (Figure 8.2).

The impact of fear on the welfare of feral cats, and on anesthetic and surgical procedures, has been a concern for many working in this field. Administration of gabapentin (50 or 100 mg) compounded into a liquid formulation and given to cats using a catheter (e.g. Tomcat catheter) attached to a syringe had beneficial effects (Pankratz et al. 2018; see Chapter 6, Figure 6.17). Feline stress scores decreased with both doses of gabapentin compared to placebo and peak effect occurred at two hours,

no adverse effects were noted (Pankratz et al. 2018). It is likely that cats would eat wet food containing gabapentin, but this should be carefully placed from outside the trap only after they are captured; food should not be baited for trapping unless traps are visited on a regular basis (e.g. two-hourly intervals), as some cats become very somnolent and could become hypothermic.

The ideal anesthetic for this situation would have a high therapeutic index or ratio, constitute a small volume, be suitable for males and females of all ages, produce a rapid onset and predictable duration of surgical anesthesia, but allow cats to recover quickly, incorporate an analgesic agent, and be cost effective (Williams et al. 2002; Harrison et al. 2011). The section on total IM anesthesia discusses several protocols that would be suited to TNR clinics, for example tiletamine/zolazepam/butorphanol/dexmedetomidine and dexmedetomidine/ketamine/butorphanol.

Monitoring Anesthetized Patients

Monitoring individual cats in large-scale clinics where the throughput can be higher than 50 cats per hour presents some unique challenges (Williams et al. 2002). The American College of Veterinary Anesthesia and Analgesia (www.acvaa.org/docs/Small_Animal_Monitoring_2009.doc) and the Association of Shelter Veterinarians (Association of Shelter Veterinarians' Veterinary Task Force to Advance et al. 2016) have crafted guidelines for monitoring of anesthetized patients, but in some situations adhering to these may not be possible. Many clinics have limited personnel and monitoring equipment. However, trained, vigilant staff and volunteers can recognize problems rapidly and intervene. Mucus membrane color and respiration can be monitored by observation. Pulse quality, rate, and rhythm can be assessed by palpation and the heart can be auscultated. Depth of anesthesia is judged on jaw

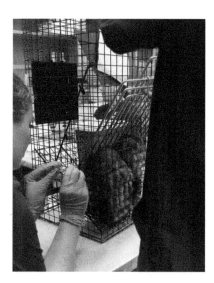

Figure 8.2 Correct restraint of an unsocialized cat within a humane trap, using a comb for intramuscular injection.

tone, eye position, and response to noxious stimuli. Purchasing of monitoring equipment is highly recommended, but it should be carefully chosen. The use of pulse oximetry is encouraged because this modality provides an objective auditory and visual means of determining the presence of a pulse, pulse rate, and adequacy of oxygenation; use of pulse oximetry monitors has been shown to decrease the risk of anesthetic death in cats (Brodbelt et al. 2007). Doppler ultrasound is also valuable as it confirms blood flow (circulation) and allows a pulse rate to be counted when placed over an artery, can be used on any size patient, and with the addition of a sphygmomanometer and blood pressure cuff allows systolic blood pressure to be measured. Further information on anesthetic monitoring can be found in Chapter 10.

References

Aleman, M., Weich, K.M., and Madigan, J.E. (2017). Survey of veterinarians using a novel physical compression squeeze procedure in the management of neonatal maladjustment syndrome in foals. *Animals (Basel)* 7: E69.

Association of Shelter Veterinarians' Veterinary Task Force to Advance, S.-N, Griffin, B., Bushby, P.A. et al. (2016). The Association of Shelter Veterinarians' 2016 veterinary medical care guidelines for spay-neuter programs. *JAVMA* 249: 165–188.

Benito, J., Monteiro, B., Lavoie, A.M. et al. (2016a). Analgesic efficacy of intraperitoneal administration of bupivacaine in cats. *J. Feline Med. Surg.* 18: 906–912.

Benito, J., Monteiro, B.P., Beaudry, F. et al. (2016b). Pharmacokinetics of bupivacaine after intraperitoneal administration to cats undergoing ovariohysterectomy. *Am. J. Vet. Res.* 77: 641–645.

Benito, J., Monteiro, B., Beaudry, F., and Steagall, P. (2018). Efficacy and pharmacokinetics of bupivacaine with epinephrine or dexmedetomidine after intraperitoneal administration in cats undergoing ovariohysterectomy. *Can. J. Vet. Res.* 82: 124–130.

Bortolami, E., Slingsby, L., and Love, E.J. (2012). Comparison of two formulations of buprenorphine in cats administered by the oral transmucosal route. *J. Feline Med. Surg.* 14: 534–539.

Bostrom, I., Nyman, G., Kampa, N. et al. (2003). Effects of acepromazine on renal function in anesthetized dogs. *Am. J. Vet. Res.* 64: 590–598.

Boveri, S., Brearley, J.C., and Dugdale, A.H. (2013). The effect of body condition on propofol requirement in dogs. *Vet. Anaesth. Analg.* 40: 449–454.

Brodbelt, D.C., Pfeiffer, D.U., Young, L.E., and Wood, J.L. (2007). Risk factors for anaesthetic-related death in cats: results from the confidential enquiry into perioperative small animal fatalities (CEPSAF). *Br. J. Anaesth.* 99: 617–623.

Brodbelt, D.C., Pfeiffer, D.U., Young, L.E., and Wood, J.L. (2008). Results of the confidential enquiry into perioperative small animal fatalities regarding risk factors for anesthetic-related death in dogs. *JAVMA* 233: 1096–1104.

Brondani, J.T., Loureiro Luna, S.P., Beier, S.L. et al. (2009). Analgesic efficacy of perioperative use of vedaprofen, tramadol or their combination in cats undergoing ovariohysterectomy. *J. Feline Med. Surg.* 11: 420–429.

Brooks, V.L. and Keil, L.C. (1994). Hemorrhage decreases arterial pressure sooner in pregnant compared with nonpregnant dogs: role of baroreflex. *Am. J. Phys.* 266: H1610–H1619.

Bruniges, N., Taylor, P.M., and Yates, D. (2016). Injectable anaesthesia for adult cat and kitten castration: effects of medetomidine, dexmedetomidine and atipamezole on recovery. *J. Feline Med. Surg.* 18: 860–867.

Bubalo, V., Moens, Y.P., Holzmann, A., and Coppens, P. (2008). Anaesthetic sparing effect of local anaesthesia of the ovarian pedicle during ovariohysterectomy in dogs. *Vet. Anaesth. Analg.* 35: 537–542.

Bushby, P.A. and Griffin, B. (2011). An overview of pediatric spay and neuter benefits and techniques. *dvm360* (1 February). http://veterinarymedicine.dvm360.com/overview-pediatric-spay-and-neuter-benefits-and-techniques.

Carpenter, R.E., Wilson, D.V., and Evans, A.T. (2004). Evaluation of intraperitoneal and incisional lidocaine or bupivacaine for analgesia following ovariohysterectomy in the dog. *Vet. Anaesth. Analg.* 31: 46–52.

Chan, M.T., Mainland, P., and Gin, T. (1996). Minimum alveolar concentration of halothane and enflurane are decreased in early pregnancy. *Anesthesiology* 85: 782–786.

Chen, X., Mao, G., and Leng, S.X. (2014). Frailty syndrome: an overview. *Clin. Interv. Aging* 9: 433–441.

Cistola, A.M., Golder, F.J., Centonze, L.A. et al. (2004). Anesthetic and physiologic effects of tiletamine, zolazepam, ketamine, and xylazine combination (TKX) in feral cats undergoing surgical sterilization. *J. Feline Med. Surg.* 6: 297–303.

Clarke, K.M. and Hall, L. (1990). A survey of anaesthesia in small animal practice. AVA/BSAVA report. *J. Vet. Anaesth.* 17: 4–10.

Cohen, A.E. and Bennett, S.L. (2015). Oral transmucosal administration of dexmedetomidine for sedation in 4 dogs. *Can. Vet. J.* 56: 1144–1148.

Davila, D., Keeshen, T.P., Evans, R.B., and Conzemius, M.G. (2013). Comparison of the analgesic efficacy of perioperative firocoxib and tramadol administration in dogs undergoing tibial plateau leveling osteotomy. *JAVMA* 243: 225–231.

De Jong, A., Futier, E., Millot, A. et al. (2014). How to preoxygenate in operative room: healthy subjects and situations "at risk". *Ann. Fr. Anesth. Reanim.* 33: 457–461.

DeClue, A.E., Cohn, L.A., Lechner, E.S. et al. (2008). Effects of subanesthetic doses of ketamine on hemodynamic and immunologic variables in dogs with experimentally induced endotoxemia. *Am. J. Vet. Res.* 69: 228–232.

Deutsch, J., Jolliffe, C., Archer, E., and Leece, E.A. (2017). Intramuscular injection of alfaxalone in combination with butorphanol for sedation in cats. *Vet. Anaesth. Analg.* 44: 794–802.

Doebeli, A., Michel, E., Bettschart, R. et al. (2013). Apgar score after induction of anesthesia for canine cesarean section with alfaxalone versus propofol. *Theriogenology* 80: 850–854.

Dyson, D.H., Maxie, M.G., and Schnurr, D. (1998). Morbidity and mortality associated with anesthetic management in small animal veterinary practice in Ontario. *J. Am. Anim. Hosp. Assoc.* 34: 325–335.

Ferreira, T.H., Rezende, M.L., Mama, K.R. et al. (2011). Plasma concentrations and behavioral, antinociceptive, and physiologic effects of methadone after intravenous and oral transmucosal administration in cats. *Am. J. Vet. Res.* 72: 764–771.

Fertziger, A.P., Stein, E.A., and Lynch, J.J. (1974). Letter: suppression of morphine-induced mania in cats. *Psychopharmacologia* 36: 185–187.

Fitzpatrick, C.L., Weir, H.L., and Monnet, E. (2010). Effects of infiltration of the incision site with bupivacaine on postoperative pain and incisional healing in dogs undergoing ovariohysterectomy. *JAVMA* 237: 395–401.

Fudge, J.M., Page, B., Mackrell, A., and Lee, I. (2019). Evaluation of targeted bupivacaine for reducing acute postoperative pain in cats undergoing routine ovariohysterectomy. *J. Feline Med. Surg.* https://doi.org/10.1177/1098612X19826700.

Gin, T. and Chan, M.T. (1994). Decreased minimum alveolar concentration of isoflurane in pregnant humans. *Anesthesiology* 81: 829–832.

Giordano, T., Steagall, P.V., Ferreira, T.H. et al. (2010). Postoperative analgesic effects of intravenous, intramuscular, subcutaneous or oral transmucosal buprenorphine administered to cats undergoing ovariohysterectomy. *Vet. Anaesth. Analg.* 37: 357–366.

Glowaski, M.M. and Wetmore, L.A. (1999). Propofol: application in veterinary sedation and anesthesia. *Clin. Tech. Small Anim. Pract.* 14: 1–9.

Gosling, L., Stavisky, J., and Dean, R. (2013). What is a feral cat? Variation in definitions may be associated with different management strategies. *J. Feline Med. Surg.* 15: 759–764.

Grint, N.J., Murison, P.J., Coe, R.J., and Waterman Pearson, A.E. (2006). Assessment of the influence of surgical technique on postoperative pain and wound tenderness in cats following ovariohysterectomy. *J. Feline Med. Surg.* 8: 15–21.

Grisneaux, E., Pibarot, P., Dupuis, J., and Blais, D. (1999). Comparison of ketoprofen and carprofen administered prior to orthopedic surgery for control of postoperative pain in dogs. *JAVMA* 215: 1105–1110.

Gunn-Moore, D.A., McVee, J., Bradshaw, J.M. et al. (2006). Ageing changes in cat brains demonstrated by beta-amyloid and AT8-immunoreactive phosphorylated tau deposits. *J. Feline Med. Surg.* 8: 234–242.

Haga, H.A., Lykkjen, S., Revold, T., and Ranheim, B. (2006). Effect of intratesticular injection of lidocaine on cardiovascular responses to castration in isoflurane-anesthetized stallions. *Am. J. Vet. Res.* 67: 403–408.

Harrison, K.A., Robertson, S.A., Levy, J.K., and Isaza, N.M. (2011). Evaluation of medetomidine, ketamine and buprenorphine for neutering feral cats. *J. Feline Med. Surg.* 13: 896–902.

Hasiuk, M.M., Brown, D., Cooney, C. et al. (2015). Application of fast-track surgery principles to evaluate effects of atipamezole on recovery and analgesia following ovariohysterectomy in cats anesthetized with dexmedetomidine-ketamine-hydromorphone. *JAVMA* 246: 645–653.

Haskins, S.C. and Patz, J.D. (1990). Ketamine in hypovolemic dogs. *Crit. Care Med.* 18: 625–629.

Hayashi, Y., Sumikawa, K., Maze, M. et al. (1991). Dexmedetomidine prevents epinephrine-induced arrhythmias through stimulation of central alpha 2 adrenoceptors in halothane-anesthetized dogs. *Anesthesiology* 75: 113–117.

Heard, D.J., Webb, A.I., and Daniels, R.T. (1986). Effect of acepromazine on the anesthetic requirement of halothane in the dog. *Am. J. Vet. Res.* 47: 2113–2115.

Hedges, A.R., Pypendop, B.H., Shilo-Benjamini, Y. et al. (2014). Pharmacokinetics of buprenorphine following intravenous and buccal administration in cats, and effects on thermal threshold. *J. Vet. Pharmacol. Ther.* 37: 252–259.

Huuskonen, V., Hughes, J.M., Estaca Banon, E., and West, E. (2013). Intratesticular lidocaine reduces the response to surgical castration in dogs. *Vet. Anaesth. Analg.* 40: 74–82.

Jimenez, C.P., Mathis, A., Mora, S.S. et al. (2012). Evaluation of the quality of the recovery after administration of propofol or alfaxalone for induction of anaesthesia in dogs anaesthetized for magnetic resonance imaging. *Vet. Anaesth. Analg.* 39: 151–159.

Johnson, R.A., Striler, E., Sawyer, D.C., and Brunson, D.B. (1998). Comparison of isoflurane with sevoflurane for anesthesia induction and recovery in adult dogs. *Am. J. Vet. Res.* 59: 478–481.

Joubert, K.E. (2007). Pre-anaesthetic screening of geriatric dogs. *J. S. Afr. Vet. Assoc.* 78: 31–35.

Joyce, A. and Yates, D. (2011). Help stop teenage pregnancy! Early-age neutering in cats. *J. Feline Med. Surg.* 13: 3–10.

Kalchofner Guerrero, K.S., Campagna, I., Bruhl-Day, R. et al. (2016). Intraperitoneal bupivacaine with or without incisional bupivacaine for postoperative analgesia in dogs undergoing ovariohysterectomy. *Vet. Anaesth. Analg.* 43: 571–578.

Kaneko, M., Nakayama, H., Igarashi, N., and Hirose, H. (1993). Relationship between the number of fetuses and the blood constituents of beagles in late pregnancy. *J. Vet. Med. Sci.* 55: 681–682.

Khenissi, L., Nikolayenkova-Topie, O., Broussaud, S., and Touzot-Jourde, G. (2017). Comparison of intramuscular alfaxalone and ketamine combined with dexmedetomidine and butorphanol for castration in cats. *J. Feline Med. Surg.* 19: 791–797.

Ko, J.C. and Berman, A.G. (2010). Anesthesia in shelter medicine. *Top. Companion Anim. Med.* 25: 92–97.

Ko, J.C.H., Thurmon, J.C., and Benson, G.J. (1993). An alternative drug combination for use in declawing and castrating cats. *Vet. Med.* 88: 1061–1065.

Koh, R.B., Isaza, N., Xie, H. et al. (2014). Effects of maropitant, acepromazine, and electroacupuncture on vomiting associated with administration of morphine in dogs. *JAVMA* 244: 820–829.

Kohrs, R. and Durieux, M.E. (1998). Ketamine: teaching an old drug new tricks. *Anesth. Analg.* 87: 1186–1193.

Kreisler, R.E., Cornell, H.N., Smith, V.A. et al. (2019). Use of nalbuphine as a substitute for butorphanol in combination with dexmedetomidine and tiletamine/zolazepam: a randomized non-inferiority trial. *J. Feline Med. Surg.* https://doi.org/10.1177/10986 12X19826715.

Kuusela, E., Raekallio, M., Vaisanen, M. et al. (2001). Comparison of medetomidine and dexmedetomidine as premedicants in dogs undergoing propofol-isoflurane anesthesia. *Am. J. Vet. Res.* 62: 1073–1080.

Lambertini, C., Kluge, K., Lanza-Perea, M. et al. (2018). Comparison of intraperitoneal ropivacaine and bupivacaine for postoperative analgesia in dogs undergoing ovariohysterectomy. *Vet. Anaesth. Analg.* 45: 865–870.

Lascelles, B.D., Cripps, P.J., Jones, A., and Waterman-Pearson, A.E. (1998). Efficacy and kinetics of carprofen, administered preoperatively or postoperatively, for the prevention of pain in dogs undergoing ovariohysterectomy. *Vet. Surg.* 27: 568–582.

Lascelles, B.D. and Robertson, S.A. (2004). Use of thermal threshold response to evaluate the antinociceptive effects of butorphanol in cats. *Am. J. Vet. Res.* 65: 1085–1089.

Lemke, K.A. (2004). Perioperative use of selective alpha-2 agonists and antagonists in small animals. *Can. Vet. J.* 45: 475–480.

Lerche, P., Muir, W.W., and Grubb, T.L. (2002). Mask induction of anaesthesia with isoflurane or sevoflurane in premedicated cats. *J. Small Anim. Pract.* 43: 12–15.

Liao, P.Y., Chang, S.C., Chen, K.S., and Wang, H.C. (2014). Decreased postoperative C-reactive protein production in dogs with pyometra through the use of low-dose ketamine. *J. Vet. Emerg. Crit. Care (San Antonio)* 24: 286–290.

Liao, P., Sinclair, M., Valverde, A. et al. (2017). Induction dose and recovery quality of propofol and alfaxalone with or without midazolam coinduction followed by total intravenous anesthesia in dogs. *Vet. Anaesth. Analg.* 44: 1016–1026.

Liu, B., Fan, L., Balakrishna, S. et al. (2013). TRPM8 is the principal mediator of menthol-induced analgesia of acute and inflammatory pain. *Pain* 154: 2169–2177.

Magnusson, K.R., Scanga, C., Wagner, A.E., and Dunlop, C. (2000). Changes in anesthetic sensitivity and glutamate receptors in the aging canine brain. *J. Gerontol. A Biol. Sci. Med. Sci.* 55: B448–B454.

Mahdmina, A., Evans, A., Yates, D., and White, K.L. (2019). Comparison of the effects of buprenorphine and methadone in combination with medetomidine followed by intramuscular alfaxalone for anaesthesia of cats undergoing ovariohysterectomy. *J. Feline Med. Surg.* https://doi.org/10.1177/10986 12X19826357.

Mama, K.R., Gaynor, J.S., Harvey, R.C. et al. (2013). Multicenter clinical evaluation of a multi-dose folrmulation of propofol in the dog. *BMC Vet. Res.* 9.

Mathews, K., Kronen, P.W., Lascelles, D. et al. (2014). Guidelines for recognition, assessment and treatment of pain: WSAVA Global Pain Council members and co-authors of this document. *J. Small Anim. Pract.* 55: E10–E68.

McKune, C.M., Pascoe, P.J., Lascelles, B.D., and Kass, P.H. (2014). The challenge of evaluating pain and a pre-incisional local anesthetic block. *PeerJ* 2: e341.

McMillan, M.W., Seymour, C.J., and Brearley, J.C. (2012). Effect of intratesticular lidocaine on isoflurane requirements in dogs undergoing routine castration. *J. Small Anim. Pract.* 53: 393–397.

McNally, E.M., Robertson, S.A., and Pablo, L.S. (2009). Comparison of time to desaturation between preoxygenated and nonpreoxygenated dogs following sedation with acepromazine maleate and morphine and induction of anesthesia with propofol. *Am. J. Vet. Res.* 70: 1333–1338.

McSweeney, P.M., Martin, D.D., Ramsey, D.S., and McKusick, B.C. (2012). Clinical efficacy and safety of dexmedetomidine used as a preanesthetic prior to general anesthesia in cats. *JAVMA* 240: 404–412.

Mellor, D.J. (2010). Galloping colts, fetal feelings, and reassuring regulations: putting animal-welfare science into practice. *J. Vet. Med. Educ.* 37: 94–100.

Mellor, D.J. and Diesch, T.J. (2006). Onset of sentience: potential for suffering in fetal and neonatal farm animals. *Appl. Anim. Behav. Sci.* 100: 45–57.

Metcalfe, S., Hulands-Nave, A., Bell, M. et al. (2014). Multicentre, randomised clinical trial evaluating the efficacy and safety of alfaxalone administered to bitches for induction of anaesthesia prior to caesarean section. *Aust. Vet. J.* 92: 333–338.

Moldal, E.R., Eriksen, T., Kirpensteijn, J. et al. (2012). Intratesticular and subcutaneous lidocaine alters the intraoperative haemodynamic responses and heart rate variability in male cats undergoing castration. *Vet. Anaesth. Analg.* 40: 63–73.

Moon, P.F., Erb, H.N., Ludders, J.W. et al. (1998). Perioperative management and mortality rates of dogs undergoing cesarean section in the United States and Canada. *JAVMA* 213: 365–369.

Muir, W.W. 3rd, Wiese, A.J., and March, P.A. (2003). Effects of morphine, lidocaine, ketamine, and morphine-lidocaine-ketamine drug combination on minimum alveolar concentration in dogs anesthetized with isoflurane. *Am. J. Vet. Res.* 64: 1155–1160.

Murrell, J. (2011). Clinical use of methadone in cats and dogs. *Companion Anim.* 16: 56–61.

Murrell, J.C. and Hellebrekers, L.J. (2005). Medetomidine and dexmedetomidine: a review of cardiovascular effects and antinociceptive properties in the dog. *Vet. Anaesth. Analg.* 32: 117–127.

Neal, J.M., Bernards, C.M., Butterworth, J.F.t. et al. (2010). ASRA practice advisory on local anesthetic systemic toxicity. *Reg. Anesth. Pain Med.* 35: 152–161.

Nejamkin, P., Cavilla, V., Clausse, M. et al. (2019). Sedative and physiologic effects of tiletamine-zolazepam following buccal administration in cats. *J. Feline Med. Surg.* https://doi.org/10.1177/1098612X19827116.

Newell, S.M., Ko, J.C., Ginn, P.E. et al. (1997). Effects of three sedative protocols on glomerular filtration rate in clinically normal dogs. *Am. J. Vet. Res.* 58: 446–450.

Nickalls, R.W. and Mapleson, W.W. (2003). Age-related iso-MAC charts for isoflurane, sevoflurane and desflurane in man. *Br. J. Anaesth.* 91: 170–174.

Niedfeldt, R.L. and Robertson, S.A. (2006). Postanesthetic hyperthermia in cats: a retrospective comparison between hydromorphone and buprenorphine. *Vet. Anaesth. Analg.* 33: 381–389.

O'Hagan, B., Pasloske, K., McKinnon, C. et al. (2012a). Clinical evaluation of alfaxalone as an anaesthetic induction agent in dogs less than 12 weeks of age. *Aust. Vet. J.* 90: 346–350.

O'Hagan, B.J., Pasloske, K., McKinnon, C. et al. (2012b). Clinical evaluation of alfaxalone as an anaesthetic induction agent in cats less than 12 weeks of age. *Aust. Vet. J.* 90: 395–401.

Pankratz, K.E., Ferris, K.K., Griffith, E.H., and Sherman, B.L. (2018). Use of single-dose oral gabapentin to attenuate fear responses in cage-trap confined community cats: a double-blind, placebo-controlled field trial. *J. Feline Med. Surg.* 20: 535–543.

Pascoe, P.J. and Moon, P.F. (2001). Periparturient and neonatal anesthesia. *Vet. Clin. North Am. Small Anim. Pract.* 31 (315–40): vii.

Perez, T.E., Grubb, T.L., Greene, S.A. et al. (2013). Effects of intratesticular injection of bupivacaine and epidural administration of morphine in dogs undergoing castration. *JAVMA* 242: 631–642.

Pettifer, G. and Dyson, D. (2000). Hydromorphone: a cost-effective alternative to the use of oxymorphone. *Can. Vet. J.* 41: 135–137.

Polson, S., Taylor, P.M., and Yates, D. (2013). Effects of age and reproductive status on postoperative pain after routine ovariohysterectomy in cats. *J. Feline Med. Surg.* 16 (2): 170–176.

Posner, L.P., Gleed, R.D., Erb, H.N., and Ludders, J.W. (2007). Post-anesthetic hyperthermia in cats. *Vet. Anaesth. Analg.* 34: 40–47.

Posner, L.P., Pavuk, A.A., Rokshar, J.L. et al. (2010). Effects of opioids and anesthetic drugs on body temperature in cats. *Vet. Anaesth. Analg.* 37: 35–43.

Pottie, R.G., Dart, C.M., and Perkins, N.R. (2008). Speed of induction of anaesthesia in dogs administered halothane, isoflurane, sevoflurane or propofol in a clinical setting. *Aust. Vet. J.* 86: 26–31.

Pozzi, A., Muir, W.W., and Traverso, F. (2006). Prevention of central sensitization and pain by N-methyl-D-aspartate receptor antagonists. *JAVMA* 228: 53–60.

Pypendop, B.H. and Ilkiw, J.E. (2008). Pharmacokinetics of tramadol, and its metabolite O-desmethyl-tramadol, in cats. *J. Vet. Pharmacol. Ther.* 31: 52–59.

Pypendop, B.H. and Ilkiw, J.E. (2014). Relationship between plasma dexmedetomidine concentration and sedation score and thermal threshold in cats. *Am. J. Vet. Res.* 75: 446–452.

Pypendop, B.H., Ilkiw, J.E., and Shilo-Benjamini, Y. (2014). Bioavailability of morphine, methadone, hydromorphone, and oxymorphone following buccal administration in cats. *J. Vet. Pharmacol. Ther.* 37: 295–300.

Pypendop, B.H., Siao, K.T., and Ilkiw, J.E. (2009). Effects of tramadol hydrochloride on the thermal threshold in cats. *Am. J. Vet. Res.* 70: 1465–1470.

Reed, R. and Doherty, T. (2018). Minimum alveolar concentration: key concepts and a review of its pharmacological reduction in dogs. Part 1. *Res. Vet. Sci.* 117: 266–270.

Ribas, T., Bublot, I., Junot, S. et al. (2015). Effects of intramuscular sedation with alfaxalone and butorphanol on echocardiographic measurements in healthy cats. *J. Feline Med. Surg.* 17: 530–536.

Robertson, S.A. and Taylor, P.M. (2004). Pain management in cats—past, present and future. Part 2. Treatment of pain—clinical pharmacology. *J. Feline Med. Surg.* 6: 321–333.

Robertson, S.A., Lascelles, B.D., Taylor, P.M., and Sear, J.W. (2005). PK-PD modeling of buprenorphine in cats: intravenous and oral transmucosal administration. *J. Vet. Pharmacol. Ther.* 28: 453–460.

Robertson, S.A., Wegner, K., and Lascelles, B.D. (2009). Antinociceptive and side-effects of hydromorphone after subcutaneous administration in cats. *J. Feline Med. Surg.* 11: 76–81.

Rodrigo-Mocholi, D., Escudero, E., Belda, E. et al. (2018). Pharmacokinetics and effects of alfaxalone after intravenous and intramuscular administration to cats. *N. Z. Vet. J.* 66: 172–177.

Sanchez, A., Belda, E., Escobar, M. et al. (2013). Effects of altering the sequence of midazolam and propofol during co-induction of anaesthesia. *Vet. Anaesth. Analg.* 40: 359–366.

Santos, L.C., Ludders, J.W., Erb, H.N. et al. (2011). A randomized, blinded, controlled trial of the antiemetic effect of ondansetron on dexmedetomidine-induced emesis in cats. *Vet. Anaesth. Analg.* 38: 320–327.

Savvas, I., Papazoglou, L.G., Kazakos, G. et al. (2008). Incisional block with bupivacaine for analgesia after celiotomy in dogs. *J. Am. Anim. Hosp. Assoc.* 44: 60–66.

Schutter, A.F., Tunsmeyer, J., and Kastner, S.B.R. (2017). Influence of tramadol on acute thermal and mechanical cutaneous nociception in dogs. *Vet. Anaesth. Analg.* 44: 309–316.

Shah, M., Yates, D., Hunt, J., and Murrell, J. (2018). Comparison between methadone and buprenorphine within the QUAD protocol for perioperative analgesia in cats undergoing ovariohysterectomy. *J. Feline Med. Surg.* 21 (8): 723–731. https://doi.org/10.1177/10986 12X18798840.

Shih, A.C., Robertson, S., Isaza, N. et al. (2008). Comparison between analgesic effects of buprenorphine, carprofen, and buprenorphine with carprofen for canine ovariohysterectomy. *Vet. Anaesth. Analg.* 35: 69–79.

Sinclair, M.D. (2003). A review of the physiological effects of alpha2-agonists related to the clinical use of medetomidine in small animal practice. *Can. Vet. J.* 44: 885–897.

Slingsby, L.S. and Taylor, P.M. (2008). Thermal antinociception after dexmedetomidine administration in cats: a dose-finding study. *J. Vet. Pharmacol. Ther.* 31: 135–142.

Slingsby, L.S., Taylor, P.M., and Monroe, T. (2009). Thermal antinociception after dexmedetomidine administration in cats: a comparison between intramuscular and oral transmucosal administration. *J. Feline Med. Surg.* 11: 829–834.

Slingsby, L.S. and Waterman-Pearson, A.E. (2000a). The post-operative analgesic effects of ketamine after canine ovariohysterectomy--a comparison between pre- or post-operative administration. *Res. Vet. Sci.* 69: 147–152.

Slingsby, L.S. and Waterman-Pearson, A.E. (2000b). Postoperative analgesia in the cat after ovariohysterectomy by use of carprofen, ketoprofen, meloxicam or tolfenamic acid. *J. Small Anim. Pract.* 41: 447–450.

Stathopoulou, T.R., Kouki, M., Pypendop, B.H. et al. (2018). Evaluation of analgesic effect and absorption of buprenorphine after buccal administration in cats with oral disease. *J. Feline Med. Surg.* 20: 704–710.

Steagall, P.V., Monteiro-Steagall, B.P., and Taylor, P.M. (2014). A review of the studies using buprenorphine in cats. *J. Vet. Intern. Med.* 28: 762–770.

Steagall, P.V., Pelligand, L., Giordano, T. et al. (2013). Pharmacokinetic and pharmacodynamic modelling of intravenous, intramuscular and subcutaneous buprenorphine in conscious cats. *Vet. Anaesth. Analg.* 40: 83–95.

Steagall, P.V., Taylor, P.M., Rodrigues, L.C. et al. (2009). Analgesia for cats after ovariohysterectomy with either buprenorphine or carprofen alone or in combination. *Vet. Rec.* 164: 359–363.

Stevens, B.J., Posner, L.P., Jones, C.A., and Lascelles, B.D. (2013). Comparison of the effect of intratesticular lidocaine/bupivacaine vs. saline placebo on pain scores and incision site reactions in dogs undergoing routine castration. *Vet. J.* 196: 499–503.

Swaffield, M.J., Molloy, S.L., and Lipscomb, V.J. (2019). Prospective comparison of perioperative wound and pain score parameters in cats undergoing flank vs midline ovariectomy. *J. Feline Med. Surg.* https://doi.org/10.1177/1098612X19837038.

Tan, E.K. and Tan, E.L. (2013). Alterations in physiology and anatomy during pregnancy. *Best Pract. Res. Clin. Obstet. Gynaecol.* 27: 791–802.

Taylor, P.M., Chengelis, C.P., Miller, W.R. et al. (2012). Evaluation of propofol containing 2% benzyl alcohol preservative in cats. *J. Feline Med. Surg.* 14: 516–526.

Taylor, P.M., Kirby, J.J., Robinson, C. et al. (2010). A prospective multi-centre clinical trial to compare buprenorphine and butorphanol for postoperative analgesia in cats. *J. Feline Med. Surg.* 12: 247–255.

Taylor, P.M., Robertson, S.A., Dixon, M.J. et al. (2001). Morphine, pethidine and buprenorphine disposition in the cat. *J. Vet. Pharmacol. Ther.* 24: 391–398.

Thies, M., Bracker, K., and Sinnott, V. (2017). Retrospective evaluation of the effectiveness of xylazine for inducing emesis in cats: 48 cats (2011-2015). *J. Vet. Emerg. Crit. Care (San Antonio)* 27: 658–661.

Tobias, K.M., Marioni-Henry, K., and Wagner, R. (2006). A retrospective study on the use of acepromazine maleate in dogs with seizures. *J. Am. Anim. Hosp. Assoc.* 42: 283–289.

Tranquilli, W.J., Thurmon, J.C., Benson, G.J., and Davis, L.E. (1986). Alteration in the arrhythmogenic dose of epinephrine (ADE) following xylazine administration to halothane-anesthetized dogs. *J. Vet. Pharmacol. Ther.* 9: 198–203.

Valverde, A., Cantwell, S., Hernandez, J., and Brotherson, C. (2004). Effects of acepromazine on the incidence of vomiting associated with opioid administration in dogs. *Vet. Anaesth. Analg.* 31: 40–45.

Wagner, A.E. (1999). Is butorphanol analgesic in dogs and cats? *Vet. Med.* 94: 346–351.

Wagner, A.E., Walton, J.A., Hellyer, P.W. et al. (2002). Use of low doses of ketamine administered by constant rate infusion as an adjunct for postoperative analgesia in dogs. *JAVMA* 221: 72–75.

Warne, L.N., Beths, T., Holm, M., and Bauquier, S.H. (2013). Comparison of perioperative analgesic efficacy between methadone and butorphanol in cats. *JAVMA* 243: 844–850.

Warne, L.N., Beths, T., Holm, M. et al. (2014). Evaluation of the perioperative analgesic efficacy of buprenorphine, compared with butorphanol, in cats. *JAVMA* 245: 195–202.

Wegner, K. and Robertson, S.A. (2007). Dose-related thermal antinociceptive effects of intravenous hydromorphone in cats. *Vet. Anaesth. Analg.* 34: 132–138.

White, S.C. (2012). Prevention of fetal suffering during ovariohysterectomy of pregnant animals. *JAVMA* 240: 1160–1163.

Willey, J.L., Julius, T.M., Claypool, S.P., and Clare, M.C. (2016). Evaluation and comparison of xylazine hydrochloride and dexmedetomidine hydrochloride for the induction of emesis in cats: 47 cases (2007–2013). *JAVMA* 248: 923–928.

Williams, L.S., Levy, J.K., Robertson, S.A. et al. (2002). Use of the anesthetic combination of tiletamine, zolazepam, ketamine, and xylazine for neutering feral cats. *JAVMA* 220: 1491–1495.

Yamashita, K., Iwasaki, Y., Umar, M.A., and Itami, T. (2009). Effect of age on minimum alveolar concentration (MAC) of sevoflurane in dogs. *J. Vet. Med. Sci.* 71: 1509–1512.

Zhang, J.H., Sampogna, S., Morales, F.R., and Chase, M.H. (2005). Age-related ultrastructural changes in hypocretinergic terminals in the brainstem and spinal cord of cats. *Neurosci. Lett.* 373: 171–174.

Zilberstein, L.F., Moens, Y.P., and Leterrier, E. (2008). The effect of local anaesthesia on anaesthetic requirements for feline ovariectomy. *Vet. J.* 178: 214–218.

Resources

Global Pain Council Guidelines: guidelines for recognition, assessment and treatment of pain. The Global Pain Treatise is a downloadable, open access practical resource to assist practitioners around the world by providing guidance in recognizing and assessing pain. It is available in multiple languages. http://www.wsava.org/WSAVA/media/Documents/Guidelines/Recognition-Assessment-and-Treatment-of-Pain-Guidelines.pdf.

2018 AAFP Feline Anesthesia Guidelines. Open access at https://catvets.com/guidelines/practice-guidelines/anesthesia-guidelines.

2015 AAHA/AAFP Pain Management Guidelines for Dogs and Cats. Open access at https://catvets.com/guidelines/practice-guidelines/pain-management-guidelines.

Association of Shelter Veterinarians' 2016 Veterinary Medical Care Guidelines for Spay-Neuter Programs. Open access at https://avmajournals.avma.org/doi/pdf/10.2460/javma.249.2.165.

9

Special Considerations for Anesthesia of Pediatric Patients

Emily McCobb and Sheilah Robertson

Neutering of dogs and cats prior to adoption and before puberty is an important strategy for controlling pet overpopulation. Thus, in many settings such as shelters or rehoming and rescue organizations, 6–16 weeks of age has become the new conventional age for ovario-hysterectomy, ovariectomy, and castration, and these procedures are no longer considered as "early-age neutering." As veterinarians become more comfortable with the concept of pediatric spaying and neutering, pet dogs and cats outside the shelter environment may also be neutered at an increasingly younger age. A discussion of the positive and potentially negative health benefits of neutering prior to puberty are discussed elsewhere in Chapter 26.

In cats and dogs, the pediatric period can be defined as the period between 6 weeks (which marks the end of the neonatal period) and 12 weeks of age (Pettifer and Grubb 2007). Puppies and kittens can be defined as dogs and cats less than six months of age. Performing elective surgery at a young age is considered sound practice due to advances in anesthesia care and our increased understanding of the unique physiology of this age group. In addition, there is some evidence, at least in cats, that it may be less painful (Polson et al. 2014). With a few simple precautions, puppies and kittens as young as six weeks can be successfully anesthetized.

Because of their relatively small size, lack of physiologic reserves, incomplete immunity,

and susceptibility to the stress of handling and separation from their dam, all puppies and kittens should be considered a special category of anesthesia patient until at least five or six months of age. The risks of anesthesia are not increased in young, healthy animals undergoing elective procedures which are performed rapidly and efficiently (Levy et al. 2017). In contrast, a large study in general veterinary practices found that the risk of anesthetic death in cats weighing less than 2 kg was over 15 times greater than that of cats between 2 and 6 kg (Brodbelt et al. 2007). In addition, the risk of anesthetic death was higher in dogs weighing <5 kg compared to dogs weighting 5–15 kg, suggesting size is a risk factor that is independent of age; these cats and dogs underwent a variety of surgical or diagnostic procedures, with duration of anesthesia being an additional risk factor (Brodbelt et al. 2008a, b). Therefore, kittens and puppies deserve special consideration both for their unique physiology and for their small size.

Characteristics of Pediatric Patients: Physiology

The unique physiologic features of pediatric cats and dogs have been reviewed (Grandy and Dunlop 1991; Pettifer and Grubb 2007). Pediatric patients have limited reserves of all body systems and a limited ability to respond to events that

High-Quality, High-Volume Spay and Neuter and Other Shelter Surgeries, First Edition. Edited by Sara White.
© 2020 John Wiley & Sons, Inc. Published 2020 by John Wiley & Sons, Inc.

challenge homeostasis. The role of a high resting basal metabolic rate in determining the pediatric patient's response to anesthesia should not be underestimated. The pediatric heart is relatively small for the size of the patient; ventricular compliance is low and stroke volume is relatively fixed. Low cardiac reserves are compounded by a high cardiac index (volume of blood pumped per minute indexed to body size: $l/min/m^2$), leading to an overall decreased ability to compensate for or respond to fluid losses and hypotension. Because the circulatory fluid volume of a pediatric patient is relatively fixed, these patients are particularly dependent on heart rate for the maintenance of cardiac output (heart rate × stroke volume) and organ perfusion (Friedman 1972; Grandy and Dunlop 1991). Any decrease in heart rate in a pediatric patient could therefore have serious consequences, and it should be noted that one of the most common causes of bradycardia is hypothermia. In addition to the lack of reserves, the autonomic nervous system, especially sympathetic control, is thought to be poorly developed in pediatric patients, leading to poor vasomotor control and responses. In particular, the baroreceptor response to hypotension may be incomplete, leading to an inadequate response in the face of a fall in blood pressure (Grandy and Dunlop 1991). Lastly, persistent fetal circulation may be present in some pediatric patients, leading to shunting and hypoxemia.

Like the pediatric cardiovascular system, the pediatric respiratory system is also characterized by a lack of reserves. While tidal volumes (TV) are similar to those of the adult animal (10–15 ml/kg), the pediatric respiratory rate (RR) must be two to three times higher in order to provide an appropriate minute ventilation (TV × RR) to meet the patient's high oxygen demand (Parot et al. 1984). An important clinical consequence of a faster RR is a shorter induction time in neonates when inhalant agents are used, although this may be counteracted by their high cardiac output and may be less obvious when using today's less soluble inhalant agents, such as isoflurane and sevoflurane. With a high resting metabolic rate, a high oxygen demand, and high baseline minute ventilation, the pediatric patient is at high risk of becoming hypoxemic and is poorly able to adapt to decreases in oxygen delivery. The heart is entirely dependent on aerobic metabolism, therefore any decrease in oxygen supply results in rapid decompensation. The nares and trachea of pediatric patients are small and susceptible to obstruction; the small airways and alveoli are also prone to collapse (Grandy and Dunlop 1991). The extremely pliant rib cage increases the work of breathing in pediatric patients, which can predispose them to ventilation fatigue and further increase the risk of hypoxemia. Ventilation of pediatric patients should be monitored and supported when necessary.

By eight weeks of age most physiologic processes related to renal and hepatic function should be relatively normal, although organ reserves may still be limited. After the age of six weeks there is no rationale for altering drug doses in animals to account for hepatic clearance (Papich 2013). However, hepatic glycogen stores are low, which increases the risk for hypoglycemia, especially if the patient is fasted for more than a short period (see section on patient preparation in this chapter).

Perhaps the single most important feature of the pediatric patient that affects anesthesia is body composition. Pediatric patients have significantly less body fat and muscle compared to adult animals and a high body water content; this may be as high as 85% in the neonate compared to 60% in mature animals (Papich 2013). These features, in addition to a high body surface area to mass ratio and a limited ability to vasoconstrict to conserve heat, contribute to a limited ability to thermoregulate, exposing them to the risks of hypothermia.

Characteristics of Pediatric Patients: Anatomy

Anatomic characteristics of puppies and kittens that are relevant to anesthesia include their high body surface areas to mass ratio and a high lean body mass compared to body fat. These features predispose the pediatric patient to hypothermia, which is perhaps the most devastating complication of anesthesia for young animals. In addition, the tissues of puppies and kittens are delicate and more friable and so gentle handling is essential. Airway anatomy can pose a challenge. The pediatric patient has small nares and the tongue is proportionally very large for the size of the mouth. Intubation can be difficult, and when performed, great care must be taken to avoid any airway trauma resulting in post-operative swelling and obstruction. However, the small trachea creates an increased resistance to airflow and intubation and ventilatory support may be necessary. Finally, the blood–brain barrier is immature in young animals and therefore profound sedative effects of drugs such as opioids and benzodiazepines may be noted.

Characteristics of Pediatric Patients: Pharmacology

While published guidelines exist for the use of medications in neonatal and pediatric human patients, there is little evidence-based guidance for pediatric dogs and cats. Many drugs commonly used in veterinary patients for anesthesia have not been approved for puppies and kittens. For example, while the non-steroidal anti-inflammatory drug (NSAID) carprofen (Rimadyl®, Zoetis, Parsippany, NJ) is labeled for dogs 12 weeks and older and robenacoxib is labeled for 16 weeks and older in cats, some other NSAIDs are not labeled for dogs or cats less than six months of age. Although NSAIDs are used to promote closure of patent ductus arteriosus in human neonates, there is concern with using them for other purposes including analgesia because of the important role of prostaglandins in the neonatal development of numerous organs and their physiologic action in sleep cycles, cerebral blood flow, and renal hemodynamics (Morris et al. 2003; Aranda et al. 2009). Data on the safety of this group of drugs

in this age group has not grown in parallel with the availability of new compounds. The use of NSAIDs for perioperative pain management continues to be evaluated (Morris et al. 2003; Aranda et al. 2009).

As mentioned, most organ function has reached adult capacity by the time many puppies and kittens undergo elective surgery (Grandy and Dunlop 1991), but there are other features of the pediatric patient that affect drug distribution, including the large percentage of body water, reduced plasma albumin levels, and lower percentage of body fat. Pediatric patients are therefore considered to be more sensitive to the effects of highly protein-bound drugs such as barbiturates or NSAIDs. Adult levels of the P-450 family of enzymes are not reached until at least five weeks of age (Debracker 1986) and therefore repeated dosing of drugs may result in accumulation of the drug in very young animals. In general, many clinicians are comfortable administering a single dose of a species-approved NSAID to a well-hydrated puppy or kitten over eight weeks old. Clinicians must use their discretion if their clinic protocol includes the off-label use of an NSAID for puppies and kittens, because of the absence of published data on NSAID use in this age group.

Patient Preparation

Pediatric patients are likely more susceptible to the effects of stress than are adults. Studies in neonatal rat pups demonstrate that the increased plasticity of the neonatal brain may increase vulnerability to stress and anxiety disorders later in life (Anand et al. 1999). Animals, particularly those living in shelters, may be presented for surgery during their critical socialization period. It is essential to protect these patients from the risk of fear imprinting, since a bad experience at the time of spay or neuter can translate to a lifetime of fearful or fractious behavior during veterinary visits. Puppies and kittens should be gently handled when they present to the spay–neuter clinic.

Table 9.1 Recommended fasting times prior to anesthesia.

Age weeks	Recommended fasting times[a] Hours
≤4	Do not fast
4–6	Maximum 1–2
6–12	Maximum 2–4
>12	Maximum 6

[a] Fasting times can be shorter if on an all milk and liquid diet.

Littermates should be housed together during transport if possible and should be kept together in the cage until the time of pre-medication. If still with their dam, they should not be separated from her. See Chapter 6 for more information about stress reduction in the spay–neuter clinic.

Fasting times for younger animals should be short to account for their decreased glycogen stores. Suggested fasting times are shown in Table 9.1. During the initial examination the puppy or kitten can be given a small amount of Nutri-Cal™ (Tomlyn, a division of Vétoquinol USA, Fort Worth, TX), or dextrose 50, which can be applied to the gums or placed under the tongue, resulting in transmucosal uptake. If dextrose is to be given peri-operatively during surgery, the concentration should be kept at 2.5% and the total rate should not exceed 0.5 g/kg/hr.

As with all surgery patients, a thorough presurgical physical exam should be conducted prior to sedation or anesthesia. It is especially important to perform a thorough auscultation in case cardiac murmurs have gone undetected. The animal should also be checked carefully for other congenital abnormalities that might affect anesthesia or surgery, such as pectus excavatum, hernias (inguinal or umbilical), and undescended testicles. Lastly, an accurate weight is very important as all drugs should be dosed on a mg/kg or mg/m² basis; "guesstimates" of weight that are off by a small amount with respect to grams can represent a

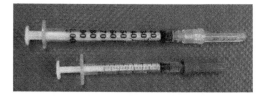

Figure 9.1 To ensure accurate dosing of drugs in small kittens and puppies, dilution of drugs and measurement with 1 ml tuberculin syringes or insulin syringes is recommended.

large percentage of a very small patient's bodyweight, resulting in drug overdose and an adverse response and outcome. To maintain dosing accuracy, drugs may need to be diluted and/or administered with insulin or 1 ml (Tuberculin-type) syringes (Figure 9.1).

Suggested Anesthetic Protocols for Puppies and Kittens

Many pediatric patients, especially kittens, may weigh 1.0 kg or less at the time of surgery, making intravenous access challenging. For this reason, many protocols have been designed so that a balanced general anesthetic can be delivered by a single intramuscular (IM) or subcutaneous (SC) injection. Balanced anesthesia provides unconsciousness, analgesia, and muscle relaxation. An "all-in-one" protocol can be valuable in many settings, as it is less time consuming so increases the number of animals that can be managed in a given period of time, requires less handling of the patient which decreases stress, requires less technical skill, and does not depend on an anesthesia machine fitted with a vaporizer. Some components of the protocol may be reversible (e.g. medetomidine and dexmedetomidine), which hastens recovery.

Alternatively, induction of anesthesia with intravenous anesthetic agents (with or without intravenous catheter placement) is used in some settings and may or may not be followed by delivery of inhalant agents by mask or endotracheal tube. Induction of anesthesia with inhalant agents delivered via a face mask, whether as a sole technique or after sedation, is not recommended due to the hazards of exposing personnel to waste anesthetic gases and the stress this technique poses to patients (also see Chapter 31 on surgeon health for more information on avoiding waste anesthetic gas). In dogs, Brodbelt et al. (2008b) reported that induction and maintenance with inhalant anesthetic agents increased the risk of peri-operative death.

Several anesthetic protocols have been described for use in pediatric patients (Fagella and Aronsohn 1993, 1994; Howe 1997; Root Kustritz 2002; Patel and Yates 2003; Robertson 2007; Joyce and Yates 2011; Polson et al. 2012; Porters et al. 2015).

Opioids and benzodiazepines (e.g. diazepam, midazolam) are generally well tolerated and have the advantage of being reversible with naloxone and flumazenil, respectively, should problems arise. Only midazolam should be used for IM injection; systemic absorption of diazepam from muscle is unreliable and injection is usually resented by the patient. Acepromazine should be used judiciously and at a lower dose (0.01–0.02 mg/kg) than normally used in adults (up to 0.05 mg/kg), as pediatric patients appear to be more sensitive to its effects, resulting in prolonged recoveries. In addition, the vasodilation produced by acepromazine may promote heat loss. Alpha$_2$-adrenergic agonists have been somewhat controversial for use in young animals because of their profound cardiac effects; however, good results have been reported with the combination of medetomidine, ketamine, and buprenorphine in healthy 7- to 12-week-old kittens (Robertson et al. 2003). A total injectable protocol which has included medetomidine and more recently dexmedetomidine in combination with ketamine and butorphanol (Bushby, personal communication, August 2, 2012; Bushby and Griffin 2011) has been used in several thousand puppies and kittens with very few anesthetic deaths. This protocol works well for kittens and puppies for ovariohysterectomy, ovariectomy, and castration surgery and results in rapid recovery to normal function, with most kittens and puppies eating within 30–60 minutes of the procedure. An alternative protocol that is very popular is "TTDex," which includes Telazol, butorphanol (or pure opioid), and dexmedetomidine. This combination is flexible and has been found to be effective and predictable for a wide variety of ages (Ko and Krimins 2019). Finally, the "quad" protocol includes midazolam, medetomidine, ketamine, and either butorphanol or buprenorphine (Polson et al. 2012), and is very popular in the UK, and is suitable for cats of all ages.

Examples of total injectable protocols are given in Tables 9.2 and 9.3.

If not using a total injectable protocol, propofol, ketamine/midazolam, or Telazol® (tiletamine and zolazepam, Zoetis) are all acceptable for induction following sedation. Alfaxalone (Alfaxan®, Jurox, Rutherford, NSW, Australia), a synthetic neuroactive steroid anesthetic, has been evaluated in pediatric cats and dogs (O'Hagan et al. 2012a, b) with good results. Examples of protocols that include sedation followed by IV induction are given in Tables 9.4 and 9.5.

Historically, anticholinergic agents (atropine, glycopyrrolate) have been used to support heart rate, especially in young human and animal patients during anesthesia (Best 2001), but have become less popular over time. The administration of atropine in conjunction with ketamine was standard of care for the sedation of pediatric patients, but critical evaluation has not found it advantageous to include an anticholinergic (Kye et al. 2012). Anticholinergic agents are generally not used in combination with an alpha$_2$-adrenergic agonist agent.

Prior to induction, pre-oxygenation is recommended due to the vulnerability of this age group to hypoxia; if using injectable-only protocols, supplemental oxygen is recommended during anesthesia. The pros and cons of intubation should be considered.

Table 9.2 Suggested total injectable protocols for puppies and kittens aged 6–16 weeks. Add 1 ml dexmedetomidine (500 µgram/ml), 1 ml ketamine (100 mg/ml), and 1 ml butorphanol (10 mg/ml) to a sterile vial, creating 3 ml of the DKB mixture. For cats and small dogs, inject in large muscle belly (of your choice). Occasionally gaseous anesthetic is needed, especially if surgery takes more than 30 minutes. Atipamezole can be used routinely or if the animal is slow to wake up (>30 minutes). Give equal volume to the dexmedetomidine in dogs and half the volume in cats.

DOGS		
Bodyweight (kg)	ml of each drug	ml of mixture
1	0.066	0.20
1.1	0.073	0.22
1.2	0.079	0.24
1.3	0.086	0.26
1.4	0.092	0.28
1.5	0.099	0.30
1.6	0.106	0.32
1.7	0.112	0.34
1.8	0.119	0.36
1.9	0.125	0.38
2	0.132	0.40
2.5	0.132	0.40
3	0.132	0.40
3.5	0.154	0.46
4	0.176	0.53
4.5	0.198	0.59
5	0.220	0.66

CATS		
Bodyweight (kg)	ml of each drug	ml of mixture
0.5	0.044	0.13
0.6	0.053	0.16
0.7	0.062	0.18
0.8	0.070	0.21
0.9	0.075	0.23
1	0.077	0.23
1.1	0.079	0.24
1.2	0.079	0.24
1.3	0.086	0.26
1.4	0.092	0.28
1.5	0.099	0.30
1.6	0.106	0.32
1.7	0.112	0.34
1.8	0.119	0.36
1.9	0.125	0.38
2	0.132	0.40
2.5	0.134	0.40
3	0.135	0.41

Table 9.3 "Quad" protocol for kittens. Use equal volumes of medetomidine (1 mg/ml), ketamine (100 mg/ml), midazolam (5 mg/ml), and buprenorphine (0.3 mg/ml). These can be mixed together in a sterile vial. Medetomidine can be substituted with dexmedetomidine (0.5 mg/ml). Administration is intramuscularly.

Bodyweight (kg)	Volume of each drug (ml)	Medetomidine (μg/kg)	Ketamine (mg/kg)	Buprenorphine (μg/kg)	Midazolam (mg/kg)
0.50	0.04	80.00	8.00	24.00	0.40
1.00	0.06	60.00	6.00	18.00	0.30
1.50	0.08	53.33	5.33	16.00	0.27
2.00	0.10	50.00	5.00	15.00	0.25
2.50	0.12	48.00	4.80	14.40	0.24
3.00	0.13	43.33	4.33	13.00	0.22

Table 9.4 Some suggested anesthetic protocols for puppies aged 6–16 weeks: pre-medication followed by induction with intravenous anesthetic agents.

Pre-medication mg/kg	Induction mg/kg	Maintenance	Analgesics mg/kg	Comments
Morphine 0.5 mg/kg IM and acepromazine 0.02–0.05 mg/kg SC or IM	Telazol 1.5 mg/kg IV	Isoflurane or sevoflurane	Meloxicam 0.1 mg/kg SC Local blocks	Humane Alliance (http://www.humanealliance.org)
Oxymorphone 0.1 mg/kg IM or hydromorphone 0.1 mg/kg IM and Acepromazine 0.02–0.05 mg/kg IM or SC	Propofol 4–6 mg/kg IV (titrate to effect) Or ketamine 5 mg/kg with midazolam or diazepam 0.25 mg/kg IV titrated to effect	Isoflurane or sevoflurane	Carprofen 2 mg/kg SC Local blocks	
Butorphanol 0.2 mg/kg IM Acepromazine 0.05 mg/kg IM Glycopyrrolate 0.01 mg/kg IM (combination known as BAG)	Either propofol or ketamine + midazolam or diazepam (see above)	Isoflurane or sevoflurane	Buprenorphine 0.01 mg/kg IV given at induction NSAIDs and local blocks as above	Useful if the practice does not have Schedule II opioid drugs

IM, intramuscularly; IV, intravenously; NSAIDs, non-steroidal anti-inflammatory drugs; SC, subcutaneously.

Intubation may not be necessary if surgery times are short (<30 minutes) and the patient is adequately ventilating. Studies that look at risks associated with anesthesia showed that, at least in cats, intubation is associated with a higher mortality rate (Brodbelt et al. 2007) for short (<30 minutes) procedures and in these cases a face mask can be used (Figure 9.2). On the other hand, because pediatric patients are poorly tolerant of hypoxemia, and because hypoventilation or apnea can occur, equipment should always be available to perform intubation if needed. When intubating small patients, it is important to take great care to

Table 9.5 Some suggested anesthetic protocols for kittens 6–16 weeks: pre-medication followed by induction with intravenous anesthetic agents.

Pre-medication All drugs are given IM	Induction mg/kg	Maintenance	Analgesics	Comments
Choose one opioid: Morphine 0.5 mg/kg Oxymorphone 0.05 mg/kg Buprenorphine 0.02 mg/kg with acepromazine 0.02–0.05 mg/kg	Propofol 4–6 mg/kg IV (titrate to effect)	Isoflurane or sevoflurane	Meloxicam 0.1 mg/kg SC or robenacoxib 1–2 mg/kg oral or 1–2 mg/kg SC Local blocks	There are no NSAIDs labeled for use in kittens under 6 months in the United States

IM, intramuscularly; IV, intravenously; NSAIDs, non-steroidal anti-inflammatory drugs; SC, subcutaneously.

avoid traumatizing the delicate airway tissues. A laryngoscope should be used to ensure excellent visualization and an adequate depth of anesthesia achieved before attempting to intubate. Puppies are intubated more commonly than kittens, but face masks are also acceptable for short procedures. All brachycephalic dogs and cats should be intubated because of the increased risk of airway obstruction.

A non-rebreathing circuit should be used for patients under 3 kg to deliver oxygen and/or inhalant anesthetic agents.

Patient Management

When the risks and benefits of intravenous catheters are weighed, most clinicians choose not to place them in healthy puppies and kittens in a high-volume spay–neuter setting, as doing so would take up valuable time. Patients may be induced using an IM combination technique or pre-medicated with an opioid and sedative combination, and then induced with an IV injection of induction agent via a syringe and needle. IV fluid support is generally not required in these patients if surgery times are short, although patients may be given SC fluids in recovery.

IV catheter placement can be greatly facilitated if topical local anesthetics are applied over the catheter site and covered with an occlusive dressing (plastic plus a flexible wrap) during the time between sedation and catheter placement (Figure 9.3). A eutectic mixture of lidocaine and prilocaine (EMLA™, 5%, AstraZeneca, Wilmington, DE; prescription only) or lidocaine topical cream (LMX 4%; Ferndale Laboratories, Ferndale, MI; over the counter) can be used, and systemic absorption is minimal (Wagner et al. 2006), although the time to onset can be up to one hour.

If IV fluids are given, crystalloids are used and administered at a rate of 3 ml/kg/h in cats and 5 ml/kg/h in dogs, in accord with the American Animal Hospital Association's fluid therapy guidelines (Davis et al. 2013).

Monitoring

Pediatric patients should be monitored while sedated and anesthetized in a similar fashion to adult patients (Griffin et al. 2016). However, what is practical, possible, and valuable should be given consideration; for example, it may not be in the best interests of the patient or the clinic's goals to spend 5 minutes instrumenting a patient for a procedure that may last less than 10 minutes. In a busy setting when it is not possible to have one person dedicated to monitoring each patient continuously, audible monitors should be used, as these will alert surgeons and other staff to a problem sooner than monitors that only have a visual display. Doppler ultrasound equipment is versatile and can be used on even the smallest of patients. A Doppler unit can be used to monitor heart rate

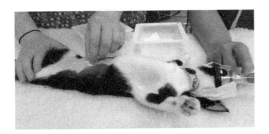

Figure 9.2 It is not recommended to intubate kittens for short (<30 minutes) procedures, but oxygen and inhalant agents can be administered using a face mask. A clear mask allows the color of the mucus membranes to be observed and the rubber diaphragm prevents leaks.

(placed directly on a shaved area over the heart; Figure 9.4), pulse rate (placed on the caudal aspect of the carpus), and blood pressure, which can be measured when the probe is placed on a limb and a blood pressure cuff applied proximally (Figure 9.5).

Pulse oximeters can also be used and decrease the risk of anesthetic-related fatalities in cats (Brodbelt et al. 2007). In dogs and cats, the preferred placement site is the hind paw (Mathews et al. 2003) and a toe can be shaved to help improve contact. The tongue is also commonly used, but may increase the risk of spreading

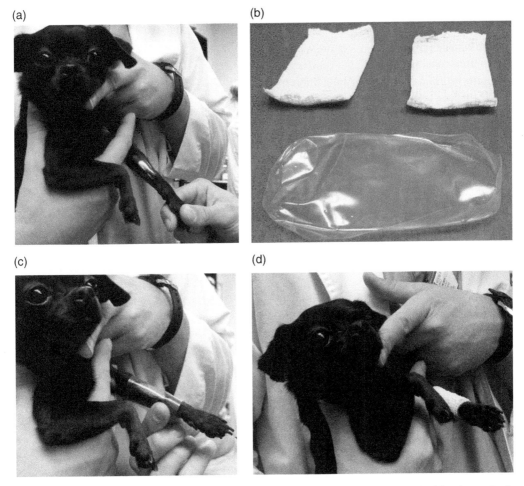

Figure 9.3 If an intravenous catheter is to be placed in a small patient, the use of topical local anesthetics is recommended. The cream is applied over the clipped and cleansed site (a); a plastic covering (e.g. cut from packaging) and a flexible wrap are then used to cover the site (b–d). After the recommended time, the wrapping is removed and the catheter can be placed with minimal response by the patient.

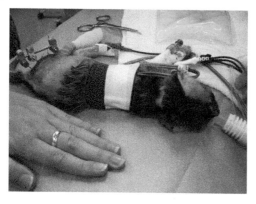

Figure 9.4 A Doppler probe can be placed directly over the heart and secured in place with flexible wrapping to provide an audible method of counting the heart rate. This kitten weighed 450 g and underwent a femur fracture repair.

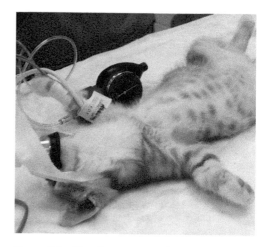

Figure 9.5 Blood pressure can be monitored in small patients by placing a Doppler probe over the digital arteries and a blood pressure cuff proximal to the probe.

infection between patients, so if this site is chosen the probe must be cleaned and disinfected thoroughly between cases. Surgery and fluorescent lighting can interfere with the functioning of pulse oximeters, so the light-emitting diode (LED) and sensor should be covered (Figure 9.6). If an electrocardiogram is used, the "alligator clips" should have their sharp edges filed down, the spring loosened, and a small square of gauze placed between the clips and the skin to avoid damage to delicate skin. The patient's color, capillary refill time, anesthetic depth, and temperature should also be assessed at five-minute intervals, as outlined in the American College of Veterinary Anesthesia and Analgesia (ACVAA) Guidelines (http://www.acvaa.org/docs/Small_Animal_Monitoring_2009.doc). Guidelines for monitoring are also available from the American Animal Hospital Association (AAHA; https://www.aaha.org/aaha-guidelines/aaha-anesthesia-guidelines-for-dogs-and-cats/anesthesia-home).

Pain Management

Contrary to earlier beliefs, young patients do experience pain and its effects may have far-reaching adverse consequences (Johnston et al.

2011). Pain experienced at a young age may lead to dynamic changes in the nociceptive pathway and result in altered responses to noxious stimuli and chronic pain later in life (Anand et al. 1999; Buskila et al. 2003; Allegaert et al. 2013). In addition to these negative effects, pain has adverse physiologic effects, resulting in tachycardia, hypertension, ileus, and immunosuppression.

A balanced anesthetic protocol including multimodal analgesia should be used in pediatric patients; the most practical and commonly used combinations are opioids and NSAIDs, and the concomitant use of these does have benefits over using either group of drug alone (Steagall et al. 2009). Opioids are generally very well tolerated in pediatric patients. As discussed earlier, the use of NSAIDs in puppies and kittens is controversial. Moreover, the available NSAIDs vary with regard to the labeled indications and some are not labeled for dogs and cats less than four to six months of age. The use of local anesthetics is encouraged; these can be injected into the testicles (Moldal et al. 2012; Huuskonen et al. 2013; Stevens et al. 2013) if large enough. In dogs, intratesticular lidocaine

(a)   (b)

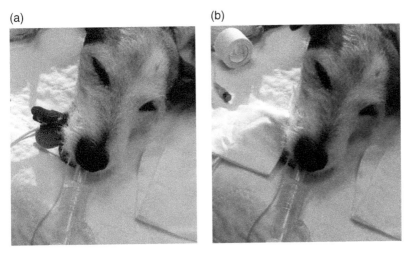

Figure 9.6   (a and b) Fluorescent or operating room lights can interfere with the function of pulse oximeters, therefore the probe should be covered; in (b) a gauze sponge is placed over the probe and this may be wetted to prevent drying of the tongue.

decreased the cardiovascular responses to castration (Huuskonen et al. 2013), but did not have an impact on post-surgery pain scores (Stevens et al. 2013). Intraperitoneal bupivacaine (2 mg/kg) was minimally absorbed into the systemic circulation and was beneficial in cats undergoing ovariohysterectomy (Benito et al. 2016, 2018).

There are several non-pharmacologic methods that can be used to address pain (Johnston et al. 2011); for example, oral sweet solutions are analgesic in pediatric humans and so human infants are often given something sugary at the time of procedures involving noxious stimuli. It is not known if this effect occurs in dogs and cats, and cats are thought not to be able to taste sweet flavors. Other non-pharmacologic strategies can be applied to veterinary patients such as cuddling or swaddling. Swaddling and contact with the mother ("kangaroo care") can diminish pain (Campbell-Yeo et al. 2011). Warmth has also shown to be analgesic in human infants (Gray et al. 2012). Pain is driven by inflammation, therefore minimizing surgical trauma and using the smallest possible incisions (Figure 9.7) will decrease pain in the post-operative period (Kristiansson et al. 1999).

Recovery

Recovery should take place in a warm, quiet, and safe environment. As soon as the puppy or kitten is awake, he or she should be placed back with his littermates and dam if applicable. In addition, the animals should be offered a small amount of soft food as soon as they can swallow. If they are slow to recover (>30 minutes), check their temperature and if this is low apply more aggressive warming strategies. If medetomidine or dexmedetomidine has been used, consider reversing it, or if atipamezole has already been given, consider a second dose. Dextrose 50% or high-fructose corn syrup (e.g. Karo Syrup, ACH Food Companies, Oakbrook Terrace, IL) can be applied to the gums or placed under the tongue, and anecdotally will often rouse puppies and kittens (Figure 9.8). However, recent research indicates that corn syrup is ineffective at raising kitten blood sugar levels and, moreover, kittens were not hypoglycemic after anesthesia that included dexmedetomidine, so routine application of corn syrup for kittens is not necessary (Cornell et al. 2018).

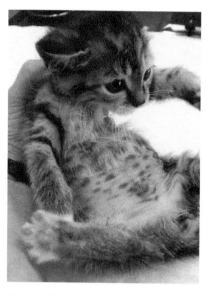

Figure 9.7 Small incisions produce less inflammation than large ones and help to decrease post-operative pain.

Prevention and Treatment of Hypothermia

The single most important thing the anesthetist can do for a pediatric patient is to avoid hypothermia. Hypothermia will decrease the patient's minimum alveolar concentration (MAC, or inhalant dose required to keep the patient unconscious) and increase the risk of inhalant anesthetic overdose. Hypothermic patients will become bradycardic, leading to decreased cardiac output and hypotension. Decreasing core temperature also increases the risk of myocardial irritability and arrhythmias. Clot formation is slower at low temperatures, potentially increasing the risk of bleeding (Taggart et al. 2012). Hypothermic patients have an increased surgical infection rate as well as a decreased immune response (Doufas 2003). Drug elimination will be prolonged and therefore recovery is delayed. Post-operative shivering in these patients increases oxygen demand and myocardial oxygen consumption.

Patient warming devices such as a forced air heating system (Warm Air Heaters, Advanced Anesthesia Specialists, Prescott, AZ) or warming blankets (Hot Dog veterinary patient

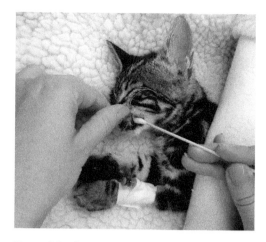

Figure 9.8 Dextrose or high-fructose corn syrup can be applied to the gums and under the tongue during recovery to prevent hypoglycemia.

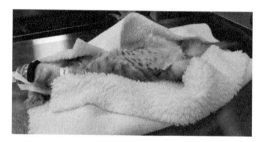

Figure 9.9 Animals should never be placed on a cold surface; a fleece blanket can be dedicated to each animal and travel with it through the clinic from start to finish.

warming system, Augustine Biomedical + Design, Eden Prairie, MN) are ideal, although recirculating warm water blankets can also be used. Kittens and puppies should never be placed on a cold surface and should be covered whenever possible; a good technique is to use one fleece blanket which travels from start to finish with the patient (Figure 9.9). A common technique is to build a "recovery beach" with blankets and a forced warm air unit, where all patients recover until they are normothermic and able to walk (Figure 9.10), as long as they appear visibly healthy. Electric blankets, warm fluid bags, heated disks, and rice bags can burn patients and should not be placed in direct contact with them. The negative effects of hypothermia are discussed fully in Chapter 7.

(a)

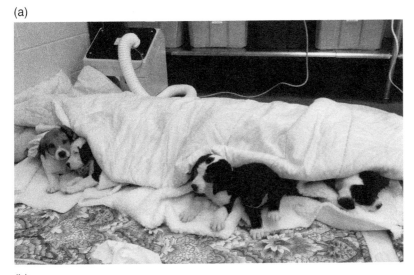

(b)

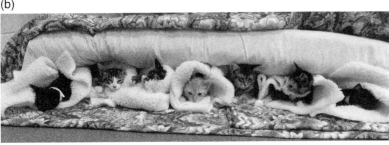

Figure 9.10   (a and b) A "recovery beach" is a set-up where kittens and puppies can recover; blankets are placed on the floor and a forced warm air system is used above the animals to rewarm them. Here they can be monitored and given dextrose or high-fructose corn syrup.

Conclusion

Surgery on puppies and kittens as young as six weeks of age is now routine in many shelter situations. The small size of these patients and their vulnerability to trauma from rough handling or fear imprinting warrant special consideration. Most notably, patients should be handled gently and every precaution should be taken to avoid hypoglycemia and hypothermia. Pediatric patients should be anesthetized using a balanced anesthetic protocol which includes multimodal analgesia. They should be monitored in a similar fashion to older animals, with special attention paid to the patient's heart rate and adequacy of ventilation. Reserves in pediatric patients are limited and the total anesthesia and surgery time should be as short as possible to avoid complications.

References

Allegaert, K., Tibboel, D., and van den Anker, J. (2013). Pharmacological treatment of neonatal pain: in search of a new equipoise. *Sem. Fetal Neonatal Med.* 18 (1): 42–47.

Anand, K.J.S., Coskun, V., Thrivikraman, K.V. et al. (1999). Long-term behavioral effects of repetitive pain in neonatal rat pups. *Physiol. Behav.* 66 (4): 627–637.

Aranda, J.V., Beharry, K.D., and Valencia, G.B. (2009). Nonsteroidal anti-inflammatory drugs (NSAIDs) in the newborn – which ones? *J. Matern. Fetal Neonatal Med.* 22 (Suppl. 3): 21–22.

Benito, J., Monteiro, B., Beaudry, F., and Steagall, P. (2018). Efficacy and pharmacokinetics of bupivacaine with epinephrine or dexmedetomidine after intraperitoneal administration in cats undergoing ovariohysterectomy. *Can. J. Vet. Res.* 82 (2): 124–130.

Benito, J., Monteiro, B., Lavoie, A.M. et al. (2016). Analgesic efficacy of intraperitoneal administration of bupivacaine in cats. *J. Feline Med. Surg.* 18: 906–912.

Best, P. (2001). Use of anticholinergics in veterinary anaesthesia. *Aust. Vet. J.* 79 (1): 22–23.

Brodbelt, D.C., Blissitt, K.J., Hammond, R.A. et al. (2008a). The risk of death: the confidential enquiry into perioperative small animal fatalities. *Veterinary Anaesthesia and Analgesia* 35 (5): 365–373.

Brodbelt, D.C., Pfeiffer, D.U., Young, L.E. et al. (2007). Risk factors for anaesthetic related death in cats: results from the confidential enquiry into perioperative small animal fatalities (CEPSAF). *Br. J. Anaesth.* 99 (5): 617–623.

Brodbelt, D.C., Pfeiffer, D.U., Young, L.E. et al. (2008b). Results of the confidential enquiry into perioperative small animal fatalities regarding risk factors for anesthetic-related death in dogs. *JAVMA* 233 (7): 1096–1104.

Bushby, P. and Griffin, B. (2011). An overview of pediatric spay and neuter benefits and techniques. *dvm360* (1 February). http://veterinarymedicine.dvm360.com/overview-pediatric-spay-and-neuter-benefits-and-techniques.

Buskila, D., Neumann, L., Ehud, Z. et al. (2003). Pain sensitivity in prematurely born adolescents. *Arch. Pediatr. Adolesc. Med.* 157 (11): 1079–1082.

Campbell-Yeo, M., Fernandes, A., and Johnston, C. (2011). Procedural pain management for neonates using non-pharmacological strategies: part 2: mother-driven interventions. *Adv. Neonatal Care* 11 (5): 312–318.

Cornell, H.N., Shaver, S.L., Semick, D.N. et al. (2018). Effect of transmucosal corn syrup application on postoperative blood glucose concentrations in kittens. *J. Feline Med. Surg.* 20 (4): 289–294.

Davis, H., Jensen, T., Johnson, A. et al. (2013). 2013 AAHA/AAFP fluid therapy guidelines for dogs and cats. *J. Am. Anim. Hosp. Assoc.* 49 (3): 149–159.

Debracker, P. (1986). Comparative neonatal pharmacokinetics. In: *Comparative Veterinary Pharmacology, Toxicology and Therapy* (eds. A.S. Van Miert, M.G. Bogaert and M. Debrackert), 161–171. Boston, MA: MTP Press.

Doufas, A.G. (2003). Consequences of inadvertent perioperative hypothermia. *Best Pract. Res. Clin. Anaesthesiol.* 17 (4): 535–549.

Fagella, A.M. and Aronsohn, M.G. (1993). Anesthetic techniques for neutering 6- to 14-week-old kittens. *JAVMA* 202 (1): 56–62.

Fagella, A.M. and Aronsohn, M.G. (1994). Evaluation of anesthetic protocols for neutering 6- to 14-week-old pups. *JAVMA* 205 (2): 308–314.

Friedman, W.F. (1972). The intrinsic physiologic properties of the developing heart. *Prog. Cardiovasc. Dis.* 15 (1): 87–111.

Grandy, J.L. and Dunlop, C.I. (1991). Anesthesia of pups and kittens. *JAVMA* 198 (7): 1244–1249.

Gray, L., Lang, C.W., and Poges, S.W. (2012). Warmth is analgesic in healthy newborns. *Pain* 153 (5): 960–966.

Griffin, B., Bushby, P.A., McCobb, E. et al. (2016). The Association of Shelter Veterinarians' 2016 veterinary medical care guidelines for spay-neuter programs. *JAVMA* 249 (2): 165–188.

Howe, L.M. (1997). Short term results and complications of prepubertal gonadectomy in cats and dogs. *JAVMA* 211 (1): 57–62.

Huuskonen, V., Huges, J.M., Banon, E. et al. (2013). Intratesticular lidocaine reduces the response to surgical castration in dogs. *Vet. Anaesth. Analg.* 40 (1): 74–82.

Johnston, C.C., Fernandes, A.M., and Campbell-Yeo, M. (2011). Pain in neonates is different. *Pain* 152: S65–S73.

Joyce, A. and Yates, D. (2011). Help stop teenage pregnancy! Early-age neutering in cats. *J. Feline Med. Surg.* 13 (1): 3–10.

Ko, J. and Krimins, R.A. (2019). Anesthesia in shelter medicine and high-volume/high quality spay neuter programs. In: *Small Animal Anesthesia and Pain Management*, 2e (ed. J.C. Ko), 419–427. Boca Raton, FL: CRC Press/Taylor and Francis Group.

Kristiansson, M., Sraste, L., Soop, M. et al. (1999). Diminished interleukin-6 and C-reactive protein responses to laparoscopic versus open cholecystectomy. *Acta Anaesthesiol Scandanavia* 43 (2): 146–152.

Kye, Y.C., Rhee, J.E., Kim, K. et al. (2012). Clinical effects of adjunctive atropine during ketamine sedation in pediatric emergency patients. *Am. J. Emerg. Med.* 30 (9): 1981–1085.

Levy, J.K., Bard, K.M., Tucker, S.J. et al. (2017). Perioperative mortality in cats and dogs undergoing spay or castration at a high-volume clinic. *Vet. J.* 224: 11–15.

Mathews, N.S., Hartke, S., and Allen, J.C. Jr. (2003). An evaluation of pulse oximeters in dogs, cats and horses. *Vet. Anaesth. Analg.* 30 (1): 3–14.

Moldal, E.R., Eriksen, T., Kirpensteijn, J. et al. (2012). Intratesticular and subcutaneous lidocaine alters the intraoperative haemodynamic responses and heart rate variability in male cats undergoing castration. *Vet. Anaesth. Analg.* 40 (1): 63–73.

Morris, J.L., Rosen, D.A., and Rosen, K.R. (2003). Nonsteroidal anti-inflammatory agents in neonates. *Paediatr. Drugs* 5 (6): 385–405.

O'Hagan, B.J., Pasloske, K., McKinnon, C. et al. (2012a). Clinical evaluation of alfaxalone as an anaesthetic induction agent in cats lets than 12 weeks of age. *Aust. Vet. J.* 90 (10): 395–401.

O'Hagen, B.J., Pasloske, K.S., McKinnon, C. et al. (2012b). Clinical evaluation of alfaxalone as an anesthetic induction agent in dogs less than 12 weeks of age. *Aust. Vet. J.* 90 (10): 346–350.

Papich, M.G. (2013). Treating animals in special situations: the old and the young: the sick and debilitated. *Proceedings of the 2013 Western Veterinary Conference*, Las Vegas Nevada (17–21 February).

Parot, S., Bonora, M., Gautier, H. et al. (1984). Developmental changes in ventilation and breathing patterns in unanesthetized kittens. *Resp. Physiol.* 58 (3): 253–262.

Patel, C.M. and Yates, D. (2003). Evaluation of an anesthetic protocol for the neutering of eight to twelve week-old puppies. *Vet. Rec.* 152 (14): 439–440.

Pettifer, G. and Grubb, T. (2007). Neonatal and geriatric patients. In: *Lumb and Jones' Veterinary Anesthesia*, 4e (eds. W.J. Tranquilli, J.C. Thurmon and K.A. Grimm), 985–991. Ames, IA: Blackwell.

Polson, S., Taylor, P.M., and Yates, D. (2012). Analgesia after feline ovariohysterectomy under midazolam-medetomidine ketamine anaesthesia with buprenorphine or butorphanol, and carprofen or meloxicam: a prospective, randomized clinical trial. *J. Feline Med. Surg.* 14 (8): 553–559.

Polson, S., Taylor, P.M., and Yates, D. (2014). Effects of age and reproductive status on postoperative pain after routine ovariohysterectomy in cats. *J. Feline Med. Surg.* 16: 170–176.

Porters, N., deRooster, H., Moons, C.P.H. et al. (2015). Prepubertal gonadectomy in cats: different injectable anesthetic combinations and comparison with gonadectomy at traditional age. *J. Feline Med. Surg.* 17 (6): 458–467.

Robertson, S.A. (2007). Anaesthesia and analgesia for kittens and puppies. European Veterinary Conference, Voorjaarsdagen, Amsterdam (27–29 April). http://www.ivis.org/proceedings/voorjaarsdagen/2007/comp_anim/Robertson3.pdf (accessed 17 August 2019).

Robertson, S.A., Levy, J., Gunkel, C. et al. (2003). Comparison of isoflurane and butorphanol with medetomidine, ketamine and buprenorphine for anesthesia of 7–12 week old kittens for surgical sterilization (abstract). *Proceedings of the Association Veterinary Anaesthetists Spring Meeting*, Doorwerth (27–30 May).

Root Kustritz, M.V. (2002). Early spay-neuter: clinical considerations. *Clin. Tech. Small Anim. Pract.* 17 (3): 124–128.

Steagall, P.V., Taylor, P.M., Rodrigues, L.C. et al. (2009). Analgesia for cats after ovariohysterectomy with either buprenorphine or carprofen alone or in combination. *Vet. Rec.* 164 (12): 359–363.

Stevens, B.J., Posner, L.P., Jones, C.A. et al. (2013). Comparison of the effect of intratesticular lidocaine/bupivacaine vs. saline placebo on pain scores and incision site reactions in dogs undergoing routine castration. *Vet. J.* 196 (3): 499–503.

Taggart, R., Austin, B., Hans, E., and Hogan, D. (2012). In vitro evaluation of the effect of hypothermia on coagulation in dogs via thromboelastography. *J. Vet. Emerg. Crit. Care* 22 (2): 219–224.

Wagner, K.A., Gibbon, K.J., Strom, T.L. et al. (2006). Adverse effects of EMLA (lidocaine/prilocaine) cream and efficacy for the placement of jugular catheters in hospitalized cats. *J. Feline Med. Surg.* 8 (2): 141–144.

10

Anesthetic Complications
Emily McCobb

The focus of this chapter is a discussion of *anesthetic* complications – their presentation, treatment, prognosis, and prevention. General anesthesia safety and monitoring are addressed in Chapter 7, and surgical complications are addressed in Chapter 17.

The risks of anesthetic death or complications in small animal patients has been described (Brodbelt et al. 2007, 2008). In the high-quality high-volume spay–neuter (HQHVSN) setting where most patients are young and healthy and procedures optimized, the risks are even lower (Levy et al. 2017). With an American Society of Anesthesiologists (ASA) status of I (see Table 7.1 in Chapter 7), patient-related risk factors should be minimal to none. However, because the overall patient-related risk in the high-volume spay–neuter clinic is so low, the expectation for a successful outcome is high and there is little tolerance for anesthetic complications. The focus of the spay–neuter team should be on the prevention of complications, and the importance of remaining vigilant and alert to potential risks cannot be overstated. Fortunately, most complications can be avoided with a little planning and attention to monitoring vital parameters and other patient needs. The reader should be directed to previous sections addressing proper protocols and monitoring for particular patients (Chapters 7 and 8). Pediatric patients, discussed in Chapter 9, older or diseased animals, and animals with a brachycephalic airway deserve special consideration in order to avoid complications.

Prevention

As in air travel, most complications occur during the induction phase (take-off) or during recovery (landing). This is not to say that complications cannot occur during anesthesia maintenance as well, but that generally we aim to reach a safe cruising altitude (a stable anesthetic plane that facilitates rapid surgery). Most peri-operative deaths have been found to occur in the early post-operative period (Brodbelt et al. 2008). Avoiding anesthetic complications requires assiduous monitoring, which will allow the anesthetist to intervene before a negative trend becomes a problem. Being prepared, verifying that equipment is well maintained and serviced, ensuring that all staff are familiar with equipment and how to use and troubleshoot the equipment, and providing adequate staffing are also useful strategies for preventing complications. In addition, when calculating drug dosages, it is important to use an accurate bodyweight and calculate doses based on that weight, particularly for very small or very large patients.

Equipment-Related Problems

Many anesthetic equipment-related problems involve the incorrect use of equipment, or equipment failure. To avoid equipment problems, it is essential to ensure that all equipment is properly maintained and is in working order. Each anesthesia machine should be checked for leaks ("pressure-checked") prior to use. Leak checks should be performed once at the beginning of every work day and again if the component parts (rebreathing bags and breathing tubes) are changed. All employees should be familiar with setting up (Food and Drug Administration 1993; ASA 2008; Mosley 2015).

Airway Management

Problems with airway management can occur after pre-medication, at induction, intraoperatively and post-operatively. Patient-related factors can also affect airway management and these will be discussed later in the chapter. Regardless of the patient, however, intubation can pose a risk of its own. For example, recently it has been found in cats that intubation was associated with an increased risk of anesthetic morbidity and mortality (Brodbelt et al. 2008). While this increase in risk could be due to the potential for damage due to improper endotracheal tube placement or overinflation of the cuff, in which case proper technique should substantially decrease or even eliminate intubation as a risk factor, we cannot conclude at this time that intubation itself is not a separate risk factor for cats, regardless of technique. Therefore, careful consideration before incorporating intubation of cats into a clinic's protocol is warranted.

Any time that the airway is manipulated there is a risk of damage to soft tissue structures, therefore great care should be taken to prevent trauma and resultant swelling, which can lead to problems in recovery. In general, the largest-bore endotracheal tube that can be safely placed should be used. This approach will decrease the work of breathing for the patient and will also decrease the risk of endotracheal tube obstruction. However, with a larger tube, the risk of injuring the laryngeal tissues is higher. In cats, care should be taken to avoid traumatizing the larynx and causing laryngospasm (Figure 10.1). The author recommends the following strategies for avoiding laryngospasm: using topical lidocaine (never setocaine) on the arytenoids prior to placing the tube, visualizing the larynx with a laryngoscope, and extubating the cat at the first signs of arousal. Should laryngospasm occur post-extubation, cats can quickly decompensate and become hypoxic. The best strategy for treatment is to sedate the cat, re-intubate, and provide supplemental oxygen therapy. The cat can often be successfully extubated once the episode has passed.

Tracheal tearing from overdistension of the endotracheal tube cuff is a reported complication for intubation of cats (Hardie et al. 1999; Mitchell et al. 2000; Hofmeister et al. 2007; Bhandal and Kuzma 2008; Bauer et al. 2009). The best cure is prevention, by taking care to inflate the cuff no more than necessary and never exceeding tracheal mucosal perfusion pressure. A proper seal can be achieved by inflating the cuff just until there is no audible leak with positive pressure ventilation to a pressure of $12\,cmH_2O$. Alternatively, a Posey Cufflator™ (Posey, Arcadia, CA, posey.com) can be used to ensure that the proper pressure is achieved.

It is equally dangerous for patients if the endotracheal tube cuff is not properly inflated. Esophageal contents can move into an unprotected airway and be aspirated. Reflux of gastrointestinal contents into the esophagus can cause an esophageal stricture, and if aspirated into the lungs could lead to pneumonia. If animals are observed to regurgitate or vomit, then the esophagus should be rinsed with warm water and suctioned. If recovering an intubated patient who has regurgitated during the procedure, extubate the patient with the cuff partly inflated in order to help to bring any liquid contents up and out of the airway. The use

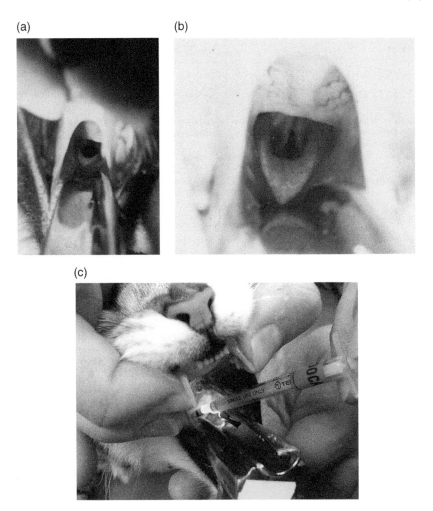

Figure 10.1 Cat airway with (a) open glottis and (b) laryngospasm. Lidocaine can be applied on the arytenoids (c) prior to intubation to reduce laryngospasm. *Source:* Photos courtesy of Cheryl Blaze.

of gastroprotectants in dogs and cats has not been shown to decrease the incidence of complications after regurgitation and is of questionable efficacy (Marks et al. 2018), although they are generally given.

While not often present in a high-volume setting, a capnograph is a very useful monitor for detecting problems with the anesthetic equipment, particularly with the airway (Figure 10.2) Failure to properly intubate the patient, leaks in the cuff, missing or stuck inspiratory one-way valves, and a disconnected or obstructed endotracheal tube are all problems that can be easily detected with the use of capnography

(Figure 10.3). This monitor will prove invaluable for improving patient safety and decreasing the risk of a serious anesthetic complication. In the absence of capnography, intubated patients should be observed carefully so that any disconnections or other problems can be detected. The patient's respiratory efforts should not be excessive and the patient should be able to move the rebreathing bag and valves easily. On 100% oxygen, the patient should saturate at 100%.

A final airway complication which can occur is the patient biting through the endotracheal tube in recovery. This problem can be avoided

Common Capnograph Waveforms

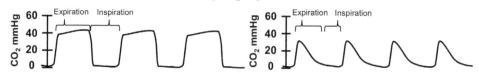

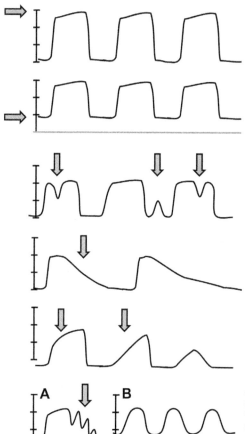

The normal capnograph on a rebreathing circuit (left) is characterized by a "square" waveform that plateaus at 30 – 40 mmHg during expiration and returns to 0 mmHg during inspiration. The capnograph on a non-rebreathing circuit (right) will have steep upslope and fall off rapidly due to dilution with high flow oxygen; the peak will be less than 30 – 40 mmHg because of sample dilution and return to 0 mmHg during inspiration.

Hypoventilation is characterized by high ETCO$_2$, indicating respiratory depression and/or inadequate ventilation. Implement treatment for hypoventilation when ETCO$_2$ is greater than 55 – 60 mmHg: decrease inhalant and/or initiate manual or mechanical ventilation.

Rebreathing of CO$_2$ is occurring when the baseline is greater than 0 mmHg. This indicates 1) malfunctioning one-way valves, 2) exhausted soda-sorb, or 3) low oxygen flow rates in a non-rebreathing circuit.

Spontaneous breathing during mechanical ventilation (i.e., patient is breathing around or "bucking" the ventilator). This occurs if ETCO$_2$ is high and/or if patient is at a light plane of anesthesia. Increase anesthetic depth to prevent spikes in pulmonary pressure from occurring.

A leak in the anesthetic circuit is indicated when the down-slope of the expiratory wave is flattened. Check the endotracheal tube cuff and common sites for leaks. This waveform may be seen with very slow respiratory rates.

Partial occlusion of the ETT or **Bronchoconstriction** are characterized by a flat or curved upslope creating the appearance of "shark fins". Give a breath and listen to the chest – do you hear gurgling of a mucus plug or wheezes associated with bronchoconstriction?

A) Cardiac oscillations. The beating heart displaces small amounts of air, resulting in small peaks in the CO$_2$ waveform coincident with heart rate. **B) Dilution of CO$_2$ sample** due to high O$_2$ flow, rapid respiratory rate or slow sampling rate; falsely low ETCO$_2$. Give a breath or sample from within the ETT to get more accurate reading.

© 2016 Veterinary Anesthesia Specialists

Figure 10.2 Common capnograph waveforms. CO$_2$, carbon dioxide; ETCO$_2$, end-tidal carbon dioxide; ETT, endotracheal tube. *Source:* Reprinted with permission from Heidi L. Shafford, Veterinary Anesthesia Specialists LLC.

by watching the patient carefully and extubating after they begin to swallow. Should the patient bite through the tube, a useful trick is to pass a second endotracheal tube of a smaller diameter into the lumen of the tube still in the trachea, inflate the cuff of the smaller tube, and then pull both tubes out together (Figures 10.4 and 10.5). It is worth mentioning that endotracheal tubes must be properly secured during anesthesia and surgery. String or rubber bands

(a)

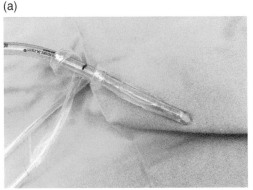

(b)

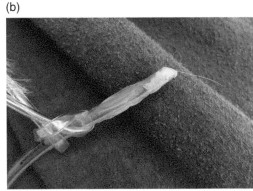

Figure 10.3 (a and b) Material such as mucous can occlude the endotracheal tube and hamper the patient's ability to ventilate. If obstruction is detected or suspected, the endotracheal tube should be immediately suctioned or, if that is not possible, replaced. *Source:* Photos courtesy of Catie Case.

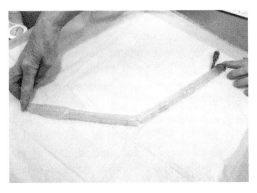

Figure 10.4 A bitten endotracheal tube. Observation of patients during recovery can prevent this complication. Patients who are observed to be chewing should be immediately extubated. *Source:* Photo courtesy of Cheryl Blaze.

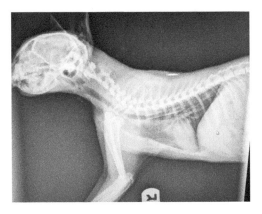

Figure 10.5 Radiograph of a kitten who bit through her endotracheal tube and swallowed the tip. Notice the tubular structure contained within the esophagus, located craniodorsal to the heart. Initially upon discovering the bitten tube, retrieval from the trachea was attempted using a Foley catheter. When that was unsuccessful, radiographs were taken which indicated the tube was esophageal. Retrieval with alligator forceps via the oral cavity was successful. *Source:* Radiographic image courtesy of Kristie Adrian.

are not recommended to use for securing the tube as there is the potential to place them too tightly and cause patient discomfort. The author recommends using used intravenous (IV) tubing instead, which can also be easily disinfected for reuse (Figure 10.6).

Airway obstruction is discussed in the section on patient-related complications later in this chapter.

Anesthetic Machine Problems

Potential problems with the anesthetic machine include improper set-up, failure of component parts, or problems with vaporizer output or carbon dioxide (CO_2) absorber. Vaporizers should be serviced periodically; while most vaporizers will remain properly calibrated for years, it is a good practice to have the vaporizer calibrated and serviced at least every five years. This servicing ensures that the vaporizer is delivering the proper output of anesthetic for the setting.

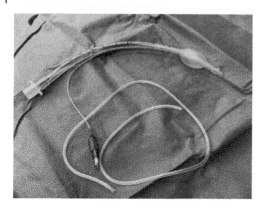

Figure 10.6 Endotracheal tubes should be properly secured. Intravenous tubing provides a soft, flexible tie that can be disinfected.

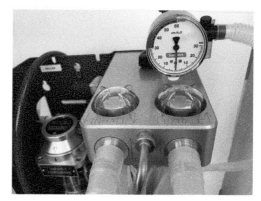

Figure 10.7 Inspiratory and expiratory valves on an anesthesia machine. These valves can accumulate moisture and stick, causing an obstruction in the anesthesia circuit. Use of capnography can aid in the early detection of this complication.

Leak checks as already described will detect most problems and prevent any danger to the patient. Leaks are most often detected at the area of the rebreathing bag or Y piece, and care must be taken to ensure that these components are replaced regularly and are secure. Another common place for leaks is the CO_2 absorber canister (Sodasorb™, Smiths Medical, Dublin, OH), particularly after it has been changed. Leaky anesthetic machines are hazardous to personnel and the environment (see Chapter 31), and if the leak is significant enough it may be difficult to provide a reliable plane of anesthesia at typical settings.

The inspiratory and expiratory one-way valves (Figure 10.7) have a tendency to stick because this area of the anesthetic circuit can accumulate moisture. A stuck valve is a threat to patient safety. Fortunately, like most equipment-related problems, a stuck valve can be detected by a characteristic pattern on the capnograph (see Figure 10.2, rebreathing of CO_2). Using a capnograph for intubated patients can alert the anesthetist to many potential problems with the machine or circuit and has been demonstrated to increase patient safety (Haskins 2015; Duke-Novakovski 2017).

Patient disconnect (the patient coming disconnected from the anesthesia machine) is a simple problem to remedy which can also be detected through monitoring capnography.

The most common and potentially catastrophic equipment-related complication is a pop-off valve that has been inadvertently left closed. In fact, a closed pop-off valve was the most common cause of veterinary anesthetic death in at least one study (Waldrop et al. 2004). This cause of arrest can be nearly eliminated through the use of push-button adjustable pressure-limiting valves (pop-off occlusion valves available from Smiths Medical, https://m.smiths-medical.com/products/veterinary/anesthesia/anesthesia-accessories/pop-off-occlusion-valve), which prevent the pop-off valve from being inadvertently screwed closed (Figure 10.8).

Failure of the oxygen delivery system can occur if pipeline pressure becomes too low (pipeline systems have alarms installed to alert users if the oxygen supply is not sufficient to supply the working pressure of 42 Psi) or for those hospitals using oxygen tanks if the tank runs empty. Failure of the oxygen supply can be avoided by checking the tank level at the beginning of the work day and rechecking it frequently. Oxygen concentrators generally can run on battery power for a number of hours (Burn et al. 2016). Patient safety can be enhanced by using a pulse oximeter. Oxygen analyzers are required by the Machine Safety Act which regulates anesthesia delivery systems for people;

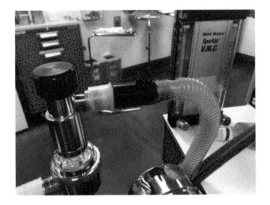

Figure 10.8 This built-in pop-off valve on an anesthesia machine, with a commercially available pop-off occlusion valve added to the expiratory limb of the anesthetic circuit (this device is also visible in Figure 10.7 behind the pressure gauge). Intermittent positive pressure ventilation can be administered to the patient by depressing the button. Using these devices prevents the need to screw closed the pop-off valve and increases safety for patients.

however, most veterinary anesthesia machines are not equipped to be able to measure the concentration of inspired oxygen.

Drug-Related Problems

Fortunately, most drugs used in spay–neuter practice are well tolerated by healthy patients. It is extremely important to screen patients prior to administration of the pre-medication. Patients who are not healthy may need a different anesthetic protocol and may not be good candidates for the high-volume setting. Another important consideration to avoid drug-related complications is to assure an accurate body-weight. All patients should be weighed prior to surgery and care should be taken by the technical staff to ensure that the recorded weight is accurate and compatible with the patient's appearance. Estimated weights are used for patients who cannot be safely handled such as feral cats; however, the use of estimated weights is one factor that will increase the risk to the patient. Drug doses should be calculated according to weight and should not be

estimated (except for drugs that are given intravenously to effect). Drug dosing charts by weight, such as those provided by the American Society for the Prevention of Cruelty to Animals (ASPCA) Spay Neuter Alliance (https://www. aspcapro.org/resource/spayneuter-clinic-drug-charts-logs), can make drug dosing by weight simple and safe.

A frequent concern in private practice is what to do with animals who are severely overweight. Dosing by the animal's measured weight can result in an overdose if the animal is obese because fatty tissue is not metabolically active. On the other hand, medications administered by injection into overweight patients are likely to remain in the fatty tissue, which can delay the onset of sedation or induction and potentially delay recovery. A reasonable compromise is to reduce the dose slightly for very overweight patients and try to avoid placing an injection into fatty tissue, by injecting a lean area such as the shoulder or triceps. Drugs that are given intravenously should be titrated to effect for overweight patients. Metabolic scaling is also useful to help avoid overdose.

While any patient can have an adverse reaction to any medication, a drug reaction to an accurate dose in a healthy patient is unlikely. Drugs that may be more likely to create adverse effects may include ketamine, alpha$_2$ agonists, and propofol. Alpha$_2$ agonists were historically thought to be associated with increased patient risk (Dyson et al. 1998). However, more recent studies of anesthetic risk do not show an increase with the use of the alpha$_2$ agonist medetomidine (Brodbelt et al. 2008), and it is likely that the early studies reflected an increased risk with the use of xylazine as compared to acepromazine. Alpha$_2$ agonists cause a profound drop in cardiac output of 40–50% (Murrell and Hellebrekers 2005). While this drop is generally well tolerated by young, healthy patients, if a patient does not appear to be doing well then the alpha$_2$ agonist should be partially or completely reversed. In a high-volume setting, the alpha$_2$ agonist is often combined with ketamine or telazol as part of a balanced anesthetic protocol, so the effects of the alpha$_2$ agonist will be less profound.

On the other hand, the use of ketamine or telazol may be associated with arrhythmias or tachycardias because of the sympathomimetic effects of these agents. These drugs are therefore best avoided in patients with underlying cardiac disease for which tachycardia might be detrimental. Tachycardia can be a particular concern if the patient has underlying hypovolemia. In such cases, after ensuring that the patient is at an adequate anesthetic plane, the judicious administration of bolus IV fluids should resolve tachycardia due to underlying hypovolemia.

Propofol is less commonly used in the high-volume setting, but may sometimes be seen. Propofol is a sedative hypnotic which has its effect at the gamma-aminobutyric acid (GABA) receptor. Propofol can cause profound cardiovascular depression and hypotension and should be used with caution in compromised patients. It can also cause apnea when administered too quickly. Intubation equipment should always be readily at hand when using propofol in order to address the respiratory depression that could occur. Propofol has a favorable profile for animals with underlying metabolic disease because of its rapid clearance.

In general, injectable agents should be used in caution in pediatric and geriatric patients, who may be more sensitive to their effects.

Acepromazine

Acepromazine is generally well tolerated in healthy patients, but side effects may be more profound in more sensitive patients. For example, in patients with pre-existing hypovolemia, vasodilation from acepromazine can result in a decrease in blood pressure and a compensatory tachycardia. For this reason, the drug should be used cautiously in patients with renal or cardiac disease. While such patients are not commonly seen in the spay–neuter setting, some patients may present with hypovolemia that is unsuspected and undetected on the pre-operative physical examination. It is important to remind owners not to pull water from patients before the morning of surgery, especially for older patients. Many canine patients will be anxious in the clinic and may suffer fluid losses due to panting.

In any patient that develops tachycardia after pre-medication with acepromazine, the administration of fluid therapy (preferably IV) should be considered. Ideally the patient should be restored to a euvolemic state prior to the administration of additional medications for induction of anesthesia. In addition to geriatric and pediatric patients, who can become quite sedate with standard dosages of acepromazine, several breeds of dogs are reportedly sensitive to the drug's effects. The boxer breed is anecdotally reported to be particularly sensitive. In addition, dogs with the MDR-1 mutation are also sensitive to the sedative effects. Collie-type dogs and other herding breeds and "big floppy" dogs such as Newfoundlands and Saint Bernards should have their dose of acepromazine reduced by half. Patients who seem excessively sedate following the administration of acepromazine can benefit from IV fluid therapy and should be monitored closely. In addition, they should be provided with heat support, as acepromazine affects the patient's ability to thermoregulate.

Patient-Related Complications

Airway Issues

Brachycephalic Breeds

Dogs and cats of brachycephalic conformation are prone to airway complications, both at the time of pre-medication and intubation and during recovery. Brachycephalic airway syndrome consists of the following features: stenotic nares, overlong soft palate, hypoplastic trachea, and everted laryngeal saccules (MacPhail 2019). Susceptible breeds include the bulldog and related breeds, as well as Persian cats, among others. Problems with anesthesia of brachycephalic breeds are very common and some high-volume programs will not accept brachycephalic breeds for surgery. Owners of brachycephalic breeds should be informed of the additional anesthetic risks at the time of admission to the clinic. While the risks of complications are certainly increased with these breeds, with proper handling they can do quite well. Clinic staff should be trained and comfortable working with them.

Brachycephalic animals may be particularly difficult to intubate. Because many brachycephalic animals have redundant soft tissues such as an overly long palate, they may have difficulty breathing once sedated. This phenomenon occurs because these individuals must actively elevate the soft tissue of the upper airway away from the trachea in order to be able to breathe. Once they are sedated, the soft tissues collapse into the airway and the patient may develop an obstruction. Changes in posture that accompany sedation, such as dropping the head and assuming a recumbent position, can exacerbate the mechanical obstruction, making the problem worse. Accordingly, brachycephalic patients should be closely observed from the time they are pre-medicated. Agents that can cause vomiting (such as morphine) should be avoided in these patients. Butorphanol pre-medication followed by buprenorphine as an analgesic should be considered. Alternatively, brachycephalic patients can be administered Cerenia® (maropitant; Zoetis, Parsippany, NJ) one hour before pre-medication with morphine or hydromorphone in order to decrease the incidence of vomiting (Hay-Kraus 2017). If the patient appears to be in distress, oxygen should be administered. Because these patients can be difficult to intubate, oxygen should be administered through a tight-fitting mask prior to induction and intubation.

Brachycephalic breeds should always be intubated for surgery, as the risk of a mechanical obstruction is too great. After pre-oxygenation, the patient should be intubated using direct observation of the larynx with a laryngoscope. The soft palate most likely will need to be gently elevated away from the larynx using the tip of the endotracheal tube or a soft-ended stylet. The patient's head and neck should be as straight and extended as possible during intubation. Most brachycephalic breeds will take a much smaller endotracheal tube than would be expected for their size. In addition, since the animal typically has a very short neck, care should be taken not pass the endotracheal tube beyond the carina and into a single bronchus. The tube should be carefully pre-measured and placed only as far as the thoracic inlet. In addition, the tube should be carefully secured to avoid inadvertent extubation due to the patient's short neck. Ideally, an end-tidal CO_2 monitor can be used to verify that the tube has been placed correctly and that it remains in place during surgery. Alternatively, signs that the tube is correctly placed include movement of the bag as the patient takes a breath, being able to hear clear lung sounds on each side of the patient's chest, and a pulse oximeter reading of 98–100%. The cuff of the endotracheal tube should be carefully inflated to prevent aspiration.

During anesthesia, the brachycephalic patient may have difficulty breathing if the portion of the endotracheal tube that extends beyond the nares is very long, as this will increase physiologic dead space. If an end-tidal CO_2 monitor is being used, this problem would be detected by noting a rise in the inspiratory CO_2 concentration, and can be avoided by not using an overly long tube or by trimming the tube so that it does not extend far beyond the patient's nares. Note that care must be used when trimming endotracheal tubes to ensure that the adaptor will still be able to fit. In addition, since many brachycephalic breeds are stocky in stature and have relatively small lung fields compared to their body size, they often need support during anesthesia to prevent hypoventilation and will benefit from gentle intermittent positive pressure ventilation (IPPV), taking care not to deliver more than $10\,cmH_2O$ to the patient's lungs.

Post-Anesthetic Airway Obstruction

Brachycephalic and other patients may suffer from airway obstruction in the post-operative period. Sometimes all that is needed is for the patient to become more alert so that they may pant. In other cases, applying dilute phenylephrine or pediatric Afrin® (Bayer, Boca Raton, FL) to the nasal passages can help relieve obstruction and allow the patient to breathe more comfortably. Oxygen support should be provided to patients that appear to be in respiratory distress. In extreme cases the patient may need to be re-sedated and re-intubated to relieve the obstruction, or a tracheostomy may need to be performed.

Respiratory Complications

Apnea

Patients in the spay–neuter clinic should be spontaneously breathing at all times. Most anesthetics and some of the sedatives and analgesics can cause respiratory depression, though this is uncommon in healthy patients who are given appropriate doses. Alpha$_2$ agonists in particular can cause respiratory depression and apnea at higher doses. Propofol, if given too rapidly, is notorious for causing apnea (Glowaski and Wetmore 1999). Ketamine can cause an altered respiratory pattern known as apneustic respiration. This can be confused with apnea, especially by lay people who may be monitoring cats in trap–neuter–release (TNR) or mobile animal sterilization hospital (MASH) settings. If there is any doubt about whether a patient is breathing, they should be immediately evaluated by the veterinarian in charge (if available) or certified veterinary technician, without waiting to verify that a problem exists. A false alarm is much better than an expired patient.

The treatment for apnea is endotracheal intubation and starting IPPV using either an Ambu bag or an anesthesia machine (if available). If an unintubated patient is not breathing, the anesthetist should check the heart rate. If the heart rate cannot be ausculted or palpated,

then cardiopulmonary resuscitation (CPR) with cardiac compressions should be instituted immediately (see Chapter 11 for CPR). If the patient's heartbeat is strong and steady but they are not breathing, then the patient should be immediately intubated and IPPV instituted. If a patient becomes apneic during a surgical procedure, IPPV should be instituted if the patient is intubated and the anesthesia should be lightened or discontinued if possible. Injectable anesthetics may need to be reversed. It is advisable for all clinics (even in a field setting) to have access to oxygen and intubation supplies in the case of a respiratory emergency.

Hypoventilation

Hypoventilation is common in the anesthetized patient, but is easily treated by supporting ventilation and possibly instituting positive pressure ventilation. The anesthetic plane can also be lightened, which should result in the patient taking deeper and more frequent breaths. Hypoventilation is readily detected with the use of capnography (the end-tidal CO_2 will increase), but may be difficult to detect otherwise.

Hypoxia

An intubated patient who is being maintained on 100% oxygen should not become hypoxic. Hypoxia might be suspected if the pulse oximetry reading is poor (less than 96%). A low pulse oximeter reading with 100% oxygen could indicate a problem with the anesthetic equipment or severe pulmonary impairment. Most commonly, however, it is rather an indication of poor perfusion. All pulse oximetry readings under 96% should be assumed to represent a problem with the patient until proven otherwise and the patient and equipment should be checked carefully until a cause is found.

Cardiovascular Complications

Cardiovascular Depression and Hypotension

Most anesthetics cause at least some degree of cardiovascular depression, which can lead to hypotension, particularly at excessive anesthetic depths. Other causes of hypotension include vasodilation (due to inhalants or acepromazine) or pre-existing hypovolemia. Hypotension can be defined as a systolic blood pressure less than 90 mmHg and or a mean blood pressure less than 60 mmHg (Clarke et al. 2014). As prolonged hypotension can result in impaired organ perfusion and function, it is prudent to consider monitoring patient blood pressure for procedures lasting longer than 20 minutes. Therefore, most, if not all, patients in the HQHVSN setting may not have their blood pressure monitored, as most procedures will be performed more quickly. Monitoring the peripheral pulse gives an indication of pulse pressure (systolic–diastolic; Clarke et al. 2014), which can be helpful in assessing patient status. While an adequate pulse pressure does not ensure that blood pressure is also adequate, weak or poorly palpable pulses could indicate a problem and should be addressed quickly. It may be advisable to monitor blood pressure for higher-risk patients, for example older dogs or cats being spayed or a dog with pyometra. Consideration should also be given to placing an IV catheter in such patients.

If low blood pressure is suspected, a blood pressure monitor (if available) should be placed for confirmation. In many cases, if the blood pressure is low other vital parameters will be affected, including heart rate and capillary refill time (CRT). As with pulse quality, a normal CRT does not ensure that perfusion is adequate, but a prolonged CRT indicates poor tissue perfusion and should be addressed promptly. If the anesthesia protocol includes alpha$_2$ agonists, it is important to keep in mind that it may be difficult or impossible to accurately assess CRT and pulse pressure due to the associated vasoconstriction.

When hypotension is suspected, the first thing to do is to adjust the patient's depth of anesthesia by reducing the vaporizer setting, lightening it as much as possible. Inhalant anesthetics reduce myocardial contractility, cardiac output, and vascular responsiveness (Haskins 2015). In addition, they cause vasodilation and reduce sympathetic tone. Lightening the anesthetic plane should be associated with improvements in cardiac function and thus blood pressure. The patient's CRT and pulse quality should improve. Bradycardia (see below) can also result in hypotension due to the decrease in cardiac output. Bradycardia resulting in suspected patient compromise or hypotension should be treated.

If lightening the anesthetic plane and or addressing any bradycardia does not result in an improved patient status, then consideration should be given to halting the procedure, reversing any reversible anesthetic drugs, and/or placing an IV catheter. Hypotension caused by hypovolemia is generally associated with tachycardia. IV fluid administration can be used to rapidly expand intravascular volume, improving cardiac output and blood pressure. If hypovolemia is suspected as a cause for hypotension or tachycardia, an IV bolus of 5–10 ml/kg of crystalloid fluid should be rapidly administered. If the patient does not respond to fluid therapy, then hypovolemia is not likely to be the primary cause of hypotension.

Occasionally sympathomimetics will need to be administered. In the author's experience, healthy patients typical of the patient population at a high-volume spay–neuter clinic almost never require sympathomimetics if the anesthetic depth is adequate and the patient is carefully monitored. Thus, many spay–neuter clinics will not stock vasopressors routinely. Dopamine is probably the most commonly used sympathomimetic in small animal anesthesia. Dopamine is a directly acting endogenous catecholamine that has dose-dependent effects on renal perfusion, cardiac contractility, and peripheral vascular tone (Clarke et al. 2014, p. 456) At low doses (1–5 µg/kg/min) dopamine causes renal vasodilation (in species with renal dopamine receptors); at mid-range doses (5–10 µg/kg/min) dopamine improves cardiac contractility by acting on myocardial

B1 receptors, leading to improved blood pressure; and at high doses (greater than 10 μg/kg/min) dopamine has vasoconstrictive effects by acting on alpha$_1$ receptors. Vasoconstriction is useful to improve blood pressure, but can also result in impaired organ perfusion.

Arrhythmias

Bradycardia Bradycardia, a decrease in heart rate, is commonly seen under anesthesia. Anesthesia can remove the patient's sympathetic drive, resulting in an increase of parasympathetic tone and vagally mediated bradycardia. Other things can also increase vagal tone, such as drugs, patient positioning (traction on the head or neck), and organ manipulation. Opioids cause a vagally mediated bradycardia and are one of the most common causes of slow heart rates in anesthetized patients. Some patients naturally have a high resting vagal tone and are prone to a slow heart rate under anesthesia. Examples of such patients include brachycephalic breeds of dogs and other breed types such as Dachsunds, West Highland White terriers, Schnauzers, and Scottish terriers, among others. Some pediatric patients will also tend to have high resting vagal tone. Other causes of bradycardia may include hypothermia, electrolyte abnormalities, or an underlying cardiac conduction abnormality.

It is important to keep in mind that the normal heart rate for an animal under anesthesia will be somewhat lower than that of the awake animal, depending of course on the anesthetic protocol that is being used. Bradycardia does not necessarily need to be treated per se, unless the associated drop in cardiac output is resulting in decreased tissue perfusion, or if the patient is experiencing long pauses and/or escape beats associated with first- or second-degree atrioventricular (AV) block. In addition, since raising the patient's heart rate will cause an increase in myocardial workload, consideration should be given to how that might adversely affect the patient. A heart rate greater than 60 beats per minute is generally adequate to maintain cardiac output for most

dogs, and a heart rate greater than 100–120 is generally adequate for most cats. If the heart rate drops below this level or the anesthetist believes the patient has hypotension that is potentiated by bradycardia or other signs of decreased perfusion, then an anticholinergic (glycopyrrolate at 0.005–0.01 mg/kg or atropine at 0.01–0.04 mg/kg) should be administered. Glycopyrrolate has a more gradual onset of action and a longer duration of action than atropine and so is generally preferred for the treatment of peri-operative bradycardias, whereas atropine is the drug of choice for CPR.

If possible, anticholinergic agents should be delivered IV. While glycopyrrolate can be given intramuscularly (IM), the onset of action with IM administration is often much longer, up to 30 minutes. In addition, while paradoxic bradycardia can be seen after any administration of an anticholinergic, it is more common to see it after IM administration.

Another common cause of bradycardia is the use of alpha$_2$ agonists in the anesthetic protocol. However, it is not generally recommended to administer anticholinergics in conjunction with alpha$_2$ agonists (Murrell and Hellebrekers 2005). If the patient is believed to be compromised due to decreased heart rate and cardiac output, reversal or partial reversal of the alpha$_2$ agonist should be considered.

Occasionally other bradyarrhythmias can be observed under anesthesia such as AV block. Most are vagally mediated and are also treated with an anticholinergic.

Tachycardias Tachycardia, or an elevated heart rate, is caused by an elevation in sympathetic tone. In general, tachycardias are usually secondary to a pre-disposing cause which is raising the sympathetic tone, and therefore initial treatment is usually directed at the underlying cause. For example, pain, hypovolemia, inadequate or excessive anesthetic depth, hypercarbia, hypoglycemia, and hypothermia are all potential causes of tachycardia. In addition, tachycardia is sometimes associated with the anesthetic ketamine because of its sympathomimetic properties. In fact, combining ketamine with an alpha$_2$ agonist is a useful way to mitigate some of the bradycardia normally seen with the use of alpha$_2$ agonists.

Tachycardia can be problematic for the patient because it will reduce the time for ventricular filling as well as increasing the overall workload of the heart. Fluid therapy (5–10 ml/kg crystalloid fluid over 10–15 minutes) is often the first line of defense for treating tachycardia, once the anesthetic depth has been determined to be adequate. Many tachycardic patients have underlying hypovolemia, which will respond to volume resuscitation. Tachycardic patients who do not respond to adjusting the anesthetic depth or to fluid therapy should be carefully evaluated for other underlying causes. In a spay–neuter clinic, the need to use other pharmacologic interventions to slow the heart rate (such as beta-blockers or calcium channel blockers, which may be used in a full-service hospital to treat supraventricular tachycardias and other tachyarrhythmias) would be very uncommon and the use of these drugs in the absence of advanced monitoring is not recommended.

Other Arrhythmias Many spay–neuter clinics do not routinely utilize electrocardiogram (EKG) monitoring due to the short length of the surgical procedures. In addition, since the electrical activity of the heart can continue well beyond the time at which effective cardiac contractions have ceased, it is not a particularly sensitive monitor for detecting a deteriorating patient under anesthesia. Nevertheless, from time to time, other atrial and ventricular arrhythmias may be observed during anesthesia and these may be difficult to troubleshoot in the absence of EKG monitoring. If an irregular heart rate is noted or dropped pulses are palpated, or there seems to be any discrepancy between the heart rate and the palpated pulse rate, the animal should be connected to an EKG monitor if one is available in the clinic. Anesthesia alters the balance between

sympathetic and parasympathetic tone, potentially resulting in arrhythmias. Other predisposing causes include underlying structural or conduction abnormalities of the heart, acid–base abnormalities, electrolyte abnormalities, hypercarbia, hypoxemia, or systemic illness. If a patient is determined to have an irregular heart rate or rhythm prior to anesthesia, then it is highly recommended that the patient not be anesthetized at the spay–neuter clinic and that the owner have the underlying cause investigated prior to spay–neuter surgery. The risk of harm to the patient must be weighed against the risk that the animal might go unaltered, and thus clear communication of anesthetic risk to the owner or agent is essential.

Patients with Murmurs

While not exactly an "anesthetic complication," cardiac murmurs or other abnormal findings are a relatively common finding during pre-anesthetic assessment, particularly in older patients. While patients with cardiac disease can be successfully anesthetized for many procedures with a good outcome (Carter et al. 2017), each spay–neuter doctor ultimately must determine which patients are safe to anesthetize in the high-volume setting. In addition, if a cardiac murmur or other finding is unexpected, the situation must be discussed with the pet owner or shelter or rescue organization. Some owners will be interested in pursuing additional diagnostic testing to further evaluation the cardiovascular system, whereas additional diagnostics such as thoracic radiographs and an EKG may be not accessible for other owners. While the presence of a murmur does not necessarily mean that an animal will have structural cardiac disease, owners should understand that additional tests would be needed to rule out the possibility. One diagnostic test that could be considered that can rule out the possibility of cardiac failure is the brain natriuretic peptide (BNP) test, which is available as a SNAP test for cats (Fox et al. 2011) and through most diagnostic laboratories for dogs. Owners should understand that if that the decision is made to carry forward with spay–neuter surgery in the absence of additional information, the animal might be at elevated anesthetic risk.

Standard spay–neuter protocols for anesthesia have an excellent safety track record; however, they are not particularly cardio friendly. Most veterinary cardiologists recommend avoiding alpha₂ agonists entirely in patients with cardiac disease, and avoiding ketamine and tiletamine in cats with hypertrophic cardiomyopathy, or in any patient for whom tachycardia has the potential to be harmful. A reasonable substitute protocol could include an opioid for pre-medication with a benzodiazepine and propofol or alfaxalone for induction, followed by intubation and maintenance on isoflurane or sevoflurane in oxygen. Judicious fluid administration, whether IV or subcutaneously (SC), is generally recommended for

patients with suspected cardiac disease. Each spay–neuter surgeon and clinic must evaluate whether such special patients can be safely accommodated in their setting or whether they would be better referred to a different facility. Whenever protocols are changed, efficiency is compromised.

Hypothermia/Hyperthermia

Temperature regulation is an important aspect of any anesthetic episode, particularly for pediatric and geriatric patients. Preventing hypothermia and hyperthermia is essential to a smooth recovery and a good post-surgical outcome. Warming devices such as recirculating warm water blankets and forced air heating units should be used. However, electric heating pads can burn patients and should never be used (Figure 10.9). Many spay–neuter clinics

(a) (b)

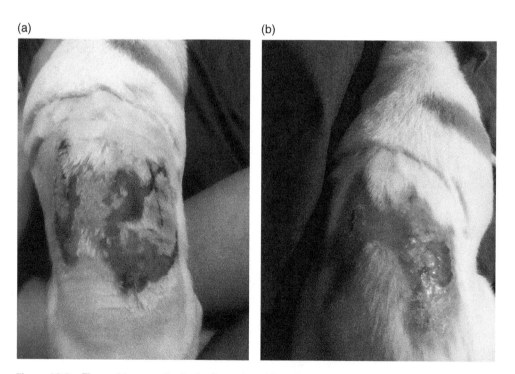

Figure 10.9 Thermal burn on the back of a patient (a) at diagnosis and (b) after several months of treatment. The burn occurred during surgery while the patient was on a v-tray with a reptile heating pad adhered to the v-tray. A blanket had been placed between the patient and the heating source, but the spay surgery was prolonged and the patient was compromised due to a necrotic fetus. *Source:* Photos courtesy of Randi Roberts.

employ heated rice bags, water bottles, or heated discs as inexpensive methods of patient warming. While these items can be useful to provide external heat, they have also been implicated in patient burns and pose a serious safety risk. If they are used, they should be wrapped with other material (like a towel or bubble wrap) and never placed directly next to patient skin. Whenever supplementary heat is provided, it is absolutely essential to monitor the patient's temperature so that overheating can also be prevented, particularly with cats.

Hypothermia

Hypothermia is one factor that can reliably decrease the minimum alveolar concentration (MAC or anesthetic requirement) of inhalant. Patients who are hypothermic can be expected to be maintained on a lower dose of inhalant. Recovery can be prolonged as the metabolism of injectable medications is slowed. Shivering is a process used by the body to warm the patient; however, shivering can lead to increased oxygen demand, which can be detrimental. Longer anesthesia and surgery times can predispose patients to hypothermia, as can the use of a high oxygen flow rate. Oxygen flow rates should be set at no more than 22 ml/kg/min for semi-closed flow and no more than 200 ml/kg/min for non-rebreathing systems. Patients who are slow to wake up from anesthesia should be assumed to be hypothermic until proven otherwise and should have their temperatures taken. Cold patients (temperatures less than 98–99 °F, 36–37 °C) should be warmed aggressively using warm water blankets or forced air heating units if they are available, although taking care not to overwarm the patient. In addition to prolonging anesthetic recovery, other adverse effects associated with peri-operative hypothermia include decreased immune function and wound healing as well as increased bleeding (Doufas 2003).

Hyperthermia

Hyperthermia can be caused by patient-related factors, but is most often iatrogenic, being caused by excessive use of warming devices or by anesthetic medications or both. Some breeds of dogs such as Greyhounds are particularly prone to hyperthermia. Appropriate precautions including low-stress handling, pre-medication with acepromazine, and the administration of IV fluids peri-operatively (when possible) can prevent problems with hyperthermia. Bulldogs and other brachycephalic breeds are also prone to hyperthermia, particularly if their ability to pant is impaired by restraint. Malignant hyperthermia-like syndromes have been reported in dogs, but occur rarely.

In the cat, several commonly used anesthetic agents have been reported to be associated with peri-operative hyperthermia. Opioid medications in particular have been implicated, as has ketamine (Posner et al. 2010). Remarkably high temperatures can be seen in cats suffering postoperative hyperthermia, with temperature readings as high as 108–109 °F (42–43 °C) having been recorded. Fortunately, morbidity is limited if the hyperthermia is caught early, and cats do not seem to suffer long-term harm from having become acutely hyperthermic. Treatment is generally symptomatic and consists of assuring vasodilation with acepromazine, administering IV or SC fluid therapy, and placing the cat on a cool surface. Cooling should be stopped when the temperature reaches about 103 °F (39.5 °C) in order to avoid overshoot. Hyperthermic cats who have been given opioid medication should have their opioids reversed. Cats should never be placed in a heated cage or warming device for recovery without the opportunity to move away from the heat source if they become uncomfortable.

Procedure-Related Problems

Hemorrhage

Acute, severe peri-operative hemorrhage is perhaps one of the most likely complications to occur in the high-volume spay–neuter setting. While it is not an anesthetic-related complication, the anesthetist must be prepared to respond rapidly to acute hemorrhage. A dropped pedicle or other source of bleeding can quickly lead to life-threatening blood loss, particularly in a very small patient. The blood volume of a canine patient is about 90 ml/kg, and the blood volume of a feline patient is about 50 ml/kg. A patient with a normal pre-operative packed cell volume (PCV) can sustain a blood loss of about 20% of total blood volume without the need for a blood transfusion. Typically blood loss of this volume or less can be replaced with crystalloid fluid administration. A spay–neuter patient who is bleeding and who does not have an IV catheter in place should have an IV placed as soon as possible. Since crystalloid fluids do not stay in the vascular space for long, two to three times the volume of blood lost is usually administered. In some settings, "low-volume" resuscitation with colloids and hypertonic saline might be instituted; however, these techniques may not be possible in an HQHVSN setting and evidence for the superior efficacy of low-volume resuscitation in veterinary patients is limited. High-volume fluid resuscitation in the face of acute hemorrhage can be life saving and is unlikely to harm a young and healthy spay–neuter patient, as long as the source of bleeding is addressed. A volume of blood loss greater than the 20% threshold or such that causes a drop in PCV below critical levels will require a blood transfusion. HQHVSN clinics could consider stocking a few units of packed red blood cells for use in the rare emergency, or could collect a unit or two from a healthy donor animal. Dogs do not form antibodies until about four days after the first transfusion and so blood typing in this setting is not necessary. Cats, on the other hand, have pre-formed antibodies and so must always be typed. A useful technique for the high-volume clinic is autotransfusion. Cell savers can be obtained from various suppliers and can easily be used to autotransfuse a patient's own blood collected from the abdominal cavity (see Chapter 17 for autotransfusion protocols).

Vagal Responses

A vagal reaction can occur suddenly, such as with traction on the abdominal organs, resulting in a rapid decrease in heart rate. Manipulation of the head and neck (such as via placement of an esophageal stethoscope) can also trigger a vagal response. Any bradycardia that appears to adversely affect cardiac output should be treated with glycopyrrolate (0.01 mg/kg) or atropine at 0.04 mg/kg. A sudden drop in heart rate or appearance of AV block or worsening AV block should also potentially be treated. An acute vagal response can progress to a cardiac arrest. Many factors can increase a patient's vagal tone, such as the use of opioid medications, hypothermia, and excessive anesthetic depth. In addition, some patients may inherently have higher resting vagal tone, such as brachycephalic breeds, little white breeds, and younger animals. In such cases the use of prophylactic anticholinergic drugs might be considered.

Pain

With a balanced anesthetic protocol and consistent surgical technique, most spay–neuter patients would not be expected to experience pain under anesthesia. However, all patients are individuals and some may react more to surgical stimulation than others. Pain should always be considered as a potential root cause, particularly for unexplained tachycardia. If pain is suspected, small doses of additional analgesics should be given and should improve the clinical picture. Small doses of dexmedetomidine (1–2 µg/kg) can be useful to smooth out the anesthesia of a patient experiencing an unexpected painful response and can be given IV, IM, or via the oral transmucosal route. In addition, local anesthetic techniques can be very useful to ensure adequate analgesia.

References

American Society of Anesthesiologists (2008). ASA recommendations for pre anesthesia checkout. http://www.asahq.org/resources/clinical-information/2008-asa-recommendations-for-pre-anesthesia-checkout (accessed 21 March 2019).

Bauer, M.D., Clark-Price, S.C., and McFadden, M.S. (2009). Anesthesia case of the month. *JAVMA* 234: 1539–1541.

Bhandal, J. and Kuzma, A. (2008). Tracheal rupture in a cat: diagnosis by computed tomography. *Can. Vet. J.* 49: 595–597.

Brodbelt, D.C., Pfeiffer, D.U., Le, Y. et al. (2007). Risk factors for anesthetic-related death in cats: results from the confidential enquiry into peri-operative small animal fatalities. *Br. J. Anaesth.* 99: 617–623.

Brodbelt, D.C., Pfeiffer, D.U., Le, Y. et al. (2008). Results of the confidential enquiry into perio-operative small animal fatalities regarding risk factors for anesthetic-related death in dogs. *JAVMA* 233: 1096–1104.

Burn, J., Caulkett, N.A., Gunn, M. et al. (2016). Evaluation of a portable oxygen concentrator to provide fresh gas flow to dogs undergoing anesthesia. *Can. Vet. J.* 57: 614–618.

Carter, J.E., Motsinger-Reif, A.A., Krug, W.V., and Keene, B.W. (2017). The effect of heart disease on anesthetic complications during routine dental procedures in dogs. *J. Am. Anim. Hosp. Assoc.* 53: 206–213.

Clarke, K.W., Trim, C., and Hall, L. (2014). *Veterinary Anaesthesia*, 11e. Cambridge: Elsevier.

Doufas, A.G. (2003). Consequences of inadvertent perioperative hypo-thermia. *Best Pract. Res. Clin. Anaesthesiol.* 17: 535–549.

Duke-Novakovski, T. (2017). Basics of monitoring equipment. *Can. Vet. J.* 58: 1200–1208.

Dyson, D.H., Maxie, M.G., and Schurr, D. (1998). Morbidity and mortality associated with anesthetic management in a small animal veterinary practice in Ontario. *J. Am. Anim. Hosp. Assoc.* 34 (4): 325–335.

Food and Drug Administration (1993). Anesthesia apparatus equipment checkout recommendations. http://vam.anest.ufl.edu/FDApreusecheck.pdf (accessed 21 March 2019).

Fox, P.R., Rush, J.E., Reynolds, C.A. et al. (2011). Multicenter evaluation of plasma N-terminal probrain natriuretic peptide (NT-pro BNP) as a biochemical screening test for asymptomatic (occult) cardiomyopathy in cats. *J. Vet. Intern. Med.* 25 (5): 1010–1016.

Glowaski, M.M. and Wetmore, L.A. (1999). Propofol: application in veterinary sedation and anesthesia. *Clin. Tech. Small Anim. Pract.* 14 (1): 1–9.

Hardie, E.M., Spodnick, G.J., Gilson, S.D. et al. (1999). Tracheal rupture in cats: 16 cases (1983–1998). *JAVMA* 214: 508–512.

Haskins, S.C. (2015). Monitoring anaesthetised patients. In: *Lumb and Jones Veterinary Anaesthesia and Analgesia*, 5e (eds. K.A. Grimm, L.A. Lamont, W.J. Tranquilli, et al.), 101. Oxford: Wiley-Blackwell.

Hofmeister, E.H., Trim, C.M., Kley, S. et al. (2007). Traumatic endotracheal intubation in the cat. *Vet. Anaesth. Analg.* 34: 213–216.

Kraus, B.L.H. (2017). Spotlight on the perioperative use of maropitant citrate. *Vet. Med. Res. Rep.* 8: 41–51.

Levy, J.K., Bards, K.M., Tucker, S.J. et al. (2017). Perioperative mortality in cats and dogs undergoing spay or castration at a high-volume clinic. *Vet. J.* 224: 11–15.

MacPhail, C. (2019). Surgery of the upper respiratory system. In: *Small Animal Surgery* (ed. T.W. Fossum), 833–883. Philadelphia, PA: Elsevier.

Marks, S.L., Kook, P.H., Papich, M.G., and Torbut, M.K. (2018). ACVIM consensus statement: support for rational administration of gastrointestinal protectants to dogs and cats. *J. Vet. Intern. Med.* 32 (6): 1823–1840.

Mitchell, S.L., McCarthy, R., Rudloff, E. et al. (2000). Tracheal rupture associated with intubation in cats: 20 cases (1996–1998). *JAVMA* 216: 1592–1595.

Mosley, C. (2015). Veterinary anesthesia apparatus checkout recommendations (table 3.4), anesthesia equipment. In: *Veterinary Anesthesia and Analgesia*, 5e (eds. K. Grimm, L. Lamont, W. Tranquilli, et al.), 63. Ames, IA: Wiley-Blackwell.

Murrell, J.C. and Hellebrekers, L.J. (2005). Medetomidine and dexmedetomidine a review of cardiovascular effects and antinociceptive properties in the dog. *Vet. Anesth. Analg.* 32 (3): 117–127.

Posner, L.P., Pavuk, A.A., Rokshar, J.L. et al. (2010). Effects of opioids and anesthetic drugs on body temperature in cats. *Vet. Anaesth. Analg.* 37: 35–43.

Waldrop, J.E., Rozanski, E.A., Swanke, E.D. et al. (2004). Causes of cardiopulmonary arrest, resuscitation management, and functional outcome in dogs and cats surviving cardiopulmonary arrest. *J. Vet. Emerg. Crit. Care* 14 (1): 22–29.

11

Cardiopulmonary Resuscitation in Shelter Animal Practice
Luisito S. Pablo

Knowledge and practice of effective cardiopulmonary resuscitation (CPR) techniques is important to veterinarians, technicians, and staff working in high-quality high-volume spay–neuter (HQHVSN) or shelter animal practice. Most patients that develop cardiac arrest in this setting are anesthetized patients. Based on clinical studies (Kass and Haskins 1992; Waldrop et al. 2004; Hofmeister et al. 2009), patients that arrested under anesthesia have a higher probability of successful resuscitation compared to those that are awake at the time of arrest. Most dogs and cats undergoing anesthesia in a shelter setting are healthy, with a potentially good outcome following an arrest, further emphasizing the importance of personnel who are well trained in resuscitation techniques.

The CPR technique performed differs among veterinary clinics due to differences in access to equipment; for example, in many shelter animal facilities an electrocardiograph (EKG) machine and electrical defibrillator will not be readily available. However, even without these tools, effective CPR can still be performed. Since ventricular fibrillation, one of the abnormal rhythms during cardiac arrest, has a low incidence in animals compared with humans (Waldrop et al. 2004; Boller et al. 2012), the absence of an electrical defibrillator will only make a small difference in the overall success rate. The most common

arrest rhythm reported in small animals is ventricular asystole (Waldrop et al. 2004).

Recognition and Treatment of Hypoventilation and/or Respiratory Arrest

Animals given injectable agents for anesthetic induction may develop apnea or respiratory arrest minutes after administration of the drug(s), during surgery, and post-operatively. Early recognition and treatment of respiratory arrest can forestall progression to cardiopulmonary arrest and avert the need for CPR.

When breathing stops for longer than 30 seconds, the pulse should be checked immediately to rule out cardiopulmonary arrest; if no pulse is identified, CPR should be initiated. If there is a pulse, immediate steps should be taken to support the ventilation of the patient. For patients who are not intubated when apnea is recognized, the mouth, pharynx, and larynx should be inspected to ensure that there is no obstruction or foreign material interfering with breathing. If the airway is clear, ventilation of the patient should be supported by intubating the patient, providing oxygen, and squeezing the bag of the anesthetic breathing circuit. If an anesthetic breathing circuit is not available, an Ambu bag can be used to support ventilation until the patient attains spontaneous breathing. If intubation is difficult, or intubation is delayed while intubation supplies are being located, ventilation by tight-fitting mask may help oxygenate the patient. If the patient continues to be apneic after about five minutes of supported ventilation, reversal agents should be administered if the patient received drugs that can be reversed. For example, atipamezole should be given if dexmedetomidine was administered. Stimulation of the patient by pinching the toe or massaging the body may help in the animal returning to spontaneous breathing.

Apneic patients who are already intubated and being maintained with inhalational agent can be easily managed by supporting or controlling ventilation. Similar to the non-intubated patients, the presence of a pulse should be confirmed. If there is no pulse, the inhalational agent should be stopped immediately and CPR initiated. The depth of anesthesia should be checked and the patient maintained in a lighter plane of anesthesia, as deep anesthesia can result in apnea. When the patient is intubated, manual ventilation can be performed using a frequency of about two to three breaths per minute. Using this slower respiratory rate allows continuous oxygen administration and a slightly higher carbon dioxide tension in the blood to stimulate breathing.

Recognition of Cardiac Arrest

Cardiac arrest is defined as the failure of the heart to pump blood, resulting in cessation of blood flow to organ systems (Macintire et al. 2005). Prompt recognition of cardiac arrest is essential for early intervention. Basic monitoring of anesthetized patients involves watching the patient breathe and feeling a peripheral pulse, but this monitoring usually only occurs intermittently. Sometimes a pulse oximeter may be available, which gives continuous information. A definitive sign of cardiac arrest is the absence of a palpable pulse or heartbeat.

Oftentimes, this is preceded by apnea. Other signs of cardiac arrest that will manifest include fixed and dilated pupils and the absence of corneal and palpebral reflexes. If the animal is not anesthetized, sudden loss of consciousness may signal that the heart has stopped. Animals with respiratory problems may manifest cyanosis and agonal breathing before developing cardiac arrest. Anesthetized patients that develop severe sinus bradycardia may progress to cardiac arrest if not treated immediately.

If an EKG machine is available, the rhythm associated with the cardiac arrest can be determined. Ventricular asystole indicates the absence of electrical activity and shows a flat or straight line on the EKG. Pulseless electrical activity will show a normal-looking EKG or a regular ventricular rhythm, but the pulse is not palpable. Ventricular fibrillation is characterized as a chaotic, irregular, and disorganized rhythm. Since this is the only rhythm that needs electrical defibrillation, it is called a shockable rhythm (Rozanski et al. 2012).

Cardiopulmonary Resuscitation Techniques

CPR can be divided into three stages: (i) basic life support, (ii) advanced life support, and (iii) post-cardiac arrest care. Of the three stages, effective basic life support is the most important in restoring spontaneous circulation (Berg et al. 2010). In humans, electrical defibrillation is part of the basic life support. For the veterinary patient in a shelter setting, success in resuscitation depends largely on immediate and effective basic life support (Boller et al. 2012) without the use of electrical defibrillation.

Basic Life Support

The primary goal of CPR is to restore perfusion to the brain and heart. Cardiac arrest develops because the heart does not have sufficient oxygen and metabolic substrates to continue its

hypotensive, administration of a positive inotrope is indicated, with dopamine being the most common agent used in small animals. The dose rate for dopamine is 5–10 ug/kg/minute. In patients with high vagal tone, administration of an anticholinergic is indicated if the patient's heart rate falls below the normal resting heart rate. Atropine or glycopyrrolate can be administered IV at a dose of 0.02–0.04 mg/kg and 0.01 mg/kg, respectively.

Body Temperature

Body temperature should be monitored post-cardiac arrest. Hyperthermia – body temperature greater than 102.5 °F (39.2 °C) for dogs and greater than 103.0 °F (39.4 °C) for cats – should be corrected by using available cooling methods. An electric fan directed at the patient will help to decrease body temperature. Cool IV fluids can also be administered. Hyperthermia is harmful because it further increases the oxygen requirements of the brain, which in turn impairs brain recovery (Peberdy et al. 2010). Mild hypothermia should not be corrected. However, close monitoring of body temperature is indicated to prevent severe hypothermia. In humans, hypothermia (body temperature of 89.6–93.2 °F, 32–34 °C) may be induced post-cardiac arrest for 12 or 24 hours (Bernard et al. 2002; Peberdy et al. 2010). This treatment requires a well-controlled environment and advanced monitoring tools because of the possible adverse effects associated with severe hypothermia. Whole-body hypothermia following cardiac arrest has not been instituted in veterinary practice. It is also important to note that when an animal arrests during anesthesia, severe hypothermia will further delay the metabolism and excretion of anesthetic drugs.

Blood Glucose Values

When compared to euglycemia, both hyperglycemia and hypoglycemia have been associated with worse outcomes in critically ill patients. It has been suggested that blood glucose levels should be maintained at between 144 and 180 mg/dl (Peberdy et al. 2010). If a glucose monitoring device is available, blood glucose should be measured post-cardiac arrest. Mild to moderate hypoglycemia can be treated using crystalloids containing 2.5–5.0% dextrose. If severe hypoglycemia is present, 50% dextrose at 1.0 ml/kg, diluted with an equal volume of 0.9% saline to prevent phlebitis, should be administered slowly (Macintire et al. 2005). In a shelter animal practice, hyperglycemia will be more difficult to manage, since this requires titrating insulin, which may not be readily available, to achieve normal blood glucose values. This also requires more intensive monitoring and can be dangerous to the patient if severe hypoglycemia results from insulin administration.

Conclusion

CPR in a shelter animal practice can be simplified without decreasing its potential for success. Effective basic life support is vital to a good outcome. Veterinarians, technicians, and staff members should master the techniques involved in basic life support. Recent recommendations have simplified CPR techniques, emphasizing the importance of basic life support and using fewer drugs. The absence of electrical defibrillators and EKG machines further simplifies CPR techniques, resulting in less confusion among resuscitators. It must be remembered that CPR is a team effort and each member should know in advance their role when a cardiac arrest occurs. Team practice should be done on a regular basis. CPR charts should be prominently displayed where they are most likely to be needed, and a CPR kit should be kept fully stocked and placed in the anesthesia and surgery area.

References

Aufderheide, T.P. and Lurie, K.G. (2004). Death by hyperventilation: a common and life-threatening problem during cardiopulmonary resuscitation. *Crit. Care Med.* 32 (Suppl): S345–S351.

Berg, R.A., Hemphill, R., Abella, B.S. et al. (2010). Part 5: adult basic life support: 2010 American Heart Association Guidelines for cardiopulmonary resuscitation and emergency cardiovascular care. *Circulation* 122 (18 Suppl. 3): S685–S705.

Berg, R.A., Sanders, A.B., Kern, K.B. et al. (2001). Adverse hemodynamic effects of interrupting chest compressions for rescue breathing during cardiopulmonary resuscitation for ventricular fibrillation cardiac arrest. *Circulation* 104: 2465–2470.

Bernard, S.A., Gray, T.W., Buist, M.D. et al. (2002). Treatment of comatose survivors of out-of-hospital cardiac arrest with induced hypothermia. *N. Engl. J. Med.* 346: 557–563.

Blecic, S., Chaskis, C., and Vincent, J.L. (1992). Atropine administration in experimental electromechanical dissociation. *Am. J. Emerg. Med.* 10: 515–518.

Boller, M., Boller, E.M., Oodegard, S. et al. (2012). Small animal cardiopulmonary resuscitation requires a continuum of care: proposal for a chain of survival for veterinary patients. *JAVMA* 240: 540–554.

Davison, R., Barresi, V., Parker, M. et al. (1980). Intracardiac injections during cardiopulmonary resuscitation. *JAMA* 244: 1110–1111.

DeBehnke, D.J., Swart, G.L., Spreng, D. et al. (1995). Standard and higher doses of atropine in a canine model of pulseless electrical activity. *Acad. Emerg. Med.* 2: 1034–1041.

DiBartola, S.P. and Batement, S. (2006). Introduction to fluid therapy. In: *Fluid, Electrolyte, and Acid-Base Disorders in Small Animal Practice*, 3e (eds. S.P. DiBartola and K.A. Grimm), 325–344. Maryland Heights, MO: Saunders Elsevier.

Feneley, M.P., Maier, G.W., Kern, K.B. et al. (1988). Influence of compression rate on initial success of resuscitation and 24 hour survival after prolonged manual cardiopulmonary resuscitation in dogs. *Circulation* 77: 240–250.

Fletcher, D.J., Boller, M., Brainard, B.M. et al. (2012). RECOVER evidence and knowledge gap analysis on veterinary CPR. Part 7: clinical guidelines. *J. Vet. Emerg. Crit. Care* 22 (Suppl. 2): S102–S131.

Gentile, N.T., Martin, G.B., Appleton, T.J. et al. (1991). Effects of arterial and venous volume infusion on coronary perfusion pressures during canine CPR. *Resuscitation* 22: 55–63.

Harrison, E.E. (1981). Intracardiac injections. *JAMA* 245: 1315.

Hofmeister, E.H., Brainard, B.M., Egger, C.M. et al. (2009). Prognostic indicators for dogs and cats with cardiopulmonary arrest treated by cardiopulmonary cerebral resuscitation at a university teaching hospital. *JAVMA* 235: 50–57.

Hopper, K., Epstein, S.E., Fletcher, D.J. et al. (2012). RECOVER evidence and knowledge gap analysis on veterinary CPR. Part 3: basic life support. *J. Vet. Emerg. Crit. Care* 22 (Suppl. 2): S26–S43.

Jespersen, H.F., Granbord, J., Hansen, U. et al. (1990). Feasibility of intracardiac injection of drugs during cardiac arrest. *Eur. Heart J.* 11: 269–274.

Kass, P.H. and Haskins, S.C. (1992). Survival following cardiopulmonary resuscitation in dogs and cats. *J. Vet. Emerg. Crit. Care* 2: 57–65.

Lemke, K.A. (2007). Anticholinergics and sedatives. In: *Lumb & Jones' Veterinary Anesthesia and Analgesia*, 4e (eds. W.J. Tranquilli, J.C. Thurmon and K.A. Grimm), 203–239. Ames, IA: Blackwell.

Lindner, K.H., Strohmenger, H.U., Ensinger, H. et al. (1992). Stress hormone response during

and after cardiopulmonary resuscitation. *Anesthesiology* 77: 662–668.

Macintire, D.K., Drobatz, K.J., Haskins, S.C. et al. (2005). *Manual of Small Animal Emergency and Critical Care Medicine.* Philadephia, PA: Lippincott Williams & Wilkins.

Maier, G.W., Newton, J.R. Jr., Wolfe, J.A. et al. (1986). The influence of manual chest compression rate on hemodynamic support during cardiac arrest: high-impulse cardiopulmonary resuscitation. *Circulation* 74: IV51–IV59.

McMichael, M. (2008). Cardiopulmonary resuscitation. In: *Small Animal Anesthesia and Analgesia* (ed. G.L. Carroll), 179–191. Ames, IA: Blackwell.

Mukoyama, T., Kinoshita, K., Nagao, K. et al. (2009). Reduced effectiveness of vasopressin in repeated doses for patients undergoing prolonged cardiopulmonary resuscitation. *Resuscitation* 80: 755–761.

Neumar, R.W. (2011). Optimal oxygenation during and after cardiopulmonary resuscitation. *Curr. Opin. Crit. Care* 17: 236–240.

Neumar, R.W., Otto, C.W., Link, M.S. et al. (2010). Part 8: adult advanced cardiovascular life support: 2010 American Heart Association Guidelines for cardiopulmonary resuscitation and emergency cardiovascular care. *Circulation* 122 (18 Suppl. 3): S729–S767.

Newton, J.R. Jr., Glower, D.D., Wolfe, J.A. et al. (1988). A physiologic comparison of external cardiac massage techniques. *J. Thorac. Cardiovasc. Surg.* 95: 892–901.

Paret, G., Vaknin, Z., Ezra, D. et al. (1997). Epinephrine pharmacokinetics and pharmacodynamics following endotracheal administration in dogs: role of volume of diluent. *Resuscitation* 35: 77–82.

Peberdy, M.A., Callaway, C.W., Neumar, R.W. et al. (2010). Part 9: post-cardiac arrest care: 2010 American Heart Association guidelines for cardiopulmonary resuscitation and

emergency cardiovascular care. *Circulation* 122 (Suppl. 3): S768–S786.

Plunkett, S.J. and McMichael, M. (2008). Cardiopulmonary resuscitation in small animal medicine: an update. *J. Vet. Intern. Med.* 22: 9–25.

Rozanski, E.A., Rush, J.E., Buckley, G.J. et al. (2012). RECOVER evidence and knowledge gap analysis on veterinary CPR. Part 4: advanced life support. *J. Vet. Emerg. Crit. Care* 22 (Suppl. 2): S44–S64.

Voorhees, W.D., Babbs, C.F., and Tacker, W.A. Jr. (1980). Regional blood flow during cardiopulmonary resuscitation in dogs. *Crit. Care Med.* 8: 134–136.

Voorhees, W.D., Ralston, S.H., Kougias, C. et al. (1987). Fluid loading with whole blood or Ringer's lactate solution during CPR in dogs. *Resuscitation* 15: 113–123.

Waldrop, J.E., Rozanski, E.A., Swanke, E.D. et al. (2004). Causes of cardiopulmonary arrest, resuscitation management, and functional outcome in dogs and cats surviving cardiopulmonary arrest. *J. Vet. Emerg. Crit. Care* 14 (1): 22–29.

Weil, M.H., Bisera, J., Trevino, R.P. et al. (1985). Cardiac output and end-tidal carbon dioxide. *Crit. Care Med.* 13: 907–909.

Wenzel, V., Krismer, A.C., Arntz, H.R. et al. (2004). A comparison of vasopressin and epinephrine for out-of-hospital cardiopulmonary resuscitation. *N. Engl. J. Med.* 350: 105–113.

Yannopoulos, D., Aufderheide, T.P., Gabrielli, A. et al. (2006). Clinical and hemodynamic comparison of 15:2 and 30:2 compression-to-ventilation ratios for cardiopulmonary resuscitation. *Crit. Care Med.* 34: 1444–1449.

Yannopoulos, D., Zviman, M., Castro, V. et al. (2009). Intra-cardiopulmonary resuscitation hypothermia with and without volume loading in an ischemic model of cardiac arrest. *Circulation* 120: 1426–1435.

Zia, A. and Kern, K.B. (2011). Management of postcardiac arrest myocardial dysfunction. *Curr. Opin. Crit. Care* 17: 241–246.

Section Three

Surgical Techniques for Spaying and Neutering

12

Dog Spay/Cat Spay
Philip Bushby and Sara White

Ovariohysterectomy is one of the most common surgical procedures performed in small animal veterinary practice. In the shelter environment, ovariohysterectomy or ovariectomy is considered a critical tool in efforts to reduce the overpopulation of unwanted dogs and cats. The basic technique for ovariohysterectomy is well documented in veterinary textbooks (Hedlund 2007; MacPhail 2013).

Descriptions of ovariohysterectomy in veterinary textbooks frequently are intended for the instruction of the beginning surgeon. Many of the specific techniques are, therefore, directed toward the surgeon with minimal experience. As veterinary surgeons gain additional experience, some of the basic techniques described can be abandoned or modified in favor of more efficient techniques that are just as safe and effective.

This chapter will describe efficient techniques for dog and cat spays, as well as several variations on these techniques.

Canine Ovariohysterectomy

The ventral abdominal skin should be clipped of hair and aseptically prepped as described in Chapter 4.

Patient Positioning

The patient should be positioned in dorsal recumbency with the front legs either left untied, secured along the sides of the lateral thoracic wall (Bushby 2013), or tied across the chest with elbows flexed. For positioning along the sides of the thoracic wall, a simple restraint device can be made from an aluminum rod and positioned under the animal to secure the legs in this position (Figure 12.1). If the surgeon is using a V-table or V-trough, the front legs can be left unrestrained. Positioning the front legs in this manner may prevent tension on the ovarian suspensory ligaments, making it easier to exteriorize the ovaries. Conversely, pulling the front legs cranially and tying them in that position, as is routinely taught, may increase tension on the ovarian suspensory ligaments, making it more difficult to exteriorize the ovaries.

Location of Incision

One key to efficient ovariohysterectomies is making appropriately placed small incisions. While surgery instructors traditionally promote long incisions and maximum exposure, lengthy incisions are considerably more time consuming to close and much more traumatic

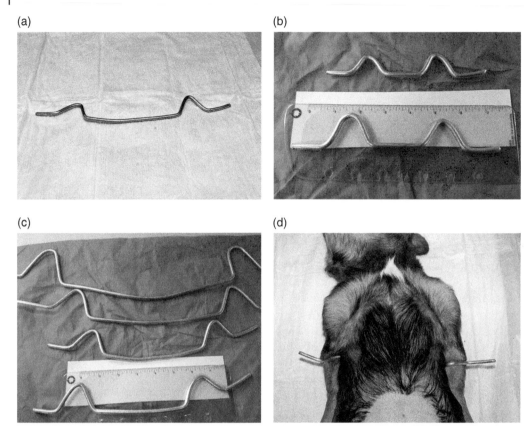

Figure 12.1 Restraint devices. (a) A simple restraint device can be made from an aluminum rod. Make various sizes for different-sized dogs and cats. (b) Cat restraint devices. (c) Dog restraint devices. (d) A dog with a restraint device. *Source:* Photos courtesy of Tom Thompson.

to the patient. Small incisions can be closed much more rapidly than long incisions and cause considerably less trauma.

The proper location of the incision is determined by which structures are more difficult to exteriorize. Accordingly, the proper location of the incision varies with the age of the patient. In the adult dog it is more difficult to exteriorize the ovaries than the uterine body, and the skin incision is on the ventral abdominal midline just caudal to the umbilicus. In the puppy (under five months of age) it is more difficult to exteriorize the uterine body, so the skin incision is made on the ventral abdominal midline a little caudal to the location of the incision in an adult dog, just cranial to the midpoint between the umbilicus and the pubis (Bushby 2013).

Abdominal Entry

Abdominal Entry through the Linea
A 1–3 cm skin incision is made on the ventral abdominal midline, located as just described. The subcutaneous tissue should be dissected to the extent necessary to visualize the linea alba. Grasp the linea alba with a thumb forceps, elevate the linea alba, and nick the linea with a scalpel blade. With the linea still elevated, extend the incision with either a scissors or a scalpel blade.

Paramedian Abdominal Entry
In the adult dog the ovaries are more difficult to exteriorize, and the right kidney and the right ovary are located further cranial in the abdomen than the left kidney and left ovary. It is, therefore, more difficult to exteriorize the

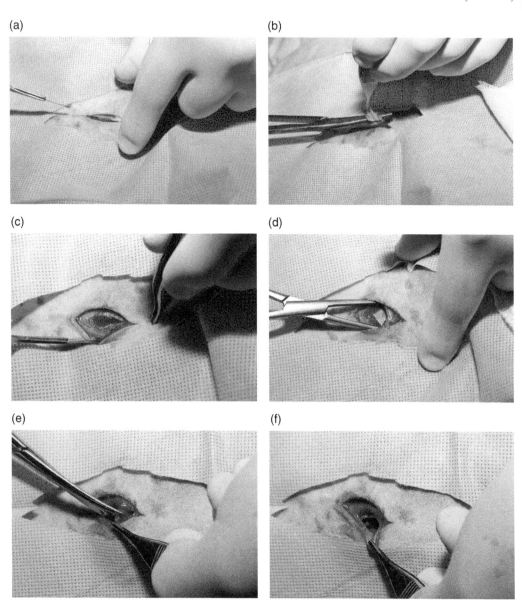

Figure 12.2 Paramedian incision. (a) Ventral midline skin incision. (b) Undermine to the right of the linea alba. (c) Incise the muscle fascia without cutting rectus muscle. (d) Bluntly separate muscle fibers. (e) Elevate and cut the peritoneum to enter the abdomen. (f) The peritoneum is incised, allowing entry into the abdomen. *Source:* Photos courtesy of Tom Thompson.

right ovary than the left ovary. To equalize the difficulty of exteriorizing the two ovaries, one of the authors (Bushby) prefers to make the entry into the abdomen through a right paramedian incision (Figure 12.2).

To perform a paramedian abdominal entry, incise the skin on the ventral abdominal midline. Undermine the subcutaneous tissue to the right of the linea alba. The external fascia is incised, being careful not to cut fibers of the rectus abdominis muscle to avoid hemorrhage. The fascial incision can be a little as 0.5 cm to the right of the linea in very small dogs and as much as 1.5 cm to the right of the linea in larger dogs. A hemostat is inserted through the rectus abdominus muscle and opened. This bluntly separates the fibers of the rectus abdominus muscle, exposing the peritoneum. The peritoneum is then grasped with a thumb forceps and cut with a Metzenbaum scissors.

Exteriorizing the Uterus and Ovaries

Upon entry into the abdominal cavity, a spay hook can be used to locate and exteriorize the first uterine horn. The spay hook should be passed into the abdominal cavity along the right abdominal wall. Upon reaching the dorsal lateral abdominal wall, the hook is then swept toward the midline and elevated out of the abdominal incision. Depending on the experience of the surgeon, it may take several passes of the spay hook to exteriorize the right uterine horn. If the right horn is not found after several passes, the surgeon may use the hook on the left side. When using a spay hook, especially on the left side, care should be taken to avoid damage to the spleen, mesentery, and other abdominal structures.

Once the uterine horn is exteriorized, gentle traction on the more cranial aspect of the uterine horn will begin to expose the ovary. Place a hemostat on the proper ligament of the ovary and apply upward tension. This tenses the suspensory ligament of the ovary, making palpation and visualization of the ligament much easier. It may also be helpful to press gently downward on the body wall at the incision to further expose the suspensory ligament. The suspensory ligament is then cut with a scissors (Figure 12.3) or a blade, or it may be torn. Tear

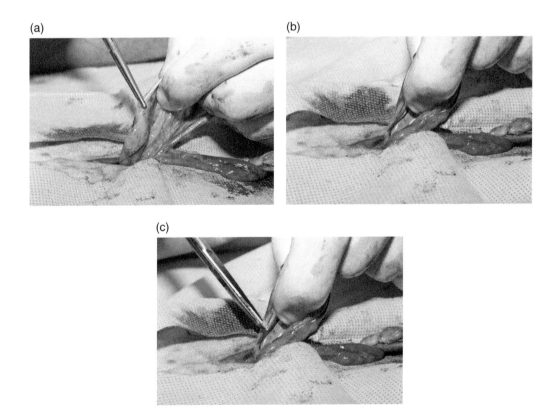

Figure 12.3 Incising the suspensory ligament. (a) Grasp the proper ligament with a hemostat. (b) Apply upward tension, exposing the suspensory ligament. (c) Cut the suspensory ligament. *Source:* Photos courtesy of Tom Thompson.

a window in the broad ligament caudal to the ovarian vessels to isolate the ovarian vessels in the ovarian pedicle.

Ovarian Pedicle Ligation

Most veterinary students are taught to double-ligate ovarian pedicles and uterine stumps and to ligate before transecting the ovarian pedicles. It is much more efficient to transect the ovarian pedicles prior to ligation and to single-ligate each pedicle (Bushby 2013). Transection prior to ligation enables the surgeon to place the ligature with minimal manipulation of the pedicle and with greater visibility when compared to ligation prior to transection. This leads to a decreased chance of damage to the pedicle during ligation or of inadvertent inclusion of inappropriate tissues in the ligature.

It is not necessary to crush the tissue that will be included in the pedicle ligation. However, it is essential to ensure that the ligature is not placed too close to the hemostat that secures the pedicle, as the "fanning out" of tissue immediately surrounding the hemostat may prevent adequate tightening of the ligature.

One of the authors (Bushby) prefers the following technique of ligating and transecting ovarian pedicles in the dog or puppy (see Figure 12.4). Place three hemostats or

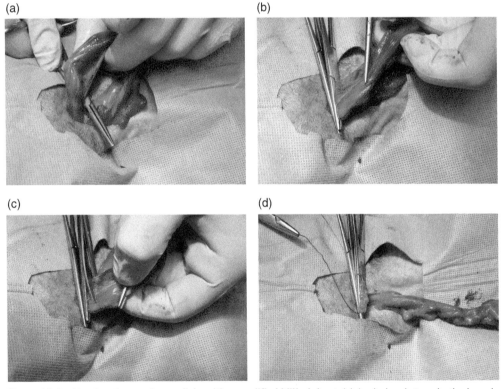

(a) (b)

(c) (d)

Figure 12.4   Ligating the ovarian pedicle with a modified Miller's knot. (a) A window is torn in the broad ligament to isolate the pedicle. (b) Three hemostats are placed: two on the pedicle, one on the proper ligament. (c) The pedicle is transected distal to the second hemostat. (d) Begin the modified Miller's knot: pass suture under the hemostat (or Carmalt). (e) Pass suture under the hemostat (or Carmalt) again, creating a loop, and pass the needle holder through the loop. (f) Wrap the long strand of suture once around the needle holder. (g) Grasp the short strand of the suture with the needle holder. (h) Pull the needle holder back out of the loop, creating the first throw of the knot. (i) Remove the most proximal hemostat (or Carmalt) and pull the first throw tight into the crushed area from the first hemostat (or Carmalt). (j) Place three or four more square knot throws, remove the remaining hemostat (or Carmalt), and check for hemorrhage.

(e)

(f)

(g)

(h)

(i)

(j)

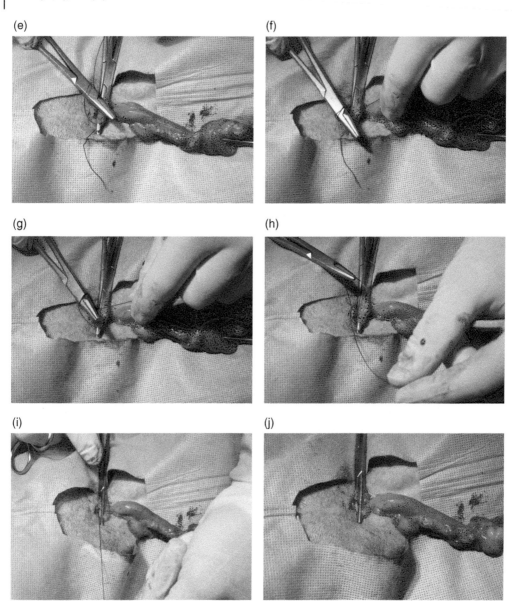

Figure 12.4 (Continued)

Carmalts, the first proximal on the ovarian pedicle, the second several millimeters distal to the first, but still proximal to the ovary, and the third on the proper ligament between the ovary and the uterine horn. Close the first hemostat one click, the second two clicks, and the third three clicks. The purpose of the 1, 2, 3 clicks is to avoid completely crushing the tissue at the most proximal clamp, which would predispose the pedicle to tearing.

Before ligating, transect the ovarian pedicle just distal to the second hemostat (between the second hemostat and the ovary). Ligate with a modified Miller's knot (see next section). Place the ligature just proximal to the most proximal hemostat and, before pulling the ligature tight, remove the most proximal hemostat. This places the ligature in the tissue compressed by the most proximal hemostat. A single ligature, appropriately placed and tied securely and tightly, is all that is necessary on ovarian pedicles.

After ligation, the transected pedicle is grasped with a thumb forceps, the clamp removed, and the pedicle observed for hemorrhage prior to returning the pedicle to the abdominal cavity.

Modified Miller's Knot

The modified Miller's knot is a very secure, self-locking knot that can be placed either with an instrument or with a hand tie (Figure 12.4). The modified Miller's knot can be used on spermatic cords, ovarian pedicles in dogs, and uterine bodies of dogs and cats (Bushby 2013). To place a modified Miller's knot, pass the suture under the tissue to be ligated, then bring the suture back over the tissue and under the tissue one more time. This creates a small loop of suture above the tissue to be ligated. Position the needle holder through that small loop, wrap the long strand once around the needle holder, grasp the short strand of suture with the needle holder, and pull the needle holder toward you while pulling the long strand of suture away from you. Gentle upward tension while pulling this knot tight facilitates even tightening of the ligature. Complete the knot by placing three or four additional square knot throws (see Figures 12.4 and 12.5).

Second Pedicle and Uterine Body Ligation

Gentle traction on the uterine horn will allow exposure of the uterine body and the second uterine horn. Caudal traction on the second uterine horn will expose the ovary. The second ovarian pedicle is ligated and transected in a manner identical to that of the first ovarian pedicle.

Following ligation and transection of both ovarian pedicles, the two uterine horns are reflected caudally, exposing the uterine body and cervix. The broad ligaments on either side of the uterine body are either torn or cut to the level of the uterine vessels. If the broad ligaments are vascular it may be necessary to ligate the broad ligaments prior to transecting them.

A single ligature with a modified Miller's knot is placed on the uterine body close to the cervix. The ligature should be tightened until tissue blanching is observed under the ligature. It is not necessary to crush the uterine tissue with a hemostat or Carmalt (see Figure 12.5); if the uterus is friable, crushing may cause tearing of the uterus. A hemostat or Carmalt is then placed distal to the ligatures and the uterine body transected between the ligatures and the hemostatic clamp, leaving several millimeters of tissue distal to the ligature to prevent slippage of the ligature.

When ligating the uterine body during ovariohysterectomy, it is not necessary to remove all uterine tissue for fear of stump pyometra, as pyometra will not occur without the presence of ovarian hormones. It is also acceptable to ligate the two uterine horns separately if the uterine body is difficult to exteriorize.

Closure

The abdomen may be closed in two or three layers. The holding layer for abdominal wall closure consists of the external rectus fascia. Selection of suture patterns and suture material is generally the surgeon's preference, and continuous, interrupted, or cruciate patterns are all acceptable. The subcutaneous tissue and the skin may be closed separately or in a single layer. It is recommended that skin closure is subcuticular such that suture removal is not required.

Aberdeen Knot

If a continuous suture line is used in any of the closure layers, an alternative knot for ending the closure is the Aberdeen knot (Figure 12.6). This knot is a self-locking knot that can be used as an alternative to a square knot at the end of any continuous suture line (Regier et al. 2015). The Aberdeen knot is equally secure to a square knot but is less bulky, thus leaving less

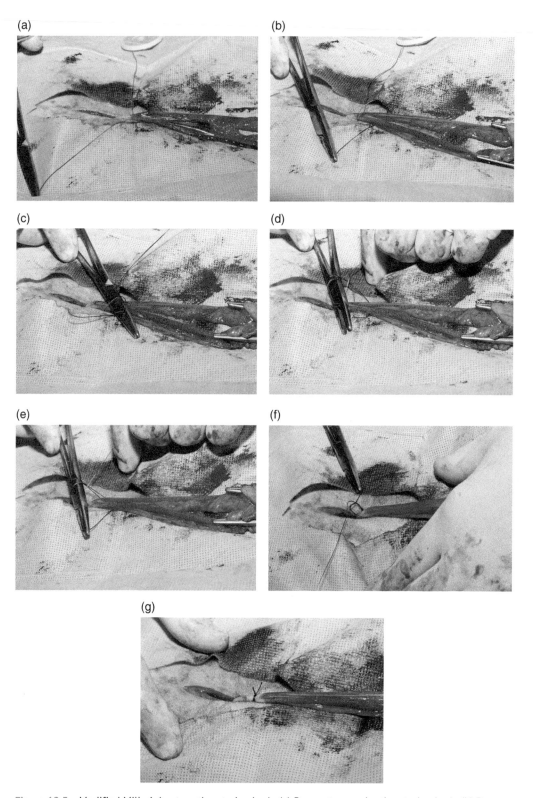

Figure 12.5 Modified Miller's knot on the uterine body. (a) Pass suture under the uterine body. (b) Pass suture under the uterine body again, creating a loop. (c) Pass the needle holder through the loop. (d) Wrap a long strand of suture around the needle holder. (e) Grasp a short strand of suture with the needle holder. (f) Pull the needle holder toward the surgeon and the long strand away from the surgeon, tightening the first throw. (g) Place three or four more square knot throws and cut the suture. *Source:* Photos courtesy of Tom Thompson.

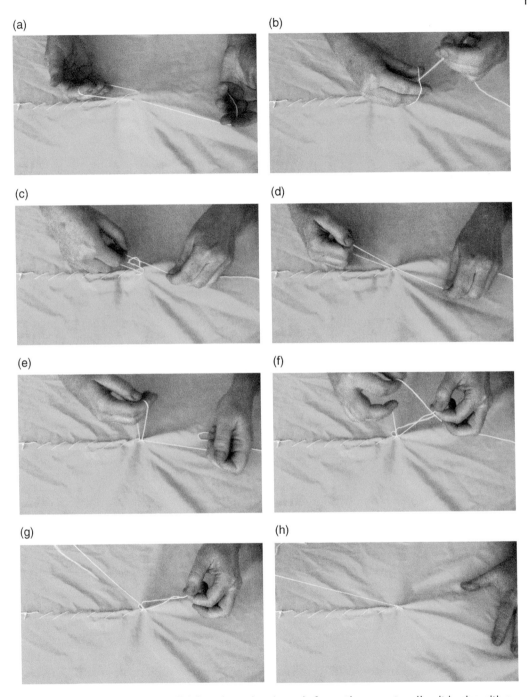

Figure 12.6   An Aberdeen knot. This knot is used at the end of a continuous suture line. It begins with a loop and an end, and can be tied with instruments or as a hand tie. A hand tie is used here for illustration purposes. (a) Pick up the last suture loop. Place the fingers of one hand through the loop while holding the needle end of the suture in the other hand. (b) Reach through the loop and grasp the suture. (c) Pull the suture through without releasing the needle end, thus creating a new loop. (d) Tighten the previous loop until it is flush with the patient. (e) Place the fingers through the new loop and repeat steps b–d at least once more. (f) To finish the knot, on the final loop, release the needle end from the other hand so that the end can be pulled through the loop. (g) Pull the end completely through the final loop. (h) Pull the end until the knot is tightened.

suture material in the wound (Stott et al. 2007). Being smaller, the Aberdeen knot may also be easier to bury at the end of a subcuticular or intradermal suture line (Thomas and Saleeby 2012; Regier et al. 2015). Figure 12.6 shows the process of constructing an Aberdeen knot. The number of throws required depends on the tissue layer, with two throws adequate for an intradermal or subcuticular closure, and three or four throws recommended for closing the linea (Stott et al. 2007; Schaaf et al. 2009).

Tattoo

Following closure, a tattoo should be placed in or near the spay incision (see Chapter 16 for information on applying a tattoo). After the tattoo is applied, skin glue may be applied to the closed incision if desired, making sure to avoid placing glue inside the wound.

Feline Ovariohysterectomy

The basic technique for ovariohysterectomy in the cat is essentially the same as that of the female dog, with the exception of the location of the incision and the autoligation technique for ovarian pedicle ligation (described below).

Preparation

The ventral abdominal skin should be clipped of hair and aseptically prepped as described in Chapter 4. The patient is positioned in dorsal recumbency with the front legs left untied, or secured along the lateral thoracic walls.

Location of Incision

In cats and kittens, the ovaries are easily exteriorized, but the uterine body is more difficult to exteriorize. The incision, therefore, should be centered at the midpoint between the umbilicus and the anterior brim of the pubis.

A 1–2 cm skin incision is made on the ventral abdominal midline at the midpoint between the umbilicus and the cranial brim of the pubis. Dissect subcutaneous tissue only to the extent necessary to visualize the linea alba. Grasp the linea alba with a thumb forceps, elevate it, and nick the linea with a scalpel blade. With the linea still elevated, extend the incision with either a scissors or a scalpel blade.

Locating the Uterus

Upon entry into the abdominal cavity, a spay hook is used to locate and exteriorize the first uterine horn. The spay hook should be passed into the abdominal cavity along the right abdominal wall. Upon reaching the dorsal lateral abdominal wall, the hook is then swept toward the midline and elevated out of the abdominal incision. Depending on the experience of the surgeon, it may take several passes of the spay hook to exteriorize the right uterine horn. If the right horn is not found after several passes, the surgeon may use the hook on the left side. When using a spay hook, especially on the left side, care should be taken to avoid damage to the spleen, mesentery, and other abdominal structures.

Pedicle Tie

In the cat spay a pedicle tie can be used for hemostasis of the ovarian vessels (Figure 12.7; Bohling et al. 2010, Griffin and Bohling 2010, Bushby 2013, Porters et al. 2014, Miller et al. 2016). The pedicle tie is a self-ligature similar to the cord tie frequently used in cat and puppy castrations. The ovarian pedicle in the cat contains very little fat, allowing exposure and isolation of the ovarian vessels. Pedicle ties are appropriate for use in cats of any age and at any stage of pregnancy or estrus. Use of the pedicle tie is only appropriate in cats. The presence of fat in the adult dog or puppy ovarian pedicle interferes with the security of the knot.

There are several variations of the pedicle tie, depending on whether the surgeon is right or left handed and on which side of the surgery table the surgeon prefers to stand. Each of the variations creates the same effect.

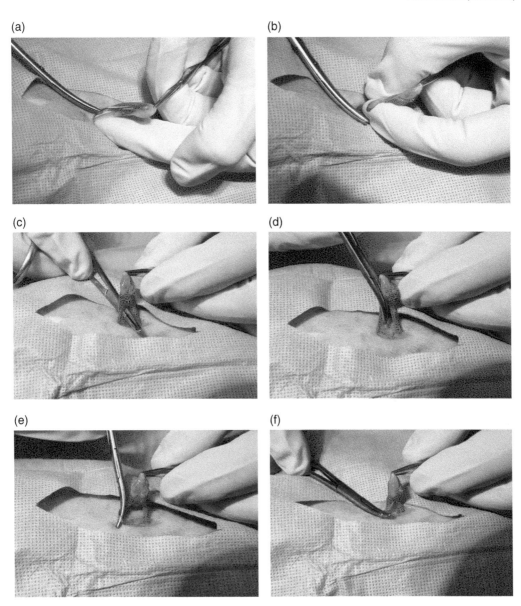

Figure 12.7 Feline ovarian ligation with pedicle tie. (a) The suspensory ligament is located and isolated from the ovarian vessels. (b) The suspensory ligament is cut. (c) A window is torn in the broad ligament caudal to the ovarian vessels, thereby isolating the vessels. (d) A curved hemostat is placed to begin the pedicle tie. The tip of the hemostat faces away from the surgeon. (e) Rotate the hemostat counterclockwise. (f) Continue to rotate counterclockwise until the hemostat faces the surgeon. (g) Open the hemostat and clamp the ovarian pedicle. (h) Transect the pedicle distal to the tip of the hemostat, leaving a few millimeters of cut end. (i) The pedicle has been transected. (j) The vessels are pushed off the end of the hemostat, tightened, and checked for hemorrhage prior to release into the abdomen.

(g)

(h)

(i)

(j)

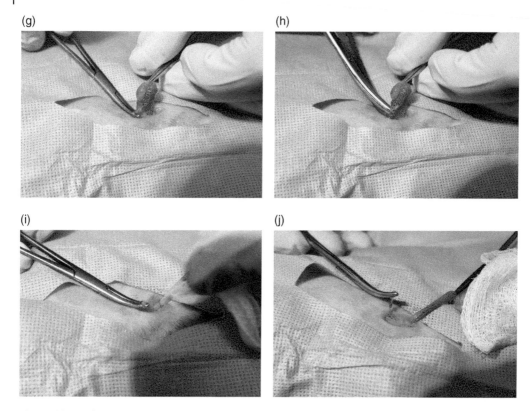

Figure 12.7 (Continued)

Preparing for the Pedicle Tie

Once the first uterine horn is exteriorized, gentle traction on the more cranial aspect of the uterine horn will begin to expose the ovary. Place a hemostat on the proper ligament of the ovary and apply upward tension. This tenses the suspensory ligament of the ovary, making visualization of the ligament much easier. It may also be helpful to press gently downward on the body wall at the incision to further expose the suspensory ligament. Placing a finger behind the pedicle may help isolate the suspensory ligament from the ovarian vessels.

The suspensory ligament is then cut with a scissors or blade, or is torn. Tear a hole in the broad ligament caudal to the ovarian vessels to isolate the ovarian vessels in the ovarian pedicle.

Performing the Pedicle Tie

With the uterine horn and ovary pulled toward the surgeon, the tip of a hemostat is crossed over the vessels and placed into the hole in the broad ligament behind the ovarian vessels. With the hemostat closed and the tip of the hemostat facing away from the surgeon, the tip of the hemostat is directed above the vessels and the hemostat is rotated counterclockwise until the tip of the hemostat faces the surgeon. This causes the ovarian vessels to be wrapped around the hemostat. The jaws of the hemostat should then be opened and used to clamp the ovarian vessels. Cut the ovarian vessels between the hemostat and the ovary and gently push the knot off the end of the hemostat. Pull the knot tight before releasing the hemostat and observe the vessels for hemorrhage.

Alternatively, the pedicle tie may be performed with the uterine horn and ovary held away from the surgeon, and the hemostat held in front of the uterine horn and placed through the hole in the broad ligament from the front.

Second Pedicle and Uterine Body Ligation

Gentle traction on the uterine horn will allow exposure of the uterine body and the second uterine horn. Caudal traction on the second uterine horn will expose the ovary. The second ovarian pedicle is ligated and transected in a manner identical to that for the first ovarian pedicle.

Following ligation and transection of both ovarian pedicles, the two uterine horns are reflected caudally, exposing the uterine body and cervix. The broad ligaments on either side of the uterine body are either torn or cut to the level of the uterine vessels. If the broad ligaments are vascular, it may be necessary to ligate the broad ligaments prior to transecting them. An autoligation similar to a pedicle tie may be used to ligate the broad ligaments.

A single ligature using a modified Miller's knot (see description in the canine ovariohysterectomy section and Figures 12.4 and 12.5) is placed on the uterine body close to the cervix. The ligature should be tightened until tissue blanching is observed under the ligature. It is not necessary to crush the uterine tissue with a hemostat or Carmalt, as in some cases crushing friable tissue may result in damage or tearing of the uterus. A hemostat or Carmalt is then placed distal to the ligatures and the uterine body transected between the ligatures and the hemostatic clamp, leaving several millimeters of tissue distal to the ligature to prevent slippage of the ligature.

When ligating the uterine body during ovariohysterectomy, it is not necessary to remove all uterine tissue for fear of stump pyometra, as pyometra will not occur without the presence of ovarian hormones. It is also acceptable to ligate the two uterine horns separately if the uterine body is difficult to exteriorize.

Closure

The abdomen may be closed in two or three layers. The holding layer for abdominal wall closure consists of the external rectus fascia.

Selection of suture patterns and suture material is generally the surgeon's preference, and continuous, interrupted, or cruciate patterns are all acceptable. The subcutaneous tissue and the skin may be closed separately or in a single layer. It is recommended that skin closure is subcuticular such that suture removal is not required.

Following closure, a tattoo should be placed in or near the spay incision (see Chapter 16 for information on applying a tattoo). After the tattoo is applied, skin glue may be applied to the closed incision if desired, making sure to avoid placing glue inside the wound.

Ovariohysterectomy via a Lateral Flank Approach

The generally accepted approach for an ovariohysterectomy in the dog and cat in the United States is through a ventral abdominal midline incision, while in many European countries an incision in the flank is the preferred approach (McGrath et al. 2004, Griffin and Bohling 2010).

There are specific situations where a flank approach for an ovariohysterectomy is indicated. Cats with mammary hyperplasia (Figure 12.8) and lactating queens or bitches are ideal candidates for flank spays (Levy and Wilford 2013). Performing a flank spay avoids damage to mammary tissue, preventing leakage

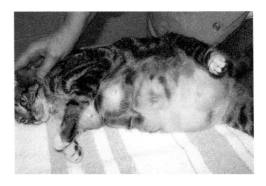

Figure 12.8 A cat with mammary hyperplasia. This cat was spayed using a flank approach. *Source:* Photo courtesy of Brenda Griffin.

of milk into the tissues. In the lactating patient a flank spay reduces the chances that nursing offspring would damage the incision site. One should also consider performing a flank spay in feral cats or dogs (Reece et al. 2012) in trap–neuter–return programs in which the patients are released back into their colony shortly after surgery. There is considerably less chance of having a surgical dehiscence through a flank incision than through a ventral midline incision (Levy and Wilford 2013).

Flank spay may be more difficult in larger, deep-bodied dogs and obese patients. It is not a recommended approach for pregnant animals or those with pyometra due to limited exposure via the flank approach. A further disadvantage of the flank approach is difficulty in retrieving dropped pedicles or achieving hemostasis if unexpected hemorrhage occurs (McGrath et al. 2004).

Flank Spay Technique

A flank spay may be performed with the patient in left or right lateral recumbency. Generally, the surgeon stands on their accustomed side of the table and the patient is positioned with feet toward the surgeon and spine away from the surgeon. This patient positioning determines the side of the approach. Left lateral recumbency may be preferable, as it minimizes the likelihood of encountering the spleen.

The skin incision may be made in a dorso-ventral direction, horizontally, or diagonally in a dorso-cranial to ventro-caudal direction. In cats, the incision is placed two-thirds to three-quarters of the way back from the last rib toward the cranial aspect of the wing of the ilium, starting approximately 2 cm ventral to the transverse spinous processes and creating a 1.5–2 cm incision (Figure 12.9; McGrath et al. 2004). In dogs, some surgeons place the incision in a proportionally similar location to cats, while other surgeons prefer to make a horizontal incision and to place the incision more ventrally, at the level of the fold of skin

connecting the stifle to the abdominal wall (Reece 2018). The incision length in dogs is typically 2–3 cm.

After making the skin incision, dissect and if necessary excise any subcutaneous fat, exposing the external abdominal oblique muscle. Bluntly separate fibers of the external abdominal oblique muscle to expose the internal abdominal oblique muscle. Muscle fibers of the internal abdominal oblique can be bluntly separated, exposing the peritoneum. Often blunt separation of the internal abdominal oblique muscle fibers penetrates the peritoneum, allowing entry into the abdominal cavity. If the peritoneum has not been penetrated, it can be cut with a scissors exposing the abdominal contents. Once the abdomen has been entered, many surgeons find it useful to grasp the transverse abdominis muscle with thumb forceps or Allis tissue forceps to retain control of the body wall (McGrath et al. 2004; Reece 2018).

If the incision is positioned properly, the right uterine horn or right ovary will be clearly visible in the cat. With the more ventral approach to the dog that has been described, these structures are likely not visible and will be located dorsal to the incision (Reece 2018). If these structures are not visible, they can be retrieved using a spay hook. Place the spay hook into the abdominal cavity at the ventral-most aspect of the incision and sweep dorsally along the body wall to the transverse spinous processes. Once the uterine horn is located, the ovaries and uterus are removed in a manner identical to that done with a ventral midline approach. The ovary can be exteriorized, the suspensory ligament torn or cut, and a pedicle tie (in cats) or a modified Miller's knot ligation (in dogs) can be performed on the ovarian vessels, with the ovarian pedicle transected between the ligation and the ovary. Gentle retraction of the uterine horn allows delivery of the uterine body into the incision, exposing the contralateral uterine horn. Traction on the uterine horn exposes the ovary, and the suspensory ligament can be torn or cut, the

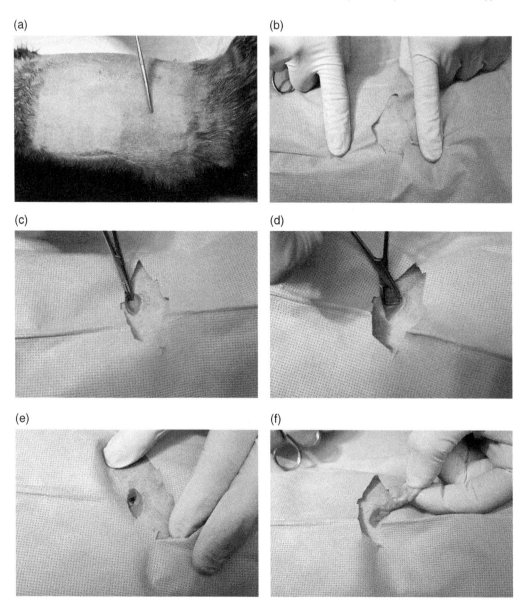

Figure 12.9   Flank spay in a cat. (a) The incision for a flank spay is made two-thirds of the way back from the last rib to the crest of the ilium and just ventral to the transverse spinous processes. (b) The surgeon palpates the locations of the last rib and iliac crest through the drape prior to placing the incision. (c) The muscle fibers of the external abdominal oblique then internal abdominal oblique are bluntly separated, not incised. First, the tip of a hemostat is placed between the muscle fibers. (d) The jaws of the hemostat are then opened to separate the fibers. (e) The appearance of the abdominal entry wound. (f) Exteriorizing the right ovary and the uterine horn.

pedicle ligated as on the first side, and the pedicle transected between the ligature and the ovary. The broad ligaments are torn or cut, allowing exposure and ligation of the uterine body with a modified Miller's knot. The uterine body is transected distal to the ligature and the stump is checked for hemorrhage and returned to the abdominal cavity.

In adult dogs, a three-layer closure is performed, suturing the internal abdominal oblique muscle, the external abdominal oblique muscle, and subcuticular tissue. In cats and puppies, three-layer closure is also common, but some surgeons choose to close all the muscle layers together in one or two simple interrupted or cruciate sutures (McGrath et al. 2004; Reece 2018). When using a three-layer closure, placement of one cruciate suture in the internal abdominal oblique muscle and one cruciate suture in the external abdominal oblique muscle, followed by two buried simple interrupted subcuticular sutures, is all that is necessary for closure.

Special Situations in Ovariohysterectomy

The Pregnant Patient

In the shelter and high-volume spay–neuter environment, surgeons may be presented with pregnant animals to spay. The technique for ovariohysterectomy in the pregnant female is virtually the same as that in the non-pregnant animal, with a few exceptions. Depending on the stage of pregnancy, the incision may need to be larger. Finding the first uterine horn in the pregnant patient is generally easier than finding the non-gravid uterus, simply because the presence of the fetuses make the uterus larger. The uterine tissue may be more friable, so the uterus must be handled with care to avoid tearing the uterine wall. This is especially important if an effort is made to exteriorize the gravid uterus though abdominal wall and skin incisions that are too small.

Special attention should be paid to hemostasis. Even though the vessels may be significantly enlarged, the pedicle tie (see Figure 12.7) is still an appropriate method for ligating the ovarian vessels in the cat. In the dog, pedicle ligation may proceed as described for routine canine ovariohysterectomy. Generally, ligation of the uterine body with a modified Miller's knot placed near the cervix with the ligature incorporating the uterine vessels on both sides

of the uterus is sufficient. If necessary, the uterine vessels can be ligated independently. Large vessels in the broad ligament can be ligated either with suture or with the pedicle tie.

What to Do with the Gravid Uterus?

Once the gravid uterus has been removed from the dam, no additional action is required to ensure fetal death without fetal suffering or consciousness (White 2012). The neurologic immaturity of fetal cats, dogs, and rabbits, combined with the high concentrations of anesthetic drugs that cross the placenta and hypoxia-induced neuroinhibitors, prevent the fetuses from becoming conscious.

The fetuses should remain in the closed uterus after uterine removal from the dam. The uterus may be simply set aside and the fetuses left undisturbed. It is not necessary to retain clamps on the uterus as long as the fetuses remain in their amniotic sacs. Some veterinarians may elect to inject euthanasia solution through the wall of the closed uterus into the fetal abdominal cavity to hasten fetal death. Although this procedure is not necessary for the prevention of fetal suffering, it has no detrimental welfare effects and may stop the spontaneous in-utero fetal movements that some veterinarians and staff find troubling.

If the gravid uterus is to be opened after ovariohysterectomy (for example, for educational purposes), it has been recommended (White 2012) that the uterus be left unopened and the fetuses undisturbed for a minimum of one hour after removal from the dam to prevent inadvertent fetal resuscitation. Fetal exposure to air prior to fetal death may lead to the stimulation of respiration, loss of neuroinhibition, exhalation of inhalant anesthetic drugs, and perhaps even the potential for fetal consciousness and suffering prior to euthanasia.

Pyometra Spay

Ovariohysterectomy is the surgical treatment for either open or closed pyometra (Hedlund 2007; MacPhail 2013). The patient with a pyometra, especially one with a closed pyometra, may present with dehydration, azotemia, and acid–base imbalances. These should be corrected prior to surgery, but without delaying surgery for more than a few hours after diagnosis.

The surgical technique for ovariohysterectomy in the patient with a pyometra is similar to that of the pregnant animal. The incision will need to be larger than usual in order to avoid damage to the uterus during exteriorization. Uterine tissue may be friable and care must be taken to prevent tearing the uterus. The uterus should be identified visually and gently elevated out of the abdominal cavity. Use of a spay hook should be avoided due to the risk of tearing friable uterine tissue. If a uterine torsion is present, do not attempt to relieve the torsion, as this could lead to a greater chance of the systemic release of bacteria or bacterial toxins.

Ligation of the ovarian pedicles can be performed as described for routine ovariohysterectomy, using a pedicle tie in cats or a modified Miller's knot in dogs. Special attention should be paid to hemostasis. Large vessels in the broad ligament can be ligated either with suture or with the pedicle tie.

In patients (especially dogs) with large or significant pyometra, prior to ligating and transecting the uterine body, sterile towels should be packed around the uterus to protect the abdominal cavity from contamination. Leakage of uterine contents can be minimized by placing a ligature at the junction of the uterine body and the cervix and occluding the uterine body with a Carmalt, then transecting between the ligature and the Carmalt. Alternatively, a ligature can be placed at the junction of the uterine body and the cervix and a second ligature on the uterine body, transecting between the two ligatures. Also, if necessary, the uterine vessels can be ligated independently. With either approach, the uterine stump should be flushed with sterile saline prior to returning it to the abdomen. Oversewing the stump is not recommended. If peritonitis is present or if abdominal contamination occurs, the abdomen should be flushed with sterile saline as well. Prior to closure of the abdomen, the sterile towels should be removed and gloves and instruments should be changed.

Uterus Unicornis

Uterus unicornis is congenital absence of one horn of the uterus, and may occur in both cats and dogs (see Chapter 2). The broad ligament and uterine vessels may be present or absent on the involved side, but both ovaries will be present in the normal location (Figure 12.10).

Often the first indications that a patient may have a unicornate uterus are either a difficulty in locating the horn of the uterus with the spay hook on the first side, or a difficulty in reaching the uterine horn bifurcation at the uterine body to access the second horn. In either case, utilize the spay hook on the second side. In the case of the difficult-to-exteriorize uterine body, using the spay hook on the second side will allow the surgeon to find the second uterine

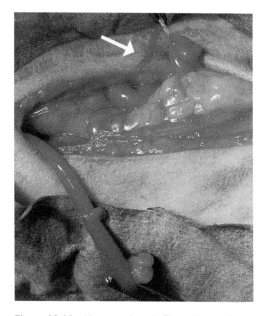

Figure 12.10 Uterus unicornis. The left ovary is located at the most cranial aspect of the left uterine horn. There is no right uterine horn, but the right ovary is present (arrow). *Source:* Photo courtesy of Julie Levy.

horn (if present) or the broad ligament (if the uterus is unicornate).

The ovary on the involved side will be in the normal location and, if a broad ligament is present, simply trace the broad ligament cranially until the ovary is encountered. If no broad ligament is present on the involved side, extend the incision and use the biologic retractors to help localize the ovary. Grasping the descending duodenum and reflecting it to the left will expose the right side, allowing visualization of the right ovary. Grasping the descending colon and reflecting it to the right will expose the left side, allowing visualization of the left ovary. It should be noted that the kidney is often absent on the same side as the missing uterine horn.

Uterine Prolapse

Spay–neuter clinics and shelter clinics may be presented with animals with uterine prolapse for "routine" spay or on an emergency basis (Figure 12.11). Uterine prolapse is rare, and occurs more frequently in cats than in dogs (Biddle and Macintire 2000). In most cases the prolapse occurs during delivery or miscarriage, or within the first 48 hours after delivery, although one case report describes prolapse three days after delivery (Sabuncu et al. 2017), and another describes prolapse in a stray cat in whom no pregnancy or delivery had been observed (Valentine et al. 2016). Some HQHVSN veterinarians have described having cats with a uterine prolapse of unknown duration and cause present via TNR programs. While uterine prolapse is considered an obstetric emergency (Biddle and Macintire 2000), some HQHVSN veterinarians have encountered cases in which the duration of the prolapse was known to have been from a few days to up to a year.

Assessment

Uterine prolapse may consist of one uterine horn (Sabuncu et al. 2017) or both horns, and may be complete or partial. If the prolapse is partial and recent, it is possible that the non-prolapsed portion of the uterus contains one or more fetuses (Uçmak et al. 2018). The prolapsed uterine tissue may be ischemic or necrotic, depending on the duration of the prolapse (Biddle and Macintire 2000). The prolapsed portion of the uterus should be palpated to assess for the presence within it of additional abdominal contents such as the urinary bladder or abdominal viscera (Deroy et al. 2015), particularly if amputation of the prolapsed tissue is being considered. If abdominal contents are present within the prolapsed uterus, open abdominal reduction will likely be necessary to return these organs to the abdomen prior to ovariohysterectomy or prolapse amputation.

The patient should be assessed and stabilized. Patients with acute uterine prolapse may be depressed, dehydrated, and in pain, may be hyper- or hypothermic, and may appear to have difficulty urinating (Deroy et al. 2015; Sabuncu et al. 2017). If the uterine or ovarian artery was torn during the prolapse, hemorrhage may have occurred and the patient may be hypovolemic or hypotensive and may require fluid support or transfusion (Biddle and Macintire 2000). In cases in which the uterus has been prolapsed for a more extended duration, the patient may be bright and alert with a normal appetite and no apparent distress resulting from the prolapse (Valentine et al. 2016).

Antibiotic therapy should be initiated at or before the time of surgery and continued during the post-operative period.

Manual Reduction and Ovariohysterectomy

If the uterus is not severely damaged, contaminated, or necrotic, the prolapsed tissue may be reduced, and a routine ovariohysterectomy can then be performed (Figure 12.12a and b). General anesthesia with or without epidural analgesia (see the anesthesia supplement to Chapter 19) will be required to replace the uterus. The prolapsed uterus should be cleaned thoroughly with an antiseptic solution and lubricated prior to attempting reduction. It may also be helpful to soak the tissue in a

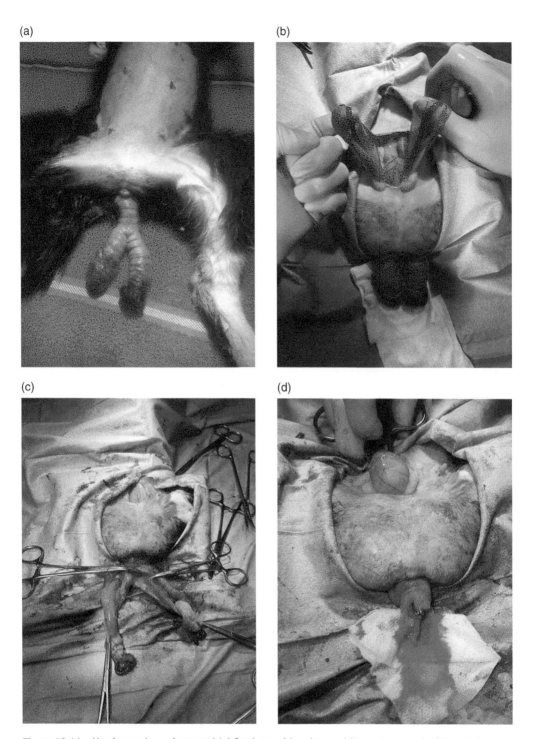

Figure 12.11 Uterine prolapse in a cat. (a) A feral cat with unknown history presented with a uterine prolapse. The cat was anesthetized, clipped, and surgically prepared from the vulva to the sternum. (b) An abdominal incision was made and the ovaries and ovarian pedicles were identified. On both sides, the suspensory ligament, pedicle, and broad ligament were each ligated using the pedicle tie technique and were transected. The tips of the uterine horns were released into the abdomen. (c) Surgery then proceeded to the prolapsed uterus. The surgeon cut along the top side of the bifurcation until the uterus could be turned inside out to access the uterine arteries. A stick tie (transfixing ligature) was placed on each uterine artery. (d) The uterine body was amputated and the uterine vessels transected distal to the ligatures. A hemostat was introduced through the abdominal incision and out of the vaginal opening to grasp the uterine stump. (e) The uterine stump was inverted and returned to the abdomen. (f) The uterine stump was double-ligated using Miller's knots. The abdomen was lavaged. Because the cat was feral and would receive no follow-up care, an incisional vaginopexy was performed to attach the uterine stump to the abdominal wall. The patient recovered well. *Source:* Photos courtesy of Brienne LeMay.

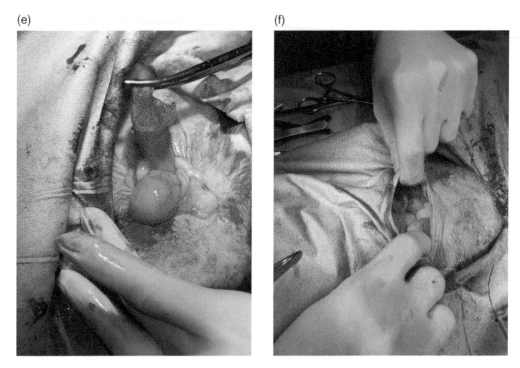

Figure 12.11   (Continued)

(a)

(b)

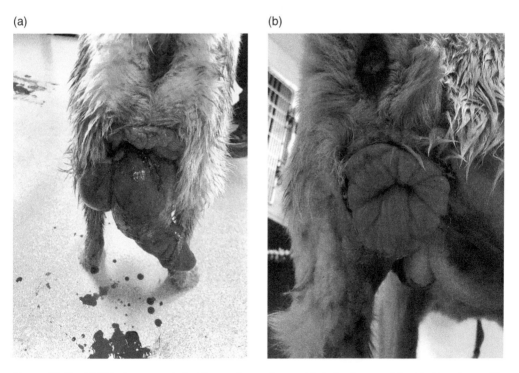

Figure 12.12   (a) This dog presented with a prolapse of a gravid uterine horn and the bladder, along with vaginal hyperplasia. The fetus was removed from the prolapsed horn and the bladder and uterine horn were returned to the abdomen, followed by a routine spay procedure. (b) The same dog during her recovery. The vaginal prolapse resolved after ovariohysterectomy without further surgical intervention (see Chapter 21 for more on treating this condition). *Source:* Photos courtesy of Patti Canchola.

hyperosmotic solution such as 50% dextrose to attempt to reduce the size of the edematous tissue before reduction. Episiotomy may also be helpful in reducing the prolapsed uterus (Biddle and Macintire 2000).

Once the uterus is reduced into the abdomen, it is possible to perform a routine ovariohysterectomy. If reduction of the uterus is not possible, prolapse amputation (external hysterectomy) and ovariectomy are indicated.

Ovariectomy and Prolapse Amputation

In cases in which the prolapsed uterine tissue is too damaged, necrotic, or edematous to return to the abdomen, it is possible to perform an ovariectomy and amputate the prolapsed uterus (see Figure 12.11). The abdominal ovariectomy (or pedicle ligation without ovariectomy) should be performed first, followed by external amputation of the uterus and reduction of the uterine stump while the abdomen remains open (Deroy et al. 2015; Valentine et al. 2016).

When pedicle ligation (with or without ovariectomy) is performed prior to uterine amputation and stump reduction, there is caudal traction on the ovaries due to the stretching resulting from the prolapsed tissues. Thus, the ovaries are located more caudally than usual and there is tension and elongation of the suspensory ligament and ovarian vessels (Deroy et al. 2015). However, a routine ovariectomy consisting of pedicle ties (in cats) or modified Miller's knots (in dogs) on the ovarian vessels and suture ligation of the uterine vessels should still be possible in these cases. Following pedicle ligation with or without ovariectomy, the tips of the uterine horns are released back into the abdomen.

When performing external amputation of the prolapsed uterus, the surgeon should ensure that the urethral opening is not damaged, removed, or ligated during the amputation. If the prolapsed tissue is not too damaged, it may be possible to identify the urethral tubercle and preserve it. Urethral catheterization may be beneficial in these cases. However, in many cases the tissue will be in poor condition, such that identification of the urethral meatus is not possible. In these cases, performing the amputation on the uterine body, between the bifurcation and the cervix, will ensure that the urethra is not damaged in the amputation.

To perform external amputation of the prolapsed uterus, the uterine body may either be ligated en bloc with a circumferential suture or modified Miller's knot, or may be opened to allow individual uterine vessel ligation prior to amputation (see Figure 12.11c). The prolapsed uterine tissue distal to the ligature(s) should be removed, and the remaining stump should be inverted and returned to the abdomen. Oversewing of the stump prior to reduction (Deroy et al. 2015) should be unnecessary, as additional transection and ligation may take place during the abdominal portion of the surgery after reduction of the stump.

Once the uterine stump is returned to the abdominal cavity, the surgery can be approached abdominally. From within the abdominal cavity, the uterine body is ligated proximal to any previously placed ligature. If tissue is friable or engorged, individual uterine vessel ligation may be indicated, if it has not already been performed. If an en bloc ligation was performed when the uterus was external, the excess uterine stump including the previous ligation is then removed (Valentine et al. 2016). As with pyometra, oversewing the stump is not recommended, but warm saline lavage of the uterine stump and abdomen is beneficial to reduce contamination prior to closing.

Post-operatively, urination should be monitored, as swelling and pain can lead to urethral obstruction (Deroy et al. 2015).

Intersex Surgery

At times, patients who have both male and female characteristics will present for surgery (see Chapter 2). While numerous variations of intersex phenotypes exist, the goal of the spay–neuter veterinarian in any case is to remove

(a)   (b)

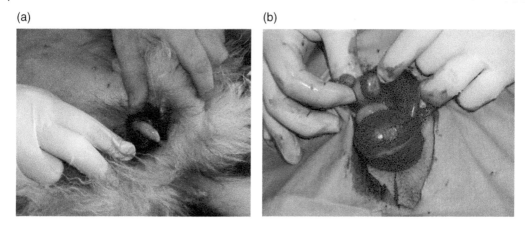

Figure 12.13   Intersex. (a) This patient presented as a female with an enlarged clitoris. (b) Ovatestes associated with a normal-appearing uterus.

the gonads, and generally to remove the tubular structures associated with them. The gonads can be located anywhere between the caudal pole of the kidneys to the inguinal area to the subcutaneous tissue in the perineum (Figure 12.13).

A fairly common intersex presentation is that of a female with an enlarged clitoris (Figure 12.13a). In this presentation, the inguinal and perineal area should be palpated carefully for the presence of gonads. If the gonads are in the perineum, the surgery is performed as a castration. If no gonads are palpated in the perineal or inguinal area, the surgery is performed as an ovariohysterectomy, as described previously (Bushby 2013).

Alternatives to Ovariohysterectomy

Ovariectomy

Ovariectomy has been described as an acceptable alternative to ovariohysterectomy (DeTora and McCarthy 2011; Peeters and Kirpensteijn 2011). In many European countries ovariectomy is considered the preferred method for surgical sterilization of the female dog, while ovariohysterectomy remains the more common technique in the United States (van Goethem et al. 2006). The Association of Shelter Veterinarians' spay neuter guidelines recognize both ovariohysterectomy and ovariectomy as acceptable techniques and simply state that "complete removal of both ovaries is required" (Griffin et al. 2016).

While some papers contend that ovariectomy is quicker than ovariohysterectomy (van Goethem et al. 2006), others document that the two techniques are similar in length of time, length of incisions, and incidence of complications (Peeters and Kirpensteijn 2011). In these authors' experience, ovariectomy involves an incision in the same location and of the same length as that in an ovariohysterectomy and the two procedures take essentially the same amount of time. Some surgeons find ovariohysterectomy to be faster than ovariectomy due to the necessity for an additional ligature during ovariectomy.

The surgical approaches for ovariectomy are the same as for ovariohysterectomy (Figure 12.14). Ovariectomy can be performed through a ventral midline, right paramedian, or flank approach. Exteriorize the first uterine horn and ovary and tear or cut the ovarian suspensory ligament. In the dog, clamp, transect, and ligate the ovarian pedicle, as described previously for canine ovariohysterectomy. In the cat, perform the pedicle tie on the ovarian pedicle, as described previously

(a)

(b)

(c)

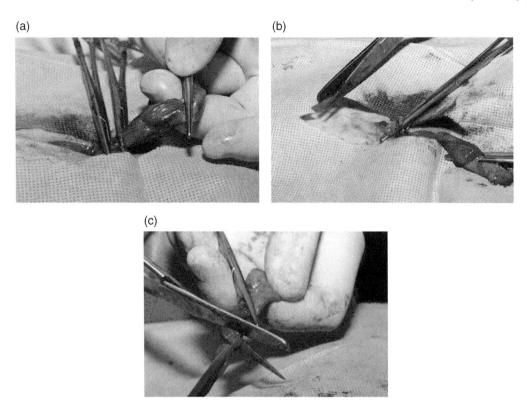

Figure 12.14 Ovariectomy. (a) Place two clamps proximal to the ovary on the ovarian pedicle and one clamp distal to the ovary, between the ovary and the uterine horn. (b) Transect the ovarian pedicle proximal to the ovary and ligate the ovarian pedicle. (c) Ligate the distal end of the uterine horn and uterine vessels and excise the ovary. *Source:* Photos courtesy of Tom Thompson.

for feline ovariohysterectomy. Next, place one hemostat or Carmalt on the proper ligament between the ovary and uterine horn. Place a ligature on the distal-most aspect of the uterine horn, proximal to the clamp, and transect between the ovary and the clamp on the uterine horn, thereby removing the first ovary. In most cases, in order to ensure that the entire ovary and fallopian tube is removed, a small portion of the tip of the uterine horn is removed as well.

Trace the first uterine horn to the uterine body to identify the second uterine horn and trace that second horn to the second ovary. The second ovary is removed and hemostasis obtained in a manner identical to the first ovary. The broad ligaments should not be incised and the uterine vessels should not be ligated.

Once both ovaries are removed, the uterine horns with their intact broad ligaments are returned to the abdominal cavity and the surgical wounds are closed, just as in the ovariohysterectomy.

Ovary-Sparing "Spay"

Hysterectomy without ovariectomy (ovary-sparing spay) has been promoted as a means to sterilize dogs while leaving reproductive hormones intact (Lissner 2013). There appears to be little interest in this option for cats, probably due to the relative lack of data related to adverse health consequences of ovary removal in cats (see Chapter 26).

In order to avoid the risk of "stump pyometra," all uterine tissue must be removed. Ligation and transection of the uterus at or proximal to the cervix are required (Mattravers 2017), necessitating a longer incision and longer surgery time than required for the typical spay. Tying off the fallopian tubes (tubal ligation) while leaving the uterus in place leaves the dog at the same risk of pyometra as if she had not been spayed, and thus is not suggested as a technique for ovary-sparing spay.

Hysterectomy may be an acceptable alternative to ovariohysterectomy for pet owners who oppose the removal of the ovaries, but do not wish for their pets to reproduce. Female dogs with hysterectomy are presumed to have the same disease risks and benefits as unaltered dogs, except for the risks of pyometra and possible complications of pregnancy, which are eliminated by hysterectomy.

Dogs who have undergone this procedure will still experience estrus cycles and demonstrate the same behaviors as intact females, a fact for which pet owners must be prepared. At this time, hysterectomy without ovariectomy has not been recommended as a technique in shelter or HQHVSN practice, due to its failure to have achieved widespread awareness and acceptance among veterinarians or pet owners.

References

Biddle, D. and Macintire, D.K. (2000). Obstetrical emergencies. *Clin. Tech. Small Anim. Pract.* 15: 88–93.

Bohling, M.W., Ridgon-Brestle, Y.K., Bushby, P.A., and Griffin, B. (2010). Veterinary seminars in spay-neuter surgeries: pediatrics. In: *Veterinary Seminars in Spay-Neuter* (ed. R.-B.Y. Karla). Asheville, NC: Humane Alliance (DVD).

Bushby, P.A. (2013). Surgical techniques for spay/neuter. In: *Shelter Medicine for Veterinarians and Staff*, 2e (eds. L. Miller and Z. Stephen), 625–646. Ames, IA: Wiley-Blackwell.

Deroy, C., Bismuth, C., and Carozzo, C. (2015). Management of a complete uterine prolapse in a cat. *J. Feline Med. Surg. Open Rep.* 1: 2055116915579681.

DeTora, M. and McCarthy, R.J. (2011). Ovariohysterectomy versus ovariectomy for elective sterilization of female dogs and cats: is removal of the uterus necessary? *JAVMA* 239: 1409–1412.

van Goethem, B., Schaefers-Okkens, A., and Kirpensteijn, J. (2006). Making a rational choice between ovariectomy and ovariohysterectomy in the dog: a discussion of the benefits of either technique. *Vet. Surg.* 35: 136–143.

Griffin, B. and Bohling, M. (2010). A review of neutering cats. In: *Consultations in Feline*

Internal Medicine, 6e (ed. J.R. August), 776–792. St. Louis, MO: Elsevier Saunders.

Griffin, B., Bushby, P.A., McCobb, E. et al. (2016). The Association of Shelter Veterinarians' 2016 veterinary medical care guidelines for spay-neuter programs. *JAVMA* 249: 165–188.

Hedlund, C.S. (2007). Surgery of the reproductive and genital systems. In: *Small Animal Surgery*, 3e (ed. T.W. Fossum), 702–720. St. Louis, MO: Mosby Elsevier.

Levy, J.K. and Wilford, C.L. (2013). Management of stray and feral community cats. In: *Shelter Medicine for Veterinarians and Staff*, 2e (ed. S.Z. Lila Miller), 669–688. Ames, IA: Wiley-Blackwell.

Lissner, E. (2013). The pros of partial spay. *Innovative Veterinary Care* (13 February). https://ivcjournal.com/the-pros-of-partial-spay (accessed 5 August 2018).

MacPhail, C.M. (2013). Surgery of the reproductive and genital systems. In: *Small Animal Surgery*, 4e (ed. T.W. Fossum), 780–855. St. Louis, MO: Mosby.

Mattravers, M. (2017). Ovary sparing spay in canines: an alternative to traditional ovariohysterectomy. https://www.parsemus. org/wp-content/uploads/2017/09/Ovary-Sparing-Spay-review-Mattravers-2017.pdf (accessed 5 August 2018).

McGrath, H., Hardie, R., and Davis, E. (2004). Lateral flank approach for ovariohysterectomy in small animals. *Compend. Cont. Educ. Pract. Vet.* 26: 922–931.

Miller, K.P., Rekers, W., Ellis, K. et al. (2016). Pedicle ties provide a rapid and safe method for feline ovariohysterectomy. *J. Feline Med. Surg.* 18: 160–164.

Peeters, M.E. and Kirpensteijn, J. (2011). Comparison of surgical variables and short-term postoperative complications in healthy dogs undergoing ovariohysterectomy or ovariectomy. *JAVMA* 238: 189–194.

Porters, N., Polis, I., Moons, C. et al. (2014). Prepubertal gonadectomy in cats: different surgical techniques and comparison with gonadectomy at traditional age. *Vet. Rec.* 175 (9): 223.

Reece, J. (2018). Ovariohysterectomy–flank approach. In: *Field Manual for Small Animal Medicine* (eds. K. Polak and A.T. Kommedal). Chichester: Wiley https://doi.org/10.1002/9781119380528.ch9b.

Reece, J., Nimesh, M., Wyllie, R. et al. (2012). Description and evaluation of a right flank, mini-laparotomy approach to canine ovariohysterectomy. *Vet. Rec.* 171: 248.

Regier, P.J., Smeak, D.D., Coleman, K., and McGilvray, K.C. (2015). Comparison of volume, security, and biomechanical strength of square and Aberdeen termination knots tied with 4–0 polyglyconate and used for termination of intradermal closures in canine cadavers. *JAVMA* 247: 260–266.

Sabuncu, A., Dal, G.E., Enginler, S.Ö. et al. (2017). Feline unilateral uterine prolapse: a description of two cases. *İstanbul Üniv. Vet. Fak. Derg.* 43: 67–70.

Schaaf, O., Glyde, M., and Day, R.E. (2009). A secure Aberdeen knot: in vitro assessment of knot security in plasma and fat. *J. Small Anim. Pract.* 50: 415–421.

Stott, P.M., Ripley, L.G., and Lavelle, M.A. (2007). The ultimate Aberdeen knot. *Ann. Royal Coll. Surg. Engl.* 89: 713–717.

Thomas, J.A. and Saleeby, E.R. (2012). The Aberdeen knot: a sliding knot for dermatology. *Dermatol. Surg.* 38: 121–123.

Uçmak, Z.G., Uçmak, M., Çetin, A.C., and Tek, Ç. (2018). Uterine prolapse in a pregnant cat. *Turk. J. Vet. Anim. Sci.* 42: 500–502.

Valentine, M.J., Porter, S., Chapwanya, A., and Callanan, J.J. (2016). Uterine prolapse with endometrial eversion in association with an unusual diffuse, polypoid, fibrosing perimetritis and parametritis in a cat. *J. Feline Med. Surg. Open Rep.* 2: 2055116915626166.

White, S.C. (2012). Prevention of fetal suffering during ovariohysterectomy of pregnant animals. *JAVMA* 240: 1160.

13

Cesarean Section

Sheilah Robertson and Sara White

In a shelter or high-quality high-volume spay–neuter (HQHVSN) clinic setting, the goal of a cesarean section (C-section) may be to save the life of the dam, the offspring, or both, and in most cases the bitch or queen will also undergo an ovariohysterectomy. The surgical technique may be a "traditional" C-section in which delivery of the puppies or kittens by hysterotomy precedes ovariohysterectomy, or be may accomplished by an en bloc C-section technique. In the latter, ovariohysterectomy is performed before hysterotomy and removal of the neonates (Robbins and Mullen 1994).

Ovariohysterectomy at the time of C-section does not affect lactation or the dam's ability to care for her litter (Onclin and Verstegen 2008).

Anesthetic Considerations

Anesthetic choices and peri-operative management require careful consideration to achieve the chosen goal. Over half of canine C-sections are emergency procedures (Moon et al. 2000), resulting in higher puppy mortality compared to an elective intervention. When labor is prolonged, dehydration, hypovolemia, sepsis, stress, exhaustion, and hypocalcemia may be present, leading to worse outcomes. Elective procedures should be considered in some dogs such as brachycephalic breeds. All animals undergoing a C-section should receive fluids and dehydration should be corrected before induction.

Maternal Considerations

Aortocaval compression in the supine position leading to maternal hypotension and fetal depression is well documented in pregnant women (Kinsella and Lohmann 1994). In dogs this may be less of a problem due to their bicornuate uterus; pregnant Beagles and Golden Retriever bitches remained normotensive in both dorsal and lateral recumbency (Probst et al. 1987; Probst and Webb 1983). However, many C-sections are performed on large or giant breed bitches (Moon et al. 1998), therefore the impact of dorsal positioning for a specific case scenario is unpredictable. A sensible approach is to do as much of the pre-incisional preparation as possible and place the bitch or queen in dorsal recumbency immediately before draping for surgery. Clipping and preparing the surgical site prior to induction of anesthesia decreases the time between induction and delivery of the offspring; during this time fluids and oxygen (see later) can be administered.

The physiologic changes associated with pregnancy influence the choice of anesthetic and analgesic drugs for C-section in queens and bitches. Although there is more information available on anesthetic protocols for C-section

High-Quality, High-Volume Spay and Neuter and Other Shelter Surgeries, First Edition. Edited by Sara White.
© 2020 John Wiley & Sons, Inc. Published 2020 by John Wiley & Sons, Inc.

and their influence on neonatal vitality and survival in dogs compared to cats, the same anesthetic management principles apply to both species. All sedative, anesthetic, and analgesic agents cross the placental barrier and reach the fetal circulation. Adjunctive agents include anticholinergics, and if these are required to treat maternal bradycardia there are two choices: one is atropine, which will cross the placenta and influence fetal heart rate; and the other is glycopyrrolate, which, due to its size and positive charge, will not enter the placental circulation.

Many clinicians are concerned that premedication causes neonatal depression. The only drug that is reported to increase maternal and/or neonatal mortality is the alpha$_2$-adrenergic agonist xylazine (Moon et al. 1998; Moon et al. 2000). Although there is no data on the effect of the newer alpha$_2$-adrenergic agonists medetomidine and dexmedetomidine on anesthetic risk associated with C-section, the potential for emesis and cardiovascular depression with their use makes them undesirable.

If properly dosed based on maternal status, pre-medicant drugs may alleviate maternal anxiety; vasoconstriction and decreased placental perfusion are more likely in an anxious dam. Pre-medicant drugs can be chosen to provide analgesia (for labor pain and surgical pain), to reduce anesthetic requirements for induction and maintenance agents, and to smooth induction and recovery. Sedation also allows clipping and administration of oxygen prior to induction of anesthesia.

When opioids are given prior to surgery, they provide preventive analgesia. It is important for the welfare of the dam and offspring that she is comfortable in the post-operative period; a mother in pain is unlikely to tend to her offspring or allow them to nurse. The administration of opioids prior to delivery has not been shown to adversely affect the outcome for the offspring (Moon et al. 2000). If opioids have been administered to the dam and the offspring are bradycardic, naloxone can be administered via the umbilical vein or sublingually. A compromise is to administer the opioid immediately after the puppies or kittens have been delivered.

Decreased gastrointestinal motility and the physical pressure from the enlarged uterus increase the risk of vomiting and aspiration. Aspiration of gastric contents is thought to contribute to maternal mortality in dogs (Moon et al. 1998). Opioids that are less likely to cause emesis – such as buprenorphine, meperidine (pethidine), and methadone – should be given to pregnant animals. Because of the risk of regurgitation, vomiting, and aspiration, intubation is recommended to protect the airway. Rapid control of the airway is essential, especially in brachycephalic breeds which commonly require C-section. Mask induction does not permit rapid control of the airway; in dogs this technique is associated with increased mortality and is not recommended (Brodbelt et al. 2008).

Due to high oxygen requirements and reduced functional residual capacity (the volume in the lungs just after passive expiration), pregnant animals are at risk for hypoxemia, which can occur rapidly during induction of anesthesia. Pre-oxygenation for three minutes using a face mask increases blood oxygen content and delays the time to desaturation (Mcnally et al. 2009). Pre-oxygenation "buys you time" if a difficult intubation is anticipated, for example in brachycephalic breeds (Figure 13.1).

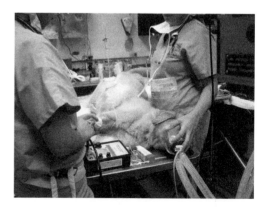

Figure 13.1 The patient is pre-oxygenated using a face mask while being prepared for surgery.

Many animals undergoing C-section are dehydrated and, even in elective situations, fluid losses can be large. Therefore, intravenous fluids are recommended and should be started prior to induction of anesthesia.

There is some controversy regarding the use of peri-operative non-steroidal anti-inflammatory drugs (NSAIDs) in dams undergoing surgery due to potential negative effects (e.g. renal development) in the offspring. Only a small percentage of the dam's dose of NSAID is secreted in milk and a single post-operative dose is regarded as a suitable compromise. NSAIDs should not be given in the face of hypovolemia and hypotension; it may not be possible to correct all fluid deficits prior to surgery and blood loss and hypotension may occur during surgery. For these reasons, if NSAIDs are used they should be given post-operatively when these issues have been addressed.

Neonatal Vitality

Luna and others (Luna et al. 2004) compared respiratory rates and neurologic reflexes of puppies born to dams that received ketamine/midazolam, thiopental, propofol, or an epidural local anesthetic. The respiratory rate was higher after epidural anesthesia and neurologic reflexes were best in the epidural group; the order of best to worst for these parameters was propofol, followed by thiopental, then ketamine/midazolam. Moon and others (Moon et al. 2000; Moon-Massat and Erb 2002) also reported that although ketamine did not increase puppy mortality, it decreased the vigor of newborn puppies; therefore, greater resuscitation efforts should be anticipated if ketamine is used. There was no difference in survival between puppies whose dams received propofol or alfaxalone (Doebeli et al. 2013). However, using a modified Apgar score (Veronesi et al. 2009), puppy vitality was found to be superior when alfaxalone was used. Induction and maintenance with alfaxalone have been compared to induction with alfax-

alone followed by isoflurane; time to recovery and suckling was significantly quicker when isoflurane was used for maintenance (Conde Ruiz et al. 2016). There is a lack of published information on kitten vitality after cesarean delivery.

Anesthetic Protocols for Cesarean Section

Different protocols for elective and emergency C-section in dogs and cats based on differences on drug availability are given in detail in the World Small Animal Veterinary Association's Global Pain Council Treatise on the recognition, assessment, and treatment of pain, released in 2014 (Mathews et al. 2014). An example of an anesthetic protocol for a C-section in a non-compromised dog or cat is given below. In this case the procedure may be planned or intervention occurs early before any physiologic deterioration occurs.

Non-compromised Dam

Pre-operative
Intramuscular (IM) or intravenous (IV) opioid (methadone 0.3–0.5 mg/kg or buprenorphine 0.02–0.03 mg/kg) ± acepromazine (lower doses of 0.01–0.03 mg/kg IM or IV are usually sufficient). An opioid normally provides adequate sedation for venous access; however, acepromazine can be used if the dam is difficult to manage and requires more sedation than an opioid alone can provide.

Induction and Maintenance of Anesthesia
IV alfaxalone to effect (3–5 mg/kg) or IV propofol to effect (3–10 mg/kg). When propofol or alfaxalone is not available, ketamine (3–5 mg/kg IV) combined with midazolam or diazepam (0.25 mg/kg for both) could potentially be used, with the understanding that this may decrease the vigor of the offspring. Midazolam is shorter acting in both dam and offspring, so

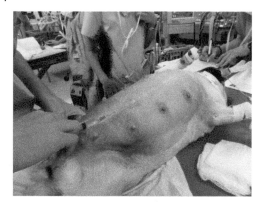

Figure 13.2   A line block is performed prior to surgery. The use of a line block helps minimize the use of general anesthetic drugs.

is preferred when available. Following intubation, anesthesia can be maintained with isoflurane or sevoflurane. Anesthesia can be maintained with repeated boluses or a continuous-rate infusion of propofol, but intubation and administration of oxygen are still required.

Additional analgesia can be provided with a pre-incisional and/or post-incisional line block (Figure 13.2) using lidocaine (1–2 mg/kg) or bupivacaine (1–2 mg/kg). Epidural morphine (0.1 mg/kg of preservative-free morphine diluted with sterile saline to a final volume of 0.2 ml/kg) can be administered pre- or post-operatively to provide up to 18–20 hours of analgesia. As discussed above, a single dose of an NSAID can be administered and the choice will depend on market authorization in the geographic location and personal preference; most NSAIDs will provide analgesia for 18–24 hours. Opioids can also be continued post-operatively.

Compromised Dam

In an emergency situation when the dam is compromised the following protocol can be used.

Pre-operative
Fentanyl IV (3–5 μg/kg). If fentanyl is unavailable, IV methadone or buprenorphine can be given.

Induction and Maintenance of Anesthesia
IV ketamine (3–5 mg/kg) plus diazepam or midazolam (0.25 mg/kg); midazolam is shorter acting in both dam and offspring, so is preferred when available. Following intubation anesthesia can be maintained with isoflurane or sevoflurane. If fentanyl was used, this can be repeated or given as an infusion due to its short duration of action. Incisional blocks with local anesthetics as described earlier can be used and, when used prior to the initial incision, can markedly reduce the inhalant anesthetic agent requirements. Additional analgesic strategies as already outlined can be used, but NSAIDs should only be considered if the bitch or queen is normovolemic and normotensive.

Epidural local anesthetic (lidocaine) can be used as a sole technique and has resulted in excellent post-delivery vitality in puppies (Luna et al. 2004); however, this technique must be used with caution. Due to the decreased size of the epidural space in pregnant animals, smaller volumes (25–30% reduction) of epidural local anesthetic drugs should be used. Epidural local anesthetics cause sympathetic blockade, resulting in vasodilation and hypotension, which can be prevented or treated with IV fluids, but could be especially detrimental in compromised dams. With this technique the dam is conscious and therefore not intubated, so there is an increased risk of aspiration; oxygen should be administered by face mask. The dam will also require to be manually restrained for surgery, which may cause her stress.

Intraoperative Anesthetic Management

The two most important functions to maintain within normal limits are maternal oxygen delivery and uterine blood flow. Since these cannot be easily measured, we rely on the assumption that adequate hematocrit, oxygen saturation of hemoglobin, heart rate, blood volume, and blood pressure will maintain these at acceptable levels. IV fluids should be administered pre-, intra-, and also post-operatively in some critical cases. Increasing the rate of fluid administration and decreasing anesthetic delivery may correct mild hypotension. The use of analgesic agents in the pre-anesthetic or intraoperative period permits a decrease in vaporizer setting and usually results in improved blood pressure. Refractory hypotension should be treated with ephedrine (0.04–0.1 mg/kg IV); this is the preferred drug for cardiovascular support in these patients, because of its ability to maintain or improve uterine blood flow despite its vasoconstrictor properties. Epinephrine will dramatically decrease uterine blood flow and should only be used to save the life of the mother in catastrophic situations such as rupture of the uterine artery. If the dam becomes bradycardic, look for an underlying cause (e.g. deep anesthesia, hypothermia, and hypoxia). If bradycardia is opioid induced, atropine should be used, as this will also maintain fetal heart rate.

Blood loss during a C-section is typically not enough to be life threatening and can be treated with crystalloid fluids (e.g. lactated Ringer's solution) given at three times the volume of estimated blood loss. However, bleeding can be rapid and severe and under emergency circumstances it is unlikely that a suitable cross-matched donor is readily available. In these situations, colloids can help to maintain circulating volume and blood pressure. Hypothermia can lead to increased bleeding and detrimental effects on the offspring include lower core body temperature and acidosis. When mothers were warmed with forced warm air systems they shivered less post-operatively, were more comfortable, and babies were warmer and had higher umbilical vein blood pH (Horn et al. 2002, 2014). Hypothermia is discussed in depth in Chapter 7.

Surgical Techniques

Surgical Technique Selection

There are three surgical options: (i) hysterotomy and removal of each fetus followed by repair of the incision (dam remains intact); (ii) hysterotomy followed by ovariohysterectomy; and (iii) en bloc technique: ovariohysterectomy is performed and the uterus handed to another team that performs a hysterotomy and removal of each fetus.

In the shelter or HQHVSN clinic setting, ovariohysterectomy is a desirable outcome for the dam. Lactation and caring for neonates are not adversely affected by ovariohysterectomy (Onclin and Verstegen 2008; Von Heimendahl and Cariou 2009; Mullen 2014). En bloc resection allows for simultaneous spay and C-section, and results in shorter surgical and anesthesia time for the dam and less chance of intraoperative contamination of the abdomen when compared to traditional C-sections (Mullen 2014). Neonatal survival rates following en bloc resection have been reported to be as good or better than neonatal survival rates following traditional C-section or natural parturition (Robbins and Mullen 1994). For these reasons, en bloc resection is strongly recommended as the usual technique for C-sections in shelter and HQHVSN settings, as well as in any other circumstance in which future litters from the dam are not desired. Other reasons for choosing en bloc resection include uterine disease (such as torsion, metritis, or fetal putrefaction), severe maternal compromise necessitating the briefest possible surgical time, and maternal morphologic abnormalities that would prevent future delivery (Von Heimendahl and Cariou 2009).

The major limitation of en bloc resection is also related to its speed, in that all fetuses are "delivered" at once so a large team of assistants (ideally, one per neonate) is required for resuscitation (Mullen 2014). Some veterinarians also report utilizing a traditional C-section technique (followed by ovariohysterectomy) if there is a fetus in the cervix or vagina that cannot be manipulated back into the uterine body prior to ovariohysterectomy. Traditional C-section is also necessary if ovariohysterectomy is not a desired outcome of the surgery.

Each technique will require more surgical instruments than the typical spay, for example many hemostats will be required both on the dam and for each umbilical cord. It is recommended that several surgery packs be made available for use during the surgery, or that additional sterilized surgical instruments are available. Laparotomy sponges and sterile isotonic fluid for lavage are also recommended supplies for either surgical technique.

Surgical Approach

Regardless of the technique chosen, the initial approach to the abdomen is the same. A ventral midline incision is made extending from near the umbilicus to the pubis. Since the linea alba is often stretched thin and the abdomen distended, the surgeon must be careful not to traumatize the uterus or other underlying organs when entering the abdomen (Gilson 2015). The uterus is carefully exteriorized, extending the abdominal wall incision if needed to exteriorize the uterus without tearing, stretching, or otherwise traumatizing the uterus. The incision is packed with moistened laparotomy sponges, and the uterine horns are laid out laterally to the incision (Mullen 2014; Gilson 2015; Figure 13.3).

En Bloc Resection

Once the uterus has been exteriorized, the suspensory ligaments should be cut or broken, but no clamps should be applied at this time

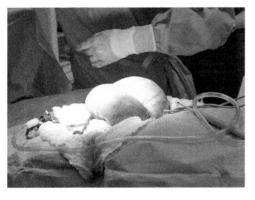

Figure 13.3 The uterus is carefully exteriorized in preparation for a cesarean section.

(Figure 13.4). Next, the broad ligaments are broken down or cut on both sides of the uterus from the ovarian pedicles to the cervix. This leaves the blood supply to the uterus and fetuses intact, but removes all uterine attachments except for the ovarian pedicles and uterine body (Mullen 2014).

Before proceeding with hemostat placement and ovariohysterectomy, the surgeon should palpate the cervix and vagina to locate any fetus that is lodged there and manipulate it back into the uterine body (Mullen 2014).

The goal now is to perform an ovariohysterectomy as rapidly as possible in order to minimize fetal hypoxia (Von Heimendahl and Cariou 2009), with a maximum time of 45–60 seconds between clamping the blood supply and delivery of the neonates. In the dog, two hemostats are placed on each ovarian pedicle, and three large hemostats (such as Carmalts) are placed across the uterine body immediately distal to the cervix. The pedicles and uterine body are divided between the hemostats, leaving one hemostat on each ovarian pedicle and two hemostats on the uterine body. The gravid uterus is handed to a team of assistants, who open the uterus and begin resuscitation (see the subsequent section on neonatal resuscitation; Mullen 2014). The ovarian pedicles and uterine stump are ligated according to the surgeon's preference; modified Miller's knots are recommended.

In the cat, the same technique is acceptable, as is pedicle tie autoligation as described in Chapter 12 (Miller et al. 2016). To use autoligation during en bloc resection, the surgeon places a clamp between the ovary and the uterus (encompassing the proper ligament and uterine vessel) on the first horn and completes the pedicle tie on the first side, then clamps between the ovary and the uterus on the second side and completes the second pedicle tie. Once both pedicle ties are completed, three clamps are placed on the uterine body and the uterus is divided between the distal two clamps and handed to the resuscitation team. The surgeon

(a)

(b)

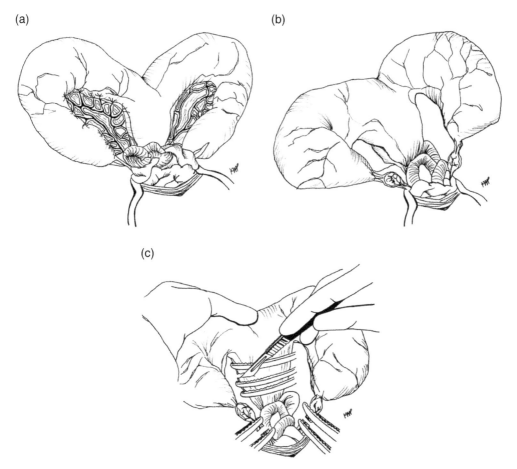

(c)

Figure 13.4   En bloc cesarean section. (a) The gravid uterus and ovaries are exteriorized and laid out laterally to the abdominal incision and (b) the suspensory ligaments are broken down and the broad ligament is divided. (c) The gravid uterus can be removed in 45–60 seconds by placing first two hemostats on each ovarian pedicle and then three clamps on the uterine body and transecting between them as shown. *Source:* Reprinted with permission from Bojrab: Current Techniques in Small Animal Surgery 5th edition, Copyright 2014, Teton NewMedia, Inc., Jackson, Wyoming.

then ligates the uterine stump using a modified Miller's knot.

When the resuscitation team receives the gravid uterus, it should immediately open the uterus with scissors or a scalpel blade, being careful to avoid cutting a fetus. The neonates should be removed rapidly and resuscitated, ideally with one assistant per neonate (Mullen 2014). Each umbilical cord should be clamped and cut approximately 2 cm from the umbilicus and resuscitation begun (see the neonatal resuscitation section later in this chapter; Von Heimendahl and Cariou 2009).

Once the ovariohysterectomy is completed, the abdomen is closed routinely as described in Chapter 12. Intradermal closure is recommended to prevent neonates causing trauma to themselves or to the incision. The skin and nipples of the ventral abdomen should be cleaned using antiseptic agents (Von Heimendahl and Cariou 2009), rinsed, and gently dried.

"Traditional" Cesarean Section and Spay

The exteriorized uterus is isolated from the abdomen with moistened laparotomy sponges to minimize contamination with fetal fluids

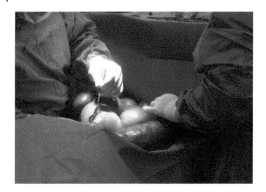

Figure 13.5 A hysterotomy incision is made in one horn of the uterus of a Golden Retriever with 12 puppies. With this large litter, multiple hysterotomy incisions will likely be required.

(Von Heimendahl and Cariou 2009; Gilson 2015). The surgeon has a choice of making a single ventral midline uterine (hysterotomy) incision (Von Heimendahl and Cariou 2009), or making multiple hysterotomy incisions along the greater curvature of the uterine horns between the locations of the placentas (Onclin and Verstegen 2008; Figure 13.5). For small litters, the single incision may be adequate, and fetuses may be manually "milked" toward the hysterotomy incision for removal. For larger litters, the use of multiple hysterotomy incisions makes access to each fetus more rapid. A disadvantage of multiple hysterotomy incisions is that, if the uterus will not be removed during the procedure (i.e. the dam will not be spayed), the multiple incisions require more time for closure (Onclin and Verstegen 2008).

To perform C-section via a single hysterotomy incision, an avascular area of the dorsal or ventral aspect of the wall of the uterine body should be tented and a longitudinal incision made with a scalpel blade and extended with scissors. The hysterotomy incision must be long enough to prevent tearing during extraction of the fetuses. Any fetus in the body of the uterus or birth canal should be removed first (Von Heimendahl and Cariou 2009). If it is difficult to mobilize fetuses to a single uterine body hysterotomy, additional hysterotomy

incisions may be made (Probst and Bebchuk 2014).

Each uterine horn is then gently squeezed to move each fetus toward the incision(s). Regardless of the number of incisions, once each fetus is manipulated toward the hysterotomy incision, the surgeon reaches into the uterus, grasps the fetus, and exerts gentle traction to exteriorize it (Gilson 2015).

The fetus may either be separated from the placenta and other fetal membranes prior to handing to resuscitation staff, or may be removed along with the placenta and intact fetal membranes and given to resuscitation staff to break the amniotic sac and clamp the umbilical cord during resuscitation (Probst and Bebchuk 2014). If the placenta separates readily from the uterus, it is the surgeon's choice whether to remove it by gentle traction along with the neonate (Gilson 2015), or to open the amniotic sac and double clamp the umbilical vessels 2–3 cm from the fetal abdominal wall using hemostats, and sever between the hemostats prior to handing off the neonate (Probst and Bebchuk 2014; Figure 13.6). After all the neonates are removed, if the dam is not being spayed the remaining placentas may be removed via gentle traction on the hemostat on the maternal portion of the umbilical cords prior to uterine closure (Onclin and Verstegen 2008). However, if the placentas are difficult to separate or if bleeding occurs when separation is attempted, they should be left in place to be passed naturally by the dam (Gilson 2015).

After removal from the uterus, each neonate is placed on a sterile towel and handed to an attendant. The amniotic sac, if intact, is broken by the assistants, the fetal fluids wiped or suctioned, and resuscitation is begun (see the later section).

Once all apparent fetuses are removed, the uterus and birth canal should be thoroughly palpated to ensure that they are clear and no fetuses remain (Gilson 2015). At this point, if the dam is to be spayed, the surgeon may proceed with a routine ovariohysterectomy, as described in Chapter 12.

(a)   (b)

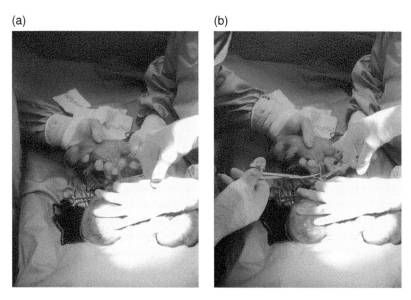

Figure 13.6 Once the amniotic sac is opened, (a) the fetus is exteriorized and the umbilical vessels are clamped 2–3 cm from the fetal abdominal wall using hemostats and (b) severed prior to handing off the neonate.

If the dam is not to be spayed, the hysterotomy incision(s) must be closed. Closure can consist of a single or double-layer continuous closure using 3-0 or 4-0 suture, even in canine patients. Recommended suture patterns include appositional patterns (Von Heimendahl and Cariou 2009), inverting patterns such as Cushings or Lambert (Onclin and Verstegen 2008), or a two-layer closure with an appositional layer followed by an inverting layer (Gilson 2015). Regardless of pattern, closure should pass through myometrium and submucosa, but avoid penetrating the lumen. The sutures should be tightened adequately to avoid leakage of uterine contents (Gilson 2015; Onclin and Verstegen 2008).

If the uterus does not begin to involute during closure or if hemorrhage is excessive, oxytocin may be injected. In dogs, 5–20 IU may be given IM, or 0.5–1 IU may be injected directly into the uterine wall musculature (Gilson 2015). Alternatively, oxytocin may be given IV at 1–5 IU per dog (Onclin and Verstegen 2008). In cats, IM oxytocin dose is approximately 2–4 IU per cat (Von Heimendahl and Cariou 2009). Beginning with the lower ends of these dose ranges is recommended and is often sufficient. Administration of oxytocin should occur while the dam is anesthetized, as administration in the awake animal and the subsequent uterine contraction can be painful.

Once the hysterotomy incisions are closed, the uterus should be lavaged with warm saline or other isotonic fluids to remove fetal fluids, blood clots, and other contaminants. If the abdomen has been contaminated, it should be lavaged copiously as well. Surgical gloves and instruments should be replaced if contaminated (Von Heimendahl and Cariou 2009). Once the lavage is complete, the abdomen may be closed routinely, as described in Chapter 12.

Intradermal closure is recommended to prevent neonates causing trauma to themselves or to the incision. The skin and nipples of the ventral abdomen should be cleaned using antiseptic agents (Von Heimendahl and Cariou 2009), rinsed, and gently dried.

Neonatal Resuscitation

Successful resuscitative efforts depend on a well-prepared and trained team. Many of the procedures recommended for neonatal puppies and kittens immediately after birth are extrapolated from human neonatal resuscitation guidelines. The latter are reviewed and updated every five years by the American Heart Association and the American Academy of Pediatrics (http://pediatrics.aappublications.org/content/126/5/e1400.full). Resuscitation protocols are available for newborn kittens and puppies (Moon et al. 2001; Traas 2008) and key points are discussed here.

As previously mentioned, keeping the dam warm during surgery will benefit the offspring. Newborn puppies and kittens should be dried immediately with warm towels and placed in a warm environment; this may be on a heated mat and/or under a warm forced-air blanket. If these are not available, a hair dryer set on "warm" can be gently moved over them to provide heat. Neonates have poor thermoregulatory mechanisms, a large surface area to bodyweight, and little insulation, therefore the ambient temperature where they are resuscitated and nursed must be high (27–32 °C, 80–90 °F; Grundy 2006). Toweling and rubbing also provide tactile stimulation which promotes spontaneous breathing. Swinging or shaking newborn animals (as previously described in the veterinary literature) is no longer recommended as it may cause head and neck injuries or intracranial hemorrhage, and is a potentially lethal practice (Grundy et al. 2009).

The nasal and oral passages must be cleared and several methods have been described, including infant nasal aspirators, DeLee mucus traps, syringes attached to syringe mounts, and syringes attached to rubber tubing or IV catheters. In a study comparing a syringe mount attached to a 1 ml syringe and a neonatal nasal aspirator for clearing nasal fluid in 171 puppies delivered by C-section, the aspirator was more practical, more efficient, and resulted in no bleeding compared to inserting the syringe

mount into the nostril (Goericke-Pesch and Wehrend 2012). A cotton-tipped swab or bulb syringe can be used to clear fetal fluids from the pharynx. Newborn animals have an irregular respiratory pattern and the pause between inspiration and expiration seen in adults is absent. If the newborn has a normal heart rate (150–220 beats/min) but is apneic, tactile stimulation (rubbing the body or "flicking" the paws) plus oxygen administration by face mask will often initiate respiration. If effective respiratory efforts do not begin within 30 seconds or the heart rate starts to decrease, positive pressure ventilation should be applied using a face mask with a rubber flange placed tightly over the nose, to expand the lungs. The head should be held in an extended position to minimize the amount of gas being forced into the stomach. The application of sufficient pressure to expand the lungs is difficult to achieve unless the mask fits tightly. Therefore, if this approach does not give adequate chest expansion within one or two attempts, the newborn should be intubated and manually ventilated until it begins to breathe on its own; intravenous catheters (14–18 gauge) can be used as endotracheal tubes. Tracheal suctioning should be attempted only if there is evidence of thick meconium staining or signs of airway obstruction.

Once ventilation has been established, cardiac compressions should begin if the newborn still has a slow, weak, or absent heartbeat. Myocardial hypoxemia is the most common cause of bradycardia or asystole, therefore it is imperative to establish respiration and oxygen delivery first. Normal neonatal heart rates range from 150 to 220 beats/minute. A Doppler flow probe held directly over the heart is helpful to monitor heart rate. In kittens and most breeds of dogs, the chest compressions should be applied across the lateral chest wall, but in some barrel-chested dog breeds such as Pugs and Bulldogs, sternal compression may be more effective.

Newborns should have a suckle reflex immediately after birth (this can be tested by placing a finger in the mouth) and they should "root," meaning that when you cup your hand over their muzzle they push. Rubbing over the lumbar area should evoke a squeal and squeezing the toes results in a head "bob." If these reflexes are weak or absent, check for the presence of hypothermia and hypoglycemia (see later in the chapter).

Drug Therapy

Epinephrine at a "low dose" (0.01–0.03 mg/kg) into the umbilical vein, via an endotracheal tube or by the intraosseous route (via placement of a hypodermic needle in the proximal humerus or femur), should be used if there is no heartbeat and there is no response to physical resuscitative efforts. The cause of bradycardia in newborn puppies and kittens is primarily myocardial hypoxemia and hypothermia, therefore the use of anticholinergics (atropine and glycopyrrolate) is not recommended as a first line of treatment. Neonates show little response to anticholinergic agents due to lack of vagal tone (Grundy 2006) and this is compounded in the face of hypothermia, which also inhibits the heart's response to atropine (Cookson and Dipalma 1955). Naloxone (0.1 mg/kg, transmucosally, IV, via an endotracheal tube, subcutaneously, IM, or by the intraosseous route) should be administered only if the puppies or kittens appear depressed and the bitch or queen received intraoperative opioids prior to delivery. The use of doxapram is controversial and its efficacy is not well established in human neonates (Henderson-Smart and Steer 2004). There are no placebo-controlled reports of its efficacy in puppies and kittens in the veterinary literature. Doxapram is thought to be a central stimulant and its efficacy is profoundly diminished when the brain is already hypoxic (Bamford et al. 1986). Given this information, doxapram is unlikely to be of much benefit in the apneic, hypoxic newborn and its routine use to stimulate respiration is not recommended.

Despite the fact that acidosis and elevated lactate levels may be present, the use of sodium bicarbonate is not advised. It is hyperosmolar and generates carbon dioxide, and if this is not expired by an increase in ventilation, respiratory acidosis leading to cerebral acidosis occurs.

Expected blood glucose values in neonates range from 2.2 to 3.3 mmol/l (40–60 mg/dl), but they have low reserves. Measurement of blood glucose is a challenge and many commercial monitors are inaccurate (Cohn et al. 2000), therefore it may be prudent to give all neonates that are slow to respond to resuscitative efforts a dose of dextrose. A 50% dextrose solution dropped under the tongue or into the cheek pouch will be absorbed through the mucus membranes; other popular choices are corn syrup and dextrose gels.

A "treatment pyramid" is shown in Figure 13.7 to emphasize the importance of each resuscitative technique.

Newborn puppy viability and short-term survival prognosis can be predicted by performing a physical examination and assigning an Apgar score (Table 13.1) that has been modified for puppies (Veronesi et al. 2009), but could also be applied to kittens. The Apgar score is based on heart rate, respiratory rate, response to a toe pinch, movement, and mucus membrane color. Assigning an Apgar score to each newborn will help identify those that need more attention. As soon as possible after the dam's recovery, the pups or kittens must be placed with her so that maternal bonding can occur and colostrum be consumed.

Neonatal Resuscitation Supplies

Figure 13.8 shows a neonatal resuscitation cart ready for use.

Supplies include:

- Warming equipment
  - Forced warm air
  - Heated mat
  - Hair dryer
- Warm towels

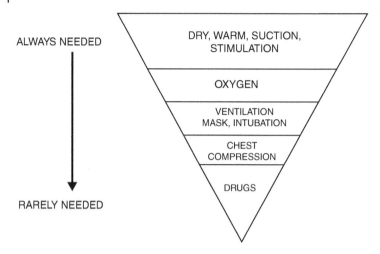

ALWAYS NEEDED

RARELY NEEDED

DRY, WARM, SUCTION, STIMULATION

OXYGEN

VENTILATION MASK, INTUBATION

CHEST COMPRESSION

DRUGS

Figure 13.7   The treatment pyramid for neonatal resuscitation.

Table 13.1   Apgar scale for puppies (Veronesi et al. 2009).

Parameter	0	1	2
Heart rate	<180 bpm	180–220 bpm	>220 bpm
Respiration	No crying, RR <6	Mild crying, RR 6–15	Crying, RR >15
Response to toe pinch	No response	Weak retraction, vocalization	Vigorous retraction, vocalizing
Movement	Flaccid	Some flexion	Active motion
Mucus membranes	Cyanotic	Pale	Pink

Interpretation: 7–10: no distress, 4–6: moderate distress, 0–3: severe distress.
All pups with scores <7 should receive intervention.
bpm, beats per minute; RR, respiration rate.

- Bulb syringes
- Cotton-tipped swabs
- Oxygen source and masks
- Dextrose or corn syrup
- Doppler and probe
- Laryngoscope
- IV catheters to use as endotracheal tubes
- Size 1 and 2 endotracheal tubes
- Insulin syringes
- Drugs
  - Epinephrine, atropine, glycopyrrolate, naloxone

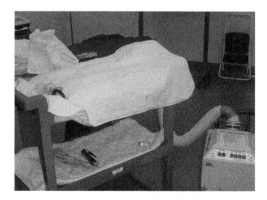

Figure 13.8   A neonatal resuscitation cart ready for use.

References

Bamford, O.S., Dawes, G.S., Hanson, M.A., and Ward, R.A. (1986). The effects of doxapram on breathing, heart rate and blood pressure in fetal lambs. *Respir. Physiol.* 66: 387–396.

Brodbelt, D.C., Pfeiffer, D.U., Young, L.E., and Wood, J.L. (2008). Results of the confidential enquiry into perioperative small animal fatalities regarding risk factors for anesthetic-related death in dogs. *JAVMA* 233: 1096–1104.

Cohn, L.A., Mccaw, D.L., Tate, D.J., and Johnson, J.C. (2000). Assessment of five portable blood glucose meters, a point-of-care analyzer, and color test strips for measuring blood glucose concentration in dogs. *JAVMA* 216: 198–202.

Conde Ruiz, C., Del Carro, A.P., Rosset, E. et al. (2016). Alfaxalone for total intravenous anaesthesia in bitches undergoing elective caesarean section and its effects on puppies: a randomized clinical trial. *Vet. Anaesth. Analg.* 43: 281–290.

Cookson, B.A. and Dipalma, J.R. (1955). Severe bradycardia of profound hypothermia in the dog. *Am. J. Physiol.* 182: 447–453.

Doebeli, A., Michel, E., Bettschart, R. et al. (2013). Apgar score after induction of anesthesia for canine cesarean section with alfaxalone versus propofol. *Theriogenology* 80: 850–854.

Gilson, S.D. (2015). Cesarean section. In: *Small Animal Surgical Emergencies* (ed. L.R. Aronson), 391–396. Chichester: Wiley-Blackwell.

Goericke-Pesch, S. and Wehrend, A. (2012). New method for removing mucus from the upper respiratory tract of newborn puppies following caesarean section. *Vet. Rec.* 170: 289.

Grundy, S.A. (2006). Clinically relevant physiology of the neonate. *Vet. Clin. North Am. Small Anim. Pract.* 36: 443–459.

Grundy, S.A., Liu, S.M., and Davidson, A.P. (2009). Intracranial trauma in a dog due to being "swung" at birth. *Top. Companion Anim. Med.* 24: 100–103.

Henderson-Smart, D. and Steer, P. (2004). Doxapram treatment for apnea in preterm infants. *Cochrane Database Syst. Rev.* (4): CD000074.

Horn, E.P., Bein, B., Steinfath, M. et al. (2014). The incidence and prevention of hypothermia in newborn bonding after cesarean delivery: a randomized controlled trial. *Anesth. Analg.* 118: 997–1002.

Horn, E.P., Schroeder, F., Gottschalk, A. et al. (2002). Active warming during cesarean delivery. *Anesth. Analg.* 94: 409–414.

Kinsella, S.M. and Lohmann, G. (1994). Supine hypotensive syndrome. *Obstet. Gynecol.* 83: 774–788.

Luna, S.P., Cassu, R.N., Castro, G.B. et al. (2004). Effects of four anaesthetic protocols on the neurological and cardiorespiratory variables of puppies born by caesarean section. *Vet. Rec.* 154: 387–389.

Mathews, K., Kronen, P.W., Lascelles, D. et al. (2014). Guidelines for recognition, assessment and treatment of pain: WSAVA Global Pain Council members and co-authors of this document. *J. Small Anim. Pract.* 55: E10–E68.

Mcnally, E.M., Robertson, S.A., and Pablo, L.S. (2009). Comparison of time to desaturation between preoxygenated and nonpreoxygenated dogs following sedation with acepromazine maleate and morphine and induction of anesthesia with propofol. *Am. J. Vet. Res.* 70: 1333–1338.

Miller, K.P., Rekers, W., Ellis, K. et al. (2016). Pedicle ties provide a rapid and safe method for feline ovariohysterectomy. *J. Feline Med. Surg.* 18: 160–164.

Moon, P.F., Erb, H.N., Ludders, J.W. et al. (1998). Perioperative management and mortality rates of dogs undergoing cesarean section in the United States and Canada. *JAVMA* 213: 365–369.

Moon, P.F., Erb, H.N., Ludders, J.W. et al. (2000). Perioperative risk factors for puppies delivered by cesarean section in the United States and Canada. *J. Am. Anim. Hosp. Assoc.* 36: 359–368.

Moon, P.F., Massat, B.J., and Pascoe, P.J. (2001). Neonatal critical care. *Vet. Clin. North Am. Small Anim. Pract.* 31: 343–365.

Moon-Massat, P.F. and Erb, H.N. (2002). Perioperative factors associated with puppy vigor after delivery by cesarean section. *J. Am. Anim. Hosp. Assoc.* 38: 90–96.

Mullen, H.S. (2014). Cesarean section by ovariohysterectomy. In: *Current Techniques in Small Animal Surgery*, 5e (eds. M.J. Bojrab, D.R. Waldron and J.P. Toombs), 527–528. Jackson, WY: Teton NewMedia.

Onclin, K.J. and Verstegen, J.P. (2008). Cesarean section in the dog. *Clinician's Brief* (May), pp. 72–78.

Probst, C.W. and Bebchuk, T.N. (2014). Cesarean section: traditional technique. In: *Current Techniques in Small Animal Surgery*, 5e (eds. M.J. Bojrab, D.R. Waldron and J.P. Toombs), 524–526. Jackson, WY: Teton NewMedia.

Probst, C.W., Broadstone, R.V., and Evans, A.T. (1987). Postural influence on systemic blood pressure in large full-term pregnant bitches during general anesthesia. *Vet. Surg.* 16: 471–473.

Probst, C.W. and Webb, A.I. (1983). Postural influence on systemic blood pressure, gas exchange, and acid/base status in the term-pregnant bitch during general anesthesia. *Am. J. Vet. Res.* 44: 1963–1965.

Robbins, M.A. and Mullen, H.S. (1994). En bloc ovariohysterectomy as a treatment for dystocia in dogs and cats. *Vet. Surg.* 23: 48–52.

Traas, A.M. (2008). Resuscitation of canine and feline neonates. *Theriogenology* 70: 343–348.

Veronesi, M.C., Panzani, S., Faustini, M., and Rota, A. (2009). An Apgar scoring system for routine assessment of newborn puppy viability and short-term survival prognosis. *Theriogenology* 72: 401–407.

Von Heimendahl, A. and Cariou, M. (2009). Normal parturition and management of dystocia in dogs and cats. *In Pract.* 31: 254.

14

Dog Neuter/Cat Neuter
Philip Bushby and Sara White

As is the case with ovariohysterectomy or ova-riectomy, castration is one of the most common surgical procedures performed in small animal veterinary practice and in shelter animal practice.

Canine and feline castration can be performed with a closed technique, not incising the parietal vaginal tunics, or with an open technique in which the parietal vaginal tunics are incised. Advantages of a closed castration include not entering the peritoneal cavity and that the ligature remains external to the inguinal canal, making it possible to retrieve it without entering the abdomen should bleeding occur intra- or post-operatively. An advantage of an open castration is the ease of exteriorizing the testicle, since the fibrous attachments of the vaginal tunic need not be broken down. Some research has shown greater risk of scrotal complications, including swelling, bruising, and pain, with the use of open castration in dogs (Hamilton et al. 2014).

Feline castrations are performed scrotally, whereas canine castrations may be performed pre-scrotally or scrotally. Scrotal castration is the preferred technique in the puppy. In adult dogs, pre-scrotal castration is the traditional technique that has been taught for many years, while scrotal castration is gaining popularity among high-quality high-volume spay–neuter (HQHVSN) veterinarians.

Canine Pre-scrotal Castration

The traditional technique for castration of the male dog is to place the animal in dorsal recumbency, clip hair and perform an aseptic surgical preparation along the ventral midline just cranial to the scrotum, and perform the castration through a pre-scrotal incision (Hedlund 2007; MacPhail 2013).

Skin Incision

With the scrotum draped out of the surgical site, one testicle is pushed cranially out of the scrotum. An incision is made in the pre-scrotal skin and subcutaneous tissue just cranial to the scrotum and over the displaced testicle. The castration is then performed using a closed or open technique.

Closed Castration

To perform a closed castration, continue the incision through the spermatic fascia without incising the parietal vaginal tunics to deliver the testicle through the incision. Using a gauze sponge, strip fat and fibrous attachments from the spermatic cord while applying traction on the testicle. This allows maximum exteriorization of the testicle. Technique for ligation of the spermatic cord is generally a matter of the

High-Quality, High-Volume Spay and Neuter and Other Shelter Surgeries, First Edition. Edited by Sara White.
© 2020 John Wiley & Sons, Inc. Published 2020 by John Wiley & Sons, Inc.

surgeon's preference. The spermatic cord can be ligated with a single ligature tied with a modified Miller's knot (see Chapter 12) or with a circumferential ligature combined with a transfixation ligature. The ligatures can be placed prior to transecting the cord or hemostats can be placed on the cord, the cord transected, and then the ligature(s) placed in the area(s) of the spermatic cord crushed by the hemostats. The second testicle is displaced forward into the surgical incision and excised in a manner identical to the first testicle.

Open Castration

Alternatively, to perform an open castration, continue the initial incision through the spermatic fascia and the parietal vaginal tunics, exposing the testicle. Placing upward tension on the testicle allows maximum exteriorization of the testicle. The ductus deferens and the pampiniform plexus are ligated separately. Some surgeons will then place a second ligature encircling both structures. The ductus deferens and pampiniform plexus are transected. The tunic is separated from the ligament of the epididymis by placing a hemostat on the tunic and applying traction on the tunic. In an open castration it might be necessary to ligate the tunic if hemorrhage is observed from the tunic. The second testicle is displaced forward into the surgical incision and excised in a manner identical to the first testicle.

Closure

Close the subcutaneous tissue with a simple continuous pattern and the skin with a subcuticular or intradermal pattern.

Scrotal Approach to Castration

Scrotal castration in the canine patient was first published in 1974 (Johnston and Archibald 1974). Since then, however, scrotal castration has fallen out of favor because of the perception

that dogs would self-mutilate if castration was performed through a scrotal incision. There is, however, no published data that confirms a greater incidence of self-trauma with scrotal castration as compared to pre-scrotal castration. In a recent study (Woodruff et al. 2015) the incidence of post-operative complications was compared between scrotal and pre-scrotal castration techniques. There was no significant difference in the incidence of post-operative swelling, hemorrhage, or pain between the two approaches. However, the incidence of self-trauma was significantly greater in dogs castrated with the pre-scrotal approach than dogs castrated with a scrotal incision (Woodruff et al. 2015).

Scrotal castration is becoming the accepted technique for castration of adult dogs in many high-volume spay–neuter clinics and can be performed more quickly and through smaller incisions than pre-scrotal castrations (Woodruff et al. 2015).

Technique in the Adult Dog

To perform a scrotal castration, carefully clip the hair on the scrotum, avoiding razor burns, and prepare the scrotum aseptically. Sterile drapes should be placed leaving only the scrotum exposed. Grasp the first testicle in one hand, elevating the testicle so it is pressed against the scrotal skin at the median raphe. Incise the skin along the median raphe over the displaced testicle. Extend the incision through the subcutaneous tissue and the spermatic fascia to exteriorize the testicle. To perform a closed castration, avoid incising the parietal vaginal tunic. For an open castration, the incision is extended through the parietal vaginal tunic, as described for open pre-scrotal castration. The tunica albuginea of the testicle should not be incised. Using gentle traction, exteriorize the testicle while stripping fat and fascia away from the spermatic cord using a gauze sponge.

In larger dogs, greater than 18 kg, one of the authors (Bushby) recommends double ligation of the spermatic cord. In dogs under 18 kg, a single ligature with a modified Miller's knot (see Chapter 12) is sufficient. To double-ligate, place three hemostats on the spermatic cord and transect the cord distal to the third hemostat. Place a ligature with a modified Miller's knot in the crushed area of the most proximal hemostat and a transfixation ligature in the crushed area of the second hemostat. To single-ligate, place two hemostats on the spermatic cord and transect distal to the second hemostat. Place a ligature with a modified Miller's knot in the crushed are of the most proximal hemostat (Figure 14.1). The spermatic cord is then replaced into the scrotum and the remaining hemostat removed.

Exteriorize the second testicle through the same scrotal incision by incising the spermatic fascia over the second testicle and stripping fat and fascia away from the spermatic cord. Ligation and transection of the second spermatic cord are performed in an identical manner as the first (Bushby 2013).

Closure

There is no common consensus on the best method for closure of a scrotal castration. Scrotal incisions can be closed completely with skin glue, closed partially with a single buried subcutaneous suture, or left open to heal by second intention (Bushby 2013). There are no research studies to date that indicate an advantage of one technique over the other. If the scrotal incision is left open or partially open, the patient's owner/caretaker should be advised to expect serosanguinous drainage for a couple of days after surgery and to take appropriate precautions.

Pediatric Canine Scrotal Castration

Scrotal castration with autoligation is the technique most commonly used in puppies, and is performed in a similar manner to feline castration.

A recent study evaluated the use of scrotal castration with autoligation in puppies aged 2–5 months and weighing 2–25 lb (0.9–11.4 kg; Miller et al. 2018). In this study, there were no major complications and only 3.5% of the puppies had minor complications, including peri-incisional dermatitis, skin bruising, or swelling. No puppies experienced intraoperative hemorrhage-related complications. In addition to the low complication rate, the study found that scrotal castration with autoligation was over three times faster than pre-scrotal castration with suture ligation.

To date there has been no published research on the maximum size or age of puppy or the size of testicle or scrotum in which the autoligation technique is appropriate. Many surgeons choose to use this technique in all puppies whose testicles are similar in size or smaller than the testicles of an adult tomcat and whose scrotum is not yet pendulous. This includes most puppies under four to five months of age, and some small breeds of dog up to about a year of age. Some veterinarians use autoligation for castration of larger, mature dogs as well (White 2018), but the outcomes of this technique in mature dogs have not been evaluated.

Technique

The puppy is placed in dorsal recumbency. The scrotum is clipped of hair and aseptically prepared. The use of sterile drapes is considered optional depending on the skill and comfort level of the surgeon (Griffin et al. 2016).

The first testicle is grasped between the surgeon's thumb and index finger (Bushby & Griffin 2011; see Figure 14.2). A scrotal incision is made over the testicle, exteriorizing the testicle with digital pressure. The castration may be performed open or closed (Miller et al. 2018). Gentle traction is applied to the testicle and spermatic cord while stripping the fat and fascia from the spermatic cord. A hemostat tie is performed just as in cats (described later) by passing the tip of the hemostat under the

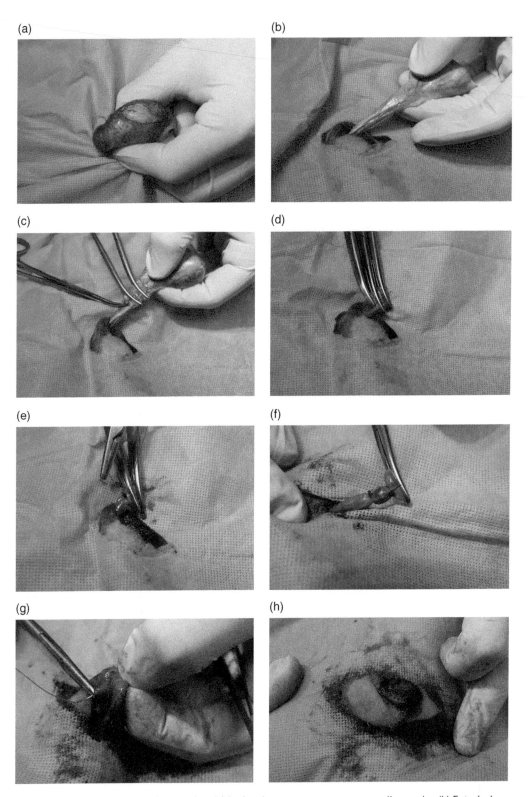

Figure 14.1 Adult dog scrotal castration. (a) Incise the scrotum on or near median raphe. (b) Exteriorize the testicle. (c) Place three clamps. (d) Transect spermatic cord distal to clamps. (e) Ligate the cord with a modified Miller's knot. (f) A second modified Miller's knot can be placed distal to the first. (g) A single buried subcutaneous suture is used for closure. (h) Appearance of the scrotum after closure.

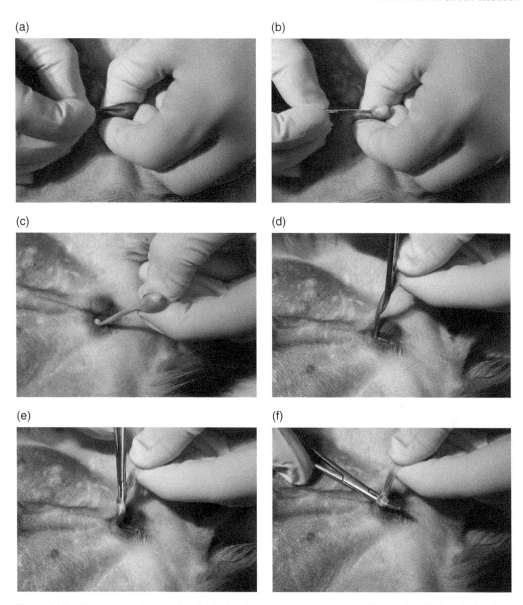

Figure 14.2 Puppy scrotal castration. (a) Incise the scrotum on or near median raphe. (b) Exteriorize the testicle. (c) Pull the testicle toward the surgeon. (d) Pass a curved hemostat over the spermatic cord and position the curved tip under the spermatic cord. (e) Rotate the hemostat counterclockwise. (f) Continue to rotate counterclockwise until the hemostat faces the surgeon. (g) Open hemostat and clamp spermatic cord. (h) Transect the cord distal to the tip of the hemostat, leaving 4–5 mm cut end. (i) The cord has been transected. (j) Slide the knot off the end of the hemostat, tighten, and check for hemorrhage before returning the spermatic cord to the scrotum. (k) The cord has been returned to the scrotum. (l) Surgical glue is applied to the scrotal skin.

(g)

(h)

(i)

(j)

(k)

(l)

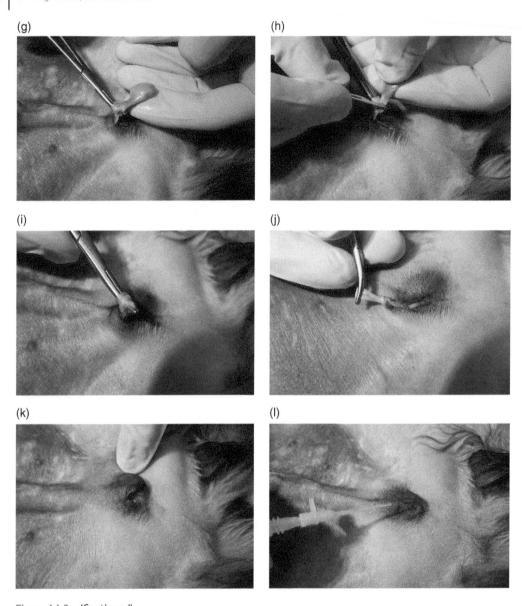

Figure 14.2 (Continued)

spermatic cord and rotating the tip around the cord. The jaws of the hemostat are opened as the distal (testicle) end of the cord is advanced around and into the hemostat jaws, and the jaws are then clamped. The cord is transected between the clamp and the testicle with a scalpel blade or scissors, leaving a tag of 4–5 mm in length to ensure that the knot does not come untied and the knot is pushed off the end of the hemostat. The knot should then be pushed off of the tip of the hemostat and tightened to ensure its security. The second testicle is pushed into the skin incision, and the same procedure is repeated. The incision is left open to heal by second intention (Bushby & Griffin 2011), or is closed with surgical glue.

Feline Castration

The technique for feline castration is identical in adult and pediatric patients (see Figure 14.3). The patient is positioned in dorsal recumbency with the rear legs pulled forward (Bushby 2013; MacPhail 2013). Scrotal hair is clipped or plucked and the scrotum is prepared aseptically. The use of sterile drapes is considered optional, depending on the skill and comfort level of the surgeon (Griffin et al. 2016).

Castration can be performed through either one incision at the median raphe, with both testicles exteriorized through that one incision, or through two separate incisions, one over each testicle. The first testicle is grasped and with gentle pressure forced against the scrotal skin. The incision should be made through the scrotal skin, subcutaneous tissue, and spermatic fascia, exteriorizing the testicle. To perform a closed castration the incision should not penetrate the parietal vaginal tunic. Gentle traction on the testicle will further exteriorize it, and the surgeon will feel two "releases" as the testicle is exteriorized. Fat and connective tissue are stripped away from the spermatic cord using a gauze sponge. Hemostasis is established by tying the spermatic cord using either the cord tie or a figure-of-eight knot. The cord tie is a self-ligature identical to the pedicle tie used in cat spays. The figure-of-eight knot is achieved by wrapping the spermatic cord once

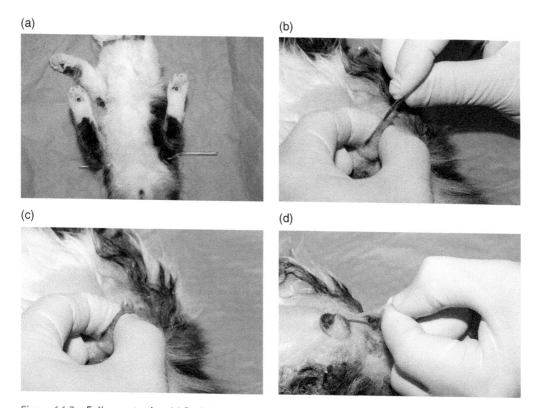

(a) (b) (c) (d)

Figure 14.3 Feline castration. (a) Position the cat with rear legs pulled forward. (b) Incise the scrotum. (c) Exteriorize the testicle. (d) Pull the testicle toward the surgeon. (e) Pass a curved hemostat over the spermatic cord and position the curved tip under the spermatic cord. (f) Rotate the hemostat counterclockwise until the hemostat faces the surgeon. (g) Open the hemostat and clamp the spermatic cord. (h) Transect distal to the tip of the hemostat leaving 4–5 mm cut end. (i) Slide the knot off the end of the hemostat, tighten, and check for hemorrhage before returning the spermatic cord to the scrotum.

(e)

(f)

(g)

(h)

(i)

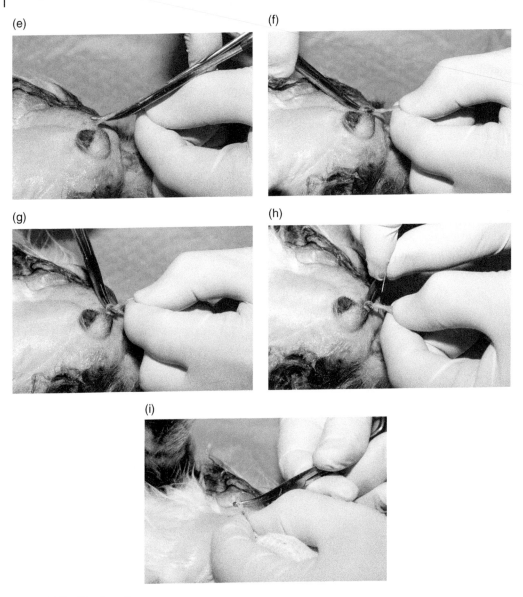

Figure 14.3 (Continued)

around the end of a hemostat and then performing the cord tie. The spermatic cord is transected distal to the hemostat, leaving a tag of 4–5 mm to ensure that the knot does not come untied and the knot is pushed off the end of the hemostat. Before removing the hemostat, the knot is tightened. After releasing the hemostat, the spermatic cord is checked for hemorrhage. The second testicle is exteriorized and the second spermatic cord is ligated and transected in an identical manner as the first (Bushby 2013).

After both testicles have been removed, the skin of the scrotum should be gently elevated to make sure the ligated spermatic cords recede into the scrotum. The scrotal incision(s) are left to heal by second intention.

Surgical Approach to Cryptorchidism

Cryptorchidism is the failure of one or both testicles to descend into the scrotum. The cryptorchid testicle can be located anywhere along the path from the area of fetal development of the gonads (just caudal to the caudal pole of the kidney) to the subcutaneous tissue between the external inguinal ring and the scrotum. Thus, a cryptorchid testicle can be located in the abdominal cavity, in the inguinal canal, or in the subcutaneous tissue between the external inguinal ring and the scrotum (Bushby 2013).

With normal development, testicles should be easily palpated in the scrotum of dogs and cats by two months of age. If both testicles are not present in the scrotum at this time, the animal should be considered cryptorchid (Birchard and Nappier 2008), and it is appropriate to perform cryptorchid neuters on patients at this age.

If one or both testicles fail to descend into the scrotum, careful palpation will generally reveal which testicle(s) are involved and if the testicle(s) are located in the subcutaneous tissue. A presumptive diagnosis of abdominal cryptorchidism is made with failure to palpate a testicle in the scrotum or the subcutaneous tissue. Palpation of the testicle in the subcutaneous tissue leads to a diagnosis of subcutaneous cryptorchidism.

Cryptorchid animals should be neutered and cryptorchid testicles should be removed due to the increased risk of neoplasia or torsion in the retained testicle and the continued production of androgens, as well as the heritable nature of cryptorchidism (Birchard and Nappier 2008). In unilateral cryptorchids, it is generally advisable to remove the cryptorchid testicle first, before proceeding with removal of the scrotal testicle (Bierbrier and Causanschi 2018). This way, in the event that the cryptorchid testicle cannot be located, the scrotal testicle can be left in place to avoid the false appearance that the animal is already neutered.

There is no benefit to removal of only the scrotal testicle while leaving the cryptorchid testicle in place, as this will only make a future veterinarian's work more difficult while providing no health benefit to the animal. If, in a young patient, the surgeon elects to wait and see if the cryptorchid testicle will descend on its own, there is no reason to remove the scrotal testicle prior to the wait.

Subcutaneous Cryptorchidism

A subcutaneous cryptorchid testicle (see Figures 14.4 and 14.5) can be excised by incising the skin directly over the testicle, dissecting through the subcutaneous tissue to expose the testicle, exteriorizing the testicle, and ligating the spermatic cord with a cord tie, figure-of-eight knot, or ligatures (Bushby 2013). Subcutaneous tissue and skin are closed routinely.

Abdominal Cryptorchidism

Locating testicles retained in the abdominal cavity is usually quite simple (Bushby 2013). Contrary to some textbook descriptions, it is not necessary to perform an exploratory laparotomy to locate the abdominal testicle(s). The anatomic factor that makes location of abdominal testicles easy is that both ductus deferens enter the urethra at the prostate. As the ductus deferens courses cranially from the prostatic urethra, it is located dorsal to the bladder. Once the ductus deferens passes the junction of the ureter and the bladder, it turns laterally on its

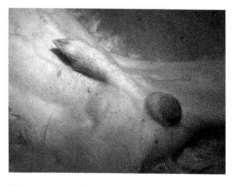

Figure 14.4 Subcutaneous cryptorchid dog. The testicle is located in the subcutaneous tissue between the scrotum and the external inguinal ring.

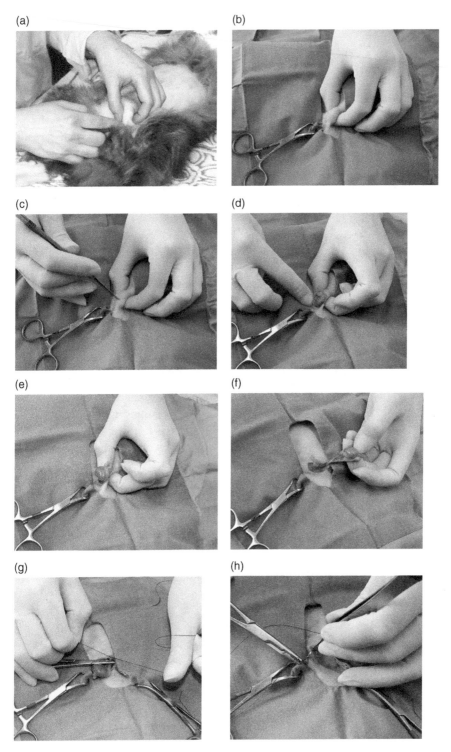

Figure 14.5 Subcutaneous cryptorchid cat. (a) Digital palpation of the cat's inguinal fat pad reveals a palpable subcutaneous testicle. (b) The testicle is isolated and held in place with the fingers of the non-dominant hand. (c) An incision is made through the overlying skin directly over the testicle. (d) Gentle digital pressure is applied to exteriorize the testicle. (e) It is sometimes necessary to bluntly or sharply dissect fat to reach the testicle at this stage. (f) The testicle is exteriorized to expose the spermatic cord. (g) The cord may be ligated with suture or via autoligation. (h) The incision is closed subcuticularly with absorbable suture. *Source:* Photos courtesy of Brenda Griffin.

course toward the inguinal canal. This anatomic feature is consistent whether the testicle(s) are descended into the scrotum or not and facilitates location of the cryptorchid testicle, either by catching the ductus deferens with a spay hook or visualizing the ductus deferens as it cross the ureter dorsal to the bladder (Boothe 1993).

Canine Abdominal Cryptorchidism

Once it is determined which testicle is cryptorchid, a skin incision is made in the caudal abdominal skin just lateral to the prepuce on the side of the cryptorchid testicle about halfway along the prepuce, or around the area of the last nipple (Bushby 2013; see Figure 14.6). With a unilateral abdominal cryptorchid testicle, the abdominal cavity is entered through a paramedian incision, incising the external rectus fascia and separating rectus abdominis muscle fibers on the appropriate side. Initially a very small incision is made in the abdominal wall and a spay hook is passed in a cranial-lateral direction, starting just lateral to the neck of the bladder. Often this maneuver will catch the ductus deferens, allowing exteriorization and excision of the testicle.

With a bilateral abdominal cryptorchid, an incision is made in the caudal abdominal skin just lateral to the prepuce, in the same location as for a unilateral cryptorchid. The subcutaneous tissue is then undermined to expose the linea alba, and the abdominal cavity is entered through an incision in the linea alba. The spay hook technique can be used on both sides of the bladder to exteriorize and excise both abdominal testicles.

In either unilateral or bilateral cryptorchid dogs, if the spay hook technique fails, extend the abdominal incision to expose and exteriorize the urinary bladder. Caudal reflection of the urinary bladder will expose the dorsal surface of the bladder, allowing visualization of both ductus deferens. Gentle retraction of the ductus of the cryptorchid testicle(s) will allow delivery of the testicle into the surgical site, ligation of the testicular vessels, and excision of the testicle (see Figure 14.7). Because this option is sometimes necessary, it is always advisable to empty the urinary bladder prior to starting surgery for the removal of an abdominal testicle.

Feline Abdominal Cryptorchidism

The technique for finding and excising the abdominal testicle(s) in the cat is essentially the same as that in the dog, except the skin incision is made in the caudal abdominal skin on the midline, about halfway between the umbilicus and the pubis (Bushby 2013). Entry into the abdomen is through an incision in the linea alba, allowing exposure of the urinary bladder.

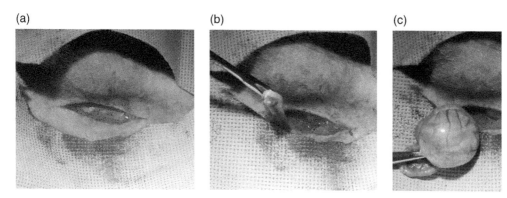

Figure 14.6 Abdominal cryptorchid – spay hook technique. (a) In the dog, paramedian in caudal abdominal skin adjacent to the prepuce. Enter the abdomen through a paramedian incision (unilateral abdominal cryptorchid) or through a linea incision (bilateral abdominal cryptorchid). (b) Pass a spay hook into the abdomen just lateral to the neck of the bladder. Sweep the spay hook in a cranial-lateral direction, exteriorizing the ductus deferens. (c) Tension on the ductus deferens exteriorizes the testicle.

(a)   (b)   (c)

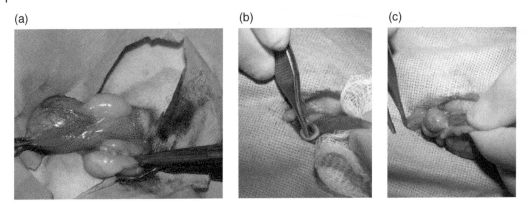

Figure 14.7 Abdominal cryptorchid – under bladder technique. (a) Exteriorize the bladder – reflecting the bladder caudally. (b) Visualize both ductus deferens dorsal to the bladder. Apply gentle traction to the ductus of the cryptorchid testicle. (c) Exteriorize the abdominal testicle.

As in the dog, using a spay hook and sweeping in a cranial-lateral direction from the neck of the bladder will often catch the ductus deferens. If this fails, caudal reflection of the urinary bladder to expose the dorsal surface of the bladder will allow visualization of both ductus deferens. Gentle retraction of the ductus of the cryptorchid testicle will allow delivery of the testicle into the surgical site, ligation of the testicular vessels, and excision of the testicle.

Failure to Find the "Abdominal" Testicle

Failure to palpate a cryptorchid testicle in the subcutaneous tissue leads to a presumptive diagnosis of abdominal cryptorchidism. The testicle, however, can be located in the abdominal cavity, trapped between the musculature of the inguinal canal, or located in the subcutaneous tissue, but not palpable. When the testicle is not found in the abdomen, gentle traction on the ductus deferens will allow visualization of the ductus deferens entering the inguinal canal. A curved mosquito hemostat can be used to gently tease the musculature of the internal inguinal ring apart, and if the testicle is trapped in the inguinal canal, gentle traction on the ductus will allow delivery of the testicle back into the abdomen for removal of the testicle as described under abdominal cryptorchid (Bushby 2013).

Cryptorchid testicles are, however, often smaller than normal and it is possible that the cryptorchid testicle is in the subcutaneous tissue, but not palpable. In this situation, surgically entering the abdomen with a presumptive diagnosis of abdominal cryptorchidism will fail to reveal the cryptorchid testicle. Further, the technique described of gently teasing apart the musculature of the internal inguinal ring and applying tension to the ductus will fail to deliver the testicle back into the abdomen.

At times, applying gentle traction on the abdominal ductus will produce visible movement or dimpling of the skin where the subcuticular testicle is located. In this case, the original skin incision may be extended or undermined, or an additional incision created to reach the testicle.

If traction fails to reveal the location of the subcutaneous testicle, undermine the skin between the skin incision and the external inguinal ring, extending the incision if necessary to allow visualization of the inguinal ring. Gentle traction on the abdominal ductus will allow the surgeon to locate the ductus deferens as it exits the inguinal canal and will lead to the cryptorchid testicle.

Once the cryptorchid testicle is located, it can be excised using any standard technique, and the abdominal and skin incisions are closed routinely.

Alternatives to Orchiectomy

Vasectomy

Vasectomy is the occlusion or removal of part of both ductus deferens. While surgical vasectomy results in sterilizing the patient by preventing the ejaculation of sperm, it does not alter male sexual characteristics and does not reduce the incidence of testosterone-dependent conditions. In the cat, vasectomy does not alter the strong odor associated with male urine. For these reasons, surgical vasectomy has had limited acceptance in veterinary medicine (Howe 2006). The one indication for vasectomy in dogs would be for those owners who refuse castration, but still desire sterilization. In cats, vasectomy has been suggested as a means of population control (Kendall 1979; McCarthy et al. 2013).

Vasectomy is performed through a 1–2 cm incision in each inguinal area in the dog and just cranial to the scrotum and prepuce in the cat (Howe 2006; MacPhail 2013). Spermatic cords are identified and isolated using a combination of blunt and sharp dissection. Identification of the spermatic cords may be facilitated by gentle manipulation of the testicles during subcutaneous dissection. Incise the tunic of each spermatic cord to expose and isolate the ductus deferens. Excise a section of each ductus deferens and ligate both proximal and distal severed ends (Howe 2006). Closure of subcutaneous tissue and skin is by a technique of the surgeon's preference.

References

Bierbrier, L. and Causanschi, H. (2018). Orchiectomy and ovariohysterectomy. In: *Field Manual for Small Animal Medicine* (eds. K. Polak and A.T. Kommedal), 201–228. Hoboken, NJ: Wiley-Blackwell.

Birchard, S.J. and Nappier, M. (2008). Cryptorchidism. *Compendium (Yardley, PA)* 30: 325–336; quiz 336–7.

Boothe, H.W. (1993). Testes and Epididymides. In: *Textbook of Small Animal Surgery*, 2e (eds. D. Slatter and E.A. Stone), 1325–1326. Philadephia, PA: Saunders.

Bushby, P.A. (2013). Surgical techniques for spay/neuter. In: *Shelter Medicine for Veterinarians and Staff*, 2e (eds. L. Miller and Z. Stephen), 625–646. Ames, IA: Wiley-Blackwell.

Bushby, P. and Griffin, B. (2011). Pediatric scrotal castration in a puppy. *dvm360* (8 February). http://veterinarymedicine.dvm360.com/pediatric-scrotal-castration-puppy (accessed 18 August 2018).

Griffin, B., Bushby, P.A., McCobb, E. et al. (2016). The Association of Shelter Veterinarians' 2016 veterinary medical care guidelines for spay-neuter programs. *JAVMA* 249: 165–188.

Hamilton, K., Henderson, E., Toscano, M., and Chanoit, G. (2014). Comparison of postoperative complications in healthy dogs undergoing open and closed orchidectomy. *J. Small Anim. Pract.* 55: 521–526.

Hedlund, C.S. (2007). Surgery of the reproductive and genital systems. In: *Small Animal Surgery*, 3e (ed. T.W. Fossum), 702–720. St. Louis, MO: Mosby Elsevier.

Howe, L.M. (2006). Surgical methods of contraception and sterilization. *Theriogenology* 66: 500–509.

Johnston, D. and Archibald, J. (1974). Male Genital System. In: *Canine Surgery*, 2e (ed. J. Archibald), 703–749. Santa Barbara, CA: American Veterinary Publications.

Kendall, T.R. (1979). Cat population control: vasectomized dominat males. *Calif. Vet.* 33: 9–12.

MacPhail, C.M. (2013). Surgery of the reproductive and genital systems. In: *Small Animal Surgery*, 4e (ed. T.W. Fossum), 780–855. St. Louis, MO: Mosby.

McCarthy, R.J., Levine, S.H., and Reed, J.M. (2013). Estimation of effectiveness of three methods of feral cat population control by use of a simulation model. *JAVMA* 243: 502–511.

Miller, K.P., Rekers, W.L., DeTar, L.G. et al. (2018). Evaluation of sutureless scrotal castration for pediatric and juvenile dogs. *JAVMA* 253: 1589–1593.

White, S. (2018). Surgery packs and suture in HQHVSN. *ergovet* (18 May). http://ergovet. com/surgery-packs-and-suture-in-hqhvsn (accessed 18 August 2018).

Woodruff, K., Bushby, P.A., Rigdon-Brestle, K. et al. (2015). Scrotal castration versus prescrotal castration in dogs. *Vet. Med.* 110 (5): 131–135.

15

Neutering Procedures and Considerations in Rabbits and Other Small Mammals

Natalie Isaza and Ramiro Isaza

Thousands of rabbits and small mammals like rats, mice, hamsters, and guinea pigs are relinquished to animal shelters every year. In addition, many of these species are readily available for purchase at local pet stores relatively inexpensively, which has led to their increasing popularity as pets. Because of this, many shelters and high-quality high-volume spay–neuter (HQHVSN) clinics must accommodate these patients.

Although rodents and other small mammals are covered in this chapter, the primary focus will be on rabbits. Because there are large numbers of rabbits routinely relinquished to animal shelters, many dedicated rabbit rescue organizations throughout the United States require that rabbits be neutered prior to placement in new homes. Rabbits have a high reproductive potential, and if unneutered animals of the opposite sex are housed together, it is inevitable that more rabbits will be born. In addition, there are medical and behavioral reasons to surgically sterilize rabbits prior to adoption, which will be discussed later in this chapter. Other topics to be covered include rabbit anatomy and reproduction, anesthetic considerations, and neutering surgical procedures.

General Considerations

Every animal, regardless of species, should be evaluated for body condition, weight, hydration, evidence of anemia, and cardiovascular status during a routine pre-anesthetic physical examination prior to performing surgery (Hanley 2013). Evidence of systemic infections, respiratory distress, and cardiovascular disease should be considered contraindications for elective surgical procedures. As rabbits and many other small mammals are obligate nasal breathers, the nares need to be assessed for patency prior to induction of anesthesia. Assessment of body condition is also important, since in an otherwise healthy rabbit or rodent, obesity can be a major surgical obstacle.

Pre-surgical fasting for elective reproductive surgeries is not recommended in rabbits and most rodents or other small mammals (Heard 2007a, b). The rationale for not fasting is based on the inability of many small mammals to vomit, the potential for the development of post-operative ileus if they are fasted, and the high caloric requirement necessary to maintain adequate blood glucose levels in these species. In general, small amounts of food should be available for one to four hours prior to anesthesia, and water should be available for at least one to two hours prior to anesthesia (Jenkins 2000).

Determining Sex Prior to Surgery

Often a careful physical examination is needed to correctly identify the sex of rabbits and other small mammal species. Confusion occasionally occurs in species like rabbits that have testicles that can be retracted into the abdomen. Similarly, species like chinchillas have a prominent female cone-shaped clitoris that can be confused with a penis. In many adults, the secondary sexual characteristics and genital anatomy are obvious on close visual inspection. Gentle manipulation of the inguinal genitalia (vulva or prepuce) in an attempt to extrude the penis can be used to differentiate the vulva from the prepuce in the rabbit (Figures 15.1 and 15.2). The determination of sex is much more challenging in neonatal and young rabbits and rodents. In these situations, the most important observation is the relative distance between the anus and the urogenital openings. As in dogs and cats, the anogenital distance is usually much shorter in females. Specifics for a particular species can be found in rabbit and rodent textbooks, as well as relevant websites that

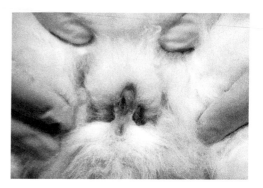

Figure 15.2 External genitalia of the male rabbit.

describe the differences in sexual morphology (Hanley 2013; Harcourt-Brown 2002; Hillyer 1994).

Age for Gonadectomy

Although many shelters and animal rescues want to spay and neuter small mammals prior to adoption, there are currently no recommendations concerning appropriate age for spay and neuter, with little to no information on the effects of pediatric gonadectomy in these species. However, it may be difficult to visualize or isolate reproductive structures in very young animals and, conversely, in older animals the structures may be buried in fat.

Anesthesia and Pain Control

The principles of analgesia and anesthetic drug selection and dosing in rabbits and small rodents are similar to domestic carnivores with some notable exceptions. The reader is advised to review more detailed chapters covering rabbit and rodent anesthesia (Flecknell 2001; Hawkins and Pascoe 2012; Heard 2007a, b; Lichtenberger and Ko 2007; Robertson 2001). Unfortunately, much of the veterinary literature contains parenteral anesthetic drug dose recommendations intended for laboratory animal procedures. These dosages are often higher than needed for routine and safe anesthesia in

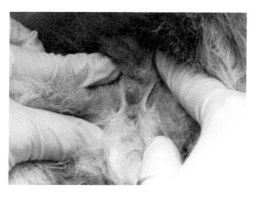

Figure 15.1 External genitalia of the female rabbit.

companion small mammals, and therefore usage of these doses should be carefully considered prior to administration. The European companion rabbit and rodent literature also tends to favor parenteral anesthetics, but generally contains lower dosage recommendations. Multiple review papers and a few studies have evaluated various parenteral drug combinations for rabbits and rodents. For example, Telazol (tiletamine/zolazepam; Zoetis, Parsippany, NJ) at high doses is associated with dose-dependent renal tubular necrosis in rabbits and should be used with caution (Brammer et al. 1991). A number of combinations of parenteral drugs have been recommended by various sources and the choice is primarily based on the clinician's preferences. Table 15.1 provides drug selections and dosages used by the authors.

Pre-medication

Sedation and pre-medication of rabbits and rodents may facilitate peri-operative physical examination and often provides smoother inductions. Intramuscular or intranasal midazolam or diazepam provides good pre-anesthetic sedation in rabbits. The routine use of parasympatholytics such as atropine is not recommended in rabbits and most other small mammals, because they can cause hypomotility of the gastrointestinal tract and may contribute to post-surgical ileus. Additionally, many rabbits have active atropine esterases that can negate the effects of atropine (Heard 2007a).

Induction

Due to their small size and temperament, options for routes of administration of induction anesthetics are often different in small mammals from those in dogs and cats. Although an intravenous (IV) catheter is ideal, placing a catheter in smaller or fractious species is often technically impossible. The use of propofol is limited to animals that have pre-placed IV or intraosseous catheters and are easily intubated so that breaths can be given during the expected period of apnea (Aeschbacher and Webb 1993). Similarly, the small body size of these patients can make intramuscular (IM) injections difficult without causing trauma to the small muscles. Both subcutaneous (SC) and IM injections of irritant drugs can cause significant self-mutilation at the injection sites. In an experimental study of rabbits, the administration of ketamine and medetomidine via IM and SC routes were found to be equally efficacious, with the SC route causing less apparent discomfort following injection (Williams and Wyatt 2007). Careful intraperitoneal injections are often a viable delivery route in very small mammals. Placement of drugs into the nares for sedation and partial induction has been recommended in rabbits, particularly prior to chamber induction (Robertson and Eberhart 1994). Direct gas induction in an anesthetic chamber that is pre-oxygenated is a common method of induction of small non-domestic mammals (Figures 15.3 and 15.4). Once the animal is placed inside the chamber, the anesthetic gas concentration is increased until the patient is in lateral recumbency and unconscious. The patient is removed from the chamber and a face mask with anesthetic gas is placed over the nose and mouth. At this point, the animal can be prepared for surgery or intubated. Direct mask induction of manually restrained, non-sedated animals is generally considered to be stressful and is not recommended for routine anesthetic induction.

Anesthesia Maintenance

Isofluorane and sevofluorane are the gas anesthetics of choice for rabbits and rodents. When used correctly they provide predictable and rapid inductions, stable maintenance, and smooth recoveries. Pre-medication with sedatives and pain medication and assisted positive pressure ventilation through an endotracheal tube improve gas-based anesthetic protocols. Consistent monitoring and recording of vital signs are important in these very small species.

Table 15.1 Drugs and drug dosages commonly used by the authors.

	Drug or combination	Rabbit	Rat	Mouse/ gerbil/ hamster	Guinea pig/ chinchilla/ degu	Prairie dog/ squirrel	Hedgehog	Sugar glider	Ferret
Sedation	Midazolam	1 mg/kg IM, SC, IN	1 mg/kg IM, SC	2 mg/kg IP, SC	1 mg/kg IM, SC	1 mg/kg IM, SC	0.3 mg/kg IM, SC	0.3 mg/kg IM, SC	0.3 mg/kg IM, SC
	Midazolam, buprenorphine	0.5 mg/kg 0.03 mg/kg IM, IN	0.5 mg/kg 0.05 mg/kg IM	1 mg/kg 0.1 mg/kg IM	0.5 mg/kg 0.05 mg/kg IM	0.5 mg/kg 0.05 mg/kg IM	0.3 mg/kg 0.02 mg/kg IM	0.3 mg/kg 0.01 mg/kg IM	0.5 mg/kg 0.02 mg/kg IM
Induction	Propofol	8 mg/kg IV, to effect	10 mg/kg IV, to effect		5 mg/kg IV, to effect	5 mg/kg IV, to effect			5 mg/kg IV, to effect
	Ketamine, midazolam	5 mg/kg 1 mg/kg IM, once	10 mg/kg 0.5 mg/kg IP, once	15 mg/kg 1 mg/kg IP, once	5 mg/kg 0.5 mg/kg IP, once	10 mg/kg 0.5 mg/kg IP, once	10 mg/kg 0.3 mg/kg IM, once	10 mg/kg 0.3 mg/kg IP, once	5 mg/kg 0.3 mg/kg IM, once
	Ketamine, dexmedetomidine	5 mg/kg 0.1 mg/kg IM, once	10 mg/kg 0.3 mg/kg IM, once	15 mg/kg 0.5 mg/kg IM, once	5 mg/kg 0.1 mg/kg IM, once	5 mg/kg 0.1 mg/kg IM, once	3 mg/kg 0.05 mg/kg IM, SC, once	3 mg/kg 0.05 mg/kg IM, SC, once	5 mg/kg 0.05 mg/kg IM, once
	Ketamine, dexmedetomidine, buprenorphine	5 mg/kg 0.1 mg/kg 0.01 mg/kg IM, once							
Local	Lidocaine	1 mg/kg SC, total	1 mg/kg SC, total	1 mg/kg SC, total	1 mg/kg SC, total	1 mg/kg SC, total	1 mg/kg SC, total	1 mg/kg SC, total	1 mg/kg SC, total
	Bupivacaine	0.5 mg/kg SC, total	0.5 mg/kg SC, total	0.5 mg/kg SC, total	0.5 mg/kg SC, total	0.5 mg/kg SC, total	0.5 mg/kg SC, total	0.5 mg/kg SC, total	0.5 mg/kg SC, total

Reversal	Atipamezole	1 mg/kg SC, once	1 mg/kg SC, once	2 mg/kg SC, once	1 mg/kg SC, once	1 mg/kg SC, once		0.3 mg/kg SC, once	1 mg/kg SC, once
	Naloxone	0.05 mg/kg SC, total					0.1 mg/kg SC, total		
Analgesia	Buprenorphine	0.03 mg/kg SC, BID	0.05 mg/kg SC, BID	0.1 mg/kg SC, BID	0.05 mg/kg SC, BID	0.05 mg/kg SC, BID	0.05 mg/kg SC, BID	0.05 mg/kg SC, BID	0.02 mg/kg SC, BID
	Meloxicam	0.3 mg/kg SC, PO SID	1 mg/kg SC, PO SID	2 mg/kg SC, PO SID	0.5 mg/kg SC, PO SID	0.5 mg/kg SC, PO SID	0.1 mg/kg SC, PO SID	0.1 mg/kg SC, PO SID	0.2 mg/kg PO SID
	Carprofen	2 mg/kg SC, PO SID	2 mg/kg SC, PO SID	4 mg/kg SC, SID	2 mg/kg SC, PO SID	2 mg/kg SC, PO SID	1 mg/kg SC, PO SID		1 mg/kg SC, PO SID

BID, twice a day; IM, intramuscular; IN, intranasal; IP, intraperitoneal; IV, intravenous; PO, oral; SC, subcutaneous; SID, once a day.

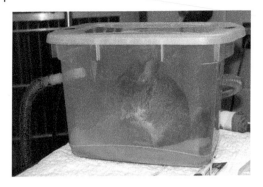

Figure 15.3 Box induction of a chinchilla following sedation.

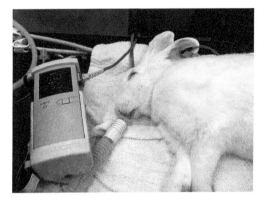

Figure 15.5 Rabbit intubated for surgical procedure.

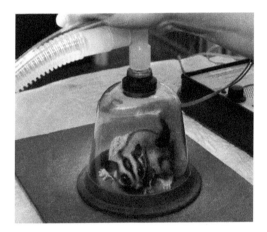

Figure 15.4 Mask induction of a sugar glider following sedation.

Intubation

In general, most anesthesiologists agree that rabbits should be intubated during most surgical procedures (Figure 15.5). However, it is recognized that rabbits are often challenging to intubate because their long narrow dental arcades, small oral cavity commissure, thick tongue base, and ventrally placed larynx impede direct visualization of the vocal folds. Iatrogenic trauma to the pharynx, larynx, and trachea from repeated and traumatic attempts at intubation can cause serious damage and result in respiratory distress during both induction and recovery (Phaneuf et al. 2006). Brodbelt et al., in a retrospective study of risks of mortality in small animals, noted an increase

in death for intubated rabbits, but did not speculate on the cause (Brodbelt et al. 2008). Intubation of rabbits for routine spay–neuter is therefore left to the discretion of the clinician.

The most common intubation method is to use a 1.5–3 mm internal diameter (ID) clear endotracheal tube using a blind technique (Flecknell 2001; Heard 2007a). The rabbit is fully induced with injectable anesthetic or gas anesthesia and placed in ventral (sternal) recumbency, with the head carefully hyperextended and the tongue gently pulled forward. Approximately 0.1 ml of 2% lidocaine is placed into the pharynx and a few minutes given to allow the larynx to become desensitized. The endotracheal tube is gently passed centrally through the oral cavity. Once at the level of the larynx, the clinician listens for breath sounds and/or looks for fogging of the inside of the endotracheal tube (Figure 15.6). The insertion of the tube is then timed to coincide with the rabbit's maximal respiratory inspiration when the larynx is open. Occasionally a slight axial twisting of the tube is needed for the tip to pass into the trachea. A strong coughing reflex is often elicited when the rabbit has been correctly intubated. Tube placement is confirmed by the passage of air with each respiration or the detection of a carbon dioxide (CO_2) wave using a capnograph.

A modification of this method is to place the rabbit in lateral recumbency with the head

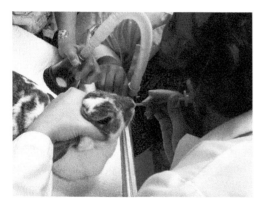

Figure 15.6 Blind intubation of a rabbit. The clinician listens for breath sounds. Insertion of the tube coincides with maximal respiration, when the larynx opens.

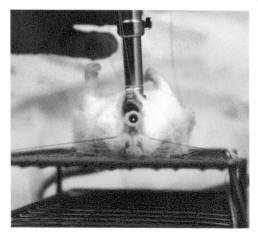

Figure 15.7 Illumination of the trachea in a small rodent through an endotracheal tube to visualize the glottis and allow correct placement of the endotracheal tube.

held in moderate hyperextension. The tube is passed through the center of the oral cavity until it is at the level of the larynx. Instead of listening for air passing during respiration, the fogging of the tube is visualized or a capnograph is placed on the tube. Again, the respirations are timed and the tube is inserted during inspiration, when the fog starts to clear from the inside of the endotracheal tube (Morgan and Glowaski 2007).

For larger rabbits, a direct visualization method is used, where a modified long, thin, pediatric laryngoscope blade is placed in the mouth to visualize the larynx. While visualizing the laryngeal opening, a thin stylet is passed into the trachea. The free distal end of stylet is then threaded into the tip of the endotracheal tube, and the endotracheal tube is passed into the trachea by following the stylet inside the endotracheal tube. Recently, laryngeal mask airway tubes originally designed for neonatal infants and now customized for rabbits and other small animals have been used successfully in rabbits (Bateman et al. 2005; Smith et al. 2004). Nasotracheal intubation has also been described, where the rabbit is placed in dorsal recumbency and a 2.0–2.5 mm ID endotracheal tube is passed through one of the nasal passages (Devalle 2009).

Tracheal intubation of rodents and other small mammals can be more challenging, but similar methods have been adapted for these species. Some practitioners have described the use of small flexible endoscopes or ridged laparoscopes as aids for intubation. A strong fiberoptic light source can be used on the ventral aspect of the cranial neck of a small rodent (Figure 15.7). The light passes through the skin and illuminates the tracheal lumen. The light exiting the larynx can be seen intraorally, and may be used to help place the endotracheal tube (Yasaki and Dyck 1991).

If tracheal intubation is not possible or is considered impractical, many small mammals can be maintained under gas anesthesia with a mask on the nose or face (Figure 15.8). Guinea pigs and chinchillas are considered particularly difficult to intubate and, unlike most other rodents, they can regurgitate food material into the oropharynx (Heard 2007b). They also have redundant pharyngeal soft tissues; specifically, the lateral aspects of the soft palate are fused to the base of the tongue, forming a palatal ostium. These species also produce copious saliva that prevents direct visualization of the larynx. Glycopyrrolate can be used pre-operatively to control excessive salivation in these species.

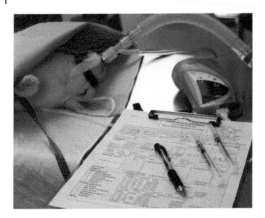

Figure 15.8   Maintenance of anesthesia in a rabbit via face mask.

Pain Control

The use of pre-operative and post-surgical multimodal analgesia is necessary in all species. Each animal should be considered individually, and utilizing several analgesic classes to prevent and treat pain is ideal. A variety of non-steroidal anti-inflammatory drug (NSAID) and narcotic drug protocols are available for small mammal species. For example, a rabbit can be given butorphanol as part of a sedative combination, low-dose ketamine as part of the induction to reduce wind-up pain, and several days of meloxicam orally during post-anesthetic recovery. Proper post-operative pain control is usually associated with return to normal feeding and drinking behavior and is an important factor in preventing post-operative ileus. In addition, regional local anesthetics can be used before the surgical incision is made or during incision closure. Examples of the types of blocks that aid in post-operative pain control are intratesticular bupivacaine or lidocaine prior to castration, intradermal injection of local anesthetic to the anticipated incision site, or splash blocks of lidocaine or bupivacaine into the ovariohysterectomy (OHE) surgical site once the body wall is closed.

Other Anesthetic Considerations

Maintenance of core body temperature is an important anesthetic consideration in small mammals, because they have a relatively large surface area that pre-disposes them to temperature changes during anesthesia. It is therefore important to monitor body temperatures during anesthesia and surgery for detection of both hypothermia and hyperthermia. Placement in a pre-warmed, thermoneutral enclosure prior to pre-medication may help maintain adequate body temperature during surgery. All animals undergoing surgery should be provided with supplemental heat and warmed fluids as necessary during the peri-operative period. During anesthesia and recovery, the animals should be wrapped in warmed towels or bubble wrap, placed under a warm air circulator, or on water-filled surgical heating blankets to help prevent heat loss during surgery. The routine use of safe heating devices listed earlier has been experimentally evaluated in rabbits (Sikoski et al. 2007). To minimize evaporative cooling, avoid soaking large areas of the animal with water, surgical scrub solutions, or alcohol. Use limited amounts of liquids to avoid excess run-off wetting the sides of the animal. In very small animals, instead of large 2×2 gauzes, smaller gauze squares or even cotton-tipped applicators in smaller species can be used for preparing the surgical site.

Many rodents have prominently placed, protruding eyes that can be exposed and injured during anesthetic procedures. Corneal ulceration as a result of traumatic injury due to exposure is a common complication in many small animals. Application of ophthalmic eye lubricants and periodic manual closing of the eyelids during surgery and recovery can minimize this problem.

General Surgical Principles and Equipment

Surgical procedures, techniques, and standards for rabbits and most other small mammals are generally similar to procedures in dogs and cats discussed throughout this book. Given the basic similarities, it is the important practical differences that the surgeon needs to be aware of prior to performing surgery (Bennett 2012a, b; Jenkins 2012; Lightfoot et al. 2012; Szabo et al. 2016). One of the most important differences between domestic carnivores and small mammals is the relative difference in body size. The body of some of the smaller rodent species complicates access to the reproductive organs and makes the anatomic details of the viscera difficult to visualize.

Surgical Instrumentation

Standard surgical instruments used in dog and cat neutering are adequate for rabbits and larger rodents. However, a set of smaller ophthalmologic or vascular instruments greatly facilitates surgery in many of the smaller species. Because of the small size of most rabbits and rodents, the use of magnification and proper illumination during the surgical procedure is highly recommended (Bennett, 2012a, b). High-quality surgical loupes with attached lighting are a good option to evaluate the tissues and assess hemostasis. Similarly, the use of an operating microscope for detailed magnification of the surgical site is recommended for very small species of animals. Small abdominal retractors are recommended to provide access and visualization to the surgical field. The use of a spay hook is not recommended in most herbivorous small mammals due to the large and delicate abdominal structures including the cecum, colon, and bladder, and the very real risk of rupturing one of these structures. Sterile surgical cotton swabs can be used to manipulate and bluntly dissect tissues.

Metal vascular clips (Ligaclip®, Ethicon, Somerville, NJ) and radiosurgical cautery (Surgitron® EMC or Dual RF, Ellman International, Oceanside, NY) are often recommended to provide quick vascular ligations and hemostasis. Regardless of the instrumentation used, it is important to minimize aggressive tissue handling and to use meticulous aseptic technique, just as with surgical procedures on any species.

Suture Selection

Synthetic monofilament suture materials (sizes 3-0 to 5-0) that are absorbed by hydrolysis are preferred in rabbits and most small rodents. Many of these species produce caseous reactions to foreign material such as catgut suture that may in turn enhance or stimulate adhesion formation (Bennett 2012a; Jenkins 2012). Inside the abdomen, synthetic absorbable monofilament suture and metal vascular clips are again preferred over catgut and braided suture materials. Synthetic monofilament suture is preferred for abdominal closure, subcutaneous tissues, and skin. Alternatively, staples and tissue adhesives can be judiciously used for skin closure.

Closing the Incision

Abdominal closure is similar to that performed in cats and dogs. For the body wall, a well-anchored and secure, simple continuous or simple interrupted suture pattern can be used. Subcutaneous tissues should be closed next, followed by an intradermal or subcuticular closure of the skin; this is preferred to eliminate the need for external skin sutures that can be chewed out post-operatively by the animal. Placement of this layer in rabbits and rodents with thin skin can be technically very challenging, but accidental external penetration of the skin should be avoided. When properly performed, an intradermal closure appears to cause minimal discomfort, and patients often seem unaware of its presence. If external skin closure is used, skin staples are preferred to prevent removal by the rodent's incisors and grooming behaviors. Appropriate post-operative pain control is important to prevent chewing and excessive grooming of the incision site.

Peri-operative Care

Housing the animal far away from other predator species like dogs and cats will decrease stress and help in pre-surgical sedation and post-anesthetic recovery. Food and water must be available very soon after surgery to stimulate digestion and prevent prolonged post-surgical anorexia and ileus. Once the animal is standing, it can be offered hay or some other appropriate food item for the species. Syringe-feeding a dilute solution of a powered herbivore diet such as Oxbow Critical Care (Oxbow Animal Health, Murdock, NE) is indicated in rabbits that do not begin eating spontaneously two to four hours after surgery. Consider the use of supplemental pain control (NSAIDs and opioids) on all animals undergoing surgery, and intestinal motility enhancers such as metoclopramide or cisapride for animals experiencing post-operative gastric hypomotility. Avoid the unnecessary use of antibiotics during the peri-operative period, as they may interfere with motility and disrupt normal intestinal flora. Monitor the recovering animal carefully to prevent licking of the surgical site, and also for signs of post-operative hemorrhage. The incision site should be monitored and the skin sutures, if present, should be removed 10–14 days following surgery. As with cats and dogs, all animals (males and females) should be tattooed following the surgical procedure to identify them as being neutered.

Peri-operative Complications

Peri-operative hemorrhage is a common and potentially fatal surgical complication. Limiting acute hemorrhage during surgery is critical in small mammals because of their body size. The blood volume of many species can be estimated to be approximately 6% of their total bodyweight. Loss of more than 20% of blood volume may result in shock and death. This corresponds to an acute blood loss of 4 ml of blood during a procedure on a 350 g rodent, or 24 ml on a 2 kg rabbit (Bennett 2012a). With these limitations in blood loss, the surgeon should use effective and secure hemostasis throughout the procedure. Similarly, the length of anesthesia and the time of surgery should be minimized to avoid sepsis, hypothermia, and anesthetic deaths. Surgical errors due

to unfamiliar anatomy are common. Inadvertent incision of gastrointestinal and urinary tract structures should be meticulously avoided. If noted during surgery, every effort should be made to repair the iatrogenic damage. The most important recommendations for surgery in these species are gentle and efficient tissue manipulation and a thorough understanding of the anatomy of the patient.

Post-operative Complications

A limited number of studies have reported the frequency of post-surgical complications and mortality associated with elective OHE or castration in rabbits and rodents. One small study of 50 rabbits described a complication rate of 24% (Millis and Walshaw 1992). These complications included self-mutilation or overgrooming of the incision site (10%), post-surgical anorexia (8%), partial incisional dehiscence (6%), and conjunctivitis or ophthalmic injuries (4%). Although all of the surgeries in this study were performed by veterinary students, these types of complications can be expected regardless of the experience of the surgeon. Larger studies with longer follow-up periods are needed to understand the long-term effects of elective reproductive surgeries on companion rabbits and rodents. Incomplete removal of the ovaries is a common error that may lead to a return of estrus cycles, pyometra, and uterine or mammary neoplasia (Hotchkiss 1995; Kottwitz 2006; Lightfoot et al. 2012).

Many small mammals, and especially rabbits, have a strong tendency to form post-surgical adhesions of their abdominal viscera. Rabbits have been used as models for studying human intraabdominal adhesions, and adhesions can develop simply by abrading the serosal surfaces of the gut by wiping them with dry surgical gauze. Although no long-term studies have been conducted on the formation of adhesions in rabbits following spay surgery, it can be assumed that routine reproductive surgeries can result in adhesions at the uterine stump, the ovarian pedicles, and the serosal surfaces of the adjacent intestines. Using talc-free surgical gloves or sterilely rinsing and wiping the surgical gloves prior to surgery may help limit the formation of adhesions. Several studies in the rabbit have evaluated different drugs and intraabdominal implants to determine if they limit the formation of intraabdominal adhesions, but none has translated to practical recommendations for use in pet rabbits (Dunn and Mohler 1993; Jenkins 2012; Legrand et al. 1995; Luciano et al. 1989; Nishimura et al. 1984; Whitfield et al. 2007).

Evidence-Based Surgical Recommendations

Numerous published articles describing the surgical procedures for neutering rabbits, as well as for a wide variety of rodent species, exist in the veterinary literature (Bennett 2012a, b; Harcourt-Brown 2002; Hillyer 1994; Idris 2012; Jenkins 2000, 2012; Olsen and Bruce 1986). These descriptions range from short and succinct descriptions to very detailed surgical descriptions with informative step-by-step photographs and illustrations. The surgeon should review these descriptions prior to attempting reproductive surgery in any unfamiliar species. It should be noted that each published description is somewhat unique, with multiple methods and variations described for each procedure and species. This lack of consensus is further confounded by the absence of any formal evaluation of the surgical recommendations. Large studies documenting complication rates, long-term survival for different surgical techniques, or biologic consequences of neutering are generally missing from the companion animal literature. A few laboratory animal studies have tracked surgical outcomes and histologic consequences, but usually only in the context of an animal model and not from the typical pet population. With only sparse relevant evidence, the surgeon is forced to make choices based primarily on anecdotal recommendations of study authors. This section will describe several of

these surgical procedures for each species type, with the most recommended method first.

Rabbit Ovariohysterectomy and Ovariectomy

The primary reason for neutering a female rabbit (*Oryctolagus cuniculus*) is to prevent unwanted reproduction. Uterine adenocarcinoma is the most common neoplasia in female rabbits, and rabbits have a high likelihood for developing uterine neoplasia if left intact (Figure 15.9). Because of this, the current recommendation is to perform OHE in all non-breeding pet rabbits. Although uterine neoplasia is often subclinical, it can be associated with reproductive failures, bloody vaginal discharge, and chronic weight loss (Tonks and Atlas 2007). If uterine neoplasia does occur, OHE is the treatment of choice if discovered before metastatic spread.

Rabbit OHE can also prevent or resolve other types of uterine pathology, including endometritis, endometrial hyperplasia, pyometra, hydrometra, and uterine aneurysms. Several studies have reviewed the range and incidence of uterine pathology from populations of rabbits (Saito et al. 2002; Walter et al. 2010). Although mammary cancer is relatively rare, there are two major types described (Toft 1992; Weisbroth 1994). The more common type is

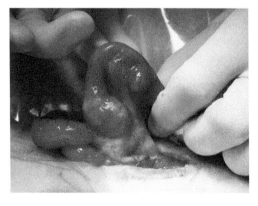

Figure 15.9 Uterine adenocarcinoma in a female rabbit.

papillary adenocarcinoma, which is usually preceded by cystic mastopathy and is often linked to uterine cancer in rabbits. The second type is medullary carcinoma arising from mammary acini.

Intact female rabbits are also prone to pseudo-pregnancy that hormonally mimics a true pregnancy. These rabbits undergo undesirable behavioral changes typically seen during pregnancy and parturition. Preemptive OHE can also decrease territorial aggression, barbering, and territorial urine-spraying behaviors in female rabbits. Although the positive effects of OHE and ovariectomy (OVE) have been documented in the literature, the negative biologic consequences of these surgeries are poorly studied.

Uterine Neoplasia in Rabbits

Current estimates of the population prevalence of uterine neoplasia vary significantly in the literature and are controversial. Several sources report that up to 80% of all rabbits will develop uterine neoplastic lesions (see Figure 15.9). Other authors more correctly state that in older rabbits the prevalence of uterine cancer can be as high as 50–80%. All of these statistical statements stem from two studies that describe the prevalence of uterine neoplasia in large laboratory rabbit populations followed for several years (Greene 1942; Ingalls et al. 1964). However, the details of these studies are often overlooked and are therefore misquoted. Both studies reported a very high prevalence of cancer in older rabbits. Greene studied one rabbit colony for nine years and reported the incidence of uterine cancer by age and other epidemiologic factors (Greene 1942). His population of rabbits was monitored throughout their natural life span; however, his monitoring began at two years of age and his study group consisted of a population that was managed with intensive selective inbreeding to study other hereditary diseases. From this group, Greene reported a prevalence of uterine cancer of 4.2% from 491 females two to

three years old, 20.8% from 259 females three to four years old, 63.3% from 71 females four to five years old, 79.1% from 24 females five to six years old, and 75% from 4 females six to seven years old. It is important to note that the high prevalence rates in the older rabbit age groups were calculated from relatively small numbers of animals surviving to the respective ages. The resulting statistics from those small denominators are artificially inflated and statistically unreliable. A similar study of another laboratory population reported 28.5% prevalence in 49 rabbits three to four years of age, and 58.9% prevalence in 73 rabbits four years or older (Ingalls et al. 1964). Both authors used these age category-based prevalence calculations to highlight that uterine cancer is correlated very strongly with age, so those rabbits surviving to old age are at higher risk for developing these cancers.

The important observation is that rabbit uterine cancer is common in most rabbit populations, but the overall prevalence may be significantly lower than the 60–80% commonly quoted in the literature for rabbits of all ages. In fact, even in the two original papers reviewed, the overall incidence of uterine cancer from the observed populations was only 17% of 849 female rabbits (Greene's population) and 20% of 1735 female rabbits (Ingall's population). Several subsequent studies of overall neoplastic incidence in rabbits reported modest prevalence of 1.3–2.6% in populations of young laboratory rabbits (Weisbroth 1994). In two veterinary teaching hospitals, only 4–6% of all rabbit admissions were due to uterine abnormalities, including adenocarcinomas (Klaphake and Paul-Murphy 2012; Paré and Paul-Murphy 2003). Unfortunately, the true prevalence of uterine neoplasia in large companion (pet) rabbit populations allowed to live their full life spans has not been reported in the literature.

Rabbit Female Anatomy

Rabbits typically reach sexual maturity between four and nine months of age, depending on the

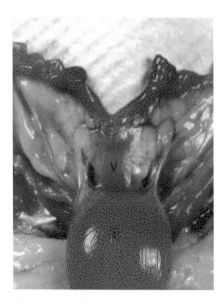

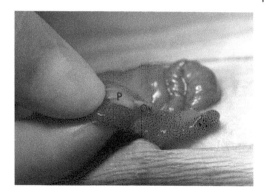

Figure 15.11   Rabbit ovary (Ov), oviduct (Od), and proper ligament (P).

Figure 15.10   Reproductive tract of the female rabbit, showing the close association between the bladder (B) and the vaginal body (V). Urine can be seen within the vaginal body.

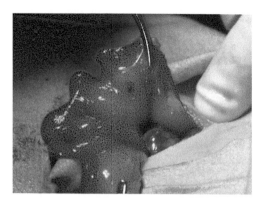

Figure 15.12   Fatty broad ligament (B) in an obese female rabbit.

adult size and breed (Hillyer 1994). Rabbits, along with most rodents, do not have overt estrus cycles. Rabbits are induced ovulators, much like the domestic cat, ovulating several hours after copulation. As in many mammals, the rabbit and rodent female reproductive tract lies partially coiled in a large loop located in the caudal abdomen. The caudal aspect of the reproductive tract originates between the colon and the urinary bladder (Figure 15.10). At the cranial end, the rabbit ovaries are not enclosed within a complete ovarian bursa. Compared to a cat, rabbits have very long fallopian tubes and shorter ovarian suspensory ligaments (Figure 15.11). These anatomic differences sometimes make elevation of the ovaries from the surgical site more difficult. In general, the tissues of the rabbit and rodent reproductive tracts are more friable than those of a domestic cat. These tissues must be handled gently and with limited traction to prevent tearing and hemorrhage.

The broad ligament is a primary fat-storage site in rabbits and most rodents. This broad ligament fat in obese pet animals can significantly complicate the visualization, isolation, and ligation of the ovarian pedicles and blood vessels supplying the uterus (Figure 15.12). Unlike the uterus in cats, the rabbit and rodent uterus has variable numbers of large vessels branching off from the main uterine arteries. A particular anatomic difference between rabbits and other mammals (including dogs and cats) is the presence of two completely separate uteruses, each with its own cervix. Thus, rabbits lack a true uterine body, with each cervix emptying directly into the vaginal vault. Different from most mammals, the urethra of the female rabbit empties directly into the caudal end of the vaginal body. In contrast to dogs and cats, the rabbit has a very long vaginal body (vaginal vestibule) that can pool urine in the caudal aspect of the vestibule during normal micturition. This pooling can be exacerbated if the urinary bladder is manually expressed while the animal is in dorsal recumbency and under anesthesia or heavy sedation.

Rabbit Ovariohysterectomy/ Ovariectomy Methods

Rabbit Ovariohysterectomy

The ventral midline approach is the most common method of performing an OHE in female rabbits (Capello 2005a; Jenkins 2012). Once anesthetized, an area of the ventral abdomen is clipped similar in size to an area prepared for a cat or kitten spay. The clipping must be done carefully, because rabbit skin is very thin and tears easily, yet fine rabbit hair is difficult to clip. Aseptically prepare the surgical site by alternating chlorhexidine or betadine scrubs with alcohol or warmed sterile water. The skin incision should be centered halfway between the umbilicus and the pubis, about 2–4 cm caudal to the umbilicus and extending 1–3 cm caudally toward the pubis. A larger incision can be made if more exposure is needed. Once the subcutaneous tissues are cleared, the ventral body wall and linea alba should be clearly identified. The body wall is elevated and an inverted scalpel (#15 blade is preferred) is used to make the first incision through the linea (Figure 15.13). This step is critical, as the thin-walled cecum and the urinary bladder of herbivorous mammals are usually located just under the abdominal wall. The linea incision should be extended far enough to provide adequate surgical access.

Generally, the rabbit uterus is easy to visualize in the caudal abdomen, just dorsal to the cranial pole of the urinary bladder with a distinctly pink coloration. Gentle retraction can be used to move the cecum or bladder aside to locate the uterus if it is not initially visualized. As mentioned previously, the use of a spay hook to locate the uterus is contraindicated in rabbits, due to the very real danger of puncturing the thin-walled cecum (Figure 15.14). Once the uterus is identified, the cranial portion is grasped with fingers or forceps and elevated out of the abdomen (Figure 15.15). In rabbits it

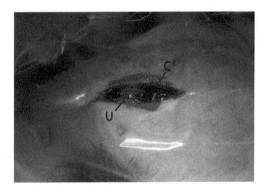

Figure 15.14 Cecum (C) and uterus (U) in the female rabbit under a plastic surgical drape.

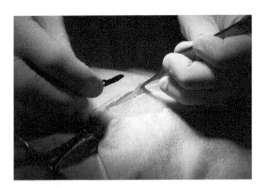

Figure 15.13 Elevation of the body wall prior to insertion of the scalpel blade is important to prevent puncture of the cecum, which lies directly beneath the abdominal wall.

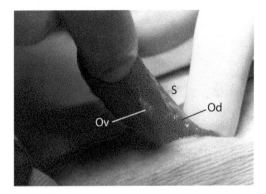

Figure 15.15 Elevation of the first uterus from the abdominal cavity in a female rabbit. The ovary (Ov), suspensory ligament (S), and oviduct (Od) are easily identified.

is usually unnecessary to actively tear the ovarian suspensory ligament, because the ovary can be successfully exteriorized without doing so most of the time. The ovary is located at the cranial end of a long and convoluted fallopian tube, and in mature rabbits is usually buried in a large amount of fat. It is critical to positively identify and remove all the ovarian tissue, as a partial OVE is a common surgical error in rabbits. The ovarian pedicle is gently elevated to provide good visualization of structures, and a small mosquito forceps is clamped across the pedicle. The pedicle is then ligated below the ovary with 3-0 or 4-0 absorbable monofilament suture or hemostatic clips (Figure 15.16). Unlike in the cat, the rabbit pedicle usually contains too much fat to make autoligation of the pedicle possible. Once ligated, the vascular ovarian pedicle is checked for hemorrhage and released into the abdomen. The uterus and ovary are then carefully elevated out of the abdomen to identify the vaginal body and the remaining uterus. During this elevation, the vessels of the mesometrium that provide blood supply to the uterus are identified and ligated as needed down to the level of the cervices (Figure 15.17). These arterial branches of the uterine artery are larger than normally seen in dogs or cats of similar size. To complicate the surgery, these vessels are usually buried in the large amount of fat associated with the broad

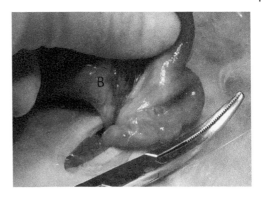

Figure 15.17 The vessels of the broad ligament (B) are identified and ligated.

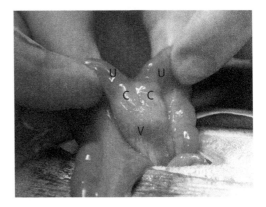

Figure 15.18 The two uteruses in the female rabbit (U), double cervices (C), and vaginal body (V).

ligament. Hemoclips can reduce the surgical time needed to elevate and ligate the vessels within the broad ligament. Once the first uterus is fully elevated, the second uterus is located and gently elevated from the other side to locate the remaining ovary. The second ovarian pedicle is ligated as previously described.

The two uteruses attached to the cranial vaginal body are then retracted caudally and elevated as a unit to provide access to the vaginal body (Figure 15.18). The two uterine arteries are located in the fat a few millimeters lateral to each side of the vaginal body. These arteries can be individually ligated if necessary, as proximal as possible to the location of the two cervixes. At this point the surgeon has a choice of four distinct ligature sites to remove the uteruses (Figure 15.19). The first is

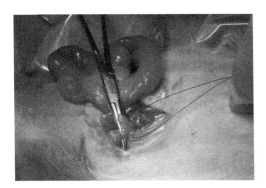

Figure 15.16 Ligation of the ovarian pedicle in a female rabbit under a plastic surgical drape. Ovarian pedicles in rabbits are very fatty, and should not be ligated via an instrument tie as in cats.

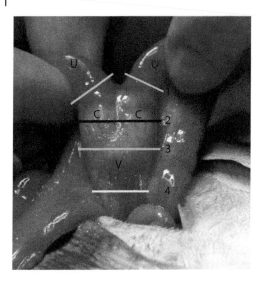

Figure 15.19 Ligature placement sites in the female rabbit reproductive tract: distal to the cervices (1); proximal to the cervices (2); through the vaginal body (3); and proximal to the vaginal body (4). C, cervix; U, uterus; V, vaginal body.

to place ligatures at the origin of each uterus just distal to their cervices. Placing the ligature at this site is technically simple and prevents leakage of urine that may have pooled in the vaginal body. The potential disadvantage of this method is that small amounts of uterine tissue remain, and have the potential to become neoplastic in the future. The second option is to place a ligature around the midsection of the two cervixes. This ligature can be transfixed into the fibrous cervical tissue to prevent slippage. This ligature location is not described often in the literature, but provides a secure ligation of the uterine stump and prevents urine leakage. Similar to the first location, this method retains some viable cervical tissue that may become neoplastic as the animal ages. The third ligation site is directly proximal to the two cervixes and around the cranial portion of the vaginal body. The vaginal body is relatively flaccid and friable, making placement of a secure ligature challenging. The vaginal body is double-ligated with transfixation ligatures. After transection, the stump of the cranial vaginal body should be examined

for possible urine leakage, and can be oversewn at the surgeon's discretion, similar to the closure of a hollow visceral structure. The advantage of placing the ligature at this site is that all the uterine structures are removed. The disadvantage is that the stump may leak urine, or result in a retrograde vaginal infection. The fourth option is to place the ligation further proximal through the central section of the vaginal body, removing approximately one-third of the vaginal body. If using this site, the surgeon must carefully identify and avoid entrapping the ureters, nerves, or vesicular arteries supplying the bladder. The advantage of this method is that it results in removal of all the uterine tissues and also removes a portion of the vaginal body that can retain urine. All four ligation sites described are acceptable choices and are described in the literature, but there are no objective studies evaluating the presumptive risks or benefits of any of the sites. Once the reproductive tract has been removed, the surgeon should check the abdomen for signs of hemorrhage. The abdomen is closed with a routine two- or three-layer closure, as described earlier.

Rabbit Ovariectomy

There is a current controversy concerning the benefits and risks of performing an OVE versus an OHE in rabbits. This is similar to the debate occurring with performing OVEs in dogs and cats. In carnivorous species, studies have shown few problems associated with OVE, although some dogs may develop pyometra if ovariectomized following sexual maturity. Extrapolating to rabbits, the complete removal of rabbit ovaries should eliminate the hormones that drive uterine pathology. Unfortunately, rabbits are not domestic carnivores and cross-species extrapolations are generally not wise. To date, no studies have been conducted in rabbit populations to follow long-term OVE versus OHE animals. Several methods of performing OVE, including midline laparotomy and laparoscopic techniques, have been published (Al-Badrany 2009; Divers 2010).

Rabbit Castration

The reasons for castrating rabbits include prevention of reproduction, with the added benefits of reduction in urine marking, reduction of urine-associated odor, and reduction of sexual or aggressive behaviors in male rabbits. Case reports of testicular diseases are relatively common and include testicular trauma, abscesses, orchitis, and neoplasia. Seminomas and interstitial cell carcinomas are the most commonly reported testicular tumors (Weisbroth 1994). They often present as a unilaterally enlarged testis with concurrent contralateral testicular atrophy.

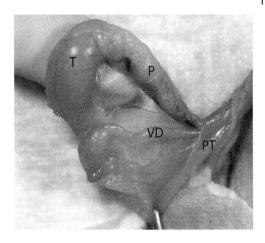

Figure 15.20   The spermatic cord of the male rabbit. Shown are the pampiniform plexus (P), testes (T), vas deferens (VD), and parietal tunic (PT).

Rabbit Male Anatomy

In the male rabbit, the testes descend into the scrotum at 10–12 weeks of age (Harcourt-Brown 2002; Hillyer 1994). Unlike most other species, the rabbit testes are located cranial to the penis, within two separate scrotal sacs. Rabbits have inguinal canals that remain open or partially open throughout their lives. The open inguinal canals allow the testicles and structures of the spermatic cord to move freely from the scrotal sacs into the abdomen. The spermatic cord is composed of arteries, veins, lymphatics, nerves, the excretory duct of the testis, and fat (Figure 15.20). The potential space of the inguinal canals is surrounded by the parietal tunic and cremaster muscle (spermatic fascia) to form a tube-shaped stalk originating from the abdomen at the inguinal ring. The inguinal canal provides a potential space connecting the abdomen and the internal scrotal sac. The epididymal fat pad prevents herniation of viscera through the inguinal ring. It is recommended that the inguinal canal is closed following castration to prevent the post-operative herniation of visceral structures such as bowel, fat, accessory sex structures, or urinary bladder.

Rabbit Castration Methods

Rabbit Scrotal Castration – Open

For scrotal castrations, the skin of both the scrotal sacs is prepared for aseptic surgery. The scrotal skin is sparsely haired and very delicate. To prevent dermal irritation that can become a focus of overgrooming post-operatively, it is necessary to carefully shave the hair and then gently prepare the skin (Figure 15.21). If the testes have been retracted into the abdomen, they can be manipulated back into the scrotum by applying a gentle rolling pressure to the caudal abdomen with the animal in dorsal recumbency. In the open castration, the testicle is gently held while the scrotal skin and the overlying inguinal canal are opened with a 1–1.5 cm incision on the ventral aspect of the scrotum (Figure 15.22). This incision must pass through both the skin and the underling parietal tunic of the testis (Figure 15.23). With gentle digital pressure, the testicle is extracted providing access to the exposed testis, epididymis, and epididymal fat pad. The ligament attaching the parietal tunic to the tail of the epididymis is severed with a dry gauze and gentle traction (Figure 15.24). The testis and epididymis are then dissected from the fat pad isolating vas deferens and testicular vessels (Figure 15.25). The vas deferens and

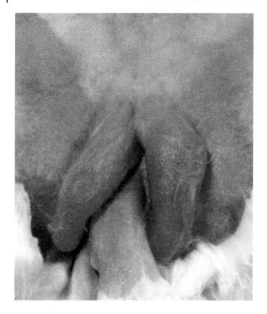

Figure 15.21   Rabbit scrotum prepared for surgery.

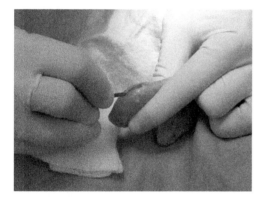

Figure 15.22   Initial incision into the rabbit scrotum.

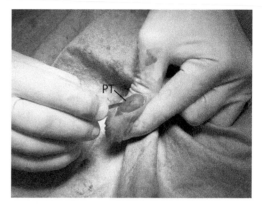

Figure 15.23   For an open castration in the rabbit, the incision must be extended through the parietal tunic (PT).

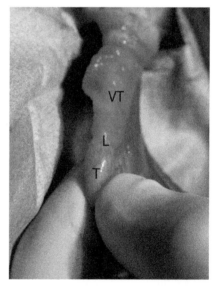

Figure 15.24   During open castration, the ligament (L) between the inverted vaginal tunic (VT) and testicle (T) must be manually broken down to expose the testicle and associated vascular structures.

the vessels of the spermatic cord are ligated and transected to remove the testicle and epididymis. An alternative method is to autoligate the spermatic cord using a mosquito hemostat, as has been described for cat castrations. The remaining fat pad and the ligated vessels are carefully replaced into the inguinal canal, which is then closed as cranially as possible by placing a ligature into the open tunics. Although some descriptions of the open castration specifically remove the epididymal fat pad, current recommendations consider the fat pad as an important structure in the inguinal ring, helping to prevent visceral herniation in both the intact and castrated male rabbit (Capello 2005b; Jenkins 2012). The skin is closed with tissue glue or left open.

Rabbit Scrotal Castration – Closed

The closed scrotal technique is similar to closed castration in cats. The rabbit is placed

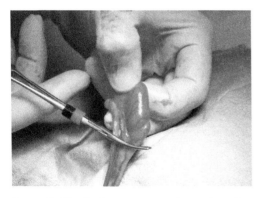

Figure 15.25 During open castration, a clamp is placed distal to the testicle across the vascular structures following separation of the testicle from the fat pad and vaginal tunic.

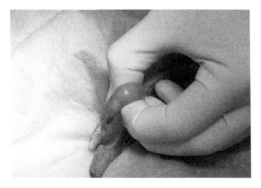

Figure 15.26 For a closed castration, the initial incision does not go through the parietal tunic, but through skin and subcutaneous structures only.

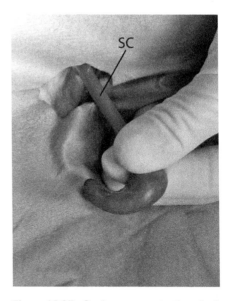

Figure 15.27 During open castration, the fascial tissue between the parietal tunic and skin is broken down to expose the spermatic cord (SC), still within the parietal tunic.

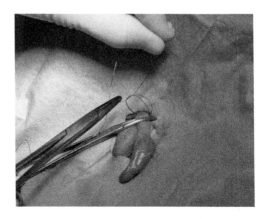

Figure 15.28 Ligature placement on the spermatic cord in a closed rabbit castration.

into dorsal recumbency and the scrotal sacs are prepared for aseptic surgery. The testicle is gently grasped and stabilized between the surgeon's fingers. A shallow 1 cm incision is made through the skin and superficial subcutaneous tissues only, and not through the parietal tunic of the testis (Figure 15.26). Once the surface of the parietal testicular tunic is identified, the tissue plane between the tunic and the subcutaneous tissue is bluntly dissected circumferentially, while the enclosed testicle and spermatic cord are elevated out of the incision and dissected free from the scrotum. These structures are elevated to help isolate the pedicle containing the spermatic cord structures within the inguinal canal that are attached to the body wall

(Figure 15.27). The pedicle containing the inguinal canal is isolated as far cranially as possible and securely ligated with a modified Miller's knot or circumferential ligature. The ligature simultaneously closes the inguinal canal and occludes the vascular supply to the testis (Figure 15.28). The isolated testicle within the inguinal canal is transected and removed. The incision through the skin of the scrotal sac is closed with surgical tissue adhesive, traditional skin sutures, or staples. The process is repeated on the other testicle (Capello 2005b). The separation of the skin from the testis is more difficult in older rabbits where these tissues are tightly attached together, potentially making the open method of castration easier to perform in these older animals.

Rabbit Pre-scrotal Castration – Closed

The pre-scrotal closed castration is similar to the scrotal castration already described, except that the location of the initial incision is different. The rabbit is placed in dorsal recumbency and the inguinal area is prepared for aseptic surgery. A single 2–3 cm skin incision is made on the ventral midline cranial to the scrotal sacs and the penis. The subcutaneous tissue around the inguinal canal is bluntly dissected to isolate the external tunics containing the spermatic cord and to allow a small curved hemostat to be placed beneath it. The blunt dissection is continued caudally so that the caudal aspect of the tunics enclosing the testicle is elevated. This process will evert the skin of the scrotal sac due to diffuse subcutaneous attachments. Once these attachments are broken down, the unopened tunics containing the spermatic cord structures and testis can be fully elevated. The scrotal sac is inverted and replaced back into its normal position. The structure consisting of the parietal tunic surrounding the spermatic cord and testicle is circumferentially ligated as cranially as possible with a securely placed ligature. This ligature simultaneously closes the inguinal canal and occludes the vascular supply to the testicle. The isolated testicle within the inguinal canal is then transected and removed. The surgical process is repeated through the same midline incision on the other testicle. Once the testicles are removed and hemostasis confirmed, the skin incision is closed in one or two layers with a combination of a subcuticular suture pattern, surgical glue, traditional skin sutures, or staples (Capello 2005b).

Rabbit Pre-scrotal Castration – Modified Open

The rabbit is placed into dorsal recumbency and the inguinal area is prepared for aseptic surgery. A 1–2 cm skin incision is made on the ventral midline cranial to the scrotum and penis. The subcutaneous tissue around the inguinal canal is bluntly dissected to isolate the intact spermatic cord and allow a small curved hemostat to be placed beneath it. Suture is grasped by the hemostat and pulled under the inguinal canal as a pre-placed ligature. The testicle is then pushed cranially into the surgical site and the parietal tunic is sharply incised to expose the testicle and epididymis. The spermatic cord is grasped, and with gentle traction the testicle and epididymis are elevated into the surgical field. As the testicle is extracted, the attachment at the tail of the epididymis is freed from the parietal tunic. The partially inverted scrotal sac is returned to the normal position and the structures of the elevated testicle are identified. The testicle and epididymis are separated from the fat pad, and the vas deferens and testicular vessels are ligated and released into the internal inguinal canal (Figure 15.29). The testicle and epididymis are removed and examined to insure complete anatomic removal. The pre-placed ligature

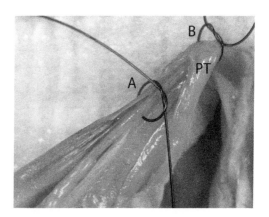

Figure 15.29 Pre-placement of a ligature (B) around the parietal tunic (PT), effectively closing the inguinal ring when tightened. A second, more distal ligature (A) ligates the vascular structures within the cord.

around the tunics of the inguinal canal is now pushed cranially toward the abdomen and tied closed. The process is repeated for the other testicle. The incision is closed in two layers. The skin is closed with a subcuticular suture pattern, surgical glue, traditional skin sutures, or staples. One common complication of this method is post-operative edema within the empty scrotal sacs. This may be due to tissue trauma to the retained parietal tunics and obstructed lymphatics caused by the surgical ligation. Generally considered a cosmetic complication, the edema usually subsides within a week (Capello 2005b).

Rabbit Abdominal Castration

Abdominal castration is possible for rabbits, but is not commonly described or recommended. The rabbit is placed in dorsal recumbency and prepared for typical midline abdominal surgery. The abdomen is entered as described for rabbit OHE, except that the incision is made closer to the pubis. The urinary bladder is gently elevated and retracted. The ductus deferens is identified dorsally, lateral to the bladder, and used to gently pull the testicle through the inguinal canal and into the abdomen. The epididymis of the testicle is freed from its distal attachment to the parietal tunic and fully elevated out of the abdomen. The structures of the spermatic cord are identified and ligated to remove the testicle and epididymis. A mattress suture is placed into the now empty opening of the inguinal canal to close the inguinal ring from inside the abdomen. The process is repeated for the other testicle and the abdomen is closed routinely (Capello 2005b).

Rodent Ovariohysterectomy and Ovariectomy

As in female rabbits, removal of the ovaries in some species of rodents may result in lower incidences of certain cancers later in life. In female domestic rats (*Rattus norvegicus*), OVE reduced the incidence of mammary tumors from 47% to less than 4%, and concurrently reduced the incidence of pituitary tumors from 66% to less than 4% (Hotchkiss 1995). These two neoplasias are consistently reported as the most common tumors in rat populations. The long-term negative consequences of OHE have not been evaluated in companion rodent populations; however, OVE of rats has been associated with bone loss and used as a reliable rodent model of post-menopausal bone loss in humans (Idris 2012).

Guinea pigs (*Cavia porcellus*) that are allowed to breed should have their first litter by six months of age to prevent the fusion of the pubic symphysis. Once fused, female guinea pigs will suffer from dystocia if allowed to give birth. Therefore, OHE or OVE can be performed in older guinea pigs to eliminate the potential for pregnancies with possibly fatal outcomes.

Female Rodent Anatomy

Rodents have variable and species-specific onset of sexual maturity, with many small species maturing quite early in life (Lennox and Bauck 2012). Most rodent species possess two uterine horns and a single cervix, similar to the female reproductive anatomy of dogs and cats. Rodents also have a shorter vaginal body than that of the rabbit. The major differences between rodents and dog and cat reproductive tracts are the small size of the reproductive structures, and the relative fragility of the reproductive tissues in rodents. As in the rabbit, the abdominal structures in obese pet rodents can be difficult to identify and isolate. The small ovaries in guinea pigs, chinchillas (*Chinchilla lanigera*), and degus (*Octodon degus*) are particularly difficult to locate in the adipose tissues. Once identified, the ovaries have relatively short ovarian suspensory ligaments that may tear easily during surgical elevation. Large, multiple ovarian cysts are a very common finding in guinea pigs, and are often the reason for performing OHE or OVE in this species. Because ovarian disease is common and uterine disease relatively rare, OVE alone can be performed. Similar to the limited studies in rabbits concerning the need for OHE to prevent uterine cancer, this recommendation for OVE has not been fully evaluated in a large population of pet guinea pigs.

Surgical Procedures for Rodent Ovariohysterectomy/Ovariectomy

Rat, Mouse, Gerbil, and Hamster Ovariohysterectomy/Ovariectomy

Because rodents are the prototypical laboratory animals, many surgeries, including OHE and OVE, have been well described in the laboratory animal medicine literature. The rat OHE and OVE will be described as a model for mice (*Mus musculus*), Mongolian gerbil (*Meriones unguiculatus*), Syrian hamster (*Mesocricetus auratus*), and other rat-like rodents.

An OHE or OVE can be performed via a ventral midline incision similar to the rabbit OHE/OVE described earlier. The incision is made through the skin from just caudal to the umbilicus to just cranial to the rim of the pubis. Rodents require relatively longer incisions to allow safe elevation of the fragile reproductive structures (Jenkins 2000). The linea alba, which is very thin, is identified and incised to enter the abdomen. The intestines are gently manipulated to the side with moistened sterile cotton swabs or a blunt surgical instrument. A sterile cotton swab can also be used to help elevate the uterus and isolate the reproductive tract. It is common for the abdomen of rats to be abundant with fat regardless of the overall size or external appearance of the animal. The ovarian vasculature is ligated using an appropriately sized hemoclip or monofilament suture material. The process is repeated on the opposite side. If performing an OHE, the junction of the uterine horns and cervix is located, elevated, and double-ligated using 4-0 absorbable monofilament suture. The abdominal wall is sutured in a simple continuous pattern, followed by a simple continuous closure of the

subcutaneous tissue (if present) and intradermal closure of the skin. Tissue adhesive may be used as an alternative to suture.

Alternatively, an OVE can be performed in rodents through a lateral flank approach. With the patient in ventral recumbency, an approximately 0.5–2 cm incision (depending on the species) is made on the midline just caudal to the last rib. The subcutaneous tissues are dissected laterally to expose the flank ventral to the lumbar musculature. The abdominal musculature is exposed and a blunt hemostat or scissor is used to spread the muscle fibers to gain entry into the abdominal cavity. The ovary is located within a bundle of fat beneath the incision and is gently exteriorized. Alternatively, the surgeon can place gentle pressure on the side of the abdomen to allow the ovary to partially exit the abdominal wall through the incision. The ovarian pedicle and uterine horn are ligated just proximal to the ovary using 4-0 absorbable monofilament suture or a hemoclip. Prior to release of the uterine horn, it is gently retracted caudally to exteriorize the contralateral horn and ovary. The same procedure is repeated on the opposite side. The muscle wall is closed with appropriately sized monofilament suture material using a cruciate or simple interrupted suture pattern (Idris 2012). The single skin incision is closed with an intradermal pattern followed by tissue adhesive. A modification of the flank approach using two separate flank skin incisions has been described (Olsen and Bruce 1986).

Guinea Pig, Degu, and Chinchilla Ovariohysterectomy/Ovariectomy

Ventral midline OHE as previously described for the rabbit has been described for guinea pigs, chinchillas, and degus, but is generally considered technically demanding due to the short, deep abdomen and large intestinal viscera that prevent easy identification of the uterine horns. This is further complicated by the relatively short suspensory ligaments and stronger mesometrium attachments to the body wall. Alternatively, bilateral OVE can be performed through small flank incisions caudal to the last rib, as described for rats. The advantages of this approach are it allows the surgeon to avoid manipulation of the organs in the gastrointestinal tract and improves access to the ovaries. The challenge is finding and identifying the normal ovaries within the abdominal fat, or removing pathologically enlarged cystic ovaries through the small incision. Skin incisions are made in the flank caudal to the last rib. Careful blunt dissection between the muscle layers provides access to the peritoneal cavity. The ovaries are usually located in the fat behind each kidney. Once the ovarian pedicle is located and elevated, ligatures can be placed around the vessels. The abdominal wall can be sutured and the skin is then closed. The process is repeated for the other side (Bennett 2012a; Capello 2006b).

Prairie Dog and Squirrel Ovariohysterectomy

Prevention of pregnancy and control of seasonal aggressive behaviors are common reasons to spay prairie dogs (*Cynomys* sp.) and squirrels (*Sciurus* sp.). Female prairie dogs tend to become obese as they get older, which complicates the identification of reproductive structures during surgery. OHE and OVE procedures are similar to those previously described for rat-like rodents.

Rodent Castration

Castration in pet rodent species is usually recommended for population control. Castrating male rodents may also result in a decrease in aggressive behavior. This is particularly true in prairie dogs and squirrels, which can develop seasonal aggressive behaviors. Castration has been used to induce an osteoporosis model in laboratory rats. The long-term effects of castration have not been studied in companion rodents.

Male Anatomy

Many rat-like rodents have inguinal rings that remain partially open throughout their lives, and have well-developed scrotums. In these species, a large fat pad is usually situated within the inguinal ring and acts to help block the inguinal canal and prevent visceral herniation. Similar to cats and dogs, the penis of rats, mice, gerbils, and hamsters is directed forward, with the prepuce opening cranial to the scrotum. In contrast, guinea pigs, chinchillas, and degus have intermediately developed scrotal sacs and relatively more mobile testes that can be easily manipulated into or out of the abdomen. Prairie dogs and squirrels lack well-developed visible scrotal sacs because the testicles are located in the inguinal canal or in the abdomen, depending on the season. Compared to other rodents, this group has larger inguinal canals and can be considered true "functional cryptorchids," with the testicles moving relatively freely between the abdomen and the scrotal sacs (Capello 2006a). This makes the risk of post-operative herniation higher in these species, and highlights the need to surgically close the inguinal canals. Many rodent species have variable testicle size and location that are influenced by their age and breeding seasonality.

Surgical Procedures

Rat, Mouse, Gerbil, and Hamster Castration

Simple, open or closed, scrotal castration can be performed on rats and other small rodents that have well-developed scrotal sacs and less mobile testes (Bennett 2012b; Idris 2012). This surgery is similar to the method of closed castration used in cats and kittens. The incisions are generally left open to heal by second intention, but this is up to the discretion of the surgeon.

Alternatively, abdominal castration can be performed on many rodent species when they are not in their breeding season or if they are sexually immature with undescended testicles. For abdominal castration, an incision is made along the ventral midline identical to OHE incision placement (Olsen and Bruce 1986). Once the abdomen has been entered, the bladder is elevated and retracted caudally to visualize the testicles and ductus deferens. The spermatic structure or epididymal fat pad is grasped and retracted out of the inguinal canal if necessary. Once isolated and identified, the testicular vessels and ductus deferens are ligated and the testicle is removed. The closure of the abdominal incision is similar to that done for the OHE.

Guinea Pig, Degu, and Chinchilla Castration

A published method for a closed castration has been described for guinea pigs (Anderson and Friomovitch 1974; Bennett 2012a). This method is identical to the closed rabbit castration described earlier. An alternative pre-scrotal castration has also been described. The animal is placed in dorsal recumbency and the inguinal area is prepared for aseptic surgery. The procedure is similar to that previously described for rabbits using the modified open technique. A single inguinal incision is made and a circumferential ligature is pre-placed on the external tunics of the cranial inguinal canal. The caudal inguinal canal is then opened to remove the testicle and epididymis. The ductus deferens and testicular vessels are ligated and released into the cranial inguinal canal. The pre-placed ligature around the external inguinal canal is pushed cranially toward the abdomen and tied closed. This ligature is necessary to close the inguinal canal and prevent post-surgical herniation (Figure 15.30). The process is repeated on the other testicle and the incision is closed with suture or tissue adhesive (Capello 2006a).

Prairie Dog and Squirrel Abdominal Castration

An abdominal castration is often selected for these species, because it avoids the loss of the testicles into the abdomen during a scrotal castration, and actually makes locating the

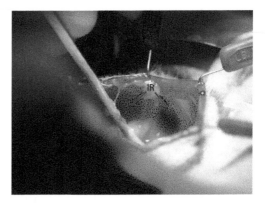

Figure 15.30 Intraabdominal view of a guinea pig castration, illustrating the large inguinal rings (IR) that must be closed following the procedure to prevent herniation.

testicles easier. If the testicle is located in the inguinal canal, it can be retracted into the abdomen by pulling gently on the ductus deferens. Once the testicle is located and elevated, the vessels and ductus deferens are ligated and cut. The opening to the inguinal canal should be closed by placing a single mattress suture through the opening. The process is repeated on the opposite side. After hemostasis has been confirmed, the closure is similar to that for an OHE.

Ferret Ovariohysterectomy

Most ferrets (*Mustela putorius furo*) destined for the pet trade in the United States have been sterilized before eight weeks of age by the breeder prior to being made available for sale (Lightfoot et al. 2012). The specific neutering method the breeders use is proprietary, but it can be assumed that it is similar to feline pediatric spay/neuter procedures. Most commercial breeders place dot tattoos in the ears of neutered ferrets, so the clinician should check the pinnae of the ears for tattoos prior to performing a neutering procedure. It has been suggested that pediatric neutering of both male and female ferrets is associated with the development of adrenocortical hyperplasia and neoplasia later in life (Bielinska et al. 2006).

Ferret Female Anatomy

The reproductive anatomy of the female ferret is similar to the cat, with the exception of the long uterine body. One difference is that adult female ferrets are induced ovulators that have a propensity to remain in heat if not stimulated to ovulate by copulation. This prolonged estrus can progress to fatal estrogen toxicity. Typical clinical signs include swollen vulva, hair loss, and significant anemia (Lightfoot et al. 2012).

Ferret Ovariohysterectomy/ Ovariectomy Methods

The adult ferret OHE is similar to the cat OHE procedure. A central midline incision through the linea alba is made about 0.5–1 cm from the umbilicus. The uterus is found in the normal position between the colon and the bladder. In fat ferrets, uterine and ovarian blood vessels can be difficult to visualize, but are in the typical location of other carnivores. Removal of the reproductive structures and closure is identical to cats of similar size (Lightfoot et al. 2012).

Ferret Castration

Most ferrets in the United States are castrated and tattooed by their breeders, as discussed for female ferrets. Intact males are more aggressive and tend to produce more body odor.

Ferret Male Anatomy

The anatomy of the male ferret is similar to that of most other domestic carnivores.

Ferret Castration Methods

The surgical castration procedure in the male ferret is similar to cat castration, with both scrotal and pre-scrotal techniques described (Lightfoot et al. 2012). The structures of the spermatic cord can be ligated with suture or autoligated using a mosquito hemostat.

Other Small Mammal Ovariohysterectomy and Ovariectomy

Hedgehog Ovariohysterectomy

In North America, African hedgehogs (*Atelerix albiventris*) are rarely presented for routine OHE because they are generally kept as solitary pets or in small breeding groups. Furthermore, they tend not to have noticeable aggressive or objectionable behaviors associated with breeding. Hedgehogs are, however, prone to uterine neoplasias, with affected females often first presenting with hematuria (Done et al. 2007). The anatomy and surgical procedure for OHE is generally similar to other small mammals; however, the uterine horns are coiled caudally, with the ovaries tucked within the coil. Attempting to remove a uterus with neoplastic changes can be difficult due to changes in the anatomy because of the neoplasia (Figure 15.31).

Sugar Glider Ovariohysterectomy

Female sugar gliders (*Petaurus breviceps*) are not commonly spayed due to their small size, challenging anatomy, and the fact that the males can be easily castrated for population control. If a spay is attempted, the female sugar

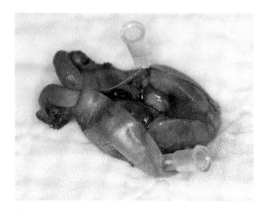

Figure 15.31 Uterine adenocarcinoma in a hedgehog.

glider reproductive anatomy is typical of marsupials and will appear very unusual for surgeons accustomed to performing OHEs in rodents and domestic carnivores (Ness and Johson-Delaney 2012). Marsupials have a single urogenital sinus that subdivides into a single central and two lateral vaginas. Each of the left and right lateral vaginas encircles a ureter and then rejoins the median vagina cranially at the opening of the two separate cervices. Attempting OHE in these species requires careful avoidance of the ureters. A midline abdominal approach is recommended; however, this approach is complicated by the ventrally located pouch. The surgeon is wise to consult anatomic descriptions and relevant literature before performing an OHE on a marsupial.

Other Small Mammal Castration

Hedgehog Castration

Companion hedgehogs are rarely castrated; however, the methods described for guinea pigs are suggested. One anatomic difference is that the penis is relatively large and must be carefully identified during surgery to avoid surgical damage.

Sugar Glider Castration

Castrating sugar gliders helps to reduce the characteristic musky male odor and decreases urine marking. It may also decrease adult-onset hair loss on the head and chest. The pendulous scrotum containing the testicles is located on the ventral abdomen cranial to the penis. The forked penis of sugar gliders can also cause confusion to someone unfamiliar with their anatomy. The long stalk of the scrotum containing the spermatic cords provides a convenient site for castration, and makes a full scrotal ablation relatively straightforward. After aseptic preparation, the distal portion of the spermatic cord

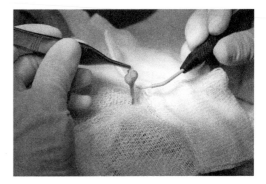

Figure 15.32 Castration and simultaneous scrotal ablation using electrocautery in a sugar glider.

can be cut with a laser or electrocautery to remove the testicles and scrotum (Figure 15.32). Alternatively, the stalk can be crushed in a hemostat and a circumferential ligature placed proximal to the crush zone to provide hemostasis. Unfortunately, sugar gliders tend to chew at their surgical sites, presenting a significant risk for self-induced post-operative trauma and hemorrhage.

Conclusions

Spay and neuter procedures in domestic rabbits, rodents, and various other small mammals are relatively similar to those performed in domestic dogs and cats. The clinician should review differences in anatomy between more exotic species if attempting surgical sterilization in these animals. As with all spay–neuter procedures, care must be taken to prevent hypothermia, hypoglycemia, and excessive blood loss. As in all animals, adequate peri-operative pain control is important in these species not only as a welfare issue, but for the prevention of post-operative complications like licking and chewing at the incision site, which may result in dehiscence or infection. With adequate preparation, rabbits, rodents, and other small animals can be safely and successfully spayed and castrated in veterinary practice.

References

Aeschbacher, G. and Webb, A.I. (1993). Propofol in rabbits, determination of an induction dose. *Lab. Anim. Sci.* 43 (4): 324–327.

Al-Badrany, M.S. (2009). Laparoscopic ovariectomy in rabbits. *Iraqi J. Vet. Sci.* 23 (2): 51–55.

Anderson, M. and Friomovitch, M. (1974). Simplified method of guinea pig castration. *Can. Vet. J.* 15 (4): 126–127.

Bateman, L., Ludders, J.W., Gleed, R.D., and Erb, H.N. (2005). Comparison between facemask and laryngeal mask airway in rabbits during isoflurane anesthesia. *Vet. Anaesth. Analg.* 32: 280–288.

Bennett, R.A. (2012a). Soft tissue surgery (guinea pigs, chinchillas, and degus). In: *Ferrets, Rabbits, and Rodents: Clinical Medicine and Surgery*, 3e (eds. K.E. Quesenberry and J.W. Carpenter), 326–338. St. Louis, MO: Elsevier Saunders.

Bennett, R.A. (2012b). Soft tissue surgery (small rodents). In: *Ferrets, Rabbits, and Rodents: Clinical Medicine and Surgery*, 3e (eds. K.E. Quesenberry and J.W. Carpenter), 373–391. St. Louis, MO: Elsevier Saunders.

Bielinska, M., Kiiveri, S., Parviainen, H. et al. (2006). Gonadectomy-induced adrenocortical neoplasia in the domestic ferret (*Mustela putorius furo*) and laboratory mouse. *Vet. Pathol.* 43 (2): 97–117.

Brammer, D.W., Doerning, B.J., Chrisp, C.E. et al. (1991). Anesthetic and nephrotoxic effects of Telazol in New Zealand White rabbits. *Lab. Anim. Sci.* 41 (4): 432–435.

Brodbelt, D.C., Blissitt, K.J., Hammond, R.A. et al. (2008). The risk of death: the confidential enquiry into perioperative small animal fatalities. *Vet. Anaesth. Analg.* 35 (5): 365–373.

Capello, V. (2005a). Surgical techniques for neutering the female pet rabbit. *Exot. DVM* 7 (5): 15–21.

Capello, V. (2005b). Surgical techniques for orchiectomy of the pet rabbit. *Exot. DVM* 7 (5): 23–31.

Capello, V. (2006a). Prescrotal approach to elective orchiectomy in guinea pigs. *Exot. DVM* 8 (5): 29–32.

Capello, V. (2006b). Flank approach to elective ovariectomy in guinea pigs. *Exot. DVM* 8 (5): 33–37.

Devalle, S.J.M. (2009). Successful management of rabbit anesthesia through the use of nasotracheal intubation. *J. Am. Assoc. Lab. Anim. Sci.* 48 (2): 166–170.

Divers, S.J. (2010). Clinical technique: endoscopic oophorectomy in the rabbit (*Oryctolagus cuniculus*): the future of preventative sterilizations. *J. Exot. Pet Med.* 19 (3): 231–239.

Done, L.B., Deem, S.L., and Fiorello, C.V. (2007). Surgical and medical management of a uterine spindle cell tumor in an African hedgehog (*Atelerix albiventris*). *J. Zoo Wildlife Med.* 38 (4): 601–603.

Dunn, R.C. and Mohler, M. (1993). Effect of varying days of tissue plasminogen activator therapy on the prevention of postsurgical adhesions in a rabbit model. *J. Surg. Res.* 54 (3): 242–245.

Flecknell, P.A. (2001). Analgesia of small mammals. *Vet. Clin. Exot. Anim. Pract.* 4 (1): 47–56.

Greene, H.S.N. (1942). Uterine adenomata in the rabbit III. Susceptibility as a function of constitutional factors. *J. Exp. Med.* 73: 273–292.

Hanley, C.S. (2013). The care of small mammals in the animal shelter. In: *Shelter Medicine for Veterinarians and Staff*, 2e (eds. L. Miller and S. Zawistowski), 185–200. Ames, IA: Wiley-Blackwell.

Harcourt-Brown, F. (2002). Urogenital diseases. In: *Textbook of Rabbit Medicine*, 1e, 348–351. Oxford: Butterworth Heinemann.

Hawkins, M.G. and Pascoe, P.J. (2012). Anesthesia, analgesia, and sedation of small mammals. In: *Ferrets, Rabbits, and Rodents: Clinical Medicine and Surgery*, 3e (eds. K.E.

Quesenberry and J.W. Carpenter), 429–451. St. Louis, MO: Elsevier Saunders.

Heard, D. (2007a). Lagomorphs (Rabbits, Hares, and Pika). In: *Zoo Animal and Wildlife Immobilization and Anesthesia* (eds. G. West, D. Heard and N. Caulkett), 647–654. Ames, IA: Blackwell Publishing.

Heard, D. (2007b). Rodents. In: *Zoo Animal and Wildlife Immobilization and Anesthesia* (eds. G. West, D. Heard and N. Caulkett), 647–654. Ames, IA: Blackwell Professional.

Hillyer, E.V. (1994). Pet rabbits. *Vet. Clin. N. Am. Small Anim. Pract* 24 (1): 25–64.

Hotchkiss, C.E. (1995). Effect of surgical removal of subcutaneous tumors on survival of rats. *JAVMA* 206 (10): 1575–1579.

Idris, A.I. (2012). Ovariectomy/Orchidectomy in rodents. In: *Bone Research Protocols, Methods in Molecular Biology*, vol. 816 (eds. M.H. Helfrich and S.H. Ralston), 545–551. Berlin: Springer Science and Business Media.

Ingalls, T.H., Adams, W.M., Lurie, M.B., and Ipsen, J. (1964). Natural history of adenocarcinoma of the uterus in the Phipps rabbit colony. *J. Nat. Cancer Inst.* 33 (5): 799–806.

Jenkins, J.R. (2000). Surgical sterilization in small mammals: spay and castration. *Vet. Clin. N. Am. Exot. Anim. Pract* 3 (3): 617.

Jenkins, J.R. (2012). Soft tissue surgery (rabbits). In: *Ferrets, Rabbits, and Rodents: Clinical Medicine and Surgery*, 3e (eds. K.E. Quesenberry and J.W. Carpenter), 269–278. St. Louis, MO: Elsevier Saunders.

Klaphake, E. and Paul-Murphy, J. (2012). Disorders of the reproductive and urinary systems. In: *Ferrets, Rabbits, and Rodents: Clinical Medicine and Surgery*, 3e (eds. K.E. Quesenberry and J.W. Carpenter), 217–231. St. Louis, MO: Elsevier Saunders.

Kottwitz, J. (2006). Stump pyometra in a chinchilla. *Exot. DVM* 8 (5): 24–28.

Legrand, E.K., Rodgers, K.E., Girgis, W. et al. (1995). Comparative efficacy of nonsteroidal anti-inflammatory drugs and anti-thromboxane agents in a rabbit adhesion-prevention model. *J. Invest. Surg.* 8 (3): 187–194.

Lennox, A.M. and Bauck, L. (2012). Basic anatomy, physiology, and clinical techniques (small rodents). In: *Ferrets, Rabbits, and Rodents: Clinical Medicine and Surgery*, 3e (eds. K.E. Quesenberry and J.W. Carpenter), 339–353. St. Louis, MO: Elsevier Saunders.

Lichtenberger, M. and Ko, J. (2007). Anesthesia and analgesia for small birds and mammals. *Vet. Clin. Exot. Anim. Pract.* 10 (2): 293–315.

Lightfoot, T., Rubinstein, J., Aiken, S., and Ludwig, L. (2012). Soft tissue surgery. In: *Ferrets, Rabbits, and Rodents: Clinical Medicine and Surgery*, 3e (eds. K.E. Quesenberry and J.W. Carpenter), 141–156. St. Louis, MO: Elsevier Saunders.

Luciano, A.A., Maier, D.B., Koch, E.I. et al. (1989). A comparative study of postoperative adhesions following laser surgery by laparoscopy versus laparotomy in the rabbit model. *Obstet. Gynecol.* 74 (2): 220–224.

Millis, D.L. and Walshaw, R. (1992). Elective castrations and ovariohysterectomies in pet rabbits. *J. Am. Anim. Hosp. Assoc.* 28: 491–498.

Morgan, T.J. and Glowaski, M.M. (2007). Teaching a new method of rabbit intubation. *J. Am. Assoc. Lab. Anim. Sci.* 46 (3): 32–36.

Ness, R.D. and Johson-Delaney, C.A. (2012). Sugar gliders. In: *Ferrets, Rabbits, and Rodents: Clinical Medicine and Surgery*, 3e (eds. K.E. Quesenberry and J.W. Carpenter), 339–410. St. Louis, MO: Elsevier Saunders.

Nishimura, K., Nakamura, R.M., and Dizerega, G.S. (1984). Ibuprofen inhibition of postsurgical adhesion formation: a time and dose response biochemical evaluation in rabbits. *J. Surg. Res.* 36: 115–124.

Olsen, M.E. and Bruce, J. (1986). Ovariectomy, ovariohysterectomy, and orchidectomy in rodents and rabbits. *Can. Vet. J.* 27 (12): 523–527.

Paré, J.A. and Paul-Murphy, J. (2003). Disorders of the reproductive and urinary systems. In: *Ferrets, Rabbits, and Rodents: Clinical Medicine and Surgery*, 2e (eds. K.E.

Quesenberry and J.W. Carpenter), 183–193. St. Louis, MO: Elsevier Saunders.

Phaneuf, L.R., Barker, S., Groleau, M.A., and Turner, P.V. (2006). Tracheal injury after endotracheal intubation and anesthesia in rabbits. *J. Am. Assoc. Lab. Anim. Sci.* 45 (6): 67–72.

Robertson, S.A. (2001). Analgesia and analgesic techniques. *Vet. Clin. N. Am. Exot. Anim. Pract.* 4 (1): 1–18.

Robertson, S.A. and Eberhart, S. (1994). Efficacy of the intranasal route for administration of anesthetic agents to adult rabbits. *Lab. Anim. Sci.* 44: 159–165.

Saito, K., Nakanishi, M., and Hasegawa, A. (2002). Uterine disorders diagnosed by ventrotomy in 47 rabbits. *J. Vet. Med. Sci.* 64 (6): 495–497.

Sikoski, P., Young, R.W., and Lockard, M. (2007). Comparison of heating devices for maintaining body temperature in anesthetized laboratory rabbits (*Oryctolagus cuniculus*). *J. Am. Assoc. Lab. Anim. Sci.* 46 (3): 61–63.

Smith, J.C., Robertson, L.D., Auhll, A. et al. (2004). Endotracheal tubes versus Laryngeal Mask Airways in Rabbit Inhalation Anesthesia: ease of use and waste gas emissions. *J. Am. Assoc. Lab. Anim. Sci.* 43 (4): 22–25.

Szabo, Z., Bradley, K., and Cahalane, A.K. (2016). Rabbit soft tissue surgery. *Vet. Clin. N. Am. Exot. Anim. Pract.* 19: 159–188.

Toft, J.D. (1992). Commonly observed spontaneous neoplasms in rabbits, rats, guinea pigs, hamsters, and gerbils. *Semin. Avian. Exot. Pet. Med.* 1 (2): 80–92.

Tonks, C.A. and Atlas, A.L. (2007). Clinical snapshot: uterine adenocarcinoma. *Compend. Cont. Educ. Vet.* 29 (1): 49–51.

Walter, B., Poth, T., Bohmer, E. et al. (2010). Uterine Disorders in 59 Rabbits. *Vet. Rec.* 166: 230–233.

Weisbroth, S.H. (1994). Neoplastic diseases. In: *The Biology of the Laboratory Rabbit*, 2e (eds. P.J. Manning, D.H. Ringler and C.E. Newcomer), 259–292. New York: Academic Press.

Whitfield, R.R., Stills, H.F., Huls, H.R. et al. (2007). Effects of peritoneal closure and suture material on adhesion formation in a rabbit model. *Am. J. Obstet. Gynecol.* 197: 644. e1–644.e5.

Williams, A.M. and Wyatt, J.D. (2007). Comparison of subcutaneous and intramuscular ketamine-medetomidine with and without reversal by atipamezole in Dutch Belted rabbits (*Oryctolagus cuniculus*). *J. Am. Assoc. Lab. Anim. Sci.* 46 (6): 16–20.

Yasaki, S. and Dyck, P.J. (1991). A simple method for rat endotracheal intubation. *Lab. Anim. Sci.* 41: 620–622.

16

Tattoo and Ear-Tipping Techniques for Identification of Surgically Sterilized Dogs and Cats

Brenda Griffin, Mark W. Bohling, and Karla Brestle

Professional Recommendations for Marking Sterilized Animals

The Association of Shelter Veterinarians' (ASV) Veterinary Medical Care Guidelines for Spay-Neuter Programs state: "Each spay-neuter program should choose a consistent, permanent means of visually identifying animals that have been neutered" (Griffin et al. 2016). Specifically, the ASV recommends application of a green linear tattoo to identify all spayed or neutered pet animals and ear-tipping to identify all community cats. According to the ASV, "Spay-neuter programs may elect to utilize more than one method of identifying individual neutered animals (ie, combining ear-tipping and tattooing or implanting microchips or using other forms of identification)." In all cases, the ASV states that neutered animals should be marked by the recommended standard means: a green linear tattoo for all pet animals and ear-tipping for all community cats. The importance of compliance with these recommendations cannot be overemphasized. This is because thousands of stray dogs and cats with unknown histories are presented to veterinarians and animal shelters for determination of sex and reproductive status each week. Obviously the presence of a distinct standard mark (i.e. a green linear tattoo or a "tipped" ear) would greatly facilitate assess-

ment of these animals. Animal welfare organizations strive to ensure that animals are spayed and neutered prior to release. When animals possess a distinct mark indicative of previous sterilization, organizations can proceed with rehoming or release of the animals without the need for further assessment of their reproductive status. This is crucial, because determining if a dog or cat has been previously sterilized can be surprisingly difficult in many cases.

The gold standard for determination of spay–neuter status is exploratory laparotomy. In a number of instances, animals undergo unnecessary anesthesia and surgery, only to reveal that previous ovariohysterectomy was performed. Obviously, this is invasive, time-consuming, expensive, stressful for the patient, and frequently frustrating for the surgeon as well. In addition to females, males may occasionally undergo unnecessary exploratory surgery. For instance, this may occur if a neutered tomcat is mistaken for a female cat. In addition, bilateral cryptorchid animals may be mistaken for neutered animals. For all of these reasons, the use of a permanent visual mark is strongly recommended to identify both female and male animals at the time of spay–neuter surgery. Chapter 1 discusses diagnostic methods for determination of spay–neuter status, which are necessary when animals are not marked.

High-Quality, High-Volume Spay and Neuter and Other Shelter Surgeries, First Edition. Edited by Sara White.
© 2020 John Wiley & Sons, Inc. Published 2020 by John Wiley & Sons, Inc.

Green Linear Tattoos for Pet Dogs and Cats

Tattooing is a useful and practical means of identifying animals as spayed and neutered. Simple tattoo techniques, which do not require special needles or instrumentation, have been developed for this purpose (Griffin et al. 2010; Bushby 2013). With these techniques, a small but distinct green line is created on the ventral abdomen to signify that the animal has been surgically sterilized. Examination for a ventral midline scar ("spay scar") is a standard practice used to aid in determination of the spay status of females, thus the presence of a tattoo in this area would be easily discovered and could verify that surgical sterilization had been performed. Even if a flank approach is used to spay a female patient, a tattoo should still be applied to the animal's ventral midline. Because neutered tomcats are sometimes mistaken for queens, placement of a ventral midline tattoo at the time of neutering is also recommended for them. For male dogs, the tattoo should be applied to the skin in the prescrotal area. The ASV's recommended standard locations for the placement of green linear tattoos on the ventral abdomen of male and female dogs and cats are illustrated in Figures 16.1–16.5 and summarized in Table 16.1 (Griffin et al. 2016).

The use of more complex tattoo designs or symbols is not recommended because they are not practical and do not offer distinct advantages over green linear tattoos. In order to create symbols or more complex tattoos, special equipment including multiple needles or a tattoo gun is required. Such equipment requires careful cleaning and disinfection between patients to prevent transmission of bloodborne pathogens, which decreases the efficiency and cost-effectiveness of a high volume spay–neuter program. Furthermore, complex tattoos often become increasingly difficult to read due to hair growth, fading, and distortion that occur over time. For all of these reasons, a

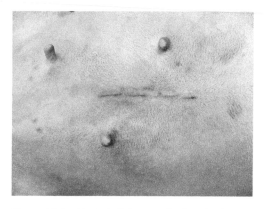

Figure 16.1 Ventral abdomen of a female dog immediately following ovariohysterectomy surgery. Note the application of a green linear tattoo near the ventral midline incision. Female cats should be similarly tattooed following ovariohysterectomy surgery.

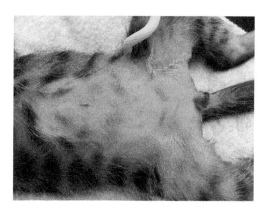

Figure 16.2 Ventral abdomen of a male cat immediately following surgical castration. Note the application of a green linear tattoo on the ventral midline. This permanent mark might one day prevent him from being mistaken for a female cat and/or undergoing an unnecessary exploratory laparotomy.

green linear tattoo is a more efficient and effective means of marking neutered animals (Griffin et al. 2010).

Tattoos have also been used for marking animals that have been sterilized via non-surgical methods. Although not currently available in the United States, a Food and Drug Administration-approved intratesticular injection of zinc gluconate neutralized with arginine

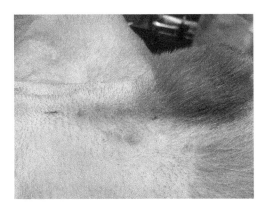

Figure 16.3 Inguinal area of a male dog immediately following surgical castration. Note the application of a green linear tattoo in the pre-scrotal area immediately lateral to the prepuce.

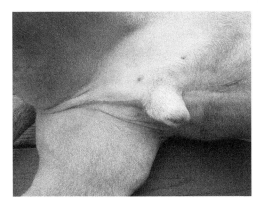

Figure 16.5 Inguinal area of a neutered male dog. Note the presence of a green linear tattoo on the ventral midline in the pre-scrotal area.

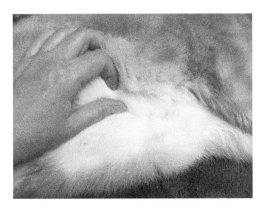

Figure 16.4 Green linear tattoo on the ventral abdomen of a cat. Depending on the individual animal's tractability and hair coat, clipping the hair over the ventral midline area may be necessary to ensure discovery and visualization of such tattoos.

marking that will be readily identifiable over time in order to ensure recognition of the animal's sterilization status and the method used (see Chapter 27 for more information on non-surgical sterilization).

Linear Tattoo Techniques

As previously stated, several simple techniques for applying green linear tattoos have been developed for use at the time of completion of

was formerly available and used by some programs for chemical castration of dogs. The product resulted in testicular atrophy and sterility in male dogs, but the testes remained present. In order to identify these dogs as non-surgically sterilized, the letter Z was tattooed in the caudolateral ventral abdomen (Griffin 2013). Since the testicles were not removed, a unique form of standard identification was essential in order to denote that the animal was non-surgically neutered. If other products become available for non-surgical sterilization in the future, it will be essential to develop simple means of permanent

Table 16.1 The Association of Shelter Veterinarians' recommendations for standard placement of green linear tattoos for identification of neutered dogs and cats (Griffin et al. 2016).

Sex and species	Location of green linear tattoo
Female dogs and cats	On or immediately lateral to the area of the ventral midline incision; if a flank approach is used to spay a female patient, the tattoo should be placed in the area where a ventral midline spay incision would have been placed
Male dogs	At the caudal aspect of the abdomen in the pre-scrotal incision or pre-scrotal area immediately lateral to the prepuce
Male cats	In the area where a ventral midline spay incision would typically be placed

spay–neuter surgery. These techniques, which do not require special equipment, have been used extensively for more than two decades by some spay–neuter programs. They utilize animal tattoo ink in the form of paste (Ketchum Manufacturing, Brockville, ON, Canada) to create a simple line on the ventral abdomen in order to mark the animal. Green paste is the recommended standard since it is easily recognizable and unlikely to be mistaken for natural pigmentation as with black ink (Griffin et al. 2016). The linear tattoo must be long enough to be readily identifiable. The authors recommend a minimum tattoo length of 1 cm. The tattoo should be shown to the owner and described in the patient's written discharge instructions to prevent unnecessary concern if the owner notices the green line.

Linear tattoo techniques include application of tattoo paste to the incision at the time of surgery ("incisional tattoo"), creation of a "scoring tattoo" adjacent to the incision, or intradermal injection of tattoo paste adjacent to the incision ("intradermal tattoo"; Griffin et al. 2010, 2016). These three techniques are described in Box 16.1. The specific tattoo technique used is according to the surgeon's preference. Incisional and scoring tattoo techniques are the most commonly used, while intradermal injection is a less widely used method. Incisional tattoos offer the advantage of clearly denoting the patient's surgical scar. Many

---

Box 16.1   Green Linear Tattoo Application Methods

Green tattoo paste is used to create a simple line on the ventral abdomen to mark the animal. Depending on the selected application method, a small dollop of paste from the tube may be deposited into a sterile syringe cap or clean contact lens case for use throughout the surgical day, taking care not to contaminate the ink between patients. Alternatively, a small amount of paste may be drawn into a syringe, with the needle changed between each patient (Figure 16.6).

Method 1: Incisional Tattoo Method (Figures 16.7–16.9)

- Apply tattoo paste directly along the cut edge of the incision after subcuticular or intradermal closure using a paper strip (such as an uncontaminated sterility indicator strip or suture packaging from the surgery pack), a sterile cotton-tipped applicator, or a needle and syringe.
- To apply the ink using a paper strip, dip the edge of the strip in ink and then gently draw it between the apposed skin edges.
- To apply the ink using a sterile cotton-tipped applicator, roll the applicator in ink

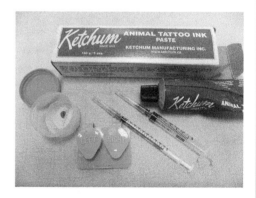

Figure 16.6   Green animal tattoo paste (Ketchum Manufacturing, Brockville, ON, Canada). A small amount of ink may be stored in a syringe cap, contact lens case, syringe, or other small sanitary container for use throughout the surgical day, taking care to prevent contamination of the ink.

and then gently draw it between the apposed skin edges.
- To apply the ink via a 3 cc syringe with a 22-gauge needle, depress the plunger of the syringe just enough to form a tiny bubble at the end of the needle, and then draw a line with it between the apposed edges of the skin incision.

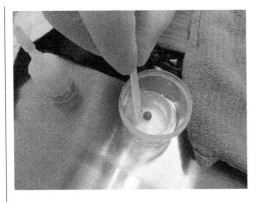

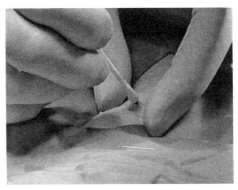

Figure 16.7 The tip of a paper sterility indicator strip from the surgical pack is dipped in tattoo ink in preparation for application to the incision. Note that only a tiny amount of ink is obtained on one corner of the end of the strip. It is desirable to avoid more liberal use of ink in order to prevent the inevitable mess that is created when ink is inadvertently deposited on the skin around the incision, which occurs when it is too heavily applied to the applicator.

Figure 16.8 Another option for applying ink to the incision is to use a sterile cotton-tipped applicator. A tiny amount of ink is retrieved with the tip of the applicator, which is then gently rolled along the cut skin edges. Note that the surgeon gently spreads the incision to ensure adequate contact of the ink with the skin edges.

(a)

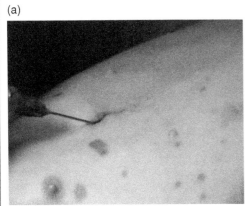

(b)

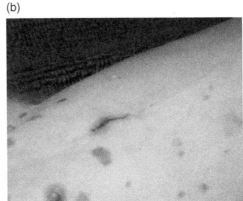

Figure 16.9 (a) A syringe and needle may also be used to deposit ink between the edges of the incision to create a linear tattoo. (b) The final appearance of the tattooed incision following application of a drop of tissue glue on top of the skin.

Method 2: Scoring Tattoo Method (Figures 16.10 and 16.11)

- Make a separate full-thickness skin incision (approximately 1.0 cm) through the dermis by scoring the skin with a scalpel blade.

- Apply a tiny drop of paste directly into this incision, as described in method 1.
- Invert the skin edges slightly and apply a drop of tissue adhesive on top of the skin for closure.

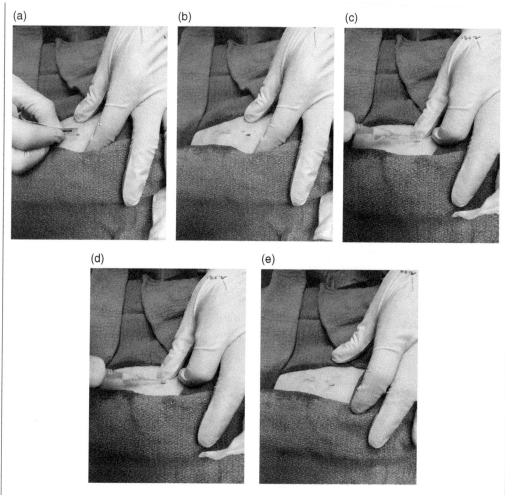

Figure 16.10 (a) Green tattoo ink is applied to a separate incision adjacent to the surgery site using a paper sterility indicator strip from the surgical pack. (b) The incision, which was made using a scalpel blade to score full thickness through the dermis, is well coated with ink. (c) The edges of the incision are gently opposed and closure is achieved using a drop of tissue glue on top of the skin. (d) Care is taken to ensure that glue is only placed on top of the opposed incision and never in the incision itself. If glue is placed in the incision itself it will act as a foreign body, delaying healing and possibly resulting in tattoo failure. (e) The final appearance of the green linear tattoo on the ventral midline adjacent to the spay incision.

Method 3: Intradermal Tattoo Method
(Figure 16.12)

- Inject ink intradermally adjacent to the incision using a tuberculin syringe with a 25-gauge needle.

- With the needle attached to the syringe, insert it intradermally to its hub, and then slowly inject ink as the needle is withdrawn.
- Use a new sterile needle for each patient.

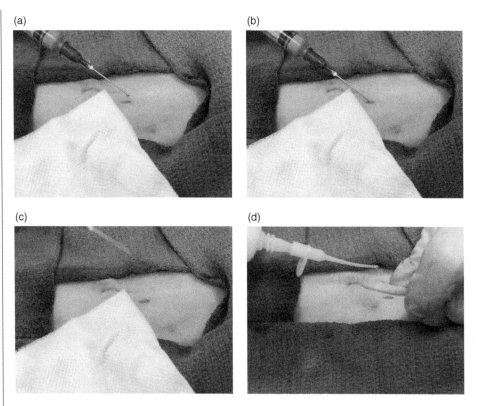

Figure 16.11 (a–d) A scoring tattoo is created using a needle and syringe to deposit the ink in the incision. Note the tiny bubble of ink at the end of the needle. This is all that is required to fully paint the inside of the small, full-thickness skin incision. Closure is achieved by applying a drop of surgical glue on top of the skin as the edges of the incision are gently held in apposition.

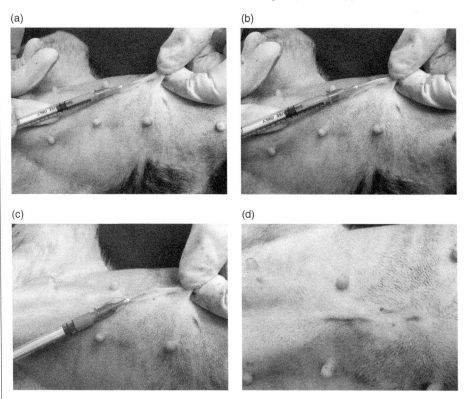

Figure 16.12 Intradermal tattoo method. (a) A 25-gauge needle is inserted intradermally adjacent to the surgical incision. (b) The needle is buried all the way to the hub. (c) A tiny amount of ink is injected as the needle is withdrawn. (d) Final appearance of the intradermal tattoo.

surgeons, however, prefer to avoid placing ink into the surgical incision itself, and elect to use the scoring tattoo technique instead.

In all cases, sterile instrumentation should be used for tattoo application. Regardless of the technique employed, many surgeons apply a small amount of tissue adhesive over the tattoo. This serves to seal the tattoo ink, preventing patients from licking it and developing a temporary case of "green tongue" following recovery. Importantly, when tissue glue is used on incisions, it should always be applied on top of the skin as the surgeon holds the edges of the incision in gentle apposition. Applying tissue glue into the incision itself must be avoided, because it will act as a foreign body, delaying healing, and may ultimately result in tattoo failure. The time and cost of incorporating these techniques for applying green linear tattoos in spay–neuter procedures are negligible, while the value of providing a permanent mark to indicate an animal's sterilization status is tremendous (Griffin et al. 2010).

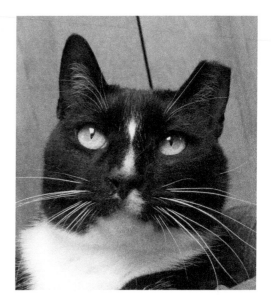

Figure 16.13   Correct appearance of a tipped ear. Ear-tipping is a standard practice for identification of community cats that have been trapped, neutered, and returned to their site of capture.

Ear-Tipping for Community Cats

"Trap–neuter–return" (TNR) is frequently used as a means of reducing birthrates and improving welfare of community cats. Ear-tipping is performed to clearly and permanently visually identify neutered, vaccinated cats that are being humanely managed by TNR. The procedure involves removal of the tip of one of the ears (or pinna) at the time of surgical sterilization and is the accepted global standard for indicating that a free-roaming community cat has been spayed or neutered (Figure 16.13). In contrast, ear-notching is not recommended because torn ear flaps are a frequent occurrence in cats as a result of fighting and are easily mistaken for surgically notched ears (Figures 16.14 and 16.15). In cold climates, mild frostbite of the ear tips is common and may be unilateral or bilateral. Frostbitten ear tips may appear to be cropped, but often have a thickened, irregular, curvilinear border (Figure 16.16). However, it is frequently

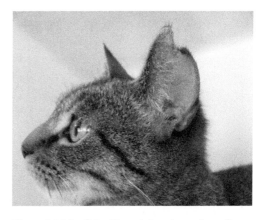

Figure 16.14   Cat with an injured ear pinna. Ears should be tipped rather than notched, because notching often occurs as the result of fighting or other injury, and can be mistaken for a sign of previous neutering.

difficult to distinguish a frostbitten pinna from a tipped pinna, especially from a distance. In such climates, some programs apply green tattoo paste to the skin margins at the ear tip site to aid in identification of neutered cats. Alley Cat Allies, a US national humane organization that serves as a resource on feral cats, recommends removal of the left ear tip. This

(a)

(b)

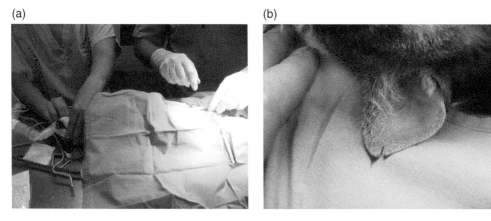

Figure 16.15 (a and b) A female cat was anesthetized for ovariohysterectomy, but exploratory surgery revealed that she was already spayed. Note the presence of a small ear notch, which unfortunately was not recognized as an identifying mark since it did not adhere to the universal standard.

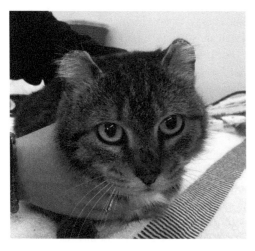

Figure 16.16 Cat with frostbitten ear tips. Frostbite may occur bilaterally or unilaterally, resulting in a cropped appearance of the ear tips. Frostbitten ears can usually be distinguished from surgically tipped ears because they tend to be thickened and irregular and maintain a curvilinear border. *Source:* Photo courtesy of Sara White.

standard is widely used in the United States; however, some organizations identify cats by removing the right ear tip, or by removing the tip on one side or the other, depending on the sex of the cat. Consistency with the standard in a given community is the best practice.

Ear-tipping is a humane procedure and provides a safe, permanent form of identification for community cats. It is often impossible to get close enough to a free-roaming cat to see a subtle mark or tattoo; thus, such methods of identification are not useful in the field because they are frequently ineffective. When cats are ear-tipped, animal control officers, shelter workers, and caregivers can easily and reliably identify cats that are spayed or neutered. This is important to ensure that all cats in a colony are humanely managed and to prevent shelter euthanasia of community cats that are part of managed colonies. Ear-tipping should be performed even in colonies of cats with dedicated caregivers who believe they "know" all of the cats in their colony by sight, because it is very common for several cats in a colony to possess similar coat colors and patterns, making it difficult, if not impossible, to distinguish which cats have already been trapped for surgery.

Ear-Tipping Techniques

Ear-tipping is a quick and simple procedure. It should be considered an antiseptic surgical procedure rather than an aseptic one. Hair removal or shaving of the pinna is unnecessary and is not recommended to avoid abrasion of the tender skin of the pinna. Antiseptic solution (such as chlorhexidine or betadine) is used to gently swab both sides of the pinna. Care should be taken to avoid introducing moisture into the ear canal, which could predispose the cat to otitis externa. There are several methods that may be used for ear-tipping. The method used is according to the surgeon's preference. In all cases, instruments used for ear-tipping must be thoroughly cleaned and disinfected or sterilized between patients to prevent the spread of pathogens, and a new pair of clean exam gloves should be worn for each patient.

A practical and commonly used method for removal of the distal tip of the pinna is simple sharp excision. In most instances, this will be performed using a pair of hemostatic forceps and scissors (Box 16.2). Scissors are preferred over a scalpel blade because their crushing action aids hemostasis. Straight scissors and straight hemostats should be used to make it easier to crop the ear in a straight line. This is very important to ensure the desired visual effect: the ear should have a distinct straight edge that is easy to recognize from a distance. If available, an electrosurgical unit or surgical laser may also be used for ear-tipping; both have the potential advantages of improved hemostasis and reduced opportunity for disease transmission via surgical instruments.

If either of these methods is employed, care must be taken to prevent collateral thermal damage to the pinna, or severe pinnal necrosis may result. This damage is usually not obvious when it is first inflicted; if anything, only mild blanching may be seen at the time of surgery. However, due to the coagulation of pinnal blood vessels, severe necrosis ensues within four to seven days, which can involve the entire pinna. The most important requirement is proper matching of energy setting to excision speed to prevent heat buildup at the excisional margin. A simple plastic spring clamp may be placed across the excised portion of the ear tip as a straight edge. This will facilitate a straight crop and make it easier to maintain adequate excision speed to minimize collateral thermal damage.

Certain patient safety measures must be taken with the use of electrosurgery. An important requirement is to ensure full contact of the patient to the passive electrode (ground plate), to prevent thermal burns on the body. These occur when the patient makes poor contact with the ground plate (usually firmly contacting only the cable connector). This allows all of the energy to be channeled into a relatively small area of skin, with resultant heat buildup.

Ear-tipping is often performed after the cat has been anesthetized and reached a surgical plane of general anesthesia, but before surgical sterilization. This sequence of events provides the advantage of allowing ample time for hemostasis to occur prior to anesthetic recovery. In contrast, some surgeons prefer to perform surgical sterilization prior to ear-tipping. The advantage of this sequence is that it avoids any instance in which a cat could be ear-tipped without undergoing surgical sterilization if the surgery had to be aborted for any reason.

Box 16.2 Procedure for Ear-Tipping Using a Straight Hemostat and Straight Scissors (Figures 16.17 and 16.18)

Use a pair of straight Mayo scissors and straight hemostatic forceps in order to create the desired visual effect. Following removal of the ear tip, the ear margin should have a distinct straight edge that is easy to recognize from a distance.

- A straight hemostat is placed perpendicular to the long axis of the pinna, exposing proportionately approximately one-third of the distal ear flap.

- Surgical scissors are used to remove the tip by cutting distally along the edge of the instrument.
- The hemostat is left in place while the cat undergoes surgery and is removed during recovery.
- Silver nitrate may be applied along the cut edge of the pinna to aid in hemostasis. Gluing or suturing the ear margin is neither necessary nor recommended.

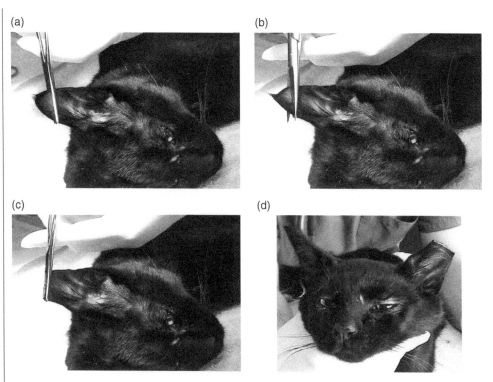

Figure 16.17   Ear-tipping procedure. (a) A straight hemostat is placed across the left pinna perpendicular to its long axis, exposing proportionately one-third of the ear tip. (b) Straight surgical scissors are used to remove the ear tip by cutting over the top of the hemostat in a straight line. (c) The hemostat is left in place to allow adequate time for hemostasis of the pinna to occur. (d) Proper appearance of the ear following removal of the hemostat. Note the distinctive straight edge that will be easily recognizable from a distance.

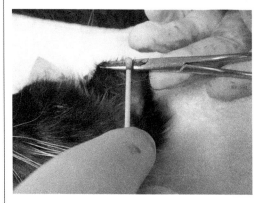

Figure 16.18   Prior to removal of the hemostat, a silver nitrate stick may be rolled over the cut surface of the pinna to aid in hemostasis.

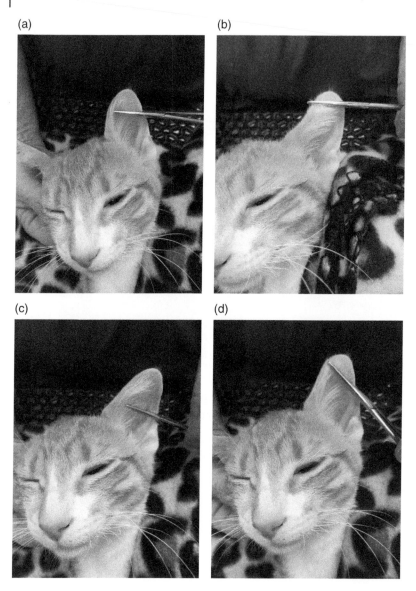

Figure 16.19 An open hemostat is gently held on various aspects of the pinna of an anesthetized cat in order to illustrate both proper and improper clamp placement for ear-tipping. (a) Proper placement of the hemostat perpendicular to the long axis of the ear, exposing proportionately one-third of the ear tip. (b) Improper placement of the hemostat: here it is placed too high, exposing less than one-third of the ear tip proportionately. Transecting the pinna here would result in an ear tip that is difficult to recognize from a distance. (c) Improper placement of the hemostat: here it is placed too low, exposing approximately half of the ear tip proportionately. Transecting the pinna here would result in skin retraction and exposure of the pinnal cartilage, prolonging healing time and predisposing to surgical site infection. (d) Improper placement of the hemostat: here it is not placed perpendicular to the long axis of the ear. Transecting the pinna here would result in a pointed ear tip, making it difficult to recognize as a tipped ear from a distance.

Most commonly, the procedure is performed by placing a straight hemostat across the designated pinna, exposing the ear tip (Box 16.2). The ASV recommends that proportionately approximately one-third of the distal pinna is removed in order to ensure a distinct and readily visible identifying mark (Griffin et al. 2016). Care must be taken to transect perpendicular to the long axis of the pinna. Straight scissors are used to excise the ear tip, leaving the hemostat in place until the cat is in recovery. While the hemostat in still in place, some surgeons apply silver nitrate to the cut surface of the pinna to aid in hemostasis (Figure 16.18). Some bleeding may occur during recovery, especially if the cat rubs or bumps the fresh clot. However, profuse, excessive, or prolonged bleeding is abnormal. Neither gluing nor suturing, nor the use of antibiotics, is necessary or recommended.

Proper placement of the hemostat on the ear tip cannot be overemphasized (Figure 16.19). It is crucial for proper healing as well as for proper appearance of the tipped ear. If the clamp is placed too high, the ear tip will be difficult to visualize and recognize from a distance. If the clamp is placed too low, skin retraction will expose the pinnal cartilage, resulting in prolonged healing and predisposition to surgical site infection. If the clamp is not placed perpendicular to the pinna long axis, the ensuing cut will cause the pinna to appear pointed from a distance, making it difficult to recognize as a tipped ear. Finally, the use of curved hemostats and/or curved scissors should be avoided. If the margin of the cropped ear is curved downward, it may be difficult to recognize as a tipped ear from a distance because the tip will appear rounded (Figure 16.20).

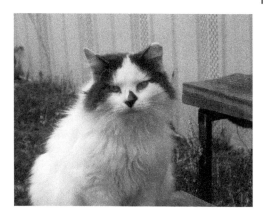

Figure 16.20   The importance of creating a distinctive straight edge at the tip of the ear cannot be overemphasized. The curvilinear appearance of this cat's tipped ear makes it quite difficult to recognize from a distance that the ear is tipped.

Conclusion

Marking animals at the time of surgery is safe, humane, and has the potential to be life-saving. When patient assessment of spay–neuter status is expedited by the presence of a standard identifying mark, it saves precious time and resources, which ultimately can be directed more effectively to help more animals. Because it can be difficult to determine the reproductive status of stray dogs and cats that are presented with little or no history, a standard mark may ultimately prevent an animal from undergoing unnecessary exploratory surgery.

References

Bushby, P.A. (2013). Surgical techniques for spay/neuter. In: *Shelter Medicine for Veterinarians and Staff*, 2e (eds. L. Miller and S. Zawistowski), 625–646. Aimes, IA: Blackwell.

Griffin, B. (2013). Nonsurgical sterilization. In: *Shelter Medicine for Veterinarians and Staff*, 2e (eds. L. Miller and S. Zawistowski), 689–696. Aimes, IA: Blackwell.

Griffin, B., Bushby, P.A., McCobb, E. et al. (2016). The Association of Shelter Veterinarians' 2016 Veterinary Medical Care Guidelines for Spay-Neuter Programs. *JAVMA* 249 (2): 165–188.

Griffin, B., DiGangi, B., and Bohling, M.A. (2010). Review of neutering cats. In: *Consultations in Feline Internal Medicine VI* (ed. J.R. August), 776–790. St. Louis, MO: Elsevier Saunders.

17

Complications in Spay and Neuter Surgery

Mark W. Bohling

The focus of this chapter is a discussion of *surgical* complications – their presentation, treatment, prognosis, and, most importantly, prevention. For a discussion of anesthetic complications, refer to Chapter 10.

Complications are "inevitable," "an unavoidable part of surgery" – or are they? The answer depends in large measure on what one accepts as inevitable and how one defines a complication. For the purposes of this chapter, we will define "surgical complications" as "*any* unexpected/unplanned/unwanted experience or outcome for the patient that causes either mortality, or sufficient morbidity to require further medical attention." With this broad definition of complications and the sheer numbers involved in high-quality high-volume spay–neuter (HQHVSN) and shelter surgery, it is easy to see the enormous potential for complications to occur and to accept a certain frequency of complications as unavoidable. Of course, the mindset of inevitability usually forms a rather poor basis for improvement – why work to improve that which we cannot influence? A better and more productive approach would be to assume that all surgical complications are at least theoretically if not actually preventable.

This mindset – the idea that complications can and should be driven down to zero, or as near to zero as possible – is particularly applicable to spay and neuter surgery in HQHVSN clinics and animal shelters, for two important reasons. The first is the widely held view that spay and neuter are "simple" surgical procedures; yet, are they really? Consider this fact: spay and neuter involve the removal of an entire endocrine organ – this aspect should alone qualify the procedures as major. The misconception of spay and neuter as simple surgery is certainly the view of the vast majority of the general public, and even within some members of the veterinary profession. After all, these procedures form the cornerstone of surgical training for veterinary students, and are described by educators as "basic" and "entry-level" skills. This terminology and attitude promote a view that spay and neuter are somehow inherently safer and less at risk for complications compared to other veterinary surgical procedures, with the implication that these procedures are somehow less demanding of excellence. This view may tend to promote a low value assignment and a careless attitude on the part of clients regarding their own pre- and post-operative responsibilities. Yet, should something go amiss, the backlash is likely to be all the more extreme – "But Doctor, how could you have anything less than a perfect result with such a simple procedure?" However, along with the negative side of this view – the promotion of a complacent attitude, inviting problems – there is also a positive side. This is the second reason: namely, that this field is ripe for improvement.

This is supported by data regarding spay and neuter complication rates. For example, in a multipractice review of electronic patient records, the following overall complication rates were reported: 21.9% for canine spay, 15.2% for canine neuter, 15.3% for feline spay, and 11.9% for feline neuter (Pollari and Bonnett 1996).

The first step toward reduction in complication rates is to know what all of the potential complications are, and their causes. With that information, one can make plans to avoid or eliminate almost all complications. For those rare instances when a complication does occur, knowledge of its cause will lead not only to the selection of an effective treatment for the patient, but, just as importantly, the implementation of the proper corrective action to prevent a recurrence.

The foundations of a plan for complication-free surgery are the same, no matter what the procedure. These foundations are (i) a complete knowledge of the condition to be surgically treated; (ii) thorough and complete familiarity with all aspects of the surgical procedure, including all relevant anatomy; (iii) a complete pre-operative surgical "game plan" that anticipates *every* eventuality and has a ready response; and (iv) a correct mindset of the surgeon. Every aspect of surgical complications – monitoring, preventive measures, management, reporting – must be assigned a central role in spay and neuter surgery, no different from any other major surgical procedure.

In order to make an organized discussion of the topic of surgical complications, they can be categorized as intraoperative complications versus post-operative complications, according to the *timeframe in which the complication first becomes evident.* This is a somewhat arbitrary categorization, as many complications that become evident in the post-operative period occur because of some error or oversight during surgery. As we proceed through the following descriptions of surgical complications of spay and neuter surgery, each complication will be discussed in terms of its recognition, cause, treatment, and prevention.

Complications of Ovariohysterectomy

Intraoperative Complications

Hemorrhage

Acute frank hemorrhage – uncontrolled bleeding during surgery or immediately after – is a potentially life-threatening complication that often on first analysis seems to occur suddenly and unpredictably. The unanticipated acute onset of a serious intraoperative bleed is often a very stressful, even frightening experience for the surgeon. However, despite the potential for disaster, acute intraoperative hemorrhage only very rarely results in serious morbidity or mortality; a review of several retrospective studies of complications of ovariohysterectomy cases revealed zero mortality in a total of 374 canine and 240 feline ovariohysterectomies, in spite of 80 cases of reported intraoperative hemorrhage (Shaver et al. 2019).

Causes of Intraoperative Hemorrhage Intraoperative hemorrhage can be divided into two categories: serious frank hemorrhage versus oozing hemorrhage. The presentation of acute serious frank hemorrhage is obvious: blood welling up into the surgical incision, visibly filling the dorsal abdomen, or the return of one or more blood-soaked gauze sponges used to check for bleeding before closure. Acute frank intraoperative hemorrhage is usually caused by a technical error of some kind. Of the possible technical errors, the two most likely to occur are tearing of the ovarian pedicle, and failure of ligation.

A proper vascular ligature must be 100% reliable in all situations; this means that it must (i) completely arrest any bleeding from the cut end of the vessel(s) in question, and (ii) remain tight and in position until no longer needed. Several aspects of surgical technique in spay will have an impact on the security of pedicle ligation and the ease of placing ligatures. Certain technical points have been identified as measures to minimize the risk of pedicular hemorrhage, and can be incorporated into the "style" of any spay surgeon. However, many experienced surgeons will have developed their own successful methods to minimize risk of hemorrhage; therefore, the following technical points should not be construed as the "best" or "proper" way to perform spay, but rather a set of guidelines for surgeons who are relatively inexperienced or for those who have had problems with operative hemorrhage.

1) Obtain an adequate length of the ovarian pedicle. An ovarian pedicle that is too short makes it more difficult to inspect the ligated pedicle, encourages excessive traction during manipulations for ligation and/or inspection, and may lead directly to a torn pedicle.
2) Place the ligature(s) far enough proximal on the pedicle so that after the pedicle is transected, several millimeters of pedicle (usually at least 5 mm) remains distal to the ligature.
3) Select the proper gauge of suture material for the ligature, neither too small nor too large. Suture material of too small a gauge may break and tend to cut through the pedicle when tightened, particularly with obese patients in which the pedicle contains a great deal of friable adipose tissue. On the other hand, a suture material of too large a gauge may exhibit poor knot security and be prone to slipping off the pedicle.
4) Utilize proper ligation technique, paying special attention to ensuring that as the second knot throw is placed, the first throw is not inadvertently loosened.
5) Post-ligation inspection of the pedicle should be gentle and minimal, and the ligature itself should never be grasped. Excessive manipulation of the pedicle after ligation may loosen a ligature, causing hemorrhage after the pedicle is returned to the abdomen. After inspection is completed, the *grasp on the pedicle should be retained as the pedicle is returned to its anatomic position* in the dorsal abdomen. It should not be merely released to fall back

into the abdomen; sometimes a small amount of subcutaneous tissue has been inadvertently incorporated into the ligature, thus the pedicle is attached both at its origin and at the subcutis and is under tension. If the pedicle is released outside the abdomen in this condition, the ligature may remain attached to the subcutis while the pedicle (now without a ligature) retracts to the dorsal abdomen.

Besides suture ligation, other options exist for hemostasis of the ovarian and uterine pedicles. One such option is the use of an electrosurgical device to coagulate the vessels before transection. Electrosurgical coagulation can be delivered via vessel-sealing devices with feedback to limit collateral thermal damage, or via conventional bipolar electrosurgical forceps. Watts (2018) reported on the use of conventional bipolar forceps in routine ovariectomy of 1406 dogs and 859 cats; in addition, the forceps were used for ovariohysterectomy for pyometra or after cesarean section in another 89 dog and 55 cats. No instances of hemorrhage were observed during or after any of the ovariectomy or ovariohysterectomy surgeries; however, skin burns from collateral heat damage were observed, mainly during the early use of the forceps, until it was found that this complication could be avoided by placement of a gauze swab between the skin and the electrosurgical forceps.

Tearing of the ovarian pedicle is the second common cause of acute intraoperative hemorrhage. Pedicular tearing has been more commonly associated with the right ovary than the left; it is hypothesized that the more cranial location of the right ovary makes exposure more difficult, requiring a greater degree of traction and thus an increased risk of tearing. The risk of tearing can be minimized by proper placement of the spay incision (not too caudal), and proper technique to rupture the suspensory ligament. "Proper technique" in this instance should not be construed to mean that there is a single best method, as a number of methods and variations exist to tear the suspensory ligament. To name a few: digital pressure ("strumming"), grasping the ligament between thumb and index finger and then turning ("twisting") the wrist, tearing the ligament with hemostats, and cutting it with scissors or electrosurgery. In a small prospective case study of 30 shelter dogs, sharp transection of the suspensory ligament was compared to digital strumming with regard to surgical time, complications, and measures of intraoperative and post-operative pain (Shivley et al. 2019). Sharp transection was found to yield a 36-second shorter overall surgical time; however, no other significant differences were noted between the two methods. Thus, it would appear that various methods for suspensory ligament transection can be performed safely when done properly, and all can cause problems when performed incorrectly. Therefore, rather than endorse one method, the author believes that the spay surgeon should become familiar with several, choose a primary method according to preference, and then become expert in the application of that method. This should then be used as one's primary method; after this expertise has been acquired, a secondary method should be similarly developed for the unusual case where the primary method is unusable or not recommended in a particular situation.

Another, much less common cause of frank intraoperative hemorrhage is the laceration of an abdominal vessel or organ. The most common abdominal organ to be unintentionally lacerated is the spleen (see Figure 17.1). Several

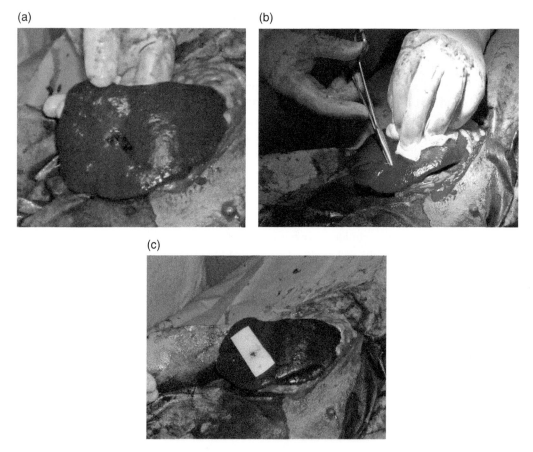

Figure 17.1 (a) Splenic laceration caused by a spay hook. (b) Suture the splenic capsule at the site of the laceration. (c) Absorbable hemostatic sponge placed over the repair.

reports of this complication are found in the literature, and the author is aware of several such cases; however, in each instance the hemorrhage was controlled with the application of pressure on minor lacerations and mattress sutures on larger ones, and no mortality was reported.

Oozing hemorrhage can also originate from errors in ligation technique: partial loosening of a ligature may result in mild oozing rather than massive bleeding. Oozing hemorrhage may also be patient related. Bitches who are either currently in heat or have recently been in heat may have deficient clotting; endogenous estrogens have been hypothesized to be at least partly responsible. Anticoagulant rodenticides may have been ingested in low doses without causing signs. These patients usually respond to empirical treatment with vitamin K. Certain breeds such as the Doberman pincher are more likely to present with inherited disorders of coagulation (von Willebrand's disease). The medical history will not always reveal these patients and screening tests (activated clotting time, buccal mucosal bleeding time) should be employed when the index of suspicion is high. Blood products should always be available. This does not necessarily mean that fresh whole blood must be kept on hand (though it may be recommended in certain situations); a supply of blood from a designated donor(s) may be perfectly adequate to meet any anticipated need, as long as blood collection materials are kept in stock and there is ready access to donors and an efficient, timely, and well-practiced protocol for blood collection. It is also wise to consider assembling an autotransfusion kit for use in cases of abdominal hemorrhage.

Managing Intraoperative Hemorrhage The vast majority of intraoperative complications will manifest as acute hemorrhage; as such, the treatment is simple: locate and correct the source of the bleeding. The following recommendations have been gleaned from the experiences of teaching spay and neuter to novice surgeons, and of having not a few complications referred for correction.

1) Obtain adequate visualization. All too often when an unexpected bleed occurs intraoperatively, the surgeon will attempt to use traction alone to locate the bleed, in an effort to avoid having to enlarge the incision. Instead, when any significantly concerning bleed occurs, the "small incision" should be abandoned and immediately converted to a large enough laparotomy to properly explore the caudal abdomen. This does not necessarily mean a full xyphoid-to-pubis incision, but rather enough of an enlargement to be able to get one's hands and eyes into the abdomen without a feeling of having to struggle for adequate room to get a good view. Most often, the time saved by not struggling for visualization will more than make up for the extra time spent in closure. More importantly, the bleeding can be quickly and definitively addressed, without creating undue risk of causing yet another unintended complication such as ureteral trauma.

2) As soon as significant uncontrolled hemorrhage is recognized intraoperatively, a scrubbed-in assistant should be utilized whenever possible. Particularly with the obese patient, an assistant can prove invaluable in aiding retraction and can also provide suction to aid visualization. Also note that the middle of a surgical emergency is a rather poor time to attempt to train an assistant in operating room technique and protocol – conduct regular training exercises with the technicians or volunteers who will be assisting you, so that they will be ready to help when you need them.

3) If a scrubbed-in assistant is not available, use self-retaining retractors. Every HQHVSN clinic and shelter operating room should have a minimum of two sets of Balfour retractors available: a large set for large and medium dogs, and a small set for small dogs and cats.

4) Surgical suction should also be available in every operating room. Sophisticated and powerful surgical suction systems, although nice to have, are not necessary. An inexpensive portable suction unit will suffice, provided it is well maintained so that it can function properly when needed. Poole and Yankauer suction tips and suction tubing should be kept on hand in sterile packaging, ready for immediate use. Suction vessels should be kept on the suction unit and tested periodically to ensure good function and absence of vacuum leaks.

5) Consider autotransfusion. Autotransfusion kits can be assembled and made available for use in cases of intraoperative or postoperative abdominal hemorrhage.

Autotransfusion Autotransfusion is a technique whereby blood salvaged from the abdominal cavity is returned to the circulatory system. In the case of spay–neuter, autotransfusion is most commonly performed in a patient with an opened abdominal cavity when blood removal is required for visualization and correction of the source of the hemorrhage. This may occur during acute massive hemorrhage during the original surgical procedure, or when a patient has returned to surgery after a post-operative hemoabdomen has been recognized. Collecting blood from the abdomen for autotransfusion can take five minutes or even less, so use of this technique should not cause a significant delay in the repair of the cause of the hemorrhage.

Using the patient's own blood to perform a transfusion offers several advantages. The first is availability: the blood is right there, and would have to be removed from the abdomen anyway in order for the surgeon to find and correct the source of the bleeding. The second is speed: it is not necessary to locate a donor animal and collect the blood from them, or to obtain blood from a blood bank, or to wait for frozen blood products to thaw. The third is avoiding transfusion reactions: returning an animal's own blood to their circulatory system can be done rapidly without risk of transfusion reaction and without

blood-typing or cross-matching (Robinson et al. 2016; Cole and Humm 2019).

There are multiple techniques published for performing autotranfusions in dogs and cats. Some involve collecting the blood in a blood collection bag with or without anticoagulant, while others simply use large syringe(s) with or without an extension set. In either case, the blood is returned intravenously to the patient through a blood filter. The use of an anticoagulant – acid citrate dextrose (ACD), citrate phosphate dextrose (CPDA-1), or other non-preservative anticoagulants – during collection is often considered unnecessary during autotransfusion, since blood that has pooled in the peritoneal cavity becomes defibrinated and does not clot (Cole and Humm 2019).

Emancipet's technique and supply list for autotransfusion appear in Figure 17.2 and Box 17.1, respectively. This technique for autotransfusion uses a blood collection bag. This is most advantageous when the patient is medium or large and more than 100 cc of free abdominal blood is anticipated. For smaller patients (cats and small dogs), two sterile 60 cc syringes should prove adequate for the anticipated volume and may be faster and easier to manage.

The following steps describe how to perform an autotransfusion:

1) Place an intravenous (IV) catheter. If additional IV fluids or medications will be given, it is ideal to have two IV catheters placed so that one can be reserved for blood administration.

2) If the autotransfusion candidate is a postoperative patient returning to surgery, reanesthetize and surgically prepare the patient. Have autotransfusion supplies ready before the abdomen is opened. This means that the sterile syringe(s) or sterile extension set should be opened and on the surgery field ready to insert into the abdomen as soon as it is opened, and any blood collection lines and bags should already be assembled and ready (see Figure 17.2).

(a)

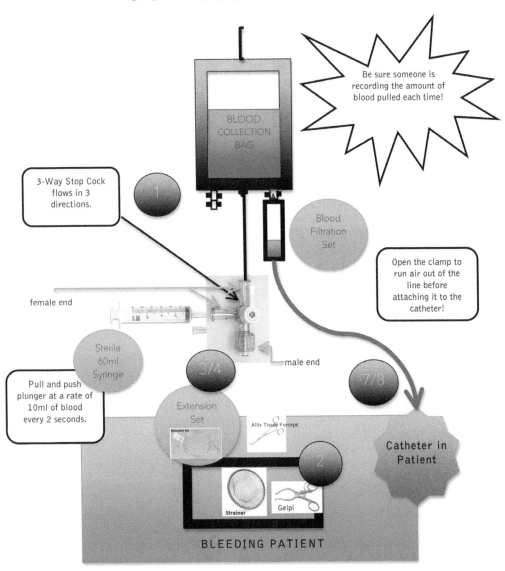

AUTOTRANSFUSION PROCEDURE

Figure 17.2   (a and b) Emancipet protocol for autotransfusion. AST, assistant surgery technician; Sx, surgery.

3) If the hemoabdomen is severe, pooled blood will flow out as soon as the abdomen is opened. Open the abdomen enough to introduce the extension set (if used) or syringe tip and begin to suction the blood. As the level of blood in the abdomen decreases, the incision can be opened more fully to provide visualization and access.

(b)

E M A N C I P E T
Autotransfusion Procedure

1. The Surgery Technician will open and hang blood collection bag. The fluid line from the blood collection bag will connect to the female end of the 3-WAY STOP COCK. *You may add an extension set to give you additional length if you need it.*
   a. Attach a 60mL SYRINGE to the middle port of the 3-WAY STOP COCK (female end). The AST will continue to hold the 60mL syringe while the SX Technician finishes setting up the equipment.
   b. Remove BLOOD FILTER DRIP SET from packaging. Make sure the CLAMP on the LINE is closed.
   c. Twist plug from the BLOOD BAG and introduce BLOOD FILTER DRIP SET.

2. Open in **STERILE** fashion and place on surgery pack:
   A. GELPI
   B. STRAINER
   C. EXTENSION SET
   d. ALLIS TISSUE FORCEPS

3. Doctor will clamp EXTENSION SET to the SURGERY DRAPE with the ALLIS TISSUE FORCEPS and drop the **female end** off the edge of the sterile drape.

4. The **surgery technician** will connect the non-sterile side (**female end**) of the EXTENSION SET to the 3-WAY STOP COCK.

5. The **surgery technician** will put on a cap, face mask, and sterile surgery gloves to be prepared to assist the surgeon to find and repair the bleed.

6. The **surgeon** will indicate when the AST can begin collecting blood from the patient.
   a. Point arrow on 3-WAY STOP COCK toward the BLOOD BAG. Pull back gently on 60mL SYRINGE.
   b. Once syringe is full, turn ARROW toward EXTENSION SET/PATIENT and push PLUNGER.
   c. Blood should flow into the BLOOD BAG. *Pull and push PLUNGER at a rate no faster than 10ml of blood every 2 seconds to ensure red blood cells are not being destroyed.*
   Be sure someone (typically the AST) is recording the amount of blood collected during this process

7. The AST will begin giving the blood back to the patient once one of the following things happens (whichever comes first):
   a. the **surgeon** instructs the **AST** to do so, or
   b. 200mls have been collected in the BLOOD BAG, or
   c. all the blood has been collected from the patient's abdomen.

8. The AST will administer the blood back to the patient through patient's established IV catheter:
   a. Squeeze the FILTER CHAMBER on BLOOD FILTER DRIP SET to fill 1/3 with blood.
   b. Flush air out of the LINE by opening the CLAMP and running all the air out of the line. RECLAMP LINE once blood reaches the line's end, careful not to waste any blood.
   c. Attach the FILTER LINE from the BLOOD FILTER DRIP SET to the patient's IV CATHETER.
   d. Start blood flow by completely opening CLAMP. Make sure the blood is flowing by monitoring your drip rate. Adjust rate per **surgeon** instructions.
   e. It is vital that the BLOOD BAG is never fully empty while the surgeon is still collecting blood from patient; this will ensure air will not get in the FILTER LINE to the patient.

Figure 17.2 (Continued)

Box 17.1   Emancipet's Autotransfusion Box Inventory List

_____ 2 – Blood collection bag: Dry 600 ml bag with Luer attachment to donor animal and single or dual "spike ports" to attach blood filtration set (for example, Jorgensen J0520C)

_____ 2 – Blood administration sets with standard blood filter (for example, Baxter 2C6700)

_____ 6 – Extension sets – 30″

_____ 2 – Three-way stopcocks with two female and one male Luer Lock fittings (for example, Jorgensen J0462)

_____ 2 – Liters NaCl (saline) 0.9% solution

_____ 2 – Sterile gauze packs

_____ 2 – Packs sterile sponges

_____ 2 – Sterile 60 cc syringes (Luer Lock)

_____ 4 – Sterile individual packets 3-0 on taper needles

_____ 2 – Sterile packages of GelFoam

_____ 2 – Gelpi retractors

_____ 2 – Allis tissue forceps

_____ 2 – Strainers (stainless-steel mesh drain strainer or tea strainer)

4) It is common for omentum and other abdominal contents to occlude the suction tip. The use of a sterilized metal tea strainer to hold back the abdominal contents while allowing the passage of blood toward the suction tip can help avoid these blockages.

5) If a blood collection bag is to be used in the process, follow the Emancipet protocol in Figure 17.2.

6) If a blood collection bag is not being used, the surgeon or an assistant can use a sterile 60 cc syringe to withdraw pooled blood from the abdomen. It may be helpful to use a sterile extension set attached to the syringe to facilitate access to areas of pooled blood deep in the body cavity. Once the syringe is full of blood or nearly so, it can be handed to a veterinary technician who then administers the blood through a blood filter (Hemo-Nate®, Jorgensen Laboratories, Loveland, CO; or other inline filter) into the IV catheter. This may be repeated as many times as necessary with new sterile syringes, although if more than two syringes of blood are salvaged from the abdomen, managing the multiple syringes will become cumbersome and use of a blood collection bag would be more appropriate.

7) Blood for autotransfusion may be administered IV at a rate of 5 ml per second, or at the speed that the filter will allow.

Iatrogenic Ureteral Trauma

This complication usually occurs during efforts to recover a dropped or torn ovarian pedicle, as the ureter is at risk for being traumatized during attempts to grasp the ovarian pedicle. As with all complications, this problem is best solved by anticipation and avoidance. Measures to ensure retention of the pedicle and to reduce the risk of tearing should be part of every surgeon's technique. Although these measures will vary to a certain extent between surgeons, all are similar in that they are readily incorporated to become a natural part of every spay–neuter surgical procedure.

Even for the highly experienced spay surgeon, a pedicle may occasionally be dropped or torn. In these instances, increasing the exposure and the availability of suction and self-retaining retractors can greatly improve visualization and help reduce the risk of ureteral trauma. Every spay–neuter surgeon should be completely conversant with the basic techniques for visualization of the ovarian pedicle via retraction of the mesoduodenum on the right side of the abdomen, and the mesocolon on the left.

Some experienced spay–neuter surgeons have described retrieving a ureter with the spay hook during routine spay, or having a ureter elevate along with a uterine horn, either during retrieval or when following the first horn past the bifurcation to the second horn. This appears to be a particular risk in some puppies, as their ureters may be less taut and more tortuous than in the adult, and they may have less retroperitoneal fat obscuring and protecting the ureter. The surgeons who have had this experience describe the tension, appearance, size, and retrieval location as being very similar to those of a uterine horn. Failure to locate an ovary at the end of the ureter reveals the error, but in some cases the ureter breaks due to the tension placed on it by the surgeon. In these cases, removal of the affected kidney (nephrectomy) is often the most viable treatment and one that can be performed in-house, whereas ureteral repair or reimplantation generally requires referral to a specialist.

Post-operative Complications

Fortunately, most post-operative complications are minor and easily handled. In this category would be minor incisional issues such as poorly coapted edges, minor contusions, local infections, exposed suture knots, and the like. Recognition and resolution of these problems should already be well within the capability of the reader and so will not be covered.

Early Post-operative Hemorrhage and Hemoabdomen

In some cases, rather than becoming apparent during the surgery, intraabdominal bleeding occurs during the recovery and post-operative period. Many of these cases become apparent within the first 12 hours after surgery: on the recovery beach, in the cage after surgery, or later the first evening, although some may take longer to become obvious. Once recognized, a patient with a serious ongoing bleed should be returned to surgery so that the source of the hemorrhage can be rectified. Once these patients return to surgery, the steps for addressing the source of the hemorrhage are the same as if the bleeding was noted during the original surgery, including the possibility for autotransfusion (see previous sections).

Recognition of post-operative abdominal bleeding is not always straightforward, and often does not result in bleeding from the incision, especially in the early stages. The index of suspicion for abdominal bleeding should be increased in patients with unusually slow recovery (recumbent for longer than expected), moderate hypothermia that is less responsive to warming than expected, an elevated heart rate without obvious other signs of pain or excitement, and pale mucous membranes. If blood pressure monitoring is available, a low blood pressure – and particularly a falling blood pressure – together with tachycardia prompts even greater suspicion of blood loss. Packed cell volume (PCV) is not a sensitive indicator of recent hemorrhage (Giger 2011), so should not be used to indicate the presence or severity of hemoabdomen during the first several hours. Blood loss into the abdomen causes hypovolemia, not hemodilution, so except when aggressive IV fluid replacement has been attempted and the intravascular volume has been restored, these patients may have minimal drop in PCV despite having lost a substantial amount of blood into the abdomen.

To assess for hemoabdomen, an abdominocentesis can be performed in the recumbent animal with a 22-gauge needle attached to a 3 cc syringe. The skin should be aseptically prepared, and the needle introduced caudal to the umbilicus near the midline or a few centimeters to the right of the midline in order to avoid puncturing the spleen. Draw back gently on the plunger of the syringe to create slight negative pressure. If the blood flows easily into the syringe, this is diagnostic for hemoabdomen; however, if the abdominocentesis does not produce blood, abdominal bleeding cannot be ruled out. In this case it is wise to continue monitoring the patient, giving fluids as needed, warming the patient, and consider repeating the abdominocentesis if clinical signs do not improve.

Dehiscence

Dehiscence (failure of the surgical closure) can have catastrophic consequences, although thankfully it usually does not. Dehiscence may involve the skin and subcutis only, the muscular body wall and its fascia, or full thickness (see Figure 17.3). A common etiology for skin dehiscence (which often progresses to full thickness) is self-trauma: the patient licks and/or chews open the skin closure. This problem in turn usually has a root cause related to technical error in suturing, as a patient will generally leave a comfortable closure alone. Skin sutures placed too tightly are commonly to blame here. When skin sutures are placed, care must be taken to avoid making them overly snug, which would cause the sutures to cut into the skin as it swells post-operatively (particularly in dogs). Because of the risks of skin sutures, and for patient comfort and client convenience, in most situations a continuous (buried) intradermal closure is the preferred method. Even with an intradermal closure, self-trauma can become a problem if the suture knot is too large (too many throws and/or too large a suture gauge) or otherwise buried too shallowly, barely beneath the epidermis. In these patients it is common for an inflammatory response to the irritation of the knot (a "suture reaction") to occur, inviting unwanted attention by the patient. Any time a patient has been demonstrated or is even suspected to be a chewing/licking risk, they should be sent home wearing an Elizabethan collar, rather than the clinic waiting for a problem and having to deal with it. These collars should be available at all times in the practice, in a proper selection of sizes for all patients. In addition, the staff must be trained how to properly fit one to the patient – few things are as discouraging as getting a dog back with a dehisced incision, wearing an Elizabethan collar that was too short.

A second common cause of skin dehiscence (particularly with continuous intradermal closures) is due to faulty knot tying technique. Body wall dehiscence is usually caused by failure to engage the external rectus sheath in each bite of the body wall closure. Long ago, research has shown that the external rectus sheath, not the

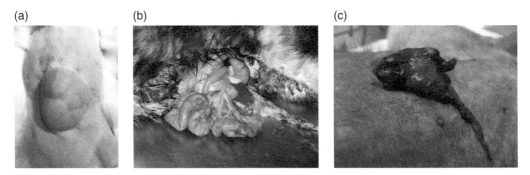

(a)　　　　　　(b)　　　　　　　　　　(c)

Figure 17.3 Dehiscence. (a) Body wall dehiscence in a cat surrendered to a shelter about 1.5 years after spay. It is unknown how long after the spay the body wall herniation occurred, but the skin appears well healed over the defect. Poor knot technique in the original surgery was suspected as the cause. *Source:* Photo courtesy of Kayla Beetham. (b) Full-thickness dehiscence in a feral cat. The dehiscence was due to poor knot technique in a simple interrupted suture closure. The cat was still in her trap when dehiscence occurred, so treatment was prompt and the cat survived. *Source:* Photo courtesy of Julie Levy. (c) Full-thickness dehiscence in a puppy one day after spay. The dehiscence occurred because the sutures that were intended to be in the linea alba were only in the subcutaneous layer, and the external rectus sheath had not been engaged. *Source:* Photo courtesy of Brian DiGangi.

peritoneum, is the strongest layer ("holding layer") in abdominal wall closure.

Repair of Dehiscence Repair of dehiscence with evisceration of abdominal contents can be successful. In a study that included eight spay dehiscences (four dogs, four cats), all survived to discharge (Gower et al. 2009). In these patients, dehiscence and evisceration had occurred a median of four days (range one to six days) post-spay. In half of the patients, the evisceration had occurred during the night when the patient was not observed; in these patients, the incision may have been open for many hours prior to repair.

To repair a dehiscence with evisceration, patients will require anesthesia, lavage of the exposed viscera, surgical exploration of the abdomen, replacement of abdominal viscera into the peritoneal cavity, and repair of the body wall. In some cases, it may be necessary to resect a portion of the intestine if damage has occurred to the intestine itself or to its blood supply. Antibiotic therapy and supportive care will also be required.

Incisional Infections

Of course surgical infections (Figures 17.4 and 17.5) occur for a variety of reasons, some of which are not under the control of the surgeon, and can occur after orchiectomy as well as after spay. Adherence to Halstead's surgical principles is the best plan for avoidance of incisional infections. This does not necessarily mean gowning and full surgical regalia, however. Attention to the creation of a healthy surgical wound (gentle tissue handling, hemostasis, minimization of dead space, reduction of anesthetic and operative time, and use of only the minimum number of sutures of the smallest possible gauge) should be the focus.

Reactions

Reaction to buried sutures and/or surgical adhesives can be seen during the weeks following surgery (Figure 17.6). Generally one of two types of problems is encountered. The first is the so-called suture reaction; the author's hypothesis is that in nearly all cases, this is not, as the name implies, an immunologic reaction to the suture material, but rather an inflammatory response to the physical characteristics of the closure. The evidence for this statement is that this problem is seen exclusively (or nearly so) at the ends of the closure, where the knots are located. Typically, a large-gauge suture of a fairly stiff, monofilament material has been used, and usually an excessive number of throws have been employed. Also it is quite common to

(a)

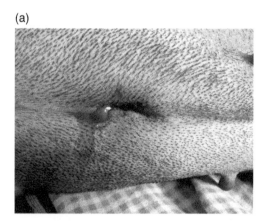

(b)

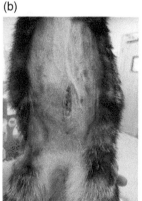

Figure 17.4   Incisional infections after spay. (a) Incision infection without skin dehiscence in a dog. *Source:* Photo courtesy of Sara White. (b) Incision infection and skin dehiscence in a cat following spay. *Source:* Photo courtesy of Brian DiGangi.

(a)   (b)   (c)

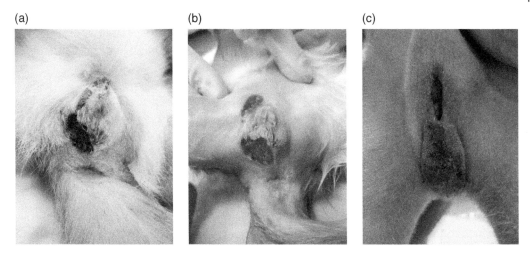

Figure 17.5   Infections following castration. (a) Infection following neutering in a cat – appearance on presentation; (b) appearance after debridement. (c) Incision infection and skin dehiscence in a dog following pre-scrotal castration. *Source:* Photos courtesy of Brian DiGangi.

find that the knot is located very superficially, and is often actually visible. Cutting off the offending knot (under appropriate sedation etc. as needed) is curative. The problem is best avoided by minimizing the amount of implanted foreign material, and ensuring that it is deeply buried. Intradermal sutures should be fine gauge: 3-0 for large dogs, 4-0 for small dogs and cats. Knots should be compact: four throws, properly applied (well tightened and not half-hitched), are more than adequate to start or finish a continuous closure. The knot should be deeply buried, by taking anchoring bites to the external rectus sheath. Polydioxanone suture, while not particularly inflammatory, is very long-lasting, and poorly buried knots often crop up later as suture granulomas.

When cyanoacrylate surgical adhesives are used, they may also be implicated in reactions. This is generally a problem stemming from misuse or misunderstanding of the proper use of these products. Cyanoacrylate can cause a profound inflammatory reaction; therefore, these products are not intended for implantation below the epidermis, and are actually intended to be used mostly as sealants on the skin surface. Whenever tissue coaptation is needed, par-

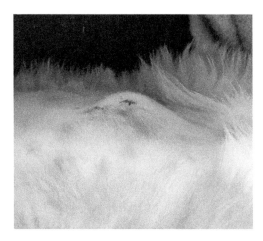

Figure 17.6   "Suture reactions" are an inflammatory response to the physical characteristics of the closure. Small suture reactions like this one resolve on their own, but may be decreased or avoided by minimizing tissue trauma, minimizing the amount of implanted foreign material, and ensuring that the knot is deeply buried. *Source:* Photo courtesy of Sandra Engelgeer.

ticularly with any closure requiring resistance to tension, surgical adhesives are a less than ideal choice, and if used at all should be considered as a supplement to suture or another tissue coaptation device such as staples.

Post-operative "Secondary" Hemorrhage

Mild, self-limiting vaginal bleeding ("spotting") is not unusual (particularly if the patient is spayed while in estrus) and is not considered to be a complication. However, serious, even life-threatening bleeding has been reported by several authors and this author has heard anecdotal reports and seen the condition. Pearson used the term "secondary hemorrhage" to describe this complication, and described 11 cases as part of a review of 72 canine cases referred for complications after ovariohysterectomy (Pearson 1973). He noted an onset from 4 to 16 days after spay, in some cases beginning with an intermittent onset which became more severe in time, while other cases presented in a more severe acute stage. Regardless of presentation, severity of bleeding could increase rapidly – to the fatal level within hours in some cases. Pearson hypothesized the cause to be erosion of the uterine vessels beneath the ligature due to infection, either pre-existent (pyometra) or from a breach of asepsis. The author's experience confirms Pearson's observation that erosion of uterine vessel(s) beneath the uterine body ligature appears to be the proximate cause of hemorrhage, but can neither confirm nor refute the claim of infection as the underlying cause of the erosion. Regardless of the cause, any serious vaginal bleed post-spay is an indication for immediate abdominal exploration. The uterine stump is re-excised and re-ligated, preferably with a Miller's knot. A two-pass uterine ligature (such as the Miller's knot or one of its modifications) will distribute the pressure beneath the ligature over a wider area of tissue. This in turn may produce less crushing and necrosis beneath the ligature and thereby reduce the risk of this complication when compared with a single-pass ligature.

Sinus Tracts and Stump Granulomas

These complications are created during surgery, due to poor aseptic technique, excess remaining stump tissue, or use of non-absorbable ligature material. Occasionally a uterine stump granuloma can become so large that it causes fecal or urinary obstruction. Sinus tracts can develop with the use of non-absorbable ligatures (particularly with a large-gauge or stiff suture material). Non-surgical ligating materials such as nylon cable ties have been demonstrated to cause fistulous tracts and should never be used, regardless of their apparent economy and/or ease of application.

While most cases of fistulous tracts or granulomas may show a transient favorable response to antibiotic administration, definitive treatment in nearly every instance requires surgical exploration of the site and correction of the cause, usually by simply removing the offending foreign material.

Ovarian Remnant Syndrome

Ovarian remnant syndrome is covered in Chapter 18.

Complications in Ovariectomy versus Ovariohysterectomy

The recent surgical trend toward minimally invasive procedures has led to a renewed interest in the potential benefits of ovariectomy as an alternative to ovariohysterectomy. Several retrospective studies have compared the two procedures in regard to post-operative morbidity and mortality. In a single small prospective, randomized study, no differences were found with regard to short-term complications (including blood loss and dehiscence), pain scores, or surgical wound scores (Peeters and Kirpensteijn 2011). Although ovariectomized patients had shorter incisions, no differences were seen in any of the surgical performance measures, including blood loss, time to close, and total surgical time. Taken as a whole, the available data does not appear to support a wholesale adoption of ovariectomy as an alternative to ovariohysterectomy at this time.

Complications in Orchiectomy

Scrotal Swelling, Contusion, and Hemorrhage

This is usually caused by oozing from small cutaneous or subcutaneous vessels rather than leakage from the testicular pedicle. In one small randomized clinical trial of 73 dogs, closed versus open orchiectomy was compared with regard to bleeding, scrotal swelling and contusion, and other early post-operative complications. Open orchiectomy was found to have a statistically greater risk of scrotal complications and higher overall complication rate (Hamilton et al. 2014). In a randomized trial of 437 dogs comparing scrotal and pre-scrotal castration in adult dogs, there was no difference in the incidence of scrotal swelling or hemorrhage between the two approaches (Woodruff et al. 2015). However, it is notable that, regardless of the surgical approach, scrotal swelling was common and was noted in over 20% of the dogs at 24 and 48 hours post-surgery (see Figure 17.7).

Scrotal swelling, scrotal and inguinal contusion, and scrotal hemorrhage can also occur after feline orchiectomy (see Figures 17.8–17.10). As with dogs, in most cases the bleeding is self-limiting and does not require that the animal return to surgery.

In terms of prevention, these complications are best avoided by attention to hemostasis and subcutaneous closure in dogs; also, a few days' post-operative exercise restriction can help reduce the incidence. If the scrotum should begin to swell, cold compresses may help reduce the severity of the problem if applied within the first 48–72 hours; after that time warm compresses should be used.

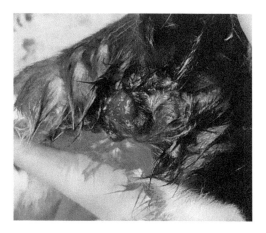

Figure 17.8   Scrotal hemorrhage in a cat several hours after scrotal castration through two skin incisions. At the time of the photo, a firm clot had formed in the scrotum and actual bleeding had ceased. No treatment was required, and the cat was observed by the owner for signs of ongoing hemorrhage. *Source:* Photo courtesy of Sara White.

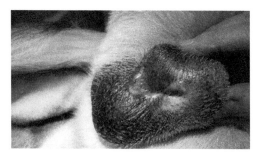

Figure 17.7   Swollen scrotum several days after scrotal castration. The scrotum is approximately the same size as prior to surgery. The incision had been closed with a single inverted subcutaneous suture in order to allow drainage, and the open ends of the incision are visible. The swelling resolved and the wound closed without treatment. *Source:* Photo courtesy of Sara White.

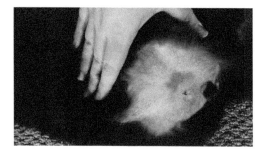

Figure 17.9   Cat several days post-operation with mild inguinal bruising near the site where a subcutaneous cryptorchid testicle was removed. *Source:* Photo courtesy of Sara White.

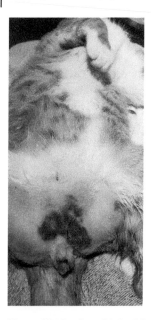

Figure 17.10 Cat with bruising in the inguinal area on the day of surgery. Cord retrieval via the scrotal incision was unsuccessful. The cat was observed overnight at an emergency clinic and required no further intervention. *Source:* Photo courtesy of Carolyn Leisz.

In some cases, bruising or swelling in the scrotal and inguinal areas may be severe, suggesting ongoing bleeding from a testicular vessel. In these cases it is advisable to return to surgery to discover and correct the source of the bleeding (see Figure 17.11). The stumps of the spermatic cords should be inspected and re-ligated if there is any evidence of bleeding or oozing (see Figure 17.12).

If the scrotum is extremely enlarged (generally, more than two to four times its size prior to castration), the surgeon may elect to perform a scrotal ablation surgery in which the scrotal sac is removed (see Figure 17.13). When performing scrotal ablation, it is necessary to ensure that adequate skin remains for the incision to close without tension.

Abdominal Hemorrhage

Abdominal bleeding is a rare complication after castration. If the spermatic cord has retracted into the abdomen, any bleeding occurring from the testicular vessels will be

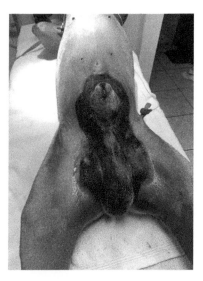

Figure 17.11 Severe inguinal and scrotal bruising and swelling in a dog 48 hours post-castration. During surgical exploration, bleeding was discovered from one of the spermatic cords. The cord was re-ligated and blood clots were removed. No additional sources of bleeding were apparent, and the dog healed well after the repair. *Source:* Photo courtesy of Heather Campbell.

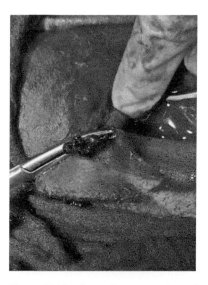

Figure 17.12 An oozing spermatic cord was located during exploratory surgery for inguinal and scrotal bruising and swelling. The cord was re-ligated. *Source:* Photo courtesy of Heather Campbell.

(a)　　　　　　　　　　　　　　(b)

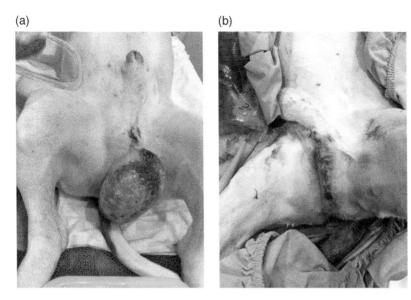

Figure 17.13 (a) Hemoscrotum approximately four hours post-castration. The scrotum is swollen to several times its pre-operative size. Surgical exploration revealed a bleeding spermatic cord, which was re-ligated. (b) A scrotal ablation was performed, and the dog was discharged the same day. *Source:* Photos courtesy of Sara White.

intraabdominal. This would be expected to occur after open castration, and could also occur if a closed castration ligature loosened or slipped. In some cases of intraabdominal bleeding after castration, inguinal and scrotal bruising or swelling may be evident, whereas in other cases there may be no external bruising or swelling.

The approach to diagnosing and resolving abdominal hemorrhage after dog castration is the same as after a spay.

Iatrogenic Urethral or Prostatic Trauma

Iatrogenic trauma to the urethra or prostate may occur during laparotomy to remove an abdominal cryptorchid testis. The complication occurs because of inadequate exposure, preventing good visualization of the testis, and/or deficient knowledge of anatomy, in which the prostate is mistaken for an abdominal testis.

Major Complications and Referral

Major complications present an entirely different set of problems, some of which may well be beyond the surgical capability of at least some animal shelters and HQHVSN clinics. Examples of these types of problems might include iatrogenic surgical trauma to the spleen, urinary tract, or gastrointestinal tract. A description of the surgical correction of these problems and others is beyond the scope of this text, partly because of the variety of potential problems that can be encountered, and partly because each complication comes with a unique set of circumstances that will dictate which remedial actions are possible, and of those possibilities, which one is the best. For example, in the case of iatrogenic ureteral trauma, possible surgical remediation options include ureteral resection and anastomosis, ureteral reimplantation, and nephrectomy. The best option would be determined by the factors in that particular situation:

patient factors, surgeon factors, and institutional factors. Therefore, in most if not all cases of major complications, it is advisable at least to consult with a surgical specialist, and in many instances to refer the case if that option is open.

Complications and the Spay–Neuter Teaching Program

No current chapter of complications in spay and neuter surgery would be complete without a discussion of complications seen during the teaching of spay and neuter to veterinary students. This is true because of two major shifts in the surgical training of veterinary students: the first being the shift to spay and neuter surgery as the primary (and in many cases the only) clinical vehicle to teach surgical skills to veterinary students; and the second, which follows logically from the first, the increasing role of animal shelters as partners with veterinary colleges and schools to provide animals, facilities, and expertise to help students acquire surgical skills. These changes mean that for many shelters, a significant proportion of the animals that are surgically sterilized are operated upon by veterinary students rather than by shelter doctor of veterinary medicine (DVM) surgeons.

Several studies have been conducted at veterinary colleges which have reported on spay and neuter complications seen with student-surgeons. In one retrospective study of shelter animals (301 cats and 201 dogs) spayed over a five-year span at a veterinary teaching hospital by third-year veterinary students, 3.3% major and 9.5% minor surgical complications were reported. The most common major complication (15/17) was abdominal wall dehiscence, and the most common minor complication was seroma formation (35/49). In another retrospective review of 1288 gonadectomies performed by second-year veterinary students, an overall rate of 8.2% of intraoperative complications, all relating to excessive hemorrhage (torn/dropped

pedicle or other causes), was reported. In canine patients the reported complication rate was 16% (Shaver et al. 2019). The complication rates reported in these studies are roughly comparable and, based on comments by the authors of the papers ("low," "very encouraging"), these rates were apparently seen in a generally positive light. However, these reported complication rates of student-surgeons do appear to be significantly higher than those seen in well-run shelter surgery programs that rely exclusively on shelter DVMs to perform all surgery.

In contrast, a large retrospective study of over 10 000 spay and neuter surgeries compared the complication rates of DVM student-surgeons and shelter veterinarians (Kreisler et al. 2018). The overall complication rates for student-surgeons (1.63%) and shelter veterinarians (1.26%) were low, and no statistical difference was seen. Careful case selection was stressed by the authors as one of the reasons for low complications among the student-surgeons in this study. Another review of 1880 spay surgeries found a direct correlation between increasing bodyweight and complication rate (Muraro and White 2014); perhaps student-surgeons should not be assigned obese patients for spay surgery, or at least not without an experienced surgeon scrubbed in to assist.

Although partnerships for student training offers benefits to the animal shelter and veterinary college (Snowden et al. 2008), such relationships also impose significant burdens and additional responsibilities on both parties (Smeak 2008; Snowden et al. 2008). While most teaching/shelter partnerships share certain common features, there are also innumerable small details that make each program unique, and broad advice is therefore of limited value. One general recommendation that can be made is that the shelter and veterinary school must make a diligent effort to discuss and agree who will train, how much intervention and when, who will treat complications, and who pays for them – and these are only a few of the details. Whether from the shelter's perspective or the veterinary school's, it is all too easy to get caught up in the perceived benefits of the relationship, and neglect to discuss and settle the negative "what ifs" beforehand. The duty to teach surgery is an enormous responsibility, because although the professional competence of the next generation of veterinary surgeons is the primary stated goal, the patient must always come first, and the balancing of these goals rests on the trainer.

Dealing with Surgical Complications – Staff and Clients

At the risk of appearing to minimize the impact of complication on the patient (always our primary concern), the impact of surgical complications *and the way they are handled with staff and clients* are almost as important and sometimes even more important to the overall mission of the animal shelter/HQHVSN clinic and its surgical sterilization program. Why is this so? Principally because in this day of universal digital photography and social media, every perceived negative outcome can be expected to be aired for all to see, inviting a rush to judgment, no matter how faulty that judgment may be. And while one could endlessly debate the pros and cons of such a level of scrutiny, the reality is that this is the environment in which veterinarians practice, and that fact is not likely to change, therefore a proactive approach is indicated. With this in mind, a few suggestions may prove useful for those who are relatively new to the field of "damage control."

First and foremost – and this really should go without saying – put the primary focus on the patient and keep it there. Make sure that everyone involved knows that the shelter or clinic is going to provide all necessary care for the patient. Sometimes this may even mean readmitting the animal to the shelter for a time, so that it can receive the care it needs. Secondly, be sympathetic and understanding in discussions with the owner/foster owner or

other caregiver – even when it is suspected that some deficiency in their care is at least partly to blame for the complication (e.g. failure to keep an Elizabethan collar on a dog, allowing self-trauma resulting in an incisional complication). Thirdly, answer any questions as fully and truthfully as possible, but do not adopt a mea culpa attitude, as if to gain sympathy. If you personally operated on the animal, you should be ready and willing to give a complete and detailed description of the procedure, including any aspects that were difficult or abnormal, and how you handled these challenges. When faced with questions about a situation in which you were not the surgeon, refuse to place blame or even speculate on potential blame. Almost always the most truthful response – "I wasn't there and I can't say" – is also the safest.

Prevention of Surgical Complications

Application of the Surgical Checklist Concept to Spay and Neuter Surgery

Recently the concept of checklists as an aid to reducing complications in surgery has gained widespread acceptance, in both human and veterinary surgery and in a number of institutions in both academia and private practice. Checklists have been proven to reduce complications in human surgical practice (Oszvald et al. 2012; Collins et al. 2014), and their efficacy at reducing perioperative and post-operative complications in veterinary medicine has also been demonstrated in the academic teaching hospital environment (Cray et al. 2018).

The basic function of a surgical checklist is to make the surgical team consciously aware of specific items relating to the procedure at hand that commonly result in complications, and ensure that the proper measures have been taken to avoid those potential problems.

There are two basic formats for checklists, the READ-DO list and the DO-CONFIRM list (Gawande 2010). The READ-DO list is administered just as the name states: each item is read from the list and then performed. This type of list is most practical when the tasks on the list are not needed until the list is read, and each task can be completed in a moment; an example would be a pre-flight checklist. The DO-CONFIRM form is appropriate when the items on the list need to be performed in advance of the time the list is read, and/or when the items take a significant amount of time to perform; this format is a more practical one for a surgical list.

The specific details of a surgical checklist will vary somewhat according to the institution; however, every well-designed checklist should have certain basic features. The checklist should be *brief*, so as not to become burdensome. In ordinary surgical situations in human medicine, it should take no more than one to two minutes to run through the checklist. In the HQHVSN or animal shelter spay–neuter scenario, with a very limited number of surgical options and rapid turnaround of cases, a more realistic time for a pre-surgical checklist would probably be closer to 30 seconds. Besides being brief, the checklist must be *relevant* – only items that will make a difference to the actions of the surgical team or that could affect the outcome are included. For example, verification of the sex of the patient is relevant, whereas exact knowledge and verification of the patient's age are probably not. The checklist must be *clear* and *simple*. Each question or statement is to worded so that it expresses a single, clear thought: What is the patient's name/ID? Do we have a signed authorization/waiver? and so on. There should be no ambiguous or open-ended questions, and most should be formatted for yes/no or other single-word responses. The checklist should be *consistent* in its administration. It should be used on every patient regardless of the perceived level of risk, just as a pre-flight checklist is used before every flight regardless of distance or flying conditions involved. The checklist should be administered by the same personnel every time. This means the same person (in most institutions probably an anesthesia technician, not the surgeon) should ask the questions, although the responses may not all come from one person.

The logical time to perform the checklist is immediately prior to an event that would be influenced by the results of the list; therefore, it is not surprising that with an important and/or complicated undertaking with multiple critical stages, more than one checklist is performed. For example, the ground crew of an aircraft will perform a final maintenance/readiness checklist before the aircraft is released to the flight crew, who in turn perform a preflight checklist before taxiing to the runway. In the same way, the benefit of checklists in a high-production surgical environment can only be maximized when a checklist is employed at each strategic juncture. For this reason, a "pre-induction" checklist should be performed just prior to induction, and then a final "pre-surgical" checklist before the actual start of the procedure.

The following is an example of the items for a pre-induction checklist for an HQHVSN clinic or animal shelter that operates an exclusively spay and neuter surgery service on a combination of client-owned and shelter-owned dogs and cats:

1) What is the name of the client and the name of the patient?
2) Has the surgical release form been signed?
3) Has the sex of the patient been verified?
4) Has the patient been fasted for the appropriate length of time (shorter for a pediatric patient)?
5) Are there any other procedures besides spay–neuter to perform, such as microchipping?
6) What is the patient's American Society of Anesthesiologists (ASA) status?
7) Are there any special anesthetic or surgical concerns or risks (e.g. cryptorchid, Doberman – Von Willebrand, etc.)?

Once the patient is on the operating table, usually after draping but before the start of the surgical procedure, a second and final checklist is performed, which may contain questions such as these or similar ones:

1) Reconfirm patient/client name? (In a large, high-volume setting with multiple patients being prepped and multiple surgeons working at the same time, this is a good idea)
2) Reconfirm procedure(s)?
3) Reproductive status (females – e.g. estrus, pregnant, pyometra)?
4) Special surgical concerns (such as unusual bleeding anticipated)?
5) Surgical gauze sponge count verified?

For convenience, both checklists can be printed on the same piece of paper. At this point it may seem redundant and burdensome to go through not one but two checklists before each surgical procedure; however, remember that the checklist is very brief, and once one is accustomed to its use, it becomes almost automatic. The author uses a similar checklist in the operating room and it takes no more than 10–15 seconds to go through the list for most patients. In a fairly busy HQHVSN surgical service in which each surgeon may perform 20–30 procedures in a day, this only adds from 3 to 7 minutes of additional time over the course of the day – a small price to pay for the security and confidence of knowing that everything is correct at the start.

Final Comments – Toward Zero Complications

This chapter began with a discussion of the incidence of surgical complications in the busy spay–neuter operating room, how the sheer volume of procedures performed virtually ensures that a certain number of complications will occur each year, and yet the perception and expectation are that nothing should ever go wrong. How does the conscientious HQHVSN surgeon reconcile these opposing positions? Through adopting a personal attitude of a continual push toward the perfect goal of zero complications, and inculcating

this culture into the clinic and shelter staff. This is not an impossible or unreasonable position. To the contrary, it is the only truly reasonable position for any veterinarian who performs surgery, for that push to perfection not only fuels improvement, but also lends significance to our work, because it is only because each outcome *is* important that we continue to strive for nothing less than a perfect outcome, every time. And this attitude in surgery can and will certainly carry over into all other aspects of the clinic or animal shelter, so that it can become what inspires an average program to become good, and a good one to become great.

How are these goals implemented? Because spay–neuter programs differ so widely with regard to the starting point in terms of performance, available resources, delivery model, and case load, the improvement program must be individualized to the individual practice. However, here are a few general suggestions:

1) Work on developing a cohesive surgical team. Hold regular short, informal meetings on relevant surgical topics – encourage everyone to contribute their thoughts. Keep it fun and positive.
2) Invest your time in training the surgical team. You are the expert, and they look to you for information and leadership.
3) Cross-train team members so that anyone can perform any function, *but* allow each staff member to find their favorite role (anesthetist, scrub nurse, post-operative care, etc.) and encourage them to develop in that area to their full potential.
4) Commit to conducting morbidity and mortality rounds on a regular schedule (monthly is good). Required attendance, DVMs and lay staff, non-punitive environment.
5) Require a post-mortem exam on any patient that dies in hospital.
6) Insist that the clinic buy excellent quality surgical instruments – the best it can afford – and then insist that everyone respect and take good care of them.

References

Cole, L.P. and Humm, K. (2019). Twelve autologous blood transfusions in eight cats with haemoperitoneum. *J. Feline Med. Surg.* 21 (6): 481–487.

Collins, S.J., Newhouse, R., Porter, J., and Talsma, A. (2014). Effectiveness of the surgical safety checklist in correcting errors: a literature review applying Reason's Swiss cheese model. *AORN J.* 100 (1): 65–79.e5. https://doi.org/10.1016/j.aorn.2013.07.024.

Cray, M.T., Selmic, L.E., McConnell, B.M. et al. (2018). Effect of implementation of a surgical safety checklist on perioperative and postoperative complications at an academic institution in North America. *Vet. Surg.* 47 (8): 1052–1065. https://doi.org/10.1111/vsu.12964.

Gawande, A. (2010). *The Checklist Manifesto: How to Get Things Right*. New York: Metropolitan Books.

Giger, U. (2011). Managing bleeding disorders (Proceedings). *dvm360* (1 October). http://veterinarycalendar.dvm360.com/managing-bleeding-disorders-proceedings (accessed 22 March 2019).

Gower, S.B., Weisse, C.W., and Brown, D.C. (2009). Major abdominal evisceration injuries in dogs and cats: 12 cases (1998–2008). *JAVMA* 234: 1566–1572.

Hamilton, K.H., Henderson, E.R., Toscano, M., and Chanoit, G.P. (2014). Comparison of postoperative complications in healthy dogs undergoing open and closed orchidectomy. *J. Small Anim. Pract.* 55 (10): 521–526. https://doi.org/10.1111/jsap.12266.

Kreisler, R.E., Shaver, S.L., and Holmes, J.H. (2018). Outcomes of elective gonadectomy procedures performed on dogs and cats by veterinary students and shelter veterinarians in a shelter environment. *JAVMA*. 253 (10): 1294–1299. https://doi.org/10.2460/javma.253.10.1294.

Muraro, L. and White, R.S. (2014). Complications of ovariohysterectomy procedures performed in 1880 dogs. *Tierarztl Prax. Ausg. K. Klientiere Heimtiere.* 42 (5): 297–302.

Oszvald, Á., Vatter, H., Byhahn, C. et al. (2012). "Team time-out" and surgical safety-experiences in 12,390 neurosurgical patients. *Neurosurg. Focus.* 33 (5): E6. https://doi.org/10.3171/2012.8.FOCUS12261.

Pearson, H. (1973). The complications of ovariohysterectomy in the bitch*. *J. Small Anim. Pract.* 14 (5): 257–266. https://doi.org/10.1111/j.1748-5827.1973.tb06457.x.

Peeters, M.E. and Kirpensteijn, J. (2011). Comparison of surgical variables and short-term postoperative complications in healthy dogs undergoing ovariohysterectomy or ovariectomy. *JAVMA* 238 (2): 189–194. https://doi.org/10.2460/javma.238.2.189.

Pollari, F.L. and Bonnett, B.N. (1996). Evaluation of postoperative complications following elective surgeries of dogs and cats at private practices using computer records. *Can. Vet. J.* 37 (6): 672–678.

Robinson, D.A., Kiefer, K., Bassett, R., and Quandt, J. (2016). Autotransfusion in dogs using a 2-syringe technique. *J. Vet. Emerg. Crit. Care* 26: 766–774.

Shaver, S.L., Larrosa, M., and Hofmeister, E.H. (2019). Factors affecting the duration of anesthesia and surgery of canine and feline gonadectomies performed by veterinary students in a year-long preclinical surgery laboratory. *Vet. Surg* https://doi.org/10.1111/vsu.13163.

Shivley, J.M., Richardson, J.M., Woodruff, K.A. et al. (2019). Sharp transection of the suspensory ligament as an alternative to digital strumming during canine ovariohysterectomy. *Vet. Surg.* 48 (2): 216–221. https://doi.org/10.1111/vsu.13121.

Smeak, D.D. (2008). Teaching veterinary students using shelter animals. *J. Vet. Med. Educ.* 35 (1): 26–30. https://doi.org/10.3138/jvme.35.1.026.

Snowden, K., Bice, K., Craig, T. et al. (2008). Vertically integrated educational collaboration between a college of veterinary medicine and a non-profit animal shelter. *J. Vet. Med. Educ.*

35 (4): 637–640. https://doi.org/10.3138/jvme.35.4.637.

Watts, J. (2018). The use of bipolar electrosurgical forceps for haemostasis in open surgical ovariectomy of bitches and queens and castration of dogs: bipolar forceps in open ovariectomy and castration. *J. Small Anim. Pract.* 59 (8): 465–473. https://doi.org/10.1111/jsap.12838.

Woodruff, K., Bushby, P.A., Rigdon-Brestle, K. et al. (2015). Scrotal castration versus prescrotal castration in dogs. *Vet. Med.* 110: 131–135.

18

Ovarian Remnant Syndrome

G. Robert Weedon and Margaret V. Root Kustritz

Ovarian remnant syndrome (ORS) is the presence of functional ovarian tissue in a previously ovariohysterectomized bitch or queen (Wallace 1991). The true incidence is not reported, likely due to subtle clinical signs in some animals, lack of pursuit of veterinary care by some owners, and lack of prospective studies. One retrospective study reported ovarian remnants in 29 of 9976 (0.3%) of feline submissions to a veterinary diagnostic laboratory and 17 of 42 401 (0.04%) of canine submissions (Miller 1995).

Causes

Reported causes are surgeon error and presence of ectopic or accessory ovarian tissue that becomes functional after removal of the main ovary; presence of such tissue has been reported in humans, cows, and cats and is considered very rare in domestic animals (McEntee 1990). However, one study (Altera and Miller 1986) reported that all of the specimens of parovarian nodules encountered during ovariohysterectomy (OHE) of 17 healthy female cats aged six months to five years were identified histologically as ectopic adrenocortical tissue (see Chapter 2), and a more recent study also failed to find any ovarian tissue in 73 feline ovarian pedicle nodules (Haase-Berglund and Premanandan 2019).

It has been demonstrated in cats that pieces of ovarian tissue sutured to the peritoneum will revascularize and become functional, causing signs of estrus (Shemwell and Weed 1970; DeNardo et al. 2001). There is no strong correlation between likelihood of ORS as a complication of OHE and years of experience of the surgeon, age of the animal at the time of OHE, or breed of the animal (Miller 1995; Ball et al. 2010). Exposure to estrogen-containing medications, including oral or topical estrogen preparations used by the owner, may cause clinical signs indicative of estrus (Schwarze and Threlfall 2008). There is one report of signs of apparent ORS due to presence of a functional adrenocortical carcinoma in a cat (Meler et al. 2011).

Avoiding Ovarian Remnant Syndrome

This condition is at its root a surgical technical problem. This complication can be avoided by obtaining adequate exposure of the ovarian pedicle to facilitate visual and/or palpable confirmation of ovarian location before ligature placement. If the surgeon has anything less than 100% certainty of complete ovarian removal, before commencing closure the removed reproductive tract should be inspected for two entire ovaries. If two complete ovaries

High-Quality, High-Volume Spay and Neuter and Other Shelter Surgeries, First Edition. Edited by Sara White.
© 2020 John Wiley & Sons, Inc. Published 2020 by John Wiley & Sons, Inc.

are not confirmed to be excised, the abdomen must be explored, beginning with the ovarian pedicles as the most likely locations. If a pedicle has been torn, an ovary or ovarian fragment may have torn free and be loose in the abdomen. Such fragments can become revascularized and cause ORS; therefore, every effort must be made to locate and remove them.

Although not technically ORS, related conditions worth noting are the rare developmental anomalies of unicornate uterus and segmental agenesis. In these patients, an isolated ovary will very likely still develop on the side which is lacking the uterine horn. This unattached ovary may be located as far cranially as the diaphragm and is easy to miss if a complete abdominal exploration is not performed.

Diagnosis

History and Physical

Duration from OHE to clinical manifestation ranges from 17 days to 9 years in cats and 1 week to 11 years in dogs (Miller 1995; Buijtels et al. 2011). The most common clinical manifestation in cats is behavioral estrus, including vocalization and lordosis, and in dogs is vulvar swelling and exudation of bloody vulvar discharge. Other reported clinical signs include mammary enlargement; pollakiuria, stranguria, or recurrent urinary tract infections; dermal hyperpigmentation, poor haircoat, or alopecia; polyuria and polydipsia; polyphagia; chronic vaginitis; and pseudopregnancy (Perkins and Frazer 1995; Pacchiana and Root Kustritz 2002; Ball et al. 2010; Gunzel-Apel et al. 2012). The month of onset may depend on the season of the year in cats; many cats first show signs of ORS starting with increasing day length in late winter or early spring, when cats at mid-latitudes resume cycling after the normal winter anestrus, an effect that becomes less evident nearer the equator.

Physical exam and history are important in the assessment of whether ORS is likely and whether further diagnostic testing and treatment are indicated. Owners or caretakers should be questioned regarding actual observed physical and behavioral signs to confirm that these signs are indicative of estrus. Not all owners are aware of the different signs of estrus in different species; for example, cat owners may believe that blood in the urine is a sign of feline estrus. Similarly, dog owners may mistake hematuria due to urinary tract infection or urolithiasis for estrus despite lack of vulvar swelling. History may also be useful in determining whether exposure to exogenous hormones is possible. Owners may be able to indicate possible sources of exposure, and may also be able to comment on the cyclicity (or lack of cyclicity) of the pet's signs of estrus.

Diagnostic Testing

Cytology

Diagnostic techniques include vaginal cytology, hormone assays, and imaging techniques. Vaginal cytology is best used when the owner perceives the bitch or queen to be in estrus. Vaginal epithelial cells can be collected with a saline-moistened cotton-tipped swab. In bitches, the swab is introduced at the dorsal commissure of the vulva and directed craniodorsally at a 45° angle. In queens, the swab is introduced to just within the lips of the vulva. The swab is rotated against the vaginal wall, withdrawn, and gently rolled onto a glass slide. The slide is stained with new methylene blue or Wright's stain. Increased serum concentrations of estrogen, produced by developing follicles on the ovarian tissue (or by exogenous sources of hormone), stimulate proliferation of stratified squamous epithelium in the vagina. Cytology representative of estrus consists of numerous cells, often clumped, the majority of which are large with irregular, folded cellular borders (Figures 18.1 and 18.2). The nuclei may be pyknotic or may fail to take up stain. Vaginal cytology has been demonstrated to be

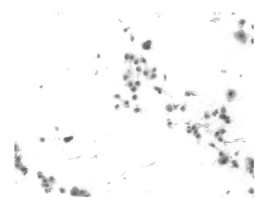

Figure 18.1 Non-cornified vaginal epithelial cells from a cat, indicative of a cat that is not under the influence of estrogen.

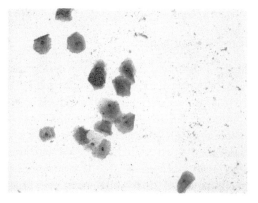

Figure 18.2 Cornified vaginal epithelial cells from a cat, indicative of a cat that is under the influence of estrogen.

supportive of the final diagnosis in a majority of animals evaluated (Wallace 1991; Perkins and Frazer 1995; Root Kustritz and Rudolph 2001; Heffelfinger 2006).

Hormone Assays

Hormones assayed include estrogen, progesterone, luteinizing hormone (LH), and anti-Mullerian hormone (AMH). Measurement of resting serum estrogen concentrations has not been consistently demonstrated to be useful. In several studies, serum estrogen concentration has been shown to be less than 20 pg/ml, the concentration indicative of functioning follicular tissue, in many animals that were

demonstrating behavioral estrus (Wallace 1991; Perkins and Frazer 1995; Ball et al. 2010). This is due to variability of sensitivity and specificity of available estrogen assays, variation in serum estrogen concentration over the estrous cycle, and relatively low absolute values even at peak serum estrogen concentrations. Vaginal cytology as a bioassay for elevated serum estrogen concentration is a more commonly used diagnostic test. Serum estrogen can be stimulated to rise in intact animals by administration of gonadotropin-releasing hormone (GnRH) or human chorionic gonadotropin (hCG). This technique is reported as a means of differentiating intact from spayed dogs and cats (Jeffcoate 1991; Jeffcoate et al. 2000; Root Kustritz and Vizecky 2002; Axner et al. 2008). There are studies demonstrating change in serum estrogen concentrations after GnRH stimulation comparing intact and spayed dogs to dogs with ORS; the rise in estrogen is lower in dogs with ORS than in intact dogs, but was considered diagnostic in some animals (Petit and Lee 1988; Ball et al. 2010).

Assay of resting progesterone concentration is not clinically useful in cats. Because cats are induced ovulators, serum progesterone concentration will not rise unless stimulated. For a progesterone assay to provide accurate assessment of presence of ovarian tissue, one must verify presence of follicular tissue by vaginal cytology, administer either GnRH (25 µg/cat intramuscularly [IM]) or hCG (50 IU/cat IM) to induce luteinization of that tissue, and assay progesterone two weeks later. Bitches are spontaneous ovulators, so stimulation testing is not required. Owners are counseled to wait until signs of estrus subside or until two to three weeks after identification of cornified vaginal epithelium by their veterinarian, and then to return the dog for serum progesterone assay. Serum progesterone concentration ≥5 ng/ml is indicative of luteal tissue and verifies the presence of ovarian tissue, which is the only tissue that can make estrogen and then make progesterone. Spontaneous or

GnRH-stimulated increase in serum progesterone concentration has been reported to be a confirmatory diagnostic test in a majority of animals in several studies (Wallace 1991; England 1997; Heffelfinger 2006).

Serum LH concentrations rise after ovariectomy and serum AMH concentrations fall after ovariectomy (Olson et al. 1992; Place et al. 2011). There is a commercially available assay for canine LH that has been demonstrated for use in differentiating intact from spayed dogs and cats (Lofstedt and VanLeeuwen 2002; Scebra and Griffin 2003). In retrospective studies, animals with ORS were documented to have serum LH concentrations greater than 1 ng/ml (Buijtels et al. 2011; Ball et al. 2010). Serum AMH assays are not readily available and results of studies to date using this technique for diagnosis of ORS are equivocal (Place et al. 2011).

Ultrasonography

Ultrasonography of the abdomen is described for diagnosis of ORS. Ovarian remnants may be visible as hyperechoic or cystic masses at the area of one or both kidneys (Sangster 2005; Ball et al. 2010). The uterine stump also should be evaluated; any increase in size suggests hormonal stimulation as would be present with a functional ovarian remnant. This technique was reported to be accurate in 9 of 12 animals in one study and in 13 of 18 dogs in another study (Ball et al. 2010; Buijtels et al. 2011). In women, ultrasonography is reported to be 93% accurate for diagnosis of ORS; this may be due to routine pre-medication with compounds that increase activity of the remnant and make it more visible (Petit and Lee 1988; Magtibay and Magrina 2006).

Treatment

ORS can be left untreated, or can be treated medically or surgically. Surgical repair is the treatment of choice.

No Treatment

Benign neglect is associated with continuing estrous cycling and associated reproductive behavior, and increased predisposition to diseases of the mammary glands and uterine stump, including stump pyometra (Demirel and Acar 2012). Historically, ovarian tissue was purposefully placed in pockets of gastric tissue in dogs to permit continuing estrus secretion without fertility (LeRoux and VanDerWalt 1977). This technique was associated with ulceration and neoplasia of tissue surrounding the implant (Davies 1989). It is possible that retention of ovarian tissue would be associated with similar sequelae.

Medical Treatment

Medical treatment consists of estrus suppression for the life of the animal. Progestogens and androgens are the classes of products most commonly described. Megestrol acetate is a progestogen and mibolerone is an androgen; these are the two products approved for estrus suppression in dogs. Neither is available as a brand-name veterinary product at this time. Megestrol acetate was never approved for long-term use in dogs. Side effects of prolonged use in dogs include polyphagia and weight gain, and mammary disease (Kutzler and Wood 2006). Megestrol acetate never was approved for estrus suppression in cats and side effects include polyphagia and weight gain, mammary hypertrophy and neoplasia, and insulin resistance and diabetes mellitus (Goericke-Pesch 2010). Side effects of prolonged use of mibolerone in dogs are clitoral hypertrophy and vaginitis, musky body odor, and mounting behavior (Kutzler and Wood 2006). Mibolerone never was approved for use in cats because the effective dose for estrus suppression nears the toxic dose, and use is associated with thyroid and hepatic disease (Burke 1978). Other non-surgical therapies that are described but are not yet readily available include use of immuno-contraceptive vaccines, treatment with GnRH agonists or antagonists, and, in cats, melatonin implants (Kutzler and Wood 2006; Goericke-Pesch 2010). Because of possible side effects associated with leaving the retained tissue in place and because there are no safe long-term medical therapies available for estrus suppression at this time, surgical therapy strongly is recommended.

Surgical Treatment

Exploratory laparotomy can be performed when the animal is in behavioral estrus, in which case the surgeon is looking for follicular tissue, or two to three weeks after spontaneous or induced luteinization, in which case the surgeon is looking for luteal tissue. The advantage of the latter is that there may be less bleeding during diestrus, due to lower serum estrogen concentrations, and corpora lutea persist longer than follicles. However, most surgeons find it much easier to locate remnant ovarian tissue when the exploratory surgery is carried out during behavioral estrus (Figure 18.3). The residual tissue almost always is at one or both ovarian pedicles (Wallace 1991; Miller 1995; Evers et al. 1996; England 1997; Sangster 2005), but may be found elsewhere in the abdomen or even in the body wall or subcutaneous layer of the original incision. If no obvious ovarian tissue is present, granulation tissue at the ovarian pedicles should be removed. Occasionally, entire ovaries may be found. Another reported finding is absence of the kidney and ureter on the same side on which an ovary or remnant is found (England 1997). Retrospective studies

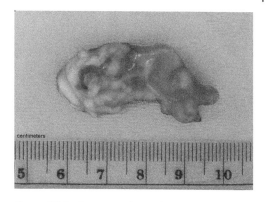

Figure 18.3 Large, cystic ovarian remnant from a cat with intermittent signs of behavioral estrus. *Source:* Photo courtesy of Brenda Griffin.

disagree as to the most common location of unilateral remnants; most studies report that unilateral ovarian remnants are found more consistently on the right side (Wallace 1991; Miller 1995; Ball et al. 2010).

All ovarian tissue removed should be submitted for histopathology. Reported findings include follicles and follicular cysts, solid and cystic corporea lutea, paraovarian cysts, and tumors including granulosa cell tumors, cystadenomas, and teratomas (Wallace 1991; Ball et al. 2010; Gunzel-Apel et al. 2012). If the uterine stump is enlarged, it also should be resected and submitted for histopathology. Reported findings at the uterine stump include cystic endometrial hyperplasia, pyometra, and neoplasia (Root Kustritz and Rudolph 2001; Ball et al. 2010; Anderson and Pratschke 2011). Prognosis for decline in clinical signs after complete removal of all abnormal tissue is excellent.

References

Altera, K.P. and Miller, L.N. (1986). Recognition of feline parovarian nodules as ectopic adrenocortical tissue. *JAVMA* 189 (1): 71–72.

Anderson, C. and Pratschke, K. (2011). Uterine adenocarcinoma with abdominal metastases in an ovariohysterectomised cat. *J. Feline Med. Surg.* 13: 44–47.

Axner, E., Gustavsson, T., and Strom Holst, B. (2008). Estradiol measurement after GnRH-stimulation as a method to diagnose the presence of ovaries in the female domestic cat. *Theriogenology* 70: 186–191.

Ball, R.L., Birchard, S.J., May, L.R. et al. (2010). Ovarian remnant syndrome in dogs and cats: 21 cases (2000–2007). *JAVMA* 236: 548–553.

Buijtels, J.J.C.W.M., DeGier, J., Kooistra, H.S. et al. (2011). The pituitary-ovarian axis in dogs with remnant ovarian tissue. *Theriogenology* 75: 742–751.

Burke, T.J. (1978). Mibolerone studies in the cat. *Proceedings, Symposium on Cheque™ for canine estrus prevention*, Augusta, MI.

Davies, N.L. (1989). Complications of ovarian autotransplantation in bitches. *J. S. Afr. Vet. Assoc.* 60: 145.

Demirel, M.A. and Acar, D.B. (2012). Ovarian remnant syndrome and uterine stump pyometra in three queens. *J. Feline Med. Surg.* 14: 913–918.

DeNardo, G.A., Becker, K., Brown, N.O. et al. (2001). Ovarian remnant syndrome: revascularization of free-floating ovarian tissue in the female abdominal cavity. *J. Am. Anim. Hosp. Assoc.* 37: 290–296.

England, G.C.W. (1997). Confirmation of ovarian remnant syndrome in the queen using hCG administration. *Vet. Rec.* 141: 309–310.

Evers, P., Kramek, B.A., and Root, M.V. (1996). Intestinal pseudodiverticulosis in a cat. *J. Am. Anim. Hosp. Assoc.* 32: 291–293.

Goericke-Pesch, S. (2010). Reproduction control in cats: new developments in non-surgical methods. *J. Feline Med. Surg.* 12: 539–546.

Gunzel-Apel, A.-R., Buschhaus, J., Urhausen, C. et al. (2012). Clinical signs, diagnostic approach and therapy regarding the ovarian remnant syndrome in the bitch. *Tierarztl. Prax.* 40 (K): 35–42.

Haase-Berglund, M.L. and Premanandan, C.L. (2019). Histologic evaluation of parovarian nodules in the cat. Submitted to *J. Feline Med. Surg.*

Heffelfinger, D.J. (2006). Ovarian remnant in a 2-year-old queen. *Can. Vet. J.* 47: 165–167.

Jeffcoate, I.A. (1991). Identification of spayed bitches. *Vet. Rec.* 129: 58.

Jeffcoate, I.A., McBride, M., Harvey, M.J. et al. (2000). Measurement of plasma oestradiol after an injection of a gonadotrophin as a test for neutered bitches. *Vet. Rec.* 146: 599.

Kutzler, M. and Wood, A. (2006). Non-surgical methods of contraception and sterilization. *Theriogenology* 66: 514–525.

LeRoux, P.H. and VanDerWalt, L.A. (1977). Ovarian autograft as an alternative to ovariectomy in bitches. *J. S. Afr. Vet. Assoc.* 48: 117–123.

Lofstedt, R.M. and VanLeeuwen, J.A. (2002). Evaluation of a commercially available luteinizing hormone test for its ability to distinguish between ovariectomized and sexually intact bitches. *JAVMA* 220: 1331–1335.

Magtibay, P.M. and Magrina, J.F. (2006). Ovarian remnant syndrome. *Clin. Obstetr. Gynecol.* 49: 526–534.

McEntee, K. (1990). The ovary. In: *Reproductive Pathology of Domestic Mammals* (ed. M. McEntee), 31–51. San Diego, CA: Academic Press.

Meler, E.N., Scott-Moncrieff, C., Peter, A.T. et al. (2011). Cyclic estrous-like behavior in a spayed cat associated with excessive sex-hormone production by an adrenocortical carcinoma. *J. Feline Med. Surg.* 13: 473–478.

Miller, D.M. (1995). Ovarian remnant syndrome in dogs and cats: 46 cases (1988–1992). *J. Vet. Diagn. Invest.* 7: 572–574.

Olson, P.N., Mulnix, J.A., and Nett, T.M. (1992). Concentrations of luteinizing hormone and follicle-stimulating hormone in the serum of sexually intact and neutered dogs. *Am. J. Vet. Res.* 53: 762–766.

Pacchiana, P.D. and Root Kustritz, M.V. (2002). Theriogenology question of the month: ovarian remnant in a dog. *JAVMA* 220: 1465–1467.

Perkins, N.R. and Frazer, G.S. (1995). Ovarian remnant syndrome in a toy poodle: a case report. *Theriogenology* 44: 307–312.

Petit, P.D.M. and Lee, R.A. (1988). Ovarian remnant syndrome. Diagnostic dilemma and surgical challenge. *Obstetr. Gynecol.* 71: 580–583.

Place, N.J., Hansen, B.S., Cheraskin, J.-L. et al. (2011). Measurement of serum anti-Mullerian hormone concentration in female dogs and cats before and after ovariohysterectomy. *J. Vet. Diagn. Invest.* 23: 524–527.

Root Kustritz, M.V. and Rudolph, K.D. (2001). Theriogenology question of the month: ovarian remnant in a cat. *JAVMA* 219: 1065–1066.

Root Kustritz, M.V. and Vizecky, K.L. (2002). Theriogenology question of the month: determination of intact status of a dog. *JAVMA* 221: 199–200.

Sangster, C. (2005). Ovarian remnant syndrome in a 5-year-old bitch. *Can. Vet. J.* 46: 62–64.

Scebra, L.R. and Griffin, B. (2003). Evaluation of a commercially available luteinizing hormone test to distinguish between ovariectomized and sexually intact queens. *Proceedings, ACVIM Forum*, Charlotte, NC. http://www.vin.com/members/proceedings/proceedings.plx?CID=advim2003&PID=pr04197&0=VIN (accessed 3 January 2013).

Schwarze, R.A. and Threlfall, W.R. (2008). Theriogenology question of the month: persistent estrus due to exposure to human topical estrogen preparation in a dog. *JAVMA* 233: 235–237.

Shemwell, R.E. and Weed, J.C. (1970). Ovarian remnant syndrome. *Obstetr. Gynecol.* 36: 299–303.

Wallace, M.S. (1991). The ovarian remnant syndrome in the bitch and queen. *Vet. Clin. N. Am. Small Anim. Pract.* 21: 501–507.

Section Four

Other Surgical Procedures

Introduction to Other Surgical Procedures

Philip Bushby

While ovariohysterectomy and castration are the mainstay of shelter surgery for the purpose of population control, many other surgical procedures may have a significant role in shelter animal care. Procedures such as enucleation, cherry eye surgery, and amputation may not only make the patient more comfortable, but may also make an unadoptable animal highly adoptable. Other procedures that can be performed in a shelter surgery setting may save the animal's life or significantly improve the animal's health.

Surgeries performed in the shelter environment must, at a minimum, meet the standards described in the Association of Shelter Veterinarians' 2016 Veterinary Medical Care Guidelines for Spay-Neuter Programs (Griffin et al. 2016). As for all surgeries, only medical-grade suture should be used and separate sterile instruments should be used for each

surgical procedure. Cold sterilization should not be used for any surgical procedure. Protocols must be in place to ensure proper cleaning and disinfection of the suite and equipment, and anesthetic and monitoring equipment appropriate for the surgeries to be performed should be functional and routinely maintained. An up-to-date crash cart should be present and staff should be fully trained in the use of emergency drugs and emergency procedures (Bushby 2013).

The types of surgeries that can be performed in the shelter environment are dependent upon the skill level of the veterinary surgeon, the specialized equipment that is available, and financial resources of the shelter. The surgeries described in the following chapters are all considered to be surgeries that can be performed in the shelter setting.

References

Bushby, P.A. (2013). Surgical techniques for spay/neuter. In: *Shelter Medicine for Veterinarians and Staff*, 2e (eds. L. Miller and Z. Stephen), 625–646. Ames, IA: Wiley-Blackwell.

Griffin, B., Bushby, P.A., McCobb, E. et al. (2016). The Association of Shelter Veterinarians' 2016 veterinary medical care guidelines for spay-neuter programs. *JAVMA* 249: 165–188.

19

Amputation
Joseph P. Weigel

Amputation for management of fracture trauma in the shelter animal is a life-saving option where primary treatment often demands resources that are not available in most shelters. While the veterinarian may prefer to treat the trauma and restore the animal to full function, the reality is that amputation has become an attractive alternative in the shelter animal, where a homeless amputee generates more compassion from the general public than for a normal animal and is therefore more likely to be adopted. However, the decision for amputation in the shelter environment still relies heavily on humane concerns and the expectation of a good quality of life. While there is increasing interest in the use of limb prostheses, the current practice of limb replacement remains experimental, so specialized amputation techniques do not apply to this discussion. Therefore, techniques described here are traditional, but are presented in a condensed format with a logical dissection sequence that conserves time and lessens post-operative complications.

Since trauma is the most likely reason for an amputation, the level of amputation is determined by convenience and cosmetics as opposed to the extent of disease. Other considerations such as the order of vessel ligation are not as important; however, as a general rule, the ligation of the arterial before the venous side allows for drainage of blood from the limb,

preserving blood volume. This can be helpful, especially if fluid loss is a potential risk. Location and resection of regional lymph nodes are not an issue in the trauma case, but may be important in the diseased or infected limb.

Gait adaptation and function in the amputee is always a concern for the veterinary surgeon. Fortunately, most animals will adapt well to a missing limb. However, this is dependent on the health of the remaining limbs. Attention to the condition of the contralateral limb is an obvious concern, but the condition of the all the limbs is important. After force platform gait analysis of dogs with an amputated rear limb, Hogy et al. found increases in the peak breaking forces in the contralateral front limb and increased propulsive forces and impulses in both the ipsilateral front limb and the remaining rear limb. Also, time to peak braking force was decreased, while the time to peak propulsive force was increased in all remaining limbs. Evaluation of spatial kinematic data by Hogy et al. on rear limb amputees demonstrated an increase in the range of motion of the remaining hock joint, the cervicothoracic and thoracolumbar spine, and an increased extension of the lumbosacral spine (Hogy et al. 2013).

In general, the loss of either a front or rear limb results in greater ground reaction force and impulse in the remaining limbs and in changes in the body's center of gravity, but

High-Quality, High-Volume Spay and Neuter and Other Shelter Surgeries, First Edition. Edited by Sara White.
© 2020 John Wiley & Sons, Inc. Published 2020 by John Wiley & Sons, Inc.

these changes are more pronounced in the amputee with a missing front limb (Kirpensteijn et al. 2000). This may be the result of the biomechanical reality that the quadruped animal is balanced on four legs, with 60% of the weight bearing focused on the front limbs (Gillette 2004). With one front limb missing, Jarvis et al. found a 14% increase in weight bearing on the remaining front limb and a combined 17% increase in weight bearing on the rear limbs (Jarvis et al. 2013). This study also described changes in the action of the other limbs, where there is increased flexion in the remaining carpus and ipsilateral hip and stifle joints, suggesting that the health of all these joints will contribute to the ability to compensate and function with a missing front limb.

Jarvis et al. also described changes in the motion of the spine, with an increase in the range of motion of the joints of the cervicothoracic and thoracolumbar spine in the sagittal plane and an increase in flexion of the lumbosacral spine. These findings would suggest that disease of the spine also has the potential to frustrate the animal's ability to compensate for a missing forelimb. With one front leg missing, the dog advances forward by first leaning back on the rear limbs and from that position propelling the trunk forward, allowing the remaining front limb to advance and catch the weight as the trunk falls back toward the ground. Increases in the vertical impulse and propulsive forces of the remaining limbs become the new normal for the remaining joints. If the remaining limbs are healthy, the adaptation is effective, but if the remaining front limb is diseased or if the rear limbs are affected by hip dysplasia, cranial cruciate instability, or patellar luxation, recovery could be prolonged and adaptation less effective. However, orthopedic disease in the remaining legs is not a certain contraindication to amputation and that each case should be evaluated on its own merits.

This chapter describes surgical techniques for amputation. For anesthetic considerations during amputation, see Chapter 19A.

Front Limb Amputation

Front limb amputation by scapular disarticulation is quicker and more cosmetic than shoulder disarticulation (Seguin and Weigel 2012). Several disadvantages to scapular disarticulation have been considered, including an increase in the vulnerability of more serious injury following blunt force trauma to the thorax, and the additional risk of inadvertent penetration of the pleural cavity during dissection over the axillary space. Over the ribs, the scapula adds an additional layer of protection to the thorax, but removal of the scapula has not been associated with increased injury to thoracic contents or death. Penetration of the pleural cavity in the axillary space during scapular disarticulation is possible; however, moderate care in the dissection should avoid this problem, and if it occurs but is promptly recognized, closure of the pleural space is not difficult.

Other options such as shoulder disarticulation and mid-humeral separations of the front leg have been reported (Leighton and Borzio 1975; Bone and Aberman 1988). The shoulder disarticulation technique is hampered by the potential for more hemorrhage due to the complexity of the vascular supply that surrounds the joint, and by additional surgical time consumed in dissecting a complex arrangement of ligaments, tendons, tendon sheaths, bursas, and synovial attachments associated with the joint. A mid-humeral amputation is simple in regard to the surgical anatomy, but the cosmetic effect for some is objectionable when a severed brachial appendage is moved about with no apparent functional purpose. However, in the cat, a mid-diaphyseal humeral amputation is sometimes functional, as the cat learns to use the foreshortened front limb during play, which for the owner lessens the emotional impact of the loss of the limb. In the final analysis, scapular disarticulation is the technique that should meet the needs of the shelter in terms of a cost-effective and time-efficient procedure resulting in an adoptable pet.

Scapular Disarticulation

The skin incision begins near the dorsal border of the scapula and follows the spine of the scapula to the level of the shoulder joint, where it swings around the limb from the cranial aspect to the medial side and then to the caudal, ending laterally where the circular incision was initiated (Figure 19.1). There is a desire in some surgeons to suspend the depth of the skin incision to the subcutaneous layer, so that the skin can be bluntly separated from the subcutaneous fascia and retracted in order to identify the deep muscles; however, this technique leaves surgical dead space immediately under the skin, which cannot be easily closed, leading to the formation of post-operative seromas. Instead, the skin incision is carried down to the deep fascia. At this depth, the subcutaneous layer can be bluntly separated from the deep fascia, which allows for visualization of the deep muscles. The resulting dead space is located between the deep fascia and the subcutaneous layers, where absorption of serous fluid is better, as opposed to the subcutaneous and skin layers, where serous fluid is more likely to accumulate and drain. An additional advantage of this approach comes with the capability of reducing skin tension by using the fascia of the subcutaneous layer to pull the skin edges together.

The amputation of a limb is a progressive dissection beginning at a starting point, traveling around the limb, and ending back at the original point. Recognizing a pattern to the execution of an amputation is a helpful concept in guiding the surgeon's progress through a complex anatomic dissection. A unique pattern for each major amputation constitutes a "road map" of the technique. In the case of scapular disarticulation, the road map covers four regions of the dissection, beginning with Phase I, the lateral dissection; continuing with Phase II, the dorsal dissection; followed by Phase III, the medial dissection; and ending with Phase IV, the ventral dissection (Figure 19.2).

Phase I: Lateral Dissection

To detach the scapula and front limb of a dog or cat, the dissection begins on the lateral side at the level of the acromion, where the

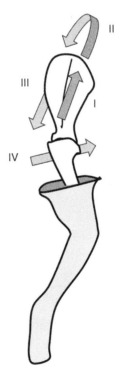

Figure 19.2 Road map for scapular disarticulation.

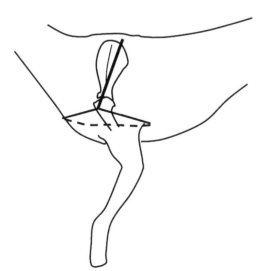

Figure 19.1 Skin incision for scapular disarticulation.

insertion of the omotransversarius muscle is incised from the spine of the scapula. This is followed by identifying and incising the insertion of the trapezius from the scapular spine (Figure 19.3).

Phase II: Dorsal Dissection

The objective of this phase is to release the dorsal border of the scapula such that it can be abducted from the chest wall, exposing the anatomy of the deep axillary space (Figure 19.4). This phase begins at the dorsal

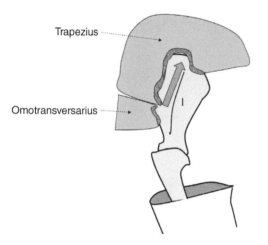

Figure 19.3   Phase I: lateral dissection for scapular disarticulation.

border of the scapula, where the insertion of the rhomboideus muscle is separated from the bone, which is followed by sub-periosteal lifting of the insertion of the serratus ventralis muscle from the medial surface of the scapula. The scapula can be abducted from the chest wall, but it is insufficient for safe dissection of the axillary space until the latissimus dorsi muscle is released several centimeters caudal to the teres tuberosity of the humerus. The dorsal border of the latissimus dorsi muscle is located caudal to the scapula and near the level of the dorsal border of the scapula. This border of the muscle is followed distally to the axillary space, where it is transected near the teres tuberosity. Technically the latissimus dorsi transection is not dorsal, but it is included in the Phase II dissection since the objective in this phase is full abduction of the scapula, which requires the distal myotomy of the latissimus dorsi muscle. Included with this myotomy is the identification of thoracodorsal artery and vein, which are ligated and divided along with the thoracodorsal nerve, which is infiltrated with local anesthetic and divided. The axillary lymph node is located in this general area and can be removed if necessary. The neurovascular structures of the axillary space are now adequately exposed for division.

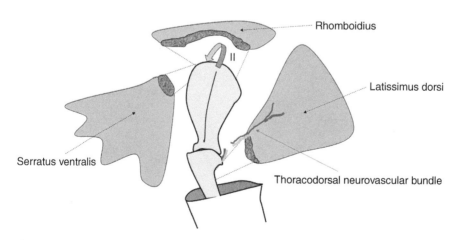

Figure 19.4   Phase II: dorsal dissection for scapular disarticulation.

Phase III: Medial Dissection

This phase involves the isolation and division of the neurovascular structures to the front limb (Figure 19.5). The major nerves from the brachial plexus are infiltrated with local anesthetic proximally and then sharply divided distal to the infiltration. The brachial artery is identified and ligated with an encircling ligature of a synthetic absorbable suture, followed just distally by a transfixing ligature. An additional encircling ligature is placed on the artery further distally. The artery is divided between this most distal ligature and the transfixing ligature. There are two major veins spanning across the axillary space, the axillobrachial and brachial veins. Each vein must be isolated, ligated, and divided. Two encircling ligatures of a synthetic absorbable suture are applied and the vein is divided between them. It is not necessary to apply transfixing ligatures to these veins.

Phase IV: Ventral Dissection

The road map for scapular disarticulation ends with incision of the insertion of the superficial and deep pectoral muscles and a mid-belly division of the brachiocephalicus muscle (Figure 19.6).

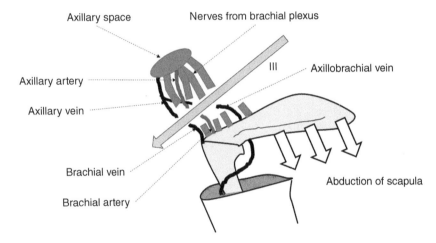

Figure 19.5   Phase III: medial dissection for scapular disarticulation.

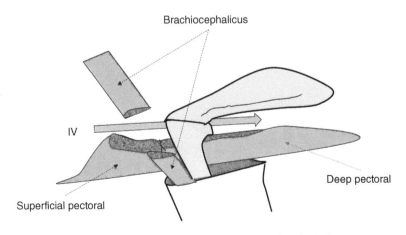

Figure 19.6   Phase IV: ventral dissection for scapular disarticulation.

Closure is preceded by a thorough inspection of the wound for any active hemorrhage. Once hemorrhage is controlled and the wound has been lightly flushed, closure begins with the objective of bringing the major muscles together closing dead space, apposing cut surfaces, and providing a tissue cushion for underlying bone and overlying skin. While the cut surfaces of the muscles are apposed for quick healing, muscular "anastomosis" is not the primary objective, because muscle function is not a consideration. Where tension is not present, the muscle can be apposed in an interrupted or continuous inverting pattern. The inverting pattern rolls the cut surface of the muscle toward the deeper aspects of the wound. Serous exudation from the raw edges of the incised muscles drains to the deeper levels of the wound, where absorption is more efficient than allowing serous fluid to drain toward the skin and the surface, where seromas form and drain through the skin incision.

Following amputation by scapular disarticulation, the closure objective is to gently pull the muscles across the axillary space, covering the severed neurovascular structures and the axillary space (Figure 19.7). This is initiated by bringing the latissimus dorsi muscle cranial and suturing it to the omotransversarius and trapezius muscles. The pectoral muscles are brought proximally and apposed to the scalenius and the available portion of the ventral border of the latissimus muscle. The remaining brachiocephalicus muscle is brought caudally and attached to the latissimus or pectoral muscles. Synthetic absorbable sutures are recommended.

The subcutaneous layer, which is still connected to the skin, is closed in the pattern intended for the skin. In the case of scapular disarticulation, the subcutaneous layer can be closed in an inverted "T" pattern that parallels the original skin incision, or as an alternative the corner of the caudal flap can be brought cranially, converting the incision into a "C"-shaped pattern. The surgeon should choose a pattern that has minimal tension and has the fewest sutured right angles (Figure 19.8).

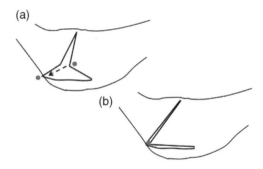

Figure 19.8 (a) The inverted "T" incision. (b) Bring the corners designated by red dots together, converting to a "C"-shaped closure.

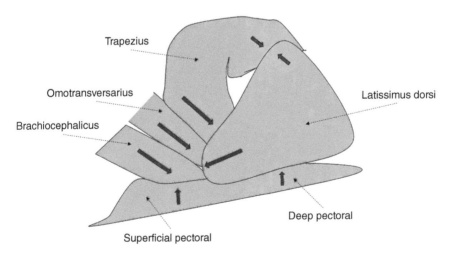

Figure 19.7 Muscle closure for scapular disarticulation.

Synthetic absorbable sutures are also recommended for this layer.

The skin can be closed with non-absorbable suture in a variety of patterns, both continuous and interrupted. Simple interrupted sutures will provide a more accurate closure of the skin and are recommended. Skin closure can also be facilitated by placing single interrupted sutures at strategic points along the incision to reduce tension, and will also help to prevent the accumulation of excess skin on one side or the other at the end of closure.

Post-operative Care/Rehabilitation

Rehabilitation of the post-operative amputee involves protection of the incision, checking for seroma formation, assisting the patient in early ambulation, maintaining hydration, and controlling pain. Cold therapy (ice packing), laser therapy, and ultrasound heat can be helpful in reducing post-operative swelling and pain. The services of a trained veterinary therapist would be advantageous to the shelter, especially if the surgery load is high. Therapists can shorten the recovery period, which can speed up the adoption process. Also, the application of body slings with handles will make movement of the animal easier and less painful. These devices also assist in early ambulation, especially in those animals that are overweight or have osteoarthritis in the other limbs. Also see chapter 19A for more information on intra- and post-operative analgesia for amputations.

Rear Limb Amputation

Amputation of the rear limb is common (Seguin and Weigel 2012), but fortunately the quadruped animal can easily adjust to a missing rear limb, especially when compared to the adjustment for a missing front limb. Division of the rear limb through the thigh is the easiest and quickest route to a functional amputation. Hip disarticulation is complicated and time consuming, carrying with it the same difficul-

ties as described for a shoulder disarticulation. Similar to the front limb, the most common indication for amputation is traumatic injury that cannot be physically repaired for reasonable pain-free function or would be cost prohibited for treatment.

In the case of a mid-thigh amputation, the femur is transected where the proximal and middle thirds of the shaft meet. This will provide sufficient structure to the stump and allow complete coverage of the bone by muscle flaps. It is also possible to extract the entire femur from the stump by advancing the dissection proximally up the shaft of the bone, severing the attachments of the adductor, gluteal, pelvic association, and quadriceps muscle groups directly from the bone. At the level of the hip joint the capsule is sharply separated from the bone, allowing the femoral head to be distracted from the acetabulum. In this position the ligament of the head of the femur can be transected by a curved Mayo blunt scissors. In the author's opinion there is no advantage to removal of the entire femur, unless there is the elimination of an abnormality that could cause persistent pain post-operatively, such as a dislocated hip.

A quadruped animal can compensate well following a single rear limb amputation, since the balance of weight bearing is located toward the front end of the body. This compensation can be so efficient that some rear leg amputees will successfully participate in canine athletic events. However, the walk remains abnormal where the contralateral rear limb "jumps" forward in order to advance the rear. This lameness is not caused by pain, but by mechanical adjustments necessary for effective motion. Compensation is not only dependent on the orthopedic soundness of the contralateral leg, but also on the soundness of the front legs. Therefore, the prognosis should be determined by an overall assessment of musculoskeletal integrity and conditioning.

The skin incision for the mid-thigh amputation is made through the skin and subcutaneous tissue, beginning in the flank, and is curved distally to the patella, along the lateral stifle, and then redirected proximally toward the tuber ischium, to end at a point at the same level as the beginning point in the flank. A medial skin incision is made as a mirror image of the lateral flap, but extending no more than halfway distal in the thigh (Figure 19.9). The lateral flap is thicker and with more hair than the medial flap and is better suited for exposure to the exterior, so the lateral flap should be long enough to be folded around the stump and sutured to the medial flap.

The road map for a mid-thigh amputation is circular, beginning on the medial side and progressing to cranial to lateral, and finally back to the medial side (Figure 19.10).

Phase I: Medial Dissection

Once the skin is incised, the leg is abducted and the medial dissection is begun. The caudal sarto-

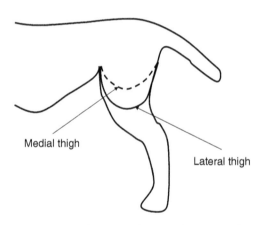

Figure 19.9   Skin incision for mid-thigh amputation.

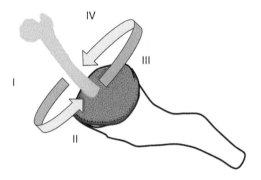

Figure 19.10   Road map for mid-thigh amputation.

rius muscle is identified and transected at the same level as the skin incision. The gracilis muscle is transected parallel to the medial skin flap, but slightly distal to the flap. The femoral artery and vein are now exposed in the femoral triangle and are ligated with an absorbable synthetic material and then divided. The artery is clamped and ligated, first with a circumferential ligature, followed by a transfixation ligature applied just distal to the original ligature. The artery is ligated again with a circumferential suture distal to the transfixing ligature and then divided between the transfixation ligature and the last, most distal ligature. The vein is similarly ligated and transected, but without the transfixation ligature. The pectineus muscle is transected through its long tendon of insertion on the femur, completing the medial dissection (Figure 19.11).

Phase II: Cranial Dissection

The caudal border of the cranial sartorius muscle is identified and followed to the patella. The stifle joint is then entered, exposing the patella and the quadriceps insertion. The insertion is incised through the parapatellar fibrocartilage immediately proximal to the bone (Figure 19.12). No muscle is cut, only the fibrous insertion. The leg is adducted and Phase III, lateral dissection, is commenced.

Phase III: Lateral Dissection

The deep incision of Phase II is continued through the biceps femoris muscle, while following the lateral skin incision to the caudal border of the thigh. The lateral tissues of the thigh, including the skin, subcutaneous layer, and the biceps femoris muscle that are proximal to the incision, are retracted proximally, exposing the sciatic nerve, which is infused with local anesthetic and transected distal to the infused region (Figure 19.13).

Phase IV: Caudal Dissection

The semitendinosus, semimembranosus, and adductor muscles are severed by a sharp

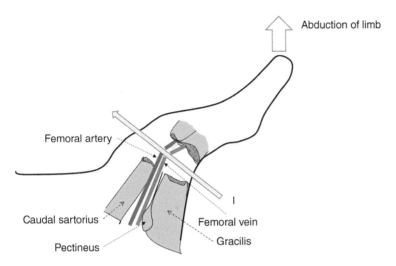

Figure 19.11   Phase I: medial dissection for mid-thigh amputation.

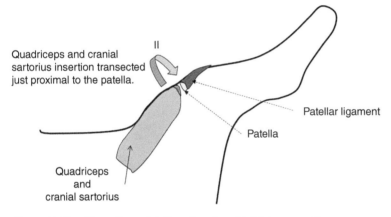

Figure 19.12   Phase II: cranial dissection for mid-thigh amputation.

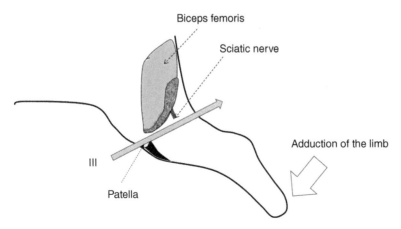

Figure 19.13   Phase III: lateral dissection for mid-thigh amputation.

incision across the muscle belly at midlevel from caudal to cranial (Figure 19.14). The adductor muscle is lifted from the proximal femur to the level of the distal extent of the greater trochanter. The remaining soft tissue is gently freed from the femur with a gauze sponge, by sliding the sponge proximally along the femur to the distal level of both the greater and lesser trochanters. At the junction of the proximal and middle thirds of the femoral shaft, a transverse osteotomy of the femur is done with a gigli wire, completing the amputation (Figure 19.15).

Closure

The quadriceps is folded in a caudal direction and sutured to the hamstring group using absorbable synthetic material (Figure 19.16). The gracilis and biceps femoris muscles are brought together and sutured in an interrupted cross-mattress pattern (Figure 19.17). The subcutaneous tissue and skin are closed in a routine fashion.

Post-operative Care/Rehabilitation

Bandages are not routinely applied. Ice packing would be helpful to prevent swelling at a

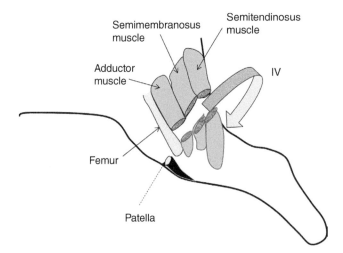

Figure 19.14 Phase IV: caudal dissection for mid-thigh amputation.

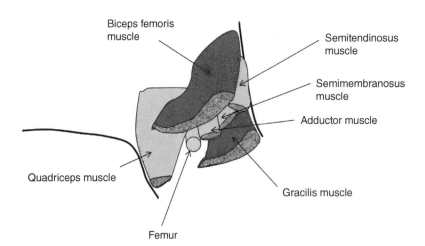

Figure 19.15 Completed dissection for mid-thigh amputation.

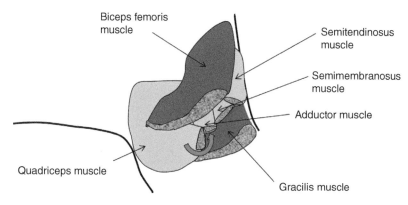

Figure 19.16   Closure is initiated by bringing the quadriceps caudally and suturing to the adductor or the semimembranosus or semitendinosus muscle.

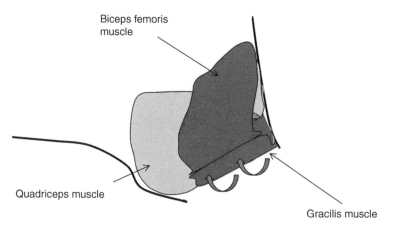

Figure 19.17   Closure is continued by bringing the gracilis to the biceps femoris muscle.

prescribed protocol of 2–3 times a day for about 10–15 minutes each time. Icing is reduced or eliminated by 3–4 days post-operatively. Heat therapy is not necessary. If the animal is overweight, then weight reduction plans should be included as part of the rehabilitation.

Amputation of the Tail

In general, the amputation of the tail should be intervertebral as opposed to transvertebral. The target disc space is identified with a hypodermic needle passed through the space. The tail is extended and a dorsal flap is prepared by beginning the skin incision on the lateral side of the tail at the level of the target disc, and proceeding in a caudodorsal direction, the

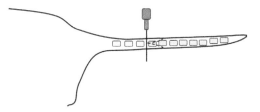

Figure 19.18   Tail amputation.

length of one vertebra to the dorsum of the tail. At the dorsum of the tail, the incision is curved and advanced in a cranioventral direction onto the contralateral side of the tail, ending at the level of the target disc. As a mirror image of the dorsal incision, a second incision is made on the ventral portion of the tail, preparing a ventral flap (Figure 19.18). The skin is not lifted from the underlying soft tissue, but the underlying soft tissue is lifted from the bone, keeping the skin naturally attached to the deep soft tissue layers. If the ventral coccygeal artery is encountered and hemorrhage cannot be controlled with cautery, a single circumferential ligature around the vessel is adequate for control. After lifting the soft tissue to the target disc space, the tail is severed through the disc. The deep tissues are gently positioned over the end of the vertebra. There should be minimal tension; however, if the tension requires mattress sutures, the amputation should be advanced to the next cranial disc space without any additional incision or removal of soft tissue. Once the soft tissue layer has been closed over the bone, the skin flaps are brought together and closed with interrupted sutures.

References

Bone, D.L. and Aberman, H.M. (1988). *Forelimb amputation in the dog. J. Am. Anim. Hosp. Assoc.* 24: 525.

Gillette, R. (2004). *Gait Analysis*. In: *Canine Rehabilitation and Physical Therapy* (eds. D. Millis, D. Levine and R.A. Taylor), 205. St. Louis, MO: Saunders.

Hogy, S.M., Worley, D.R., Jarvis, S.L. et al. (2013 Sep). *Kinematic and kinetic analysis of dogs during trotting after amputation of a pelvic limb. Am. J. Vet. Res.* 74 (9): 1164–1171.

Jarvis, S.L., Worley, D.R., Hogy, S.M. et al. (2013 Sep). *Kinematic and kinetic analysis of dogs during trotting after amputation of a thoracic limb 2nd. Am. J. Vet. Res.* 74 (9): 1155–1163.

Kirpensteijn, J., van den Bos, R., van den Brom, W.E., and Hazewinkel, H.A. (2000 Feb 5). *Ground reaction force analysis of large breed dogs when walking after the amputation of a limb. Vet. Rec.* 146 (6): 155–159.

Leighton, R.L. and Borzio, F. (1975). *Amputation of the foreleg of the dog*. In: *Current Techniques in Small Animal Surgery* (ed. Bojrab MJ), 491. Philadelphia, PA: Lea and Febiger.

Seguin, B. and Weigel, J.P. (2012). *Amputations*. In: *Veterinary Surgery Small Animal* (eds. K.M. Tobias and S.A. Johnston), 1031–1034. St. Louis, MO: Saunders.

19A

Amputation: Anesthesia Supplement
Lydia Love

Amputation of a limb or the tail may be indicated following traumatic injury to soft tissue or bone, as a result of severe congenital deformity, or in the treatment of certain neoplastic diseases. These procedures are invasive, painful, and can be associated with clinically significant fluid and blood losses. Injuries requiring amputation may be accompanied by damage to other organ systems and trauma patients may require stabilization prior to anesthesia. Pre-anesthetic evaluation of the patient should include rigorous examination of the cardiac, respiratory, and nervous systems, as well as assessment of fluid balance and the patient's level of pain. Suggested minimum baseline hematologic information should include packed cell volume and total protein concentration. If possible, a platelet count (or subjective evaluation of a blood smear) should be performed and electrolyte concentrations evaluated. If neoplasia is the reason for amputation or the patient is aged, more extensive diagnostics and clinical staging should be considered.

Anesthetic Concerns for Limb and Tail Amputation

Peri-operative concerns for limb and tail amputation center on appropriate monitoring and supportive care. General anesthesia frequently results in hypotension, hypoventilation, and hypothermia, unless supportive measures are taken to counteract these adverse events. Fluid shifts associated with amputation can be dramatic, especially with the removal of a limb, and clinically significant hemorrhage can also occur. With forelimb amputation, the possibility of hemorrhage into the chest cavity from the brachial artery should be considered. A balanced isotonic fluid should be infused intravenously and blood pressure monitored and maintained (mean arterial pressure >60 mmHg). Any blood loss should be estimated and acute hemorrhage (≥20% of calculated blood volume) may require transfusion of blood products, in addition to crystalloid and artificial colloid administration (Table 19.1). The most accurate method for assessing blood loss is actually measuring volume and weighing blood-soaked gauzes (1 ml of blood weighs ~1 g). However, a blood-soaked 4 in. × 4 in. (10 cm × 10 cm) gauze will hold 10–20 ml of blood and a laparotomy sponge can absorb 50–100 ml.

The recovery period following limb or tail amputation requires close monitoring for fluid and electrolyte balance and adequacy of analgesia. Packed cell volume and total solids should be compared to pre-operative values and intravenous fluids should be continued until the animal is eating and drinking. Placement of a closed urinary collection system for the first 12–24 hours will prevent urine soiling in animals that are not yet able to walk.

High-Quality, High-Volume Spay and Neuter and Other Shelter Surgeries, First Edition. Edited by Sara White.
© 2020 John Wiley & Sons, Inc. Published 2020 by John Wiley & Sons, Inc.

Table 19.1 Estimated blood volumes in a variety of species.

Species	Estimated blood volume
Dog	80–90 ml/kg
Cat	40–50 ml/kg
Ferret	70–80 ml/kg
Rabbit	50–60 ml/kg

Analgesic Concerns for Limb and Tail Amputation

Amputation of a limb or the tail is associated with considerable pain, and management of the patient's pain is essential on humane grounds and to ensure a rapid recovery. Conditions that lead to the need for amputation (e.g. trauma, neoplasia) often involve pre-existing pain, and evidence from several species indicates that greater than expected post-operative pain and the development of persistent pain syndromes are linked to the presence of pre-amputation pain (Katz et al. 1991; Hanley et al. 2007; Sommer et al. 2010). A balanced analgesic technique should be incorporated and a dynamic interactive pain scoring system should be used frequently in the post-operative period.

Opioids

Systemic administration of opioids is the foundation of peri-operative pain management. Opioids can be administered as intermittent injections, although this results in fluctuating plasma concentrations and possibly periods of under- or overtreatment. Constant- and adjustable-rate infusions may help obtain steady plasma concentrations and analgesic effects, and can be inexpensively administered by adding the desired analgesics to the bag of intravenous fluids (see www.vin.com or www.vasg.org for details). Opioids can also be administered into the epidural space. Full mu-agonist opioids (e.g. morphine) should be considered due to the invasive nature of amputation procedures, and several inexpensive and effective choices are available (Table 19.2).

Non-steroidal Anti-Inflammatory Drugs

Non-steroidal anti-inflammatory drugs (NSAIDs) dampen peripheral and central nociception,

Table 19.2 Opioids for systemic analgesia in cats and dogs (N.B. high end of dosing ranges for full mu agonists are used during general anesthesia with ability to control ventilation).

Opioid	Bolus dose	Intravenous (IV) infusion dose	Expense
Morphine	0.25–1.0 mg/kg q1–4 h (give slowly IV)	0.1–0.5 mg/kg/h	$
Hydromorphone	0.05–0.2 mg/kg q2–6 h	0.01–0.05 mg/kg/h	$
Fentanyl	2–10 µg/kg	2–20 µg/kg/h	$$
Oxymorphone	0.05–0.1 mg/kg q2–6 h	0.01–0.025 mg/kg/h	$$$
Methadone	0.1–0.5 mg/kg	0.03–0.15 mg/kg/h	$$$
Meperidine	2–10 mg/kg q1–2 h (not administered IV due to histamine release)	Not administered IV due to histamine release	$$
Buprenorphine	0.01–0.03 mg/kg q4–8 h	Not used as infusion due to pharmacokinetics	$$
Butorphanol	0.2–0.4 mg/kg q1–4 h	0.05–0.2 mg/kg/h	$$
Nalbuphine	0.1–0.5 mg/kg q1–4 h	Use as CRI not described	$$

CRI, constant-rate infusion; q, every.

reducing the need for post-operative opioid administration (Michelet et al. 2012), and should be used in the peri-operative period if possible. Patients that are volume depleted or hypotensive should not be administered NSAIDs, because prostaglandins help to maintain renal blood flow in the face of renal hypoperfusion (Henrich et al. 1978; Khan et al. 1998). In addition, because general anesthetics can cause vasodilation and relative hypovolemia, administration of NSAIDs may be safest if confined to the post-operative period. Multiple studies have not demonstrated renal injury when label doses of NSAIDs are administered to healthy dogs prior to anesthesia, as determined by creatinine and blood urea nitrogen concentrations, urine-specific gravity, or glomerular filtration rate (Ko et al. 2000; Crandell et al. 2004; Kay-Mugford et al. 2004; Bergmann et al. 2005). However, these parameters do not directly measure the effects of acute changes in renal blood flow, unless the clinical outcome is disastrous. In cats, clinical studies indicate similar uneventful renal outcomes when NSAIDs are administered prior to anesthesia (King et al. 2016); however, anecdotal evidence suggests that cats may be more sensitive to the renal effects of cavalier NSAID administration and caution is warranted. The peri-operative use of NSAIDs requires careful consideration in animals with pre-existing renal disease and may be best avoided.

Grapiprant is a relatively new anti-inflammatory agent labeled for control of osteoarthritis-related pain and inflammation in dogs. This drug is an antagonist at the EP4 receptor, the natural ligand of which is prostaglandin E_2. It has been suggested that the side effect profile is less severe than traditional NSAIDs due to fact that production of prostaglandins is not inhibited. Evidence from laboratory species suggests that grapiprant is effective in reducing surgically induced acute pain and it may be a reasonable analgesic/anti-inflammatory choice in the peri-operative time period. Safety and efficacy studies in cats and rabbits are available, but the drug has not yet been marketed for these species (Rausch-Derra and Rhodes 2016; De Vito et al. 2017)

Local Anesthetics

Local anesthesia added to general anesthesia decreases the peri-operative stress response (Teyin et al. 2006), reduces the incidence of chronic pain (Kairaluoma et al. 2006), decreases post-operative opioid requirements (Paul et al. 2010), improves patient satisfaction as reported by humans (Jeske et al. 2011), and may decrease the metastasis and recurrence of certain tumors (Gottschalk et al. 2012). In addition, effective local or regional anesthesia can reduce inhalational requirements, thereby improving cardiopulmonary function during general anesthesia. Provision of local anesthesia provides excellent analgesia in instances where access to opioid analgesics is restricted. Fortunately, local anesthetics are inexpensive and the drugs are not controlled.

There are several local anesthetic techniques for amputation of the hindlimb and tail, whereas those for the forelimb are more limited. In the caudal half of the body, lumbosacral epidural placement of local anesthetics is effective and easily performed. More advanced techniques include lumbar and sacral plexus blocks using a nerve locator, ultrasound visualization, or the combination of both tools to avoid entry into the central nervous system and allow the clinician to produce unilateral motor blockade. Motor blockade of the limbs can be avoided for tail amputations by accessing the epidural space at the sacrocaudal junction, rather than at the lumbosacral space (see also Chapter 21A: Rectal and vaginal prolapse anesthesia supplement). For the forelimb, there are fewer described local anesthetic techniques, though a cervical paravertebral brachial plexus block can provide anesthesia distal to the shoulder joint.

Application of local anesthetics directly to the nerves intraoperatively or at the site of the surgical wound may be the simplest method of local anesthesia for the forelimb and can also be applied for hindlimb and tail amputations. Intraoperative placement of a wound catheter is easy, inexpensive, and effective (see later; Abelson et al. 2009). Repository, liposomal bupivacaine placed in all layers of the wound during closure provides up to 72 hours of analgesia. This product, Nocita® (Aratana Therapeutics, Leawood, KS), is labeled for cruciate surgery in dogs and onychectomy in cats, but is widely used off-label in a variety of orthopedic (and soft tissue) procedures in both species.

Toxicity of local anesthetics is additive, varies with conditions of use (e.g. in conscious versus anesthetized patients), and among species. Doses of lidocaine ≤4–5 mg/kg and bupivacaine under 2 mg/kg are considered safe in dogs and cats.

Epidural

Lumbosacral epidural injections can be performed with the patient in sternal or lateral recumbency and the hindlimbs flexed alongside the body. The lumbosacral space is shaved and surgically scrubbed. With sterile gloves, the iliac crests are palpated with the thumb and middle finger of the non-dominant hand. The index finger is used to identify the dorsal spinous process of L7 and the lumbosacral space immediately caudal. The dominant hand directs the spinal needle perpendicular to the skin, with the bevel pointing cranially (Figure 19.19). The spinal needle is advanced slowly until penetration of the ligamentum flavum and entry into the epidural space is indicated by a "popping" sensation. A syringe is attached and negative pressure applied to check for aspiration of blood or cerebrospinal fluid (CSF). If CSF is aspirated, the subarachnoid space has been entered and drug doses should be reduced to at least one-half to one-quarter of that planned for epidural administration. If blood is seen in the syringe, the

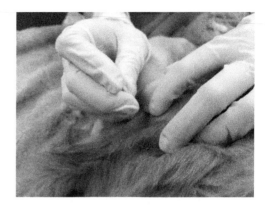

Figure 19.19 Lumbosacral epidural placement of local anesthetics and opioids will provide regional anesthesia to the pelvis and hind limbs.

needle should be withdrawn and another attempt should be made.

Injection into the epidural space should be easy and the "loss of resistance" technique is commonly used to identify correct positioning. The epidural space can also be accessed at the sacrococcygeal or C1–C2 space for anesthesia of the tail and perineal region without loss of motor function in the limbs (see Chapter 21; O'Hearn and Wright 2011). Drugs for epidural injection are shown in Table 19.3.

Wound Catheters

Wound, or "soaker", catheters are commercially available, can be fashioned from red rubber catheters and gas sterilized (Figure 19.20), or made on demand with the help of an assistant intraoperatively. The distal end of a 5–8 Fr red rubber catheter is cut off and sealed using a hemostat that has been heated in the flame of a lighter (do not apply the flame directly to the red rubber catheter as it may melt, char, or catch fire). The proximal end of the catheter is cut to accept an IV catheter injection cap. After closure of the distal end and fitting of the catheter cap to the proximal end, an air-filled syringe is used to ascertain that the catheter does not leak. A small, for example 27-gauge

Table 19.3   Drugs for epidural dosing.

Drug	Dose	Can be combined with	Comments
Lidocaine	2 mg/kg	An opioid	~45–180 min of motor blockade
Bupivacaine	0.5 mg/kg	An opioid	~60–240 min of motor blockade
Morphine	0.1 mg/kg	A local anesthetic	Preservative-free formulations preferred but intravenous solutions less expensive
Hydromorphone	0.02 mg/kg	A local anesthetic	Shorter-acting than morphine
Dexmedetomidine	2 µg/kg	A local anesthetic	Expect systemic cardiovascular effects

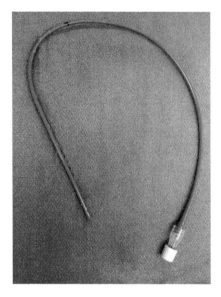

Figure 19.20   A homemade wound or soaker catheter. The distal end of a 5-Fr red rubber urinary catheter was sealed with a heated hemostat and a catheter cap was attached to the proximal end. A 27-gauge needle was used to make holes to allow local anesthetic to be delivered directly into the surgical site.

needle, such as those attached to an insulin syringe, is then used to make holes in the distal end to the desired length; the catheter is filled with local anesthetic and placed in the wound during closure. All holes in the catheter should be placed within the wound, and this is easiest if the beginning of the "soaker section" is marked with a permanent marker. The catheter should be placed in the deepest layer of closure, preferably close to transected nerves, but must be easy to remove. Lidocaine infusions can be used, but this requires an infusion pump. Bolus injection of bupivacaine (1–2 mg/ kg) every six to eight hours is commonly employed.

Anti-hyperalgesics

Various IV and oral drugs (Table 19.4) can be used peri-operatively to reduce wind-up, central sensitization, and development of chronic and persistent post-operative pain. Strong evidence for the effectiveness of these strategies is lacking in veterinary medicine, but studies are generally more encouraging in human patients. IV lidocaine infusions in particular can improve recovery and immediate post-operative analgesia, as well as the incidence of chronic pain (Grigoras et al. 2012; Sun et al. 2012); however, IV infusions of lidocaine should be used cautiously in cats due to the risk of cardiovascular depression at high doses (Pypendop and Ilkiw 2005).

Table 19.4   Anti-hyperalgesics for peri-operative use in dogs and cats.

Drug	Dose	Expense
Ketamine CRI	2–20 µg/kg/min	$
Lidocaine CRI	10–100 µg/kg/min (used cautiously if at all in cats)	$
Amantadine	3–5 mg/kg PO q24 h	$$$
Gabapentin	5–20 mg/kg PO q8 h	$

CRI, constant-rate infusion; PO, orally; q, every.

References

Abelson, A.L., McCobb, E.C., Shaw, S. et al. (2009). Use of wound soaker catheters for the administration of local anesthetic for post-operative analgesia: 56 cases. *Vet. Anaesth. Analg.* 36 (6): 597–602.

Bergmann, H.M., Nolte, I.J., and Kramer, S. (2005). Effects of preoperative administration of carprofen on renal function and hemostasis in dogs undergoing surgery for fracture repair. *Am. J. Vet. Res.* 66 (8): 1356–1363.

Crandell, D.E., Mathews, K.A., and Dyson, D.D. (2004). Effect of meloxicam and carprofen on renal function when administered to healthy dogs prior to anaesthesia and painful stimulation. *Am. J. Vet. Res* 65: 1384–1390.

De Vito, V., Salvadori, M., Poapolathep, A. et al. (2017). Pharmacokinetic/pharmacodynamic evaluation of grapiprant in a carrageenan-induced inflammatory pain model in the rabbit. *J. Vet. Pharmacol.* 40 (5): 468–475.

Gottschalk, A., Brodner, G., Van Aken, H.K. et al. (2012). Can regional anaesthesia for lymph-node dissection improve the prognosis in malignant melanoma? *Br. J. Anaesth.* 109 (2): 253–259.

Grigoras, A., Lee, P., Sattar, F. et al. (2012). Perioperative intravenous lidocaine decreases the incidence of persistent pain after breast surgery. *Clin. J. Pain* 28 (7): 567–572.

Hanley, M.A., Jensen, M.P., Smith, D.G. et al. (2007). Preamputation pain and acute pain predict chronic pain after lower extremity amputation. *J. Pain* 8: 102–109.

Henrich, W.L., Anderson, R.J., Berns, A.S. et al. (1978). The role of renal nerves and prostaglandins in control of renal hemodynamics and plasma renin activity during hypotensive hemorrhage in the dog. *J. Clin. Invest.* 61 (3): 744–750.

Jeske, H.C., Kralinger, F., Wambacher, M. et al. (2011). A randomized study of the effectiveness of suprascapular nerve block in patient satisfaction and outcome after arthroscopic subacromial decompression. *Arthroscopy* 27 (10): 1323–1328.

Kairaluoma, P.M., Bachmann, M.S., Rosenberg, P.H. et al. (2006). Preincisional paravertebral block reduces the prevalence of chronic pain after breast surgery. *Anesth. Analg.* 103 (3): 703–708.

Katz, J., Vaccarino, A.L., Coderre, T.J. et al. (1991). Injury prior to neurectomy alters the pattern of autotomy in rats. Behavioral evidence of central neural plasticity. *Anesthesiology* 75 (5): 876–883.

Kay-Mugford, P.A., Grimm, K.A., Weingarten, A.J. et al. (2004). Effect of preoperative administration of tepoxalin on hemostasis and hepatic and renal function in dogs. *Vet. Ther.* 5 (2): 120–127.

Khan, K.N., Venturini, C.M., Bunch, R.T. et al. (1998). Interspecies differences in renal localization of cyclooxygenase isoforms: implications in nonsteroidal antiinflammatory drug-related nephrotoxicity. *Toxicol. Pathol.* 26 (5): 612–620.

King, S., Roberts, E.S., and King, J.N. (2016). Evaluation of injectable robenacoxib for the treatment of post-operative pain in cats: results of a randomized, masked, placebo-controlled clinical trial. *BMC Vet. Res.* 12 (1): 215.

Ko, J.C., Miyabiyashi, T., Mandsager, R.E. et al. (2000). Renal effects of carprofen administered to healthy dogs anesthetized with propofol and isoflurane. *JAVMA* 217 (3): 346–349.

Michelet, D., Andreu-Gallien, J., Bensalah, T. et al. (2012). A meta-analysis of the use of nonsteroidal antiinflammatory drugs for pediatric postoperative pain. *Anesth. Analg.* 114 (2): 393–406.

O'Hearn, A.K. and Wright, B.D. (2011). Coccygeal epidural with local anesthetic for catheterization and pain management in the treatment of feline urethral obstruction. *J. Vet. Emerg. Crit. Care* 21 (1): 50–52.

Paul, J.E., Arya, A., Hurlburt, L. et al. (2010). Femoral nerve block improves analgesia outcomes after total knee arthroplasty: a meta-analysis of randomized controlled trials. *Anesthesiology* 113 (5): 1144–1162.

Pypendop, B.H. and Ilkiw, J.E. (2005). Assessment of the hemodynamic effects of lidocaine administered IV in isoflurane-anesthetized cats. *Am. J. Vet. Res.* 66 (4): 661–668.

Rausch-Derra, L.C. and Rhodes, L. (2016). Safety and toxicokinetic profiles associated with daily oral administration of grapiprant, a selective antagonist of the prostaglandin E2 EP4 receptor, to cats. *Am. J. Vet. Res.* 77 (7): 688–692.

Sommer, M., de Rijke, J.M., van Kleef, M. et al. (2010). Predictors of acute postoperative pain after elective surgery. *Clin. J. Pain* 26 (2): 87–94.

Sun, Y., Li, T., Wang, N. et al. (eds.) (2012). Perioperative systemic lidocaine for postoperative analgesia and recovery after abdominal surgery: a meta-analysis of randomized controlled trials. *Dis. Colon Rectum* 55 (11): 1183–1194.

Teyin, E., Derbent, A., Balcioglu, T. et al. (2006). The efficacy of caudal morphine or bupivacaine combined with general anesthesia on postoperative pain and neuroendocrine stress response in children. *Paediatr. Anaesth.* 16 (3): 290–296.

20

Surgery of the Eye
Susan Nelms

Many eye disorders can be painful, vision threatening, or lead to an undesirable appearance of the eye that may render a shelter pet unadoptable or less likely to be adopted. The following eye surgeries can be done in a shelter setting and at the time of spay or neuter surgery. These ophthalmic surgeries can enhance the adoptability of a shelter pet. This chapter covers surgical techniques. For anesthesia and analgesia during eye surgery, see Chapter 20A.

Enucleation

Enucleation is removal of the globe, third eyelid, conjunctiva, and eyelids (Miller 2008, Ramsey and Fox 1977).

Indications

This surgery is indicated to provide comfort for a blind, painful eye or removal of an eye with intraocular neoplasia that is not amenable to medical or other surgical treatments (Miller 2008, Ramsey and Fox 1977). Enucleation is indicated for the following eye conditions: chronic glaucoma, severe penetrating or blunt trauma, traumatic proptosis with optic nerve avulsion or scleral rupture, uncontrollable endophthalmitis, or panophthalmitis (Ramsey and Fox 1977; Miller 2008; Speiss 2007). Enucleation may be indicated for phthisis bulbi,

as some animals will develop discomfort from chronic ocular discharge, secondary entropion, and chronic periocular dermatitis. The phthisical globe can serve as a nidus for chronic ocular inflammation (Ramsey and Fox 1977). In addition, these conditions can result in an undesired cosmetic appearance (Figure 20.1). In cats, phthisis bulbi can lead to traumatic sarcoma later in life. Because of this potential but rare risk, enucleation is indicated for all blind cat eyes with phthisis bulbi (Zeiss et al. 2003; Figure 20.2).

Intraorbital Prosthesis

Following removal of the globe, an intraorbital prosthesis may be placed to improve the cosmetic appearance post-operatively (Hamor et al. 1993; Nasisse et al. 1988). Providing a space filler to take up the place of the enucleated globe prevents a "sunken" appearance post-operatively (Figures 20.3 and 20.4). Implantation of a silicone orbital prosthesis has been shown to be safe and inexpensive (Hamor et al. 1993) and improves the cosmetic appearance post-enucleation. Enucleation in a young animal slows the growth of the orbit, as the orbital contents stimulate normal growth (Miller 2008). Replacement of orbital volume with a prosthesis tends to result in an orbit that more closely approximates normal size (Miller 2008).

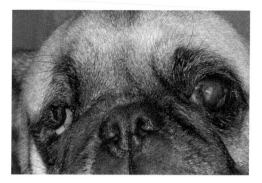

Figure 20.1 Phthisis bulbi OD (right eye) in a pug resulting in chronic inflammation, ocular discharge, secondary entropion, and an unattractive cosmetic appearance.

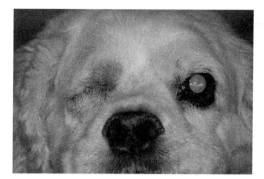

Figure 20.4 Post-operative appearance with silicone orbital prosthesis.

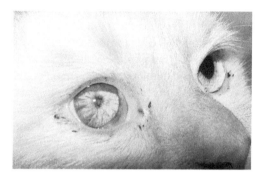

Figure 20.2 Phthisis bulbi OD (right eye) in a cat. Even though this cat is not showing signs of discomfort, enucleation is indicated for this blind eye.

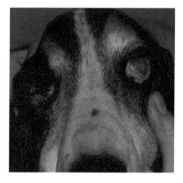

Figure 20.3 Post-operative orbital depression following enucleation surgery.

Surgical Technique

Subconjunctival Enucleation

This approach is most common and is recommended, as more soft tissue is left in the orbit and it provides the greatest exposure of the optic nerve (Martin 2005; Miller 2008; Ramsey and Fox 1977).

1) Perform a lateral canthotomy with scissors, 1–2 cm in length (Figures 20.5a and 20.6).
2) Grasp the conjunctiva near the limbus and make a 360° perilimbal incision with scissors (Figure 20.5b and 20.7).
3) Separate the conjunctiva from the sclera with blunt dissection and sever the extraocular muscles close to their attachment to the sclera (Figures 20.5c and 20.7).
4) Gently rotate the globe medially, but do not put rostral traction on the globe (Figure 20.8).
5) Sever the optic nerve with scissors. Approach from the lateral aspect of the globe (Figure 20.5c).
   a) Do not place traction on the optic nerve and do not twist the optic nerve, as this can cause optic nerve trauma to the chiasm and blindness in the contralateral eye, especially in cats (Stiles 1993). Cats are at increased risk due to the shorter distance of the optic nerve to the chiasm.
   b) Control hemorrhage in the orbit with compression. The orbit can be packed with gauze sponges for approximately three to five minutes. Alternatively, the tissues in the orbital cone can be closed with a ligature. It is not necessary to ligate the optic nerve in dogs and cats (Miller 2008). Applying pressure with

(a)

(b)

(c)

(d)

(e)

(f)

(g)

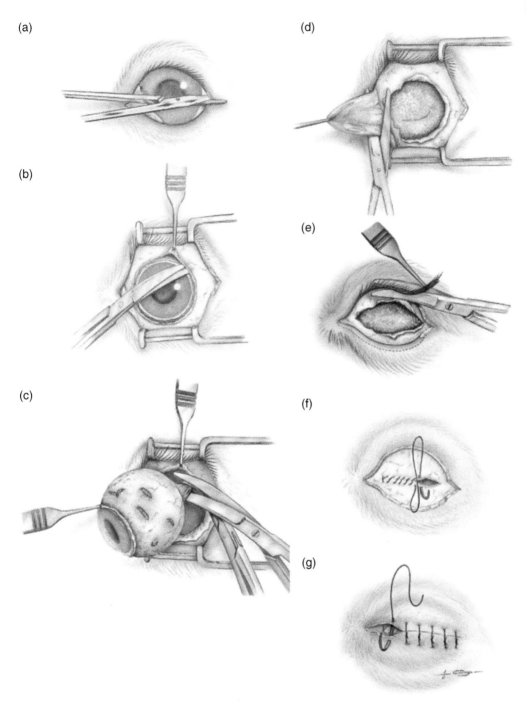

Figure 20.5 Subconjunctival enucleation. *Source:* Miller (2008, p. 367), reproduced with permission of Elsevier.

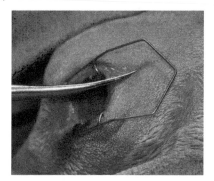

Figure 20.6   Lateral canthotomy.

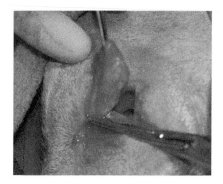

Figure 20.9   Third eyelid and gland excised.

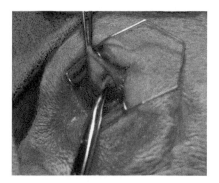

Figure 20.7   Perilimbal incision with dissection of conjunctiva from sclera and severing of extraocular muscle attachments to sclera.

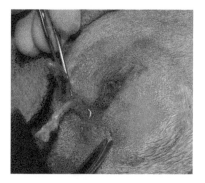

Figure 20.10   Orbit packed with gauze sponges to control hemostasis. (Sponges removed prior to closure.) The eyelid margins are removed with scissors.

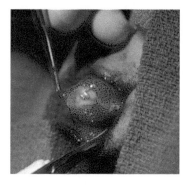

Figure 20.8   Gentle rotation of globe medially. Optic nerve severed.

surgical sponges or temporarily packing the orbit should achieve hemostasis. A ligature can be placed around the vessels in the muscle cone if needed after the globe is removed. Closure will form a seal, controlling hemorrhage.

6) Excise the third eyelid and gland (inspect the lid to be sure the entire gland was excised; Figures 20.5d and 20.9).

7) Remove 2–3 mm of the eyelid margins with scissors, starting at the lateral aspect and cutting toward the medial canthus (Figures 20.5e and 20.10).

8) Remove conjunctival epithelium by gently dissecting the tissue away from the underlying Tenon's capsule. Tenon's capsule is the thick fibrous tissue underlying the conjunctiva and is the holding layer for the orbital prosthesis and should not be removed.

9) Remove the medial canthal tissue (the caruncle, or fleshy tissue at the canthus).

10) Place an intraorbital prosthesis if elected or begin closure (see below for prosthesis selection).

11) Close tissues in three layers (Figure 20.5f and g; Figures 20.11–20.13):

a) Periorbita/Tenon's capsule should be tightly apposed with 4-0 to 5-0 absorbable suture in an interrupted or continuous pattern.

b) Subcutaneous tissue with 4-0 to 5-0 absorbable suture in a continuous pattern.

c) Eyelids with 4-0 to 5-0 nylon or polypropylene in an interrupted pattern.

Ideally, all enucleated globes should be submitted for histopathology, but this may not be practical for all patients in a shelter situation.

Orbital Prosthesis Selection (if Elected)

Autoclavable silicone or methyl methacrylate spheres (Figure 20.14) may be placed in the orbit to prevent post-operative orbital depression (Hamor et al. 1993, Nasisse et al. 1988). The size of the implant needed can be estimated in surgery based on the depth and diameter of the orbit. Most cats and dogs will require a 16–22 mm sphere (Hamor et al. 1993; Miller 2008; Nasisse et al. 1988; Ramsey and Fox 1977). For puppies and kittens, the prosthesis size should be selected to approximate the mature size of the animal eye, not the size of the contralateral eye (Miller 2008).

Post-operative Care/Pain Management

Post-operative swelling and bruising should be expected (Figure 20.13). There may be slight

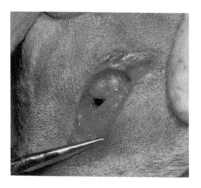

Figure 20.11 Intraorbital prosthesis placed (optional step). Closure of periorbita with 4-0 to 5-0 absorbable suture in an interrupted pattern. The closure is the same with or without a prosthesis.

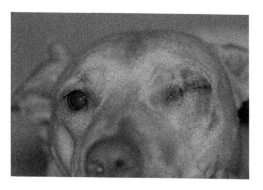

Figure 20.13 Immediate post-operative appearance with silicone orbital prosthesis.

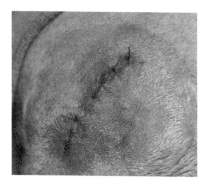

Figure 20.12 Appearance after placement of an orbital prosthesis and three-layer closure.

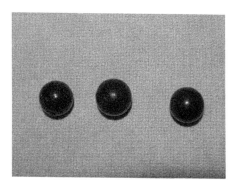

Figure 20.14 Silicone orbital prostheses. Most common sizes required for dogs and cats range from 16 to 22 mm.

bleeding from the incision or nose for a day or two. Post-operative treatment may include:

1) Broad-spectrum oral antibiotic.
2) Oral non-steroidal anti-inflammatory drugs (NSAIDs).
3) Oral tramadol or injectable butorphanol or buprenorphine.
4) Feed soft food for a few days as chewing may cause discomfort.
5) Suture removal in 10–14 days.
6) Elizabethan collar if needed to prevent rubbing/trauma to surgery site.

Complications

The most common complication of enucleation surgery is hemorrhage with post-operative swelling (Martin 2005; Speiss 2007). Draining tracts or serous discharge accumulation within the orbit can occur if there is incomplete excision of the secretory tissues during surgery (Martin 2005; Miller 2008; Ramsey and Fox 1977; Speiss 2007; Ward and Neaderland 2011). Infection of the orbit is an uncommon post-operative complication and most cases can be managed with systemic antibiotics. In brachycephalic breeds, orbital emphysema, a rare complication, can occur if air leaks into the orbit via the nasolacrimal duct (Bedford 1979; Martin 1971). Orbital depression or an undesired cosmetic appearance is common, especially for shorthaired animals. This can be avoided by placement of an intraorbital prosthesis, as already discussed. Complications of orbital implant placement are uncommon and surgical infection and dehiscence rates are no greater in implanted orbits than in general surgical wounds (Hamor et al. 1993). Enteral or parenteral antibiotic therapy is recommended to reduce the risk of infection post-operatively in all enucleation patients. Infection can also lead to implant extrusion (Hamor et al. 1993). Table 20.1 summarizes enucleation complications.

Table 20.1 Post-operative enucleation complication causes and treatments.

Post-operative enucleation complication	Cause	Treatment
Hemorrhage and swelling	Poor hemostasis intraoperatively	Cold compresses/ice pack Sedation
Serous draining tract	Failure to remove third eyelid gland, conjunctival epithelium, or caruncle	Explore surgery site for tissue remnants
Infection	Contamination of orbit due to infection at time of surgery	Systemic antibiotics Consider drain placement (rarely needed)
Contralateral vision loss	Traction of optic nerve with damage to optic chiasm	None
Depressed orbit (cosmetic complication)	Lack of orbital implant	Place orbital prosthesis
Extrusion of orbital implant	Failure to adequately close Tenon's capsule/periorbita Infection Neoplasia	If no infection or neoplasia can replace implant If infection/neoplasia present, biopsy tissue, do not replace implant
Orbital emphysema	Air leakage into orbit due to patent nasolacrimal duct	Explore surgery site and close nasolacrimal puncta

Surgical Repair of Prolapsed Third Eyelid Gland, "Cherry Eye"

Indications

The prolapsed third eyelid gland should be surgically replaced and never excised (Maggs 2008a; Martin 2005; Moore and Constantinescu 1997; Morgan et al. 1993). This gland contributes a large portion of the tear film. Excision of the gland commonly results in keratoconjunctivitis sicca (KCS; Helper 1970; Helper et al. 1974), often years later, especially in breeds that are genetically prone (Morgan et al. 1993). Replacing the prolapsed gland does not eliminate the chance of developing KCS, but can delay the onset and the severity. Left untreated, the prolapsed third eyelid gland can develop chronic inflammation, secondary infection, and an undesirable cosmetic appearance. There is a higher incidence of KCS in patients with untreated third eyelid gland prolapse compared with patients who have the gland replaced (Morgan et al. 1993). Surgical replacement of the prolapsed third eyelid gland in the shelter dog will improve adoptability by improving cosmetic appearance and decreasing the chance of developing KCS and the need for ongoing medical treatment.

Cherry eye is most commonly a disease of dogs less than one year of age. An older animal presenting with a cherry eye should be evaluated very carefully for orbital disease or neoplasia.

Surgical Technique

Several techniques have been described for replacement of the prolapsed third eyelid gland and are either "anchoring" or "pocket" techniques. Anchoring techniques are associated with a high rate of re-prolapse of the gland post-operatively as well as decreased mobility of the third eyelid (Morgan et al. 1993). The Morgan pocket-flap technique is recommended, as it has the highest success rate, most cosmetic outcome, and is easy to perform (Maggs 2008a; Morgan et al. 1993; Figure 20.15).

Morgan "Pocket-Flap" Technique

1) The third eyelid is retracted away from the globe to expose the posterior surface (Figure 20.16).
2) Two incisions are made on the posterior surface of the third eyelid, parallel to the free margin on either side of the prolapsed gland (Figure 20.17):
   a) The first incision is made 2–3 mm from the free margin.
   b) The second incision is made 6–7 mm toward the base of the third eyelid.
   c) The incision length is approximately 1 cm.

Figure 20.15 Morgan pocket-flap technique. *Source:* Maggs (2008a, p. 154), reproduced with permission of Elsevier.

(a)   (b)

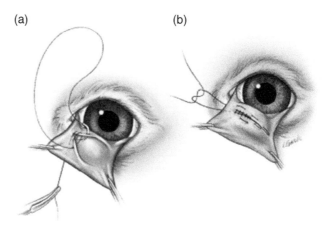

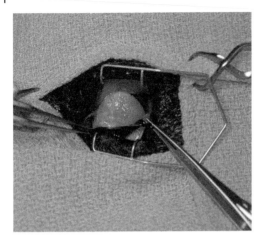

Figure 20.16   Retraction of third eyelid to expose the posterior surface.

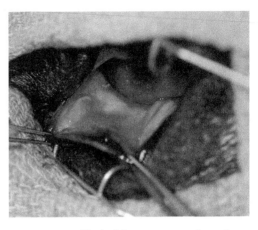

Figure 20.18   The incisions are sutured together in a continuous pattern.

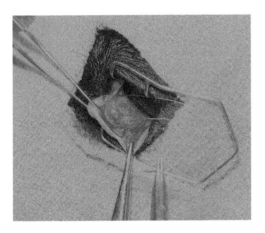

Figure 20.17   Parallel incisions are made on either side of the prolapsed gland.

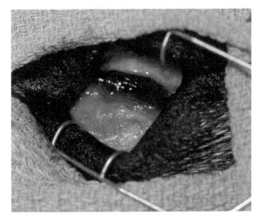

Figure 20.19   The final anchoring knot can be placed on the anterior surface of the third eyelid.

3) The outer edges of the two incisions are sutured together with 5-0 or 6-0 braided polyglycolic acid suture in a continuous pattern (Figure 20.18 and Figure 20.15a):
   a) Openings are left at the lateral and medial aspects of the incision to allow flow of secretions.
   b) Care is taken to bury the suture knots.
   c) The final anchoring knot is placed on the anterior surface of the third eyelid by passing the needle through the body of the third eyelid to the conjunctival fornix to avoid corneal irritation (Figures 20.19 and 20.15b).

Post-operative Care

1) Topical antibiotic or antibiotic-steroid ointment.
2) Elizabethan collar.
3) Oral NSAIDs for analgesia.

Complications

Re-prolapse of the gland occurs in approximately 6% of cases (Morgan et al. 1993). A common reason for re-prolapse, in the author's experience, is the presence of conjunctivitis at the time of surgery. These cases can be treated

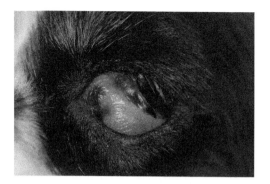

Figure 20.20 Failure to leave the conjunctival incision ends open can result in retention cyst formation following the pocket-flap technique.

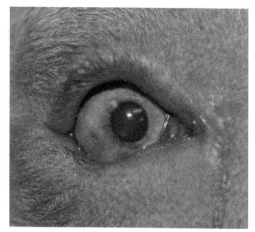

Figure 20.21 Entropion of the lower eyelid causing corneal ulceration and vascularization.

pre-operatively with topical steroids and post-operatively with a topical antibiotic-steroid, and most will have a successful second surgery.

Corneal ulceration can occur due to suture knot trauma to the cornea. This can be avoided by taking care to bury the initial knot within the conjunctiva and tying off the final suture knot on the anterior surface of the third eyelid. Alternatively, both the beginning and ending suture knots can be tied on the anterior surface of the third eyelid. A retention cyst can form if the incisions are closed completely, allowing tears to accumulate (Figure 20.20). This rare complication can be treated by creating a stoma, allowing the tears to escape (Hendrix 2007).

Markedly enlarged third eyelid glands can be more difficult to replace. In order to improve the surgical outcome, treat conjunctivitis with a topical antibiotic-steroid to reduce swelling prior to surgery. In addition, the conjunctival incision can be reinforced with a second layer of continuous Connell–Cushing suture pattern placed with bites parallel to the conjunctival incision and the knots buried on the anterior surface of the third eyelid (Maggs 2008a).

Entropion Repair

Entropion repair involves either temporary or definitive surgical techniques to evert the eyelid.

Indications

Entropion is "rolling in" or inversion of the eyelid toward the eye (Martin 2005). As the lid rolls inward, hair and lashes can contact the globe (Figure 20.21). It is very common in dogs and less common in cats. Surgical correction is indicated for most cases of entropion (Miller and Albert 1988). Blepharospasm with absence of the normal hairless eyelid margin against the cornea is diagnostic (Martin 2005; Stades and Gelatt 2007).

There are three forms of entropion and the surgical indications vary with type. Spastic entropion is secondary to a painful ocular condition such as a corneal ulcer, ectopic cilia, distichia, or KCS. A cycle of irritation and blepharospasm develops (Miller and Albert 1988). If the underlying pain is removed early on, the entropion often resolves. If the irritation–blepharospasm cycle becomes established, the entropion becomes permanent and surgical correction is warranted, but should not be undertaken without specific treatment of the cause (Miller and Albert 1988). Spastic entropion is the most common form in cats and the cause tends to vary with age. For young cats, entropion occurs secondary to irritation from conjunctivitis or corneal ulceration; and for older cats, entropion occurs secondary to enophthalmos resulting from loss of orbital fat and subsequent lid laxity (Williams and Kim 2009). Conformational entropion is the most common form in dogs, and many breeds have a genetic predisposition. Cicatricial entropion occurs secondary to an injury or contact with a caustic chemical that results in scarring and lid contracture.

Entropion causes pain and can lead to vision-threatening complications such as corneal ulceration, secondary infection, corneal pigmentation, and scarring, therefore surgical repair is indicated for shelter dogs and cats that are affected.

Surgical Technique

Eyelid Tacking

Eyelid tacking is indicated for temporary relief in puppies less than 12 weeks (most commonly Shar Pei and Chow Chow, but any breed can be affected). This may be curative, allowing the puppy to "outgrow" the entropion, or the tacking will provide relief from pain and corneal injury until the puppy is more mature and a permanent surgery can be done. Temporary eyelid tacking is also indicated for patients with spastic entropion that is likely to be transient. This procedure involves temporarily everting the eyelid margin with vertical mattress sutures (Johnson et al. 1988). The sutures are left in place as long as needed and may need to be replaced at two to four week intervals, as they may break down as the puppy grows (Figures 20.22 and 20.23).

1) Use 3-0 to 5-0 nylon or other non-absorbable suture.
2) Place the needle 2–3 mm from the lid margin for the first bite.
3) Engage 2–3 mm of skin and subcutaneous tissue in the first bite.
4) Start the second bite 1–2 cm from the lid margin and incorporate the same amount of tissue.
5) Tie the knot, applying enough tension to evert the lid margin.
6) Place sutures to evert all areas of the lids that are affected.
7) Place as many sutures as needed to establish a normal to slightly overcorrected lid conformation.

(a)   (b)

(c)

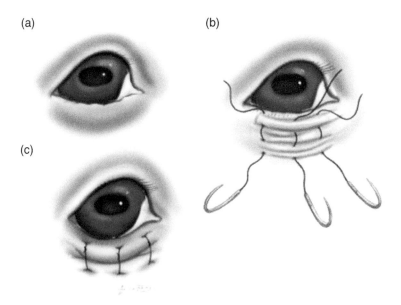

Figure 20.22   Temporary "tacking" sutures to correct entropion in an immature animal or animals with a transient cause for entropion. *Source:* Maggs (2008b, p. 117), reproduced with permission of Elsevier.

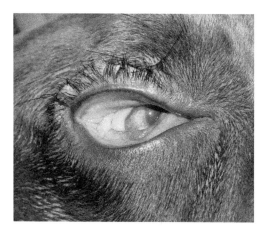

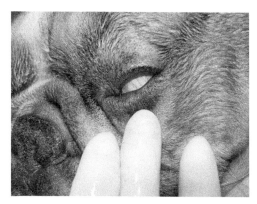

Figure 20.23 Temporary "tacking" sutures everting the upper eyelid in a Mastiff puppy. Note that these temporary sutures are placed to "overcorrect" the entropion.

Figure 20.24 "Rule of thumb" for estimating the amount of tissue to excise for the Hotz–Celsus procedure. The distance the thumb is moved to expose the lid margin is the depth of the widest portion of skin excision.

Another temporary eyelid tacking procedure has been described using surgical staples instead of suture material, but it is considered unpredictable, irritating, and animal-unfriendly (Stades and Gelatt 2007).

Modified Hotz–Celsus

Established entropion requires surgical correction (Martin 2005). The Hotz–Celsus procedure is a simple, definitive entropion repair that can be used to treat most cases of entropion. This procedure involves excising a crescent of skin from the entropic portion of the eyelid (Hamilton et al. 2000; Miller and Albert 1988; Moore and Constantinescu 1997).

There are three different methods that can help to estimate the amount of tissue to resect in the Hotz–Celsus procedure (Miller and Albert 1988; Stades and Gelatt 2007). The skin can be marked just along the edge of the inverted lid, after the first incision has been made. This will determine the placement of the second elliptical incision. The "rule of thumb" can be applied by placing digital pressure on the lid skin and pulling down until the free lid margin is exposed (Figure 20.24). The distance that the thumb moves is the widest portion of the crescent of skin to be excised. Finally, the skin can be grasped with a tissue

forceps or mosquito hemostat until the lid returns to the normal position (Hamilton et al. 2000). The resulting fold of skin is removed by cutting with scissors. This "pinch" technique may provide the easiest method for less experienced surgeons to estimate the amount of tissue to excise (Hamilton et al. 2000). In general, the maximum amount of tissue that would be resected is no greater than 5–6 mm at the widest part of the ellipse (Martin 2005).

Pre-operative considerations are as follows:

1) Eliminate other causes of spastic entropion before deciding on the extent of surgical resection. Applying a drop of topical proparacaine can help to distinguish conformational component from secondary spastic or pain contribution to the entropion (Stades and Gelatt 2007).
2) Assess the degree of skin resection prior to sedation.
3) Undercorrection with the need for a second surgery is preferable to overcorrection, except in cats where slight overcorrection is required or recurrence is common (Williams and Kim 2009).

The Hotz–Celsus procedure:

1) Stabilize the eyelid with a Jaeger lid plate placed in the conjunctival fornix (Figures 20.25a, 20.26).

(a)

(b)

(c)

(d)

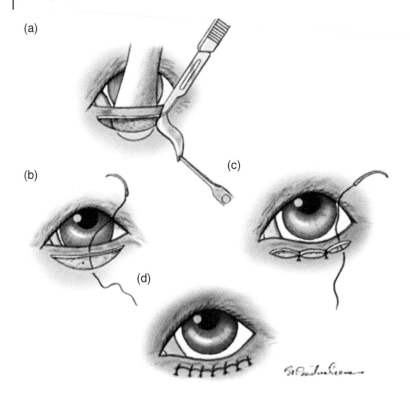

Figure 20.25 Hotz–Celsus procedure. *Source:* Maggs (2008b, p. 118), modified from Moore and Constantinescu (1997). Reproduced with permission of Elsevier.

2) Incise the lid 2–3 mm from the lid margin with a #15 Bard Parker blade (Figure 20.25a):
   a) Placement of this incision too far from the lid margin is a common error that will not allow the eversion desired.
   b) Placement of this incision too close to the lid margin will make closure difficult.
3) The incision is extended parallel to the lid margin for the length of the entropion (lid inversion).
4) A second incision is made to create a crescent shape and tapered laterally and medially to meet the first incision (Figures 20.25a, 20.26).
5) The distance between the two incisions forming the crescent is estimated to correct the degree of entropion present:
   a) It is better to err on the side of undercorrection (except in cats where slight overcorrection is needed).

   b) The widest portion of tissue resection should be planned for the most inverted area of eyelid (Maggs 2008b).
6) The incised strip of skin is removed by sharp dissection.
7) It is not necessary to remove the orbicularis muscle, and the conjunctiva should not be incised (however, if these tissues are accidently incised, proceed with skin closure as described and the surgical wound should heal without complication).
8) The defect is closed with 4-0 to 6-0 suture in an interrupted pattern (non-absorbable or absorbable suture may be used; Figure 20.27). The author prefers absorbable suture, as it is less irritating if a suture tag were to contact the cornea. Also, the sutures do not have to be removed if the patient is fractious.
9) The central aspect of the incision is closed first using a split-thickness technique (the

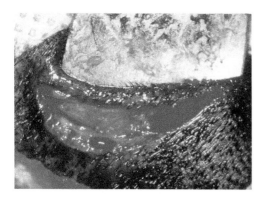

Figure 20.26 Crescent-shaped area of skin is excised.

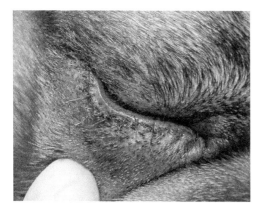

Figure 20.27 Appearance after closure with interrupted absorbable sutures.

depth of the suture bites approximates half the depth of the skin on each side of the incision) with sutures spaced 2–3 mm apart (Figure 20.25b).

10) Additional sutures are placed by splitting the distance of the unsutured spaces until the wound closure is complete (Figure 20.25c and d).

Post-operative Care

1) Topical antibiotic ointment.
2) Oral NSAIDs for analgesia.
3) Elizabethan collar.
4) Suture removal in 10–14 days; absorbable sutures may be removed at this time or may be left alone to dissolve.

Complications

Complications include overcorrection or undercorrection, leading to a need for additional surgical repair and possible undesirable cosmetic appearance (Figure 20.28). Wound infection or dehiscence is uncommon with appropriate aftercare.

Wedge Resection for Eyelid Tumor Removal

Eyelid tumors are common in older dogs and most are benign (Roberts et al. 1986). Lid tumors can cause ocular irritation and undesired cosmetic appearance that may hinder adoption. Eyelid tumors are rare in cats and squamous cell carcinoma is most common (Martin 2005).

Indications

Eyelid tumors involving up to one-third of the eyelid margin may be excised by full-thickness wedge resection (Maggs 2008b). Tumors involving greater than one-third of the eyelid margin will require more extensive excision and likely reconstructive techniques, therefore referral may be indicated.

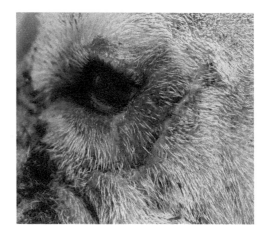

Figure 20.28 Incorrect suture placement (too far from the lid margin), failing to evert the lid and necessitating additional surgery.

Surgical Technique

1) The lid is stabilized with a Jaeger lid plate or chalazion forceps.
2) Skin incisions are made with a #15 Bard Parker scalpel blade:
   a) A "wedge" or "triangle" of skin is incised.
   b) The "wedge" should include the tumor plus 1–2 mm of normal tissue on each side of the mass.
3) Subcutaneous tissues and conjunctiva are cut with Stevens tenotomy scissors, completely excising the tissue wedge (Figure 20.29a).
4) Standard two-layer closure (described in the following).

Standard Two-Layer Closure for Eyelid Wounds

This technique is used for all eyelid wounds or incisions that involve the eyelid margin (Maggs 2008b). All injuries that involve the eyelid margin should be surgically repaired to avoid scarring that could lead to corneal irritation.

Indications

Eyelid lacerations or eyelid injuries involving up to one-third of the eyelid margin or eyelid tumors removed by wedge resection should be closed with a two-layer closure to achieve precise apposition of the eyelid margin and a stable repair, with minimal chance of ocular irritation from suture knots (Moore and Constantinescu 1997).

Surgical Technique

1) 5-0 to 6-0 absorbable suture is buried in a mattress pattern in the subcutaneous tissue without penetrating the skin or conjunctiva. This buried suture may be continued from the eyelid margin to the apex of the

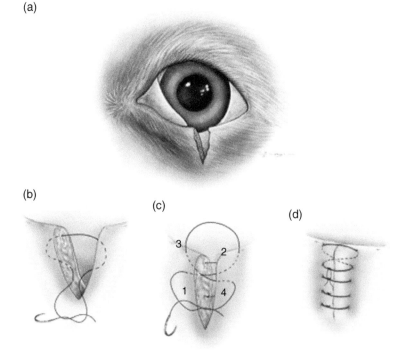

(a)

(b)

(c)

(d)

Figure 20.29 Two-layer closure technique for repair of all eyelid wounds or incisions that involve the eyelid margin. *Source:* Maggs (2008b, p. 112), reproduced with permission of Elsevier.

incision/wound in a continuous pattern if necessary to close the subcutaneous tissue (Figure 20.29b).

2) The skin is closed with 5-0 to 6-0 absorbable or non-absorbable suture:

   a) A figure-of-eight suture is used at the eyelid margin, with the knot being tied 3–4 mm from the eyelid margin (Figure 20.30). This suture pattern provides good eyelid margin apposition to insure a cosmetic outcome and minimal chance of corneal injury (Figure 20.29c).

   b) The rest of the skin is closed with simple interrupted sutures (Figures 20.29d, 20.31).

Post-operative Care/Pain Management

1) Topical antibiotic ointment.
2) Oral NSAIDs for analgesia.
3) Oral antibiotics may be indicated in select cases.
4) Elizabethan collar.
5) Suture removal in 10–14 days; absorbable sutures may be removed at this time or may be left alone to dissolve.

Complications

Possible complications include infection, surgical dehiscence, corneal irritation, or ulceration due to suture knot trauma or inadequate eyelid margin apposition.

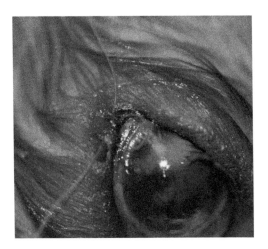

Figure 20.30   Figure-of-eight suture showing placement of suture. When the suture ends are tied the suture knot will be 3–4 mm from the eyelid.

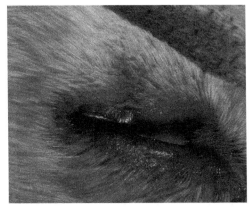

Figure 20.31   Appearance of eyelid after V-lid resection for eyelid tumor removal and closure of eyelid margin with figure-of-eight suture. The rest of the skin was closed with interrupted sutures. This closure provides minimal chance of corneal injury, as the suture knot is several millimeters from the eyelid margin. This pattern can be used to close any type of wound involving up to one-third of the eyelid margin.

References

Bedford, P.G. (1979). Orbital pneumatosis as an unusual complication to enucleation. *J. Small An. Pract.* 20: 551–555.

Hamilton, H.L., Whitley, R.D., McLaughlin, S.A. et al. (2000). Diagnosis and blepharoplastic repair of conformational eyelid defects. *Compend. Cont. Educ. Pract. Vet* 22: 588–599.

Hamor, R.E., Roberts, S.M., and Severin, G.A. (1993). Use of orbital implants after enucleation in dogs, horses, and cats: 161 cases (1980–1990). *JAVMA* 203 (5): 701–706.

Helper, L.C. (1970). The effect of lacrimal gland removal on the conjunctiva and cornea of the dog. *JAVMA* 157: 72–75.

Helper, L.C., Magrane, W.G., Koehm, J. et al. (1974). Surgical induction of keratoconjunctivitis sicca in the dog. *JAVMA* 165: 172–174.

Hendrix, D.V. (2007). Canine conjunctiva and nictitating membrane. In: *Veterinary Ophthalmology*, 4e (ed. K.N. Gelatt), 675–689. Ames, IA: Blackwell.

Johnson, B.W., Gerding, P.A., McLaughlin, S.A. et al. (1988). Nonsurgical correction of entropion in Shar Pei puppies. *Vet. Med.* 83: 482–483.

Maggs, D.J. (2008a). Third eyelid. In: *Slatter's Fundamentals of Veterinary Ophthalmology*, 4e (eds. D.J. Maggs, P.E. Miller and R. Onfri), 151–156. St. Louis, MO: Saunders Elsevier.

Maggs, D.J. (2008b). Eyelids. In: *Slatter's Fundamentals of Veterinary Ophthalmology*, 4e (eds. D.J. Maggs, P.E. Miller and R. Onfri), 107–134. St. Louis, MO: Saunders Elsevier.

Martin, C.L. (1971). Orbital emphysema: a compilcation of ocular enucleation in the dog. *Vet. Med. Small Anim. Clin.* 66: 986.

Martin, C.L. (2005). *Ophthalmic Disease in Veterinary Medicine*. London: Manson Publishing/Veterinary Press.

Miller, P.E. (2008). Orbit. In: *Slatter's Fundamentals of Veterinary Ophthalmology*, 4e (eds. D.J. Maggs, P.E. Miller and R. Onfri), 352–373. St. Louis, MO: Saunders Elsevier.

Miller, W.M. and Albert, R.A. (1988). Canine entropion. *Compend. Cont. Educ.* 10 (4): 431–438.

Moore, C.P. and Constantinescu, G.M. (1997). Surgery of the adnexa. *Vet. Clin. N. Am. Small Anim. Pract.* 27 (5): 1052–1058.

Morgan, R.V., Duddy, J.M., and McClurg, K. (1993). Prolapse of the third eyelid in dogs: a retropspective study of 89 cases (1980–1990). *J. Am. Anim. Hosp. Assoc.* 29: 56–61.

Nasisse, M.P., van Ee, R., and Munger, R. (1988). Use of methyl methacrylate orbital prostheses in dogs and cats: 78 cases (1980–1986). *JAVMA* 192: 539–542.

Ramsey, D.T. and Fox, D.B. (1977). Surgery of the orbit. *Vet. Clin. N. Am. Small Anim. Pract.* 27 (5): 1247–1261.

Roberts, S.M., Severin, G.A., and Lavach, J.D. (1986). Prevalence and treatment of palpebral neoplasms in the dog: 200 cases (1975–1983). *JAVMA* 189: 1355.

Speiss, B.M. (2007). Diseases and surgery of the canine orbit. In: *Veterinary Ophthalmology*, 4e (ed. K.N. Gelatt), 539–562. Ames, IA: Blackwell Publishing.

Stades, F.C. and Gelatt, K.N. (2007). Diseases and surgery of the canine eyelids. In: *Veterinary Ophthalmology*, 4e (ed. K.N. Gelatt), 563–617. Ames, IA: Blackwell Publishing.

Stiles, J., Buyukmihci, N.C., and Hacker, D.V. (1993). Blindness from damage to optic chiasm. *JAVMA* 202: 1192.

Ward, A. and Neaderland, M. (2011). Complications from residual adnexal structures following enucleation in three dogs. *JAVMA* 239: 1580–1583.

Williams, D.L. and Kim, J. (2009). Feline entropion: a case series of 50 affected animals (2003–2008). *Vet. Ophthalmol.* 12 (4): 221.

Zeiss, C.J., Johnson, E.M., and Dubielzig, R.R. (2003). Feline intraocular tumors may arise from transformation of lens epithelium. *Vet. Pathol.* 40: 355–363.

20A

Surgery of the Eye: Anesthesia Supplement
Lydia Love

Anesthetic Concerns for Ocular and Adnexal Surgery

In addition to the common complications of general anesthesia including hypoventilation, hypotension, and hypothermia, ocular surgery may precipitate the oculocardiac reflex (OCR). The OCR is a component of the trigeminocardiac reflex, and similar hemodynamic events may occur with nasal and palatal stimulation. Stimulation of the ophthalmic branch of the trigeminal nerve activates the trigeminal sensory nucleus, which in turn communicates with vagal efferents that reach the myocardium, resulting in bradycardia or asystole. This reflex occurs more commonly in the face of hypoxemia, hypercapnia, or under a light plane of general anesthesia and with the use of potent opioids (Bohluli et al. 2009, Lubbers et al. 2010). Although the OCR is a rare event in dogs and cats, it occurs more frequently in the young and in brachycephalic dog breeds, in which it may be a result of higher resting vagal tone (Schaller 2004). It is often recommended that anticholinergic drugs (e.g. glycopyrrolate or atropine) be administered to all veterinary patients undergoing ocular surgery to prevent the OCR. An alternative preventive measure is local anesthesia of the efferent pathway (see later discussion of local anesthetic techniques). In children undergoing strabismus surgery, the use of ketamine reduced the occurrence of the OCR (Choi et al. 2007). However, no technique is 100% reliable at preventing the OCR, therefore monitoring heart rate continuously during ocular procedures, preferably with an audible device, is important. Reduction in heart rate may be mild to moderate and treatment in these cases consists of stopping ocular traction or pressure. More severe cases may require atropine 0.04 mg/kg intravenously (IV) and, in the event of a cardiac arrest, resuscitative efforts (see Chapter 11).

Patients that have sustained ocular trauma may have other cranial injuries, including brain trauma, and should be evaluated carefully prior to anesthesia. A high level of monitoring (e.g. blood pressure and end-tidal carbon dioxide) and supportive care are required during anesthesia for patients with neurologic deficits secondary to head trauma. During enucleation, hemorrhage may occur from the ophthalmic artery during, or occasionally after, surgery. Strict hemostasis is required and if hemorrhage occurs, blood loss should be estimated (see Chapter 19A) and blood products administered if necessary.

Vomiting, coughing, struggling, and jugular occlusion should be avoided in patients for whom increases in intraocular pressure could be problematic, including those with deep corneal ulcers or glaucoma.

High-Quality, High-Volume Spay and Neuter and Other Shelter Surgeries, First Edition. Edited by Sara White.
© 2020 John Wiley & Sons, Inc. Published 2020 by John Wiley & Sons, Inc.

Analgesic Concerns

Most ocular surgeries will result in mild to moderate pain. Additionally, some patients requiring enucleation will present with pre-existing pain (e.g. glaucoma, severe corneal ulceration, neoplasia), which may increase the risk of developing chronic pain following surgery. In a Danish study, about a quarter of human patients that underwent invasive ocular surgeries experienced post-operative phantom pain, and about a third of these patients reported phantom pain every day (Rasmussen 2010).

Assessment of pain in veterinary patients can be difficult. In a clinical trial of 22 dogs undergoing enucleation, owner-evaluated pain scores were decreased in the post-operative period from initial presentation, regardless of the analgesic strategy (hydromorphone alone or hydromorphone plus carprofen), suggesting either that termination of the disease process significantly alleviated pain independently of the analgesic regimen (Bentley 2011), or that the additional benefit of the non-steroidal analgesic was not detectable in these circumstances. Regardless, multimodal peri-operative analgesia is highly recommended for the aforementioned procedures.

In addition to systemic opioids and non-steroidal anti-inflammatory drugs, local anesthesia should be employed for cases of enucleation. The simplest method is to splash the orbit with 1–2 mg/kg of bupivacaine before closure or to place bupivacaine-soaked gel foam in the orbital space, but these techniques do not provide pre-emptive analgesia or allow for a reduction in inhalant requirements intraoperatively. Retrobulbar (Figure 20.32) or peribulbar blocks can be performed prior to surgery and reduce the need for post-operative analgesia (Myrna et al. 2010). These simple regional anesthetic techniques target cranial nerves III, IV, V, and VI, resulting in analgesia and akinesia of the eye. Several approaches have been reported in the literature for retrobulbar placement of local anesthetics, but the inferior-temporal approach

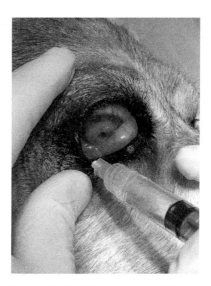

Figure 20.32 Placement of an inferior-temporal retrobulbar local anesthetic block prior to enucleation. *Source:* Photo courtesy of Dr. Brad Holmberg.

has been identified as the most satisfactory one in dogs (Accola et al. 2006). A 1.5 in. (3.8 cm), 22-gauge needle is bent approximately 20° at its midpoint. With the bevel facing slightly medially, the needle is inserted through the inferior lid at the junction of the middle and outer third along the orbital rim. A similar approach is typically used in cats and puppies, though a shorter needle may be chosen.

A popping sensation may be felt as the orbital fascia is entered and the needle is advanced about 1 cm further. The syringe should be aspirated before injection to ensure that a vessel has not been pierced. Possible complications of retrobulbar local anesthesia include inadvertent intravenous or subarachnoid injection, perforation of the globe, retrobulbar hemorrhage, infection, systemic toxicity, and initiation of the OCR. One case report of subarachnoid spread of local anesthesia and brain-stem anesthesia resulting in transient respiratory arrest and neurologic signs has been reported in a cat (Oliver and Bradbook 2012). Bupivacaine at 1–2 mg/kg diluted to a volume of 1 ml/10 kg should produce adequate spread of local anesthetic within the retrobulbar space and also cause slight proptosis of the intact globe, providing improved surgical exposure.

Peribulbar placement of local anesthetics has largely replaced retrobulbar techniques in human ocular surgery due to an improved safety profile and has been described in dogs and cats (Shilo-Benjamini et al. 2014, 2018). With this approach, a larger volume of local anesthetic is deposited outside of the extraocular muscle cone, avoiding possible needle-based trauma of the sensitive structures therein. A 25 g 5/8 in. needle is inserted at the superior temporal aspect of the orbital rim and advanced along the wall of the orbit to its full length. The syringe is aspirated to ascertain that the injection will not be into a vessel and 0.7–1 ml/kg of diluted bupivacaine (maximum total dose ~2 mg/kg) is administered. In dogs, the total local anesthetic dose is split between a superior temporal and inferior lateral injection for more reliable clinical effect.

References

Accola, P.J., Bentley, E., Smith, L.J. et al. (2006). Development of a retrobulbar injection technique for ocular surgery and analgesia in dogs. *JAVMA* 229 (2): 220–225.

Bentley, E. (2011). Pain management in ocular disease. Western Veterinary Conference, Las Vegas, NV (20–24 February).

Bohluli, B., Ashtiani, A.K., Khayampoor, A. et al. (2009). Trigeminocardiac reflex: a MaxFax literature review. *Oral Surg. Oral Med. Oral Pathol. Oral Radiol. Endodontol.* 108 (2): 184–188.

Choi, S.H., Lee, S.J., Kim, S.H. et al. (2007). Single bolus of intravenous ketamine for anesthetic induction decreases oculocardiac reflex in children undergoing strabismus surgery. *Acta Anaesthesiologica Scandanavica* 51 (6): 759–762.

Lübbers, H.T., Zweifel, D., Grätz, K.W. et al. (2010). Classification of potential risk factors for trigeminocardiac reflex in craniomaxillofacial surgery. *J. Oral Maxillofac. Surg.* 68 (6): 1317–1321.

Myrna, K.E., Bentley, E., and Smith, L.J. (2010). Effectiveness of injection of local anesthetic into the retrobulbar space for postoperative analgesia following eye enucleation in dogs. *JAVMA* 237 (2): 174–177.

Oliver, J.A. and Bradbrook, C.A. (2012). Suspected brainstem anesthesia following retrobulbar block in a cat. *Vet. Ophthalmol.* 16 (3): 225–228.

Rasmussen, M.L. (2010). The eye amputated – consequences of eye amputation with emphasis on clinical aspects, phantom eye syndrome and quality of life. *Acta Ophthalmologica* 88 (Thesis 2): 1–26.

Schaller, B. (2004). Trigeminocardiac reflex. A clinical phenomenon or a new physiological entity? *J. Neurol.* 251 (6): 658–665.

Shilo-Benjamini, Y., Pascoe, P.J., Maggs, D.J. et al. (2014). Comparison of peribulbar and retrobulbar regional anesthesia with bupivacaine in cats. *Am. J. Vet. Res.* 75 (12): 1029–1039.

Shilo-Benjamini, Y., Pascoe, P.J., Maggs, D.J. et al. (2018). Retrobulbar vs peribulbar regional anesthesia techniques using bupivacaine in dogs. *Vet. Ophthalmol.* 22 (2): 183–191.

21

Rectal and Vaginal Fold Prolapse
Kimberly Woodruff

This chapter covers diagnosis and treatment; for anesthetic concerns see Chapter 21A, and for uterine prolapse see Chapter 12.

Vaginal Fold Prolapse

Vaginal fold prolapse is the protrusion of vaginal mucosa through the vulva due to edematous hypertrophy of the vaginal tissue (Fossum 2002). Previous names for this condition include vaginal prolapse, vaginal hypertrophy, vaginal hyperplasia, estral hypertrophy, vaginal eversion, and vaginal protrusion (Nelissen 2015). Vaginal fold prolapse can be categorized into three categories. Type I involves slight eversion of the vaginal floor without complete protrusion. Type II involves prolapse of the cranial floor and lateral walls of the vagina. In type III prolapse, the entire vaginal circumference protrudes through the vulva and causes the distinct doughnut-shaped appearance (Figure 21.1; Johnston et al. 2001). Type III often involves exteriorization of the urethral orifice.

Vaginal fold prolapse is an uncommon condition, but most commonly occurs at predictable phases in the estrous cycle, usually proestrus and estrus, or shortly after parturition, as progesterone levels decline and estrogen levels increase (Johnston et al. 2001; Fossum 2002). It is normal for vaginal mucosa to become hyperemic, edematous, and keratinized during estrus, but when these effects are accentuated, vaginal fold prolapse may result. There have also been reports of vaginal fold prolapse during diestrus and normal pregnancy, but this is extremely rare (Johnston et al. 2001).

True vaginal prolapse, involving the entire vaginal wall (Nelissen 2015), leads to 360° protrusion of the vaginal mucosa as with Type III vaginal fold prolapse, but may also encompass other organs, including the urinary bladder, uterine body, or distal colon (McNamara et al. 1997). Some cases of complete vaginal prolapse may involve the cervix as well (Fossum 2002). Vaginal fold prolapse may also be caused by vaginal tumors or trauma (Arbeiter and Bucher 1994; Williams 2005). Trauma may include forced separation during mating, and difference between size of breeding animals (Purswell 2000).

Although vaginal fold prolapse can be seen in any breed of dog, large breed and brachycephalic dogs seem to be at an increased risk (McNamara et al. 1997). Occurrence is most common in dogs under the age of two years, especially during their first three estrus cycles. Clinical signs at presentation may include a mass protruding from the vulva, vulvar discharge, or vulvar bleeding. There may also be other signs including pollakiuria, dysuria, or signs of vaginal/perineal discomfort such as licking or chewing (Fossum 2002).

Other diseases with signs similar to vaginal fold prolapse should be ruled out. These most

High-Quality, High-Volume Spay and Neuter and Other Shelter Surgeries, First Edition. Edited by Sara White.
© 2020 John Wiley & Sons, Inc. Published 2020 by John Wiley & Sons, Inc.

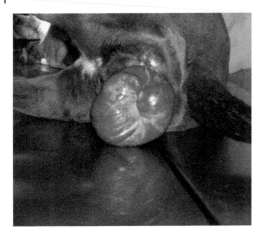

Figure 21.1 Vaginal fold prolapse. Note the distinct "doughnut" appearance. *Source:* Photo courtesy of Jack Smith, DVM, DACT. Mississippi State University College of Veterinary Medicine.

commonly include uterine prolapse and vaginal tumors. Vaginal tumors may include fibroleiomyoma, lipoma, leiomyosarcoma, squamous cell carcinoma, and transmissible venereal tumor. Most vaginal tumors occur in older, intact females. Other conditions to rule out include vaginal cysts, septa, and congenital malformations (Fossum 2002).

Treatment

Mild to moderate cases of vaginal fold prolapse, those that are not fully circumferential, spontaneously regress during diestrus (McNamara et al. 1997; Fossum 2002). Conversely, more severe cases have the potential for necrosis in the absence of proper medical attention (McNamara et al. 1997).

Everted tissue should be lavaged with warm saline or water. In cases of mild to moderate prolapse, the mass may be manually reduced into the vagina.

Medical management may be an option for mild cases. Administration of gonadotropin-releasing hormone (GnRH, 50 µg/40 lb) or human chorionic gonadotropin (HCG, 500–1000 IU, intramuscularly) can shorten the estrus phase and induce ovulation (Fossum 2002). These drugs will cause decreasing estrogen levels and may lead to spontaneous regression of the edematous

tissue (Johnston et al. 2001). Recurrence after spontaneous regression, in the absence of an ovariohysterectomy, is common.

Surgical correction is warranted in prolapses with severe edema, necrotic tissue, or those that fail to regress spontaneously. It is important to determine the extent of involvement of the urethral opening. If the urethra is involved, the opening can be found on the ventral surface of the prolapsed tissue and should be catheterized before surgical correction (see Figure 21.2a; Fossum 2002). Surgical options include purse-string sutures, hysteropexy, circumferential excision of the prolapsed tissue (Figure 21.2), and episiotomy (Figure 21.3; Johnston et al. 2001). Hysteropexy is not a common surgical treatment for vaginal fold prolapse, but has been successfully performed in cases of true vaginal prolapse (Memon et al. 1993). Circumferential excision may be required for type II or III vaginal fold prolapse, as well as in those cases with necrotic tissue. Reduction can be maintained by placing two to three horizontal mattress sutures between the vulvar lips (Fossum 2002).

Episiotomy

In some cases, an episiotomy may be needed in order to replace or resect prolapsed tissue. An episiotomy is an incision in the vulvar orifice that allows better access to the vagina (Figure 21.3). For this procedure the animal is placed in a perineal position. In this position, the patient is placed in ventral recumbency with the hind legs over the end of the table. The tail can be tied away from the surgical site by gauze or a comparable material. Doyen intestinal clamps are placed on each side of the perineal midline along the shaft of the vagina. A midline skin incision is made through the dorsal commissure of the vulvar lips and extends to just distal to the external anal sphincter muscle (Figure 21.4). The incision is then extended to the rectal sphincter using Metzenbaum scissors (Figure 21.5). Two to three horizontal mattress stay sutures are placed through the skin and vaginal mucosa on both sides of the incision (Figure 21.6). The stay sutures allow for retraction of the vaginal

(a)

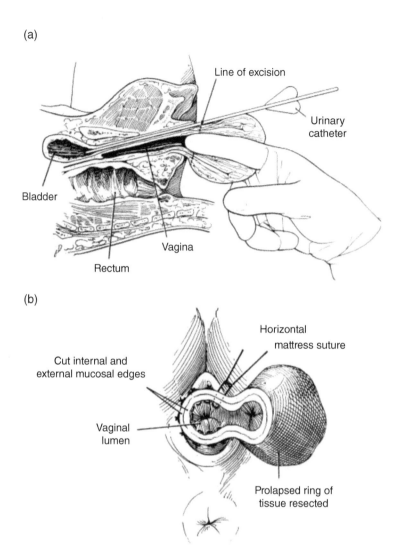

Line of excision

Urinary
catheter

Bladder

Vagina

Rectum

(b)

Horizontal
mattress suture

Cut internal and
external mucosal edges

Vaginal
lumen

Prolapsed ring of
tissue resected

Figure 21.2 Surgical treatment for a Type III vaginal fold prolapse. (a) The dog is placed in dorsal recumbency and a urethral catheter is placed. A finger can be inserted into the center of the prolapsed tissue. The dashed line indicates the intended line of resection. (b) A full-thickness circumferential incision is made in a stepwise manner through the vaginal wall. Horizontal mattress sutures are placed to close the incisional edges. *Source:* Nelissen (2015), reproduced with permission of John Wiley and Sons.

folds. The vagina is manually replaced or, if manual replacement is not possible, the prolapsed tissue may be amputated. The episiotomy incision is closed with a three-layer closure (Figure 21.7; Fossum 2002). Ovariectomy or ovariohysterectomy should be performed to reduce the recurrence rate (Morrow 1986; Fossum 2002).

Post-operatively, patients should be supported with analgesics and may need fluid therapy. Cold compresses to the surgical site should be applied intermittently for 24 hours following surgery. Warm compresses should be applied intermittently starting 24 hours postoperatively. An Elizabethan collar or other method should be used to avoid self-trauma. The vulvar sutures should be removed five to seven days following prolapse repair if the tissue eversion and edema have regressed significantly (Fossum 2002).

(a) (b) (c)

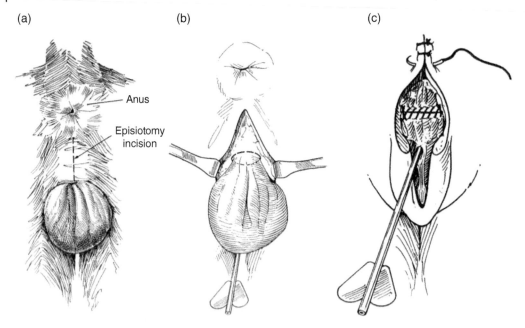

Figure 21.3 Surgical treatment for a Type II vaginal fold prolapse. (a) Location of episiotomy incision for better exposure to treat vaginal fold prolapse. (b) The tissue is lifted off the vestibular floor for catheterization of the urethra. A transverse elliptical incision is made at the base of the mass. Care is taken to avoid the urethral tubercle. (c) The defect in the vaginal wall is closed with a continuous suture using absorbable material. The episiotomy incision is closed. *Source:* Nelissen (2015), reproduced with permission of John Wiley and Sons.

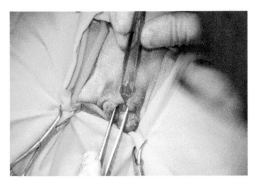

Figure 21.4 Episiotomy. A midline skin incision is made through the dorsal commissure of the vulvar lips and extends to just distal to the external anal sphincter muscle. *Source:* Photo courtesy of Cory Fisher, DVM, MS, DACVS. Mississippi State University College of Veterinary Medicine.

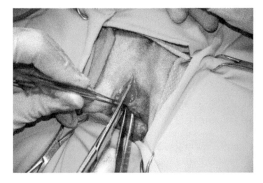

Figure 21.5 Episiotomy. The incision is then extended to the rectal sphincter using Metzenbaum scissors. *Source:* Photo courtesy of Cory Fisher, DVM, MS, DACVS. Mississippi State University College of Veterinary Medicine.

Prognosis

Medical or surgical management in conjunction with ovariohysterectomy provides the best long-term prognosis (Johnston et al. 2001). Vaginal fold prolapse carries an excellent prognosis following an ovariohysterectomy. Conversely, recurrence is common in those animals that do not undergo ovariohysterectomy (Fossum 2002).

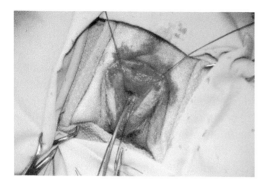

Figure 21.6 Episiotomy. Note placement of urethral catheter to mark urethral orifice and placement of stay sutures placed near the urethral papilla. *Source:* Photo courtesy of Cory Fisher, DVM, MS, DACVS. Mississippi State University College of Veterinary Medicine.

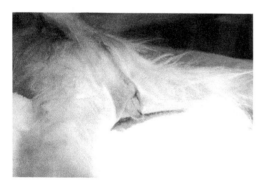

Figure 21.7 Episiotomy closure. *Source:* Photo courtesy of Cory Fisher, DVM, MS, DACVS. Mississippi State University College of Veterinary Medicine.

Rectal Prolapse

Although uncommon, rectal prolapse is documented in both dogs and cats and is more common in young animals. There does not appear to be any breed predisposition. Some resources argue that rectal prolapse may occur more commonly in Manx cats due to breed-associated anal laxity (Fossum 2002).

Rectal prolapse must be differentiated from intussusception. To differentiate between the two, a probe such as a thermometer or tubing should be gently inserted between the prolapsed tissue and the rectal wall. If the mass is the result of an intussusception, the probe can be easily passed. Conversely, if the mass is due to a rectal prolapse, it will not be possible to insert the probe (Fossum 2002).

Animals that present with rectal prolapse usually have a history of dyschezia or tenesmus, heavy parasite burden, or other colonic inflammatory condition. There have also been reports of rectal prolapse following antibiotic use (Marjani et al. 2009). In older animals, rectal prolapse may be associated with tumors or perineal hernias (Fossum 2002).

Prolapse may be classified as complete, circumferentially involving all layers of the rectal wall, or incomplete, involving only the mucosa. Once the prolapse occurs, the involved tissue layers continue to become increasingly edematous and may progress to excoriation, bleeding, and necrosis (Fossum 2002).

Medical Management

An important step in any treatment, medical or surgical, is the identification of the underlying cause (Popovitch and Holt 1994; Sherding and Johnson 2006). Identification of the primary cause may also help determine the prognosis for recovery without recurrence.

Medical management is an option for treatment, especially in mild cases of prolapse, or with acute prolapse. Following lavage with warm saline and lubrication, manual reduction and subsequent placement of a purse-string suture around the anus may be adequate to prevent recurrence. The purse-string suture should be tight enough to prevent recurrence, while allowing the passage of soft stool (Fossum 2002). Low-fiber diets and stool softeners are indicated while the purse-string suture is in place. The suture may be removed three to five days following manual reduction.

Surgical Management

Surgical treatment is warranted if the prolapse is non-reducible or if the tissue involved in the prolapse is severely traumatized. In this case, the traumatized tissue should be amputated (Fossum 2002).

Prior to surgery, the perianal area should be clipped and aseptically prepped. As with manual reduction, the everted tissue should be lavaged and lubricated. The animal should be placed in ventral recumbency with the hind legs over the end of the table to allow easiest access to the prolapse, and gauze or similar material should be used tie the tail over the back, away from the surgical site (Fossum 2002).

A probe should be inserted into the rectal lumen and horizontal mattress sutures should be placed in the rectal tissue cranial to the surgical site at the 12, 5, and 8 o'clock positions. The sutures should pass through all layers of the prolapse and enter the lumen to the point that they are deflected off the probe. Following the placement of the stay sutures, the traumatized tissue can be transected caudal to the sutures. It is recommended that the transection be done in sections, with each section then being apposed at the cut edge with simple interrupted sutures approximately 2 mm apart. Once the entire circumference of the prolapse has been transected and anastomosed, the stay sutures can be removed and the tissue can be placed back into the pelvic canal. In some cases an anal purse-string suture may be indicated, especially if the underlying cause of the prolapse involved tenesmus (Fossum 2002).

For pain control, opioid epidurals may help to decreased or eliminate tenesmus. Systemic analgesics should be given as needed. If a purse-string suture is placed, a low-fiber diet is indicated post-operatively. Stool softeners should be administered for at least two weeks following amputation and resection. The purse-string suture can be removed two days following resection. The anastomosis site should be monitored for leakage following surgery (Fossum 2002).

Colopexy

Colopexy is indicated if the prolapse recurs following manual reduction or amputation and resection (Fossum 2002). This surgery should create an adhesion between the serosal surface of the colon and the abdominal wall. Two techniques are described, incisional and non-incisional, and both are considered to be effective.

For either technique, an incision is made on the midline caudal to the umbilicus to expose the abdomen. The descending colon is delivered through the incision and manipulated cranially to reduce the prolapse. The anus should be visibly inspected to ensure that the prolapse is sufficiently reduced.

For the incisional approach, a 3–5 cm incision is made longitudinally along the antimesenteric border of the distal colon through the serosal and muscularis layers. Care must be taken not to penetrate the lumen of the colon. An incision is made on the interior surface of the abdominal wall approximately 2.5 cm (or less, relative to the size of the animal) left of the midline. The incision should extend through the peritoneum and into the underlying muscle layer. The respective edges of the incision in the colon and the abdominal incision should be apposed and sutured using non-absorbable sutures in simple continuous or simple interrupted patterns.

For a non-incisional approach, an 8–10 cm area on the antimesenteric border of the distal colon should be scraped with a scalpel blade or abraded with a gauze sponge. The same should be done to the abdominal wall 2.5 cm left of the midline. Horizontal mattress sutures should be pre-placed between the two areas and the sutures should be tied to appose the scored surfaces (Fossum 2002). A 1994 study of 14 dogs and cats comparing the incisional and non-incisional methods found that there was no significant clinical difference in outcome between the two procedures (Popovitch and Holt 1994).

A laparoscopic technique has been described in which a 10/11 mm trocar-cannula unit was placed on the midline 2.5–5 cm caudal to the umbilicus. A second trocar-cannula unit was placed 2.5 cm to the right of the midline to allow for laparoscopic forceps and exteriorization of the descending colon. The incisions as previously described were utilized (Zhang et al. 2012).

Prognosis

The prognosis for rectal prolapse is good, assuming that the primary cause of straining is identified and successfully treated.

References

Arbeiter, K. and Bucher, A. (1994). Traumatically caused perineal prolapse of the vagina followed by a retroflexion of the urinary bladder in the bitch. *Tierärztl. Prax.* 22: 78–79.

Fossum, T.W. (2002). *Small Animal Surgery*, 2e, 619–620. St. Louis, MO: Mosby.

Johnston, S., Kustritz, M.V., and Olson, P. (2001). *Canine and Feline Theriogenology*. Philadelphia, PA: W.B. Saunders.

Marjani, M., Ghaffari, M.S., and Moosakhani, F. (2009). Rectal prolapse secondary to antibiotic-associated colitis in a dog. *Comp. Clin. Pathol.* 18: 473–475.

McNamara, P.S., Dykes, N., and Harvey, H.J. (1997). Chronic vaginocervical prolapse with visceral incarceration in a dog. *J. Am. Anim. Hosp. Assoc.* 33: 533–536.

Memon, M.A., Pavletic, M.M., and Kumar, M.S. (1993). Chronic vaginal prolapse during pregnancy in a bitch. *JAVMA* 202: 295–297.

Morrow, D.A. (ed.) (1986). *Current therapy in theriogenology: Diagnosis, Treatment, and Prevention of Reproductive Diseases in Small and Large Animals*, 2e. Philadelphia, PA: Saunders.

Nelissen, P. (2015). Uterine and vaginal prolapse. In: *Small Animal Surgical Emergencies* (ed. L.R. Aronson), 420. Hoboken, NJ: Wiley.

Popovitch, C.A. and Holt, D. (1994). Colopexy as a treatment for rectal prolapse in dogs and cats: a retrospective study of 14 cases. *Vet. Surg.* 23: 115–118.

Purswell, B.J. (2000). Vaginal disorders. In: *Textbook of Veterinary Internal Medicine: Diseases of the Dog and Cat*, vol. 1 and 2 (eds. S.J. Ettinger and E.C. Feldman), 1566–1571. Philadelphia, PA: W.B. Saunders.

Sherding, R.G. and Johnson, S.E. (2006). *Diseases of the Intestines*. Philadelphia, PA: Elsevier.

Williams, J.M. (2005). Disorders of the perineum and anus. In: *BSAVA Manual of Canine and Feline Gastroenterology* (eds. J.E. Hall, J.W. Simpson and D.A. Williams), 213–221. Quedgeley: British Small Animal Veterinary Association.

Zhang, S., Zhang, J., Zhang, N. et al. (2012). Comparison of laparoscopic-assisted and open colopexy in dogs. *B. Vet. I. Puawy* 56: 415–417.

21A

Rectal and Vaginal Fold Prolapse: Anesthesia Supplement
Lydia Love

Rectal prolapse may occur as a result of gastrointestinal or urogenital disease and subsequent straining. The condition may be managed by manual reduction of the prolapsed tissue and placement of a purse-string suture. Severe cases, or those in which conservative management fails, will require a colopexy. Animals should be carefully assessed to rule out concurrent perineal hernias.

The list of differential diagnoses for a mass protruding from the vulva includes vaginal hyperplasia, vaginal fold prolapse, uterine prolapse, or neoplasia. Vaginal hyperplasia (edema of the vaginal wall mediated by estrogen) is common in certain breeds of dog, including Staffordshire Terriers and pugs, and also occurs in cats. Treatment consists of reducing the tissue and ovariohysterectomy (OHE) or ovariectomy. True vaginal fold prolapse is uncommon in dogs and cats and may require resection of the prolapsed tissue in addition to OHE/ovariectomy. Uterine prolapse is rare in dogs and cats and usually occurs post-parturition (see Chapter 12). In all cases, urethral patency must be assessed and the urethra should be catheterized to reduce the likelihood of surgical trauma.

Anesthetic Concerns

Pediatric cats and dogs with gastrointestinal parasite infestations may be the most common patients presenting with rectal prolapse in the shelter setting; however, older patients may also suffer from rectal prolapse secondary to diseases such as prostatitis, cystitis, and related to dystocia. General anesthetic considerations for neonatal and pediatric patients are presented in Chapter 15. Older patients should be carefully screened for concurrent systemic disease prior to general anesthesia.

Most cases of vaginal fold prolapse will require standard monitoring and supportive care during anesthesia. Uterine prolapse patients may be nursing and many drugs will be excreted in the milk. Use of non-steroidal anti-inflammatory drugs (NSAIDs) should be limited in nursing patients; however a single post-operative dose of injectable NSAIDs is generally regarded as safe (Mathews 2005).

Analgesic Concerns

In addition to systemic analgesics including opioids and NSAIDs, epidural administration of analgesics should be considered for reduction of rectal and vaginal fold prolapses. Local anesthetics placed into the epidural space will provide analgesia as well as motor blockade that may facilitate reduction of the prolapse. Epidural local anesthetic administration will prevent straining and may allow manual reduction of a prolapse without general anesthesia.

High-Quality, High-Volume Spay and Neuter and Other Shelter Surgeries, First Edition. Edited by Sara White.
© 2020 John Wiley & Sons, Inc. Published 2020 by John Wiley & Sons, Inc.

A lumbosacral approach to the epidural space is most commonly employed in dogs and cats, and would be indicated for prolapses that require an abdominal approach for OHE/ovariectomy or colopexy (see Chapter 19, amputation anesthesia supplement). However, a sacrocaudal (or coccygeal) epidural approach may be considered in addition to or in place of general anesthesia for reduction of rectal and vaginal fold prolapses. This technique is routinely used in standing ruminants for similar procedures, and has recently been described for urethral catheterization of conscious, but mildly sedated, cats (O'Hearn and Wright 2011). With the patient positioned in sternal recumbency, the injection site is located by palpating the first moveable vertebral joint at the base of the tail as it is moved up and down. A 4×4 cm square area is clipped and prepared using an aseptic technique. In the conscious patient, 0.25–0.5 ml lidocaine should be injected into the subcutaneous tissues. A 25-gauge, 1 in. (3.8 cm) hypodermic needle is inserted at a 30–45° angle with the bevel facing cranially. A pop may be felt as the needle penetrates the ligamentum flavum and the needle will feel

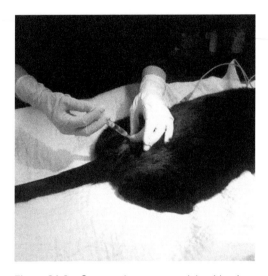

Figure 21.8 Coccygeal or sacrocaudal epidural placement of local anesthetics will provide anesthesia to the external genitalia, perineum, rectum, tail, and a portion of the pelvic viscera.

firmly seated in the tissues (Figure 21.8). The syringe should be aspirated to ensure that intravenous injection will be avoided and 2–4 mg/kg of 2% lidocaine or 1–2 mg/kg of 0.5% bupivacaine is then injected. There should be no resistance to injection.

References

Mathews, K.A. (2005). Analgesia for the pregnant, lactating and neonatal to pediatric cat and dog. *J. Vet. Emerg. Crit. Care* 15 (4): 273–284.

O'Hearn, A.K. and Wright, B.D. (2011). Coccygeal epidural with local anesthetic for catheterization and pain management in the treatment of feline urethral obstruction. *J. Vet. Emerg. Crit. Care* 21 (1): 50–52.

22

Dental Extractions in a Shelter Environment
Diana L. Eubanks and Lydia Love

Dental disease is a common source of pain in middle-aged and older animals, and is frequently encountered in the shelter environment. Animals in pain may become listless or aggressive, or exhibit other behaviors that significantly decrease their adoptability. For example, many cats with tooth resorption will react negatively to any form of touch, earning them a label of "aggressive" or "unfriendly" when they may simply need analgesics and oral healthcare. Animals that are pain free will be more interactive and less stressed, thus healthier and overall more adoptable.

Most facilities will be able to provide anesthesia, but may not have dental and oral radiology equipment. For those fortunate enough to have the proper instruments and equipment, dentistry can often offer an excellent return on investment.

Advanced procedures such as root canal treatment and crown placement are available to save animals' teeth. Lack of resources and difficulty with adequate follow-up care make advanced procedures a less viable option for shelter practices. However, cats and dogs generally manage quite well with the proper removal of teeth, and many can live comfortable lives with few or no teeth at all. Removal of a tooth generally results in a gap in the dentition that is rarely a problem and canine and feline teeth do not often suffer from "dental drift," a potential consequence of tooth extraction in human dentistry. Failure to treat a painful tooth will lead to continued pain for the animal. Proper pain management and extraction of diseased teeth, however, can be accomplished successfully in the shelter environment.

This chapter will cover the basics of proper extraction technique, dental instrumentation, and pain management in the oral cavity.

Indications and Equipment

Persistent primary (deciduous) teeth, periodontal disease, and endodontic disease are the most common indications for extraction of a tooth. Persistent primary teeth (Figure 22.1) should be extracted as soon as the permanent tooth begins to erupt, in order to reduce the likelihood of a developmental malocclusion and prevent periodontal disease associated with crowding. Additionally, any tooth that is fractured with pulp exposure should be treated, if not endodontically, then by extraction (Figure 22.2). It is no longer acceptable practice to leave these teeth and "see what happens." Invariably "what happens" is that they abscess and become painful. Many owners and veterinarians see these teeth months or years after the initial trauma. They do not appear painful at that point, but many have gone through an acutely painful process that has subsequently become a chronic low-grade pain and source of infection.

High-Quality, High-Volume Spay and Neuter and Other Shelter Surgeries, First Edition. Edited by Sara White.
© 2020 John Wiley & Sons, Inc. Published 2020 by John Wiley & Sons, Inc.

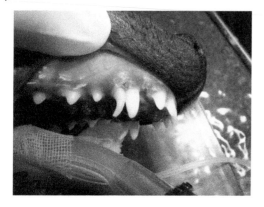

Figure 22.1 A young adult dog with a persistent primary (deciduous) tooth. This tooth should be carefully extracted in order to prevent periodontal disease and possible displacement of the successional adult tooth, although in this case the adult tooth is nearly completely erupted. Ideally, this persistent primary tooth should have been identified much earlier.

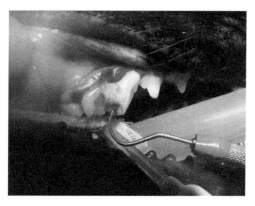

Figure 22.2 A dog with a fractured tooth. The pulp exposure necessitates either extraction or possible root canal procedure.

A proper pre-extraction plan should include pain management and pre- and post-operative intraoral radiographs.

Safe and effective dentistry requires general anesthesia. Dental instruments are equipped with water irrigation systems, necessitating that general anesthesia and a cuffed endotracheal tube be used in all patients in order to protect the airway from water, blood, tooth particles, calculus, and other debris. Further, any sudden movement of a conscious patient could result in tissue damage, including severed arteries or a broken mandible. There is no way to perform a safe dental procedure without anesthesia.

Instrumentation

Many of the instruments used for oral surgery are the same as those used for other soft tissue procedures (needle holders, scalpel handles, blades, forceps, straight and curved scissors). Additionally, special dental instruments are needed.

Periodontal elevators (Figure 22.3) are used to cut/break down the periodontal ligament with a combination of apical pressure and leverage. Periodontal elevators are also used as a wedge between the segments of an individual tooth, between two teeth, or between tooth and alveolar bone. Controlled force is applied in an attempt to fatigue the periodontal ligament and "elevate" the tooth out of the alveolus (bony socket).

Dental luxators have a thinner working end than elevators and may also be used to sever the periodontal ligament. They should not be used for leverage, as they may break. Dental luxators and elevators come in a variety of sizes. An appropriately sized elevator should "hug" the tooth. Smaller elevators are useful for cat and small dog teeth. Larger ones are available for use with larger animals. Most of these instruments are available as a set of four or five, suitable for most small animal dental extractions.

Periosteal elevators are used in open (surgical) extractions, where access to the tooth roots requires the lifting of a mucoperiosteal flap and subsequent removal of alveolar bone. In closed (simple) extraction, the periosteal elevator can be used to "free up" the gingival margins and facilitate a tension-free closure. A quality periosteal elevator is invaluable in allowing the practitioner to gently elevate the mucoperiosteal tissues without significant damage. The importance of this becomes apparent when closing the flap. A healthy, properly elevated flap is much easier to work with than one that has been damaged in the initial phases of handling.

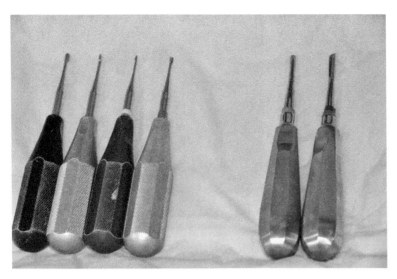

Figure 22.3 Periodontal elevators.

Extraction forceps are used in the final extraction of the tooth. There is an old adage that says "the only extraction forceps needed are your fingers," which emphasizes the fact that the tooth must be very loose prior to using these forceps. Crowns are easily snapped off when forceps are used improperly or with excessive force. A forceps that properly fits onto the crown should be used to gently grasp the crown and slightly rotate the tooth or tooth segment while applying gentle, controlled traction. As with other surgical instruments, all dental instruments should be sterilized prior to use.

The typical dental unit (or "cart") can be stationary (mounted on the table or wall), or can be an actual cart that allows the user to move it about in the clinic. A dental unit should include a low-speed handpiece (for polishing), a high-speed handpiece (for bone removal during surgical extractions), an air/water syringe, and a scaler. Follow manufacturer's directions for maintenance of equipment.

Extraction Technique

First, the epithelial attachment is severed using a scalpel blade (#11 or #15; Figure 22.4a).

Access to the tooth is important. If needed, mesial and/or distal releasing incisions are made in the gingiva, extending beyond the mucogingival junction (Figure 22.4b). The gingival flap is then gently raised using a periosteal elevator. (A flap may not be needed in all extractions; Figure 22.5a.) A pair of scissors can be used to help undermine the flap and release tension (Figure 22.5b).

Access to the tooth root can be obtained by removing buccal alveolar bone using a round bur on a high-speed handpiece with water cooling (Figure 22.6). Care should be taken to remove bone only and not tooth material. When dealing with a multirooted tooth, the tooth must be sectioned, starting at the furcation and moving toward the crown (Figure 22.7).

By working on alternating surfaces of the tooth and using various techniques, the periodontal ligament is fatigued and the tooth can be lifted out of the alveolus. A periodontal elevator is introduced into the periodontal ligament space. Careful, controlled force is applied in an apical direction (toward the root) around the entire tooth. Additionally, an elevator may be introduced perpendicular to the axis of the tooth and between two adjacent portions of the sectioned tooth. Using gentle pressure, the

(a) (b)

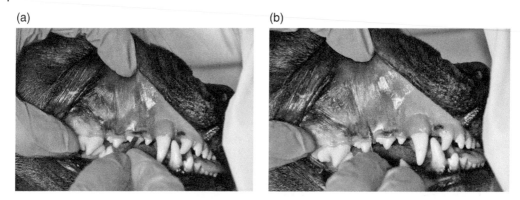

Figure 22.4 A scalpel blade is used to severe the epithelial attachment (a). Releasing incisions can be made perpendicular to the sulcus and aid in releasing tension on the flap (b).

(a) (b)

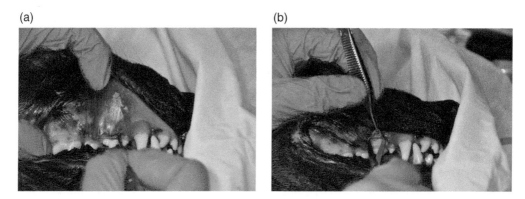

Figure 22.5 A periosteal elevator is used to gently lift a full-thickness flap from the underlying alveolar bone. Care must be taken to preserve the integrity of the flap, as it will be used to cover the defect (a). Scissors may also be used to facilitate the release of tension on the flap (b).

(a) (b)

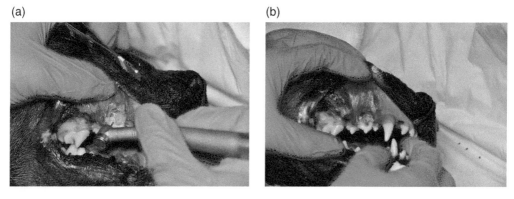

Figure 22.6 A high-speed handpiece (a) equipped with a bur can be used to remove buccal alveolar bone in order to expose the tooth root surfaces (b).

elevator can be rotated until the two segments become loosened (Figure 22.8). One of the authors (Eubanks) prefers a winged elevator for the first approach and a regular or non-winged elevator for placing between adjacent tooth segments.

The extraction site is curetted free of debris and the alveolar edges are smoothed using a round or

(a)

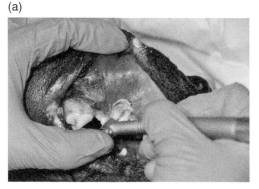

(b)

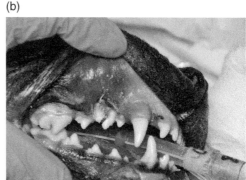

Figure 22.7   (a and b) Multirooted teeth are sectioned to facilitate removal.

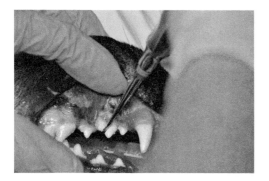

Figure 22.8   A non-winged periodontal elevator being used to stretch the periodontal ligament.

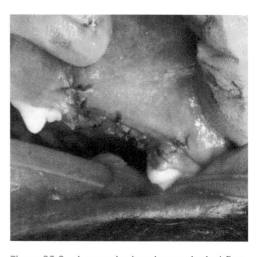

Figure 22.9   A properly closed mucogingival flap.

diamond bur on a high-speed handpiece. Some cases may require the use of a synthetic bone material in the empty socket. Synthetic bone material is best placed along the mandible, for instance when removing a first mandibular molar, and in areas of significant bone loss such as occurs in the mandibular incisor region. Extractions in the upper arcade that result in oronasal fistulation are not good candidates for placement of synthetic bone material. Regardless, a blood clot should be left in place and simple interrupted sutures placed to close the defect.

4-0 or 5-0 absorbable suture is used in a simple interrupted pattern to close the flap. The type of suture depends on the surgeon's preference, but common choices are monofilament synthetic suture materials. Additional undermining may be necessary to "free up" the flap. Periosteal fibers may need to be severed, taking care not to tear the flap (Figure 22.9). There is no substitute for experience. Therefore, it is recommended

that extractions be practiced on cadaver heads to allow the veterinarian to develop a "feel" for the amount of pressure and tension that can be applied while performing the procedure. Many frustrating situations such as fractured tooth roots and dehiscence of flaps can be prevented by proper practice of the procedures. Also, in most states in the United States, the extraction of teeth is considered "oral surgery" and as such is *not* a procedure that can be legally performed by even certified veterinary technicians.

Principles to keep in mind for flap closure include:

1) The flap should be under absolutely no tension.
2) The sutures should, if possible, be placed over solid bone rather than directly over a void.

3) Sutures should be placed 2mm apart. Simple continuous suture patterns are rarely recommended for oral surgery.
4) The base of the flap should be at least as large as the apex (or larger) to preserve blood supply.
5) Place edges of fresh epithelium adjacent to fresh epithelium (bleeding edges) with no overlap or gaps.
6) The caretaker should check the area daily, but should be cautious about putting tension on the flap.

Deciduous teeth can be approached in much the same manner as adult teeth. They often have long, slender roots that may break easily (especially deciduous canines). If a deciduous canine tooth is not mobile, bone must be removed on the buccal aspect in order to prevent the tooth from "snapping off" and leaving root behind. Every effort should be made to remove all of the tooth material and to avoid damaging the underlying permanent tooth bud.

Feline teeth may also present a challenge as they can be quite fragile, especially when they are affected by tooth resorption. Buccal bone removal will facilitate fracture-free extractions. In any species, care should be taken when working on the mandibular teeth not to cause an iatrogenic fracture, either at the mandibular body or the symphysis. Pre-operative radiographs can help to identify osteomyelitis and areas of significant bone loss that may predispose a patient to fracture.

If a root breaks, additional alveolar bone can be removed in an effort to reveal the root segment and make retrieval easier. Dental radiographs can be of great value in this situation.

Anesthetic Concerns

Standard peri-anesthetic concerns apply to oral surgical procedures, including the need to prevent, monitor for, and respond to hypothermia, hypotension, and hypoventilation. In addition, patients with retained deciduous teeth are often small brachycephalic breed dogs that require extra care related to maintaining a patent airway, especially in the recovery period. Small patients are more likely to lose body heat precipitously and close attention should be paid to active warming measures.

The use of mouth gags has been linked to the occurrence of post-anesthetic blindness and other neurologic deficits following anesthesia in cats (Stiles et al. 2012; de Miguel Garcia et al. 2013). The maxillary artery, a branch of the external carotid artery, is responsible for perfusion of the retina, inner ear, and much of the cerebral cortex in cats, and spring-loaded mouth gags can attenuate maxillary artery blood flow during anesthesia (Barton-Lamb et al. 2013). Spring-loaded mouth gags should be avoided and, in adult cats when the mouth is held open by any type of device, the intergingival distance between the upper and lower canine teeth should be less than 42mm (Martin-Flores et al. 2014). Vigilance in monitoring blood pressure and oxygenation is also required, as hypotension and hypoxemia may compromise oxygen delivery to the retina and brain even without the use of mouth gags.

Analgesic Concerns

Dental extractions range in invasiveness and degree of post-operative pain. Systemic analgesia in the form of opioids and non-steroidal anti-inflammatory drugs (NSAIDs) should be available for all patients undergoing invasive procedures. Generally, opioids are administered in the immediate peri-operative period, and may be continued post-operatively if invasive procedures including extractions are performed. NSAIDs should also be considered for post-operative administration, once it is established that renal function is normal and the patient is volume replete.

Local anesthesia is easy to provide and extremely effective. Complete blockade of pain impulses in the periphery reduces the amount of inhalant anesthetic required (Snyder and Snyder 2013), thereby improving cardiovascular parameters, as well as reducing the need for analgesics in the post-operative period.

When performing a nerve block, a small volume of local anesthetic is placed in close proximity to the nerve, using anatomic landmarks. Oral nerve blocks are easy to learn, inexpensive to perform, have a relatively rapid onset of effect, and should be included in every balanced anesthetic protocol where potentially painful dental procedures are to be performed.

Anesthetic Agents

Choice of local anesthetic determines onset and length of anesthesia (Table 22.1). Lidocaine and bupivacaine are the two most commonly used local anesthetics in veterinary dental procedures, though mepivacaine, ropivacaine, levobupivacaine, and articaine are also employed. Lidocaine and mepivacaine are short-acting agents that, when administered alone, are typically effective for 1–2 hours. Bupivacaine, and its enantiomer levobupivacaine, have an onset of action of around 10 minutes and effects can last for 3–6 hours. Bupivacaine is available in a variety of concentrations and in a long-acting DepoFoam® formulation (Pacira BioSciences, San Diego, CA) that can provide up to 72 hours of analgesia (Nocita®, Aratana Therapeutics, Leawood, KS). The local anesthetic articaine is available in dental cartridges mixed with epinephrine (Septocaine®, Septodont, Louisville,

CO) to prolong anesthesia. This local anesthetic has gained widespread acceptance in humans for dental procedures because of its reported superiority in penetration of bony structures and lower risk of systemic toxicity. However, enhanced effectiveness may be site dependent (mandibular versus maxillary nerve blockade) and controversy exists as to whether paresthesias may be more common with articaine (Yapp et al. 2011).

Mixtures of short-acting and long-acting local anesthetics have been advocated to provide short onset time and longer-lasting anesthesia. However, multiple studies, mostly in humans, indicate that the combination of short- and long-acting local anesthetics provides minimal advantage in terms of speed of onset and actually decreases the length of anesthesia, compared to the long-acting anesthetic alone (Lawal and Adetunji 2009; Gadsden et al. 2011).

Duration of efficacy of local anesthetics can be extended by the use of various adjuncts, including vasoconstrictors (such as epinephrine), opioids, and alpha$_2$ agonists (Table 22.2).

Adverse effects of local anesthesia can be systemic or local. Systemic toxicity includes neurologic (drowsiness, seizures) and cardiovascular complications (hypotension, dysrhythmias, cardiac arrest). Attention must be paid to total local anesthetic dose and it should be noted when using combinations of local anesthetics that toxicity is additive. In addition, aspiration of the syringe before injection should always be performed to avoid

Table 22.1 Local anesthetics commonly used in veterinary dental nerve blocks.

Local anesthetic	Speed of onset	Duration	Suggested maximum dose
Lidocaine	2–5 min	1–2 h	6 mg/kg
Mepivacaine	2–5 min	1–2 h	6 mg/kg
Articaine	1–3 min	2–4 h	7 mg/kg
Bupivacaine	5–10 min	3–6 h	2 mg/kg
Levobupivacaine	5–10 min	3–6 h	2 mg/kg
Ropivacaine	5–10 min	3–6 h	3 mg/kg

Table 22.2 Adjuvants to local anesthetics used in veterinary dental nerve blocks.

Drug	Suggested dose	Comments
Buprenorphine	3–4 µg/kg	May interact with peripheral opioid receptors
Dexmedetomidine	0.5–1 µg/ml of local anesthetic	Vasoconstrictor; may also have direct effects on local ion currents
Epinephrine	1 : 200 000 (5 µg/ml of local anesthetic)	Vasconstrictor
Sodium bicarbonate	1 part NaHCO$_3$ to 9 parts local anesthetic	Excessive alkalinization of local anesthetics will cause precipitation

inadvertent intravascular injection. Local adverse effects of local anesthetic blocks include temporary or permanent paresthesias, infection, or hemorrhage. Dental blocks may cause loss of sensation to the tongue or lips, resulting in self-mutilation, though this is not common (Beckman 2006). Other rare complications include direct nerve trauma, anaphylactic or anaphylactoid reactions to the agent, and local hematoma formation.

Materials

The materials needed to perform a nerve block are a 1–3 ml syringe and a 25–27-gauge × 0.75–1.5 in. (1.9–3.8 cm) needle. Flexible intravenous (IV) catheters may be used for some dental blocks.

Technique

The oral mucosa at the needle entry site should be gently stretched to stabilize the tissue. The needle is placed into the tissue with bevel side facing bone and advanced to the target area. Cats typically will receive 0.1–0.5 ml at each injection site and dogs 0.25–1 ml, depending on body size (Beckman and Legendre 2002).

Infraorbital Nerve Block

The infraorbital foramen is located on the maxilla dorsal to the distal root of the third premolar (PM3) in dogs or the PM2 in cats. The caudal extent of the canal is located at the

medial canthus of the eye and the needle should never be advanced beyond this point (a special concern in brachycephalic breeds and all cats; Figure 22.10).

Palpate the infraorbital foramen as a depression in the alveolar mucosa apical to the distal root of PM3 (Figures 22.10–22.12). While holding the syringe and needle parallel to the nose, advance the needle into the canal. In brachycephalic dogs and cats, the angle of approach toward midline is much greater than in dolicocephalic or mesaticephalic breeds (45° vs. 10–20°). In addition, it is important in brachycephalic animals to keep the needle flat in the dorsoventral plane to avoid entering the globe or retrobulbar space. For a cranial infraorbital nerve block, the needle should not be advanced deeply. After injection, apply digital pressure to the rostral opening of the canal for one minute (Rochette 2005; Reuss-Lamky 2007).

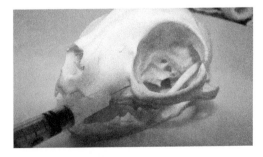

Figure 22.10 A feline skull used to demonstrate placement of an anesthetic in the infraorbital foramen. It should be noted that the canal in cats and brachycephalic dogs is very near the orbit and extreme caution should be observed.

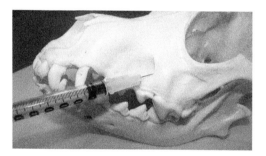

Figure 22.11 A canine skull used to demonstrate placement of an anesthetic in the infraorbital foramen.

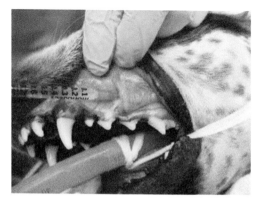

Figure 22.12 Placement of local anesthetic at the infraorbital canal can provide anesthesia to the ipsilateral premolars, incisors, canines, and soft tissue. Advancement of the needle deep into the canal can block the maxillary nerve, providing anesthesia to the entire hemimaxilla. *Source:* Photo courtesy of Dr. Carlos Rice.

Nerves blocked include the infraorbital nerve, and the rostral and middle maxillary alveolar nerves. Structures affected are as follows: ipsilateral canine, incisors and first two premolars, maxilla and intraoral soft tissues, nose, upper lip, and skin ventral to infraorbital foramen (Rochette 2005; Reuss-Lamky 2007).

Maxillary Nerve Block

The maxillary nerve is blocked as it enters the maxillary foramen at the rostral aspect of the pterygopalatine fossa and can be approached intra- or extraorally. In dogs, this block is performed intraorally by inserting the needle immediately caudal to the last upper molar.

The needle is then advanced dorsally just beyond the root tips of the last molar. In cats, the needle is placed just medial to the caudal root tips of the fourth upper premolar. Landmarks for the extraoral approach include the rostroventral aspect of the zygomatic arch, the caudal portion of the maxilla, and the coronoid process of the mandible. The needle is inserted perpendicular to the skin surface and advanced toward the pterygopalatine fossa (about 0.5–1 cm in cats and up to 3 cm in large dogs). Another extraoral approach (also referred to as a caudal infraorbital block) is commonly used, wherein an IV catheter or 27-gauge needle is advanced into the infraorbital canal to the level of the medial canthus.

The entire hemimaxilla, including the teeth, bone, and skin, as well as the soft tissues of the ipsilateral nose, cheek, and upper lip, can be desensitized by a properly performed maxillary nerve block (Rochette 2005; Reuss-Lamky 2007; Figures 22.13 and 22.14).

Mental Nerve Block

In the dog, the middle mental foramen is located ventral to the mesial root of the PM2, immediately caudal to the fleshy mandibular labial frenulum. The needle should be directed in a rostral to caudal direction into the foramen if possible, but not advanced very deeply. Nerves blocked include the mental nerve and mandibular ipsilateral canine and incisor teeth. Advancement of the needle into the foramen and application of digital pressure after injection may increase the desensi-

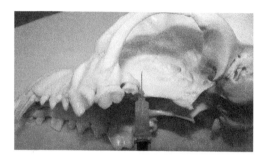

Figure 22.13 A canine skull used to demonstrate the maxillary nerve block.

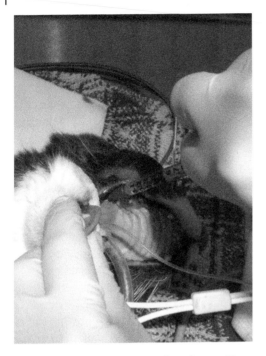

Figure 22.14   Intraoral approach to the maxillary nerve to provide anesthesia to the ipsilateral hemimaxilla.

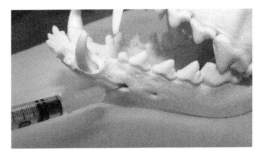

Figure 22.15   A canine skull used to demonstrate placement of an anesthetic in the middle mental foramen. The needle need not be advanced into the canal.

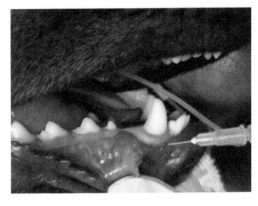

Figure 22.16   Injection of local anesthetic at the entrance of the middle mental foramen to provide anesthesia to the distal soft tissues. *Source:* Photo courtesy of Dr. Carlos Rice.

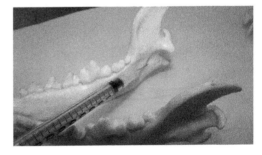

Figure 22.17   A canine mandible used to demonstrate placement of an anesthetic near the inferior alveolar nerve as it enters the mandibular canal.

tized area to include the incisors and possibly the canine teeth. However, one study in dogs demonstrated disappointingly variable anesthesia of the incisors and soft tissue distal to the foramen (Krug and Losey 2011). The foramen can be somewhat difficult to locate in cats and small dogs. In these cases, use of the mandibular nerve block may be more successful (Rochette 2005; Reuss-Lamky 2007; Figures 22.15 and 22.16).

Mandibular or Inferior Alveolar Block

The mandibular foramen is on the medial side of the ramus of the mandible at the base of the coronoid process (Figures 22.17 and 22.18). The mandibular nerve fossa can be palpated via an intraoral approach and is located on a line extending caudally from the last molar. With the mouth open, the needle is advanced at a 30° angle to the junction of the rostral aspect of the coronoid process with the horizontal segment of the mandible, just caudal to the last molar. The inferior alveolar branch of the mandibular

nerve is desensitized, preventing sensation to the entire mandible (right or left).

An extraoral technique is also described and may be preferred by some practitioners. The

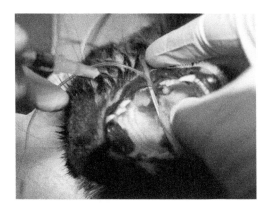

Figure 22.18 Performance of an intraoral mandibular nerve block in a cat. This technique can provide anesthesia to the entire hemimandible. *Source:* Photo courtesy of Dr. Carlos Rice.

vascular notch located on the medial aspect of the ventral mandible can be palpated with the non-dominant hand. The needle is inserted along the medial aspect of the ramus of the mandible and the needle tip is palpated as it is advanced toward the foramen beneath the oral mucosa, blocking the nerve before it enters the canal. The bevel should face the foramen to increase the likelihood that the agent will enter the canal (Figure 22.19).

When performing an inferior alveolar nerve block, it should be noted that the lingual nerve branches from the inferior alveolar nerve immediately before it enters the foramen, and

inclusion of the lingual nerve can desensitize the tongue, resulting in tongue and lip chewing on recovery. This complication has been reported, but is not common. For this reason, lower concentrations (e.g. 0.25% bupivacaine) and volumes of local anesthetics should be considered for this block, especially when completed bilaterally. Proper supervision during the recovery stage should prevent significant trauma.

Major Palatine Nerve Block

The palate and palatal gingiva at and mesial to the fourth upper premolar can be desensitized by blocking the major palatine nerve. This nerve cannot be palpated due to the thickness of the palatine mucosa. An imaginary line is drawn connecting the maxillary first molars in the dog (and the maxillary fourth upper premolars in the cat). The major palatine foramen is located midway between the dental arcade and the palatal midline along this imaginary line (Figure 22.20). The major palatine nerve lies in a trough superficial to the palatal bone and deep to the hard palate. This nerve block is reserved for surgical procedures of the hard and soft palate.

Alveolar/Intraosseous Block

Individual alveoli may be desensitized by insertion of a 25–27-gauge needle into the soft tissue/periodontal ligament space and slowly injecting local anesthetic. In humans, this block may fail in the mandible because the cortical bone is too dense for adequate diffusion to occur, though the use of articaine may improve efficacy (Meechan 2011; Rochette 2005).

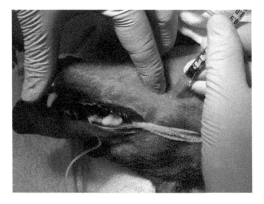

Figure 22.19 The extraoral approach to the mandibular nerve for anesthesia of the entire hemimandible. *Source:* Photo courtesy of Dr. Carlos Rice.

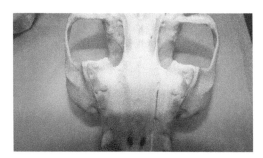

Figure 22.20 A feline skull demonstrating the location of the palatine foramen.

References

Barton-Lamb, A.L., Martin-Flores, M., Scrivani, P.V. et al. (2013). Evaluation of maxillary arterial blood flow in anesthetized cats with the mouth closed and open. *Vet. J.* 196 (3): 325–331.

Beckman, B.W. (2006). Pathophysiology and Management of Surgical and Chronic Oral Pain in dogs and cats. *J. Vet. Dent.* 23 (1): 50–60.

Beckman, B. and Legendre, L. (2002). Regional nerve blocks for oral surgery in companion animals. *Compendium* 24 (6): 439–444.

de Miguel Garcia, C., Whiting, M., and Alibhai, H. (2013). Cerebral hypoxia in a cat following pharyngoscopy involving use of a mouth gag. *Vet. Anaesth. Analg.* 40 (1): 106–108.

Gadsden, J., Hadzic, A., Gandhi, K. et al. (2011). The effect of mixing 1.5% mepivacaine and 0.5% bupivacaine on duration of analgesia and latency of block onset in ultrasound-guided interscalene block. *Anesth. Analg.* 112 (2): 471–476.

Krug, W. and Losey, J. (2011). Area of desensitization following mental nerve block in dogs. *J. Vet. Dent.* 28 (3): 146–150.

Lawal, F.M. and Adetunji, A. (2009). A comparison of epidural anaesthesia with lignocaine, bupivacaine and a lignocaine-bupivacaine mixture in cats. *J. S. Afr. Vet. Assoc.* 80 (4): 243–246.

Martin-Flores, M., Scrivani, P.V., Loew, E. et al. (2014). Maximal and submaximal mouth opening with mouth gags in cats: implications for maxillary artery blood flow. *Vet. J.* 200 (1): 60–64.

Meechan, J.G. (2011). The use of the mandibular infiltration anesthetic technique in adults. *J. Am. Dent. Assoc.* 142 (Suppl 3): 19S–24S.

Reuss-Lamky, H. (2007). Administering dental nerve blocks. *J. Am. Anim. Hosp. Assoc.* 43: 298–305.

Rochette, J. (2005). Regional Anesthesia and analgesia for Oral and dental procedures. *Vet. Clin. N. Am. Small Anim. Pract.* 35: 1041–1058.

Snyder, C.J. and Snyder, L.B. (2013). Effect of mepivacaine in an infraorbital nerve block on minimum alveolar concentration of isoflurane in clinically normal anesthetized dogs undergoing a modified form of dental dolorimetry. *JAVMA* 242 (2): 199–204.

Stiles, J., Weil, A.B., Packer, R.A. et al. (2012). Post-anesthetic cortical blindness in cats: twenty cases. *Vet. J.* 193: 367–373.

Yapp, K.E., Hopcraft, M.S., and Parashos, P. (2011). Articaine: a review of the literature. *Br. Dent. J.* 210 (7): 323–329.

Part Two

Fundamentals of HQHVSN

23

Fundamentals of HQHVSN
Sara White

This book is about high-quality, high-volume spay–neuter (HQHVSN). The first part of the book has discussed clinical knowledge and procedures focused on the individual patient, while this second part focuses on the HQHVSN program as a whole. The anesthetic and surgical procedures described in this book need not be done in high-volume settings, but the high-volume surgical setting is a special organizational and logistical challenge that this book seeks to address and explain. A successful HQHVSN program is more than just the sum of its parts and requires more than the knowledge of how to perform successful anesthetic and surgical procedures: it requires planning, strategies, and protocols. This chapter introduces the core components of HQHVSN programs and serves as a guide to Part Two of this textbook.

HQHVSN

Throughout this book, authors have used the acronym HQHVSN when talking about good practices for programs focused on spaying and neutering, and procedures performed by those programs. More specifically, the Association of Shelter Veterinarians (ASV) "defines HQHVSN services as efficient surgical initiatives that meet or exceed veterinary medical standards of care in providing accessible, targeted sterilization of large numbers of cats and dogs to reduce their overpopulation and subsequent euthanasia" (Griffin et al. 2016).

In order to understand more about HQHVSN, we need to consider several of the terms used in this definition. We need to understand the meanings and implications of "high volume," "accessible," and "targeted."

What Is "High Volume"?

The ASV task force that defined HQHVSN chose not to place a number on how many surgeries are required to count as "high volume." This was to take into account the many different models for providing efficient spay and neuter services. Some high-volume clinics operate daily, while others may operate only one day a month, and still others, like "in-clinic clinics" (see Chapter 36), may only operate for a few hours a week within an existing full-service veterinary practice. This variability made it impossible to choose a daily, weekly, monthly, or annual number of surgeries that would be required to qualify as high volume.

The more salient and distinctive characteristics that define the "high-volume" in HQHVSN are the singular focus and efficient flow of the high-volume surgery day. In veterinary general practice, spaying and neutering may be interspersed with other procedures and outpatient visits, and staffing and protocols reflect this broad emphasis. In HQHVSN, protocols, staffing, and workflow are optimized to provide safe and efficient spay–neuter services.

What Is High-Volume Flow?

What does high-volume flow look like and how does it happen? When an HQHVSN provider talks about clinic flow, what they mean is the coordination of tasks from intake through pre-op, surgery, post-op, and discharge (Hwang et al. 2011; Griffin et al. 2016). Good clinic flow is not only efficient, it also has the potential to result in reduced errors and improved outcomes.

In surgery, flow refers not only to efficient surgical procedures (as described in Part One of this book), but also and perhaps more importantly to the efficient transitions from one surgical procedure to the next. For example, "good flow requires the next patient already in place on the second table, prepped for surgery, at the time the current surgery is being closed. This enables the veterinarian to change gloves and begin the next surgery with no downtime in between" (ASPCAPro 2018).

Good flow in surgery relies upon good flow throughout the clinic, which in turn requires adequate staffing. When clinics with one staff member per veterinarian were compared to those with two, three, or four or more, each addition of a staff member led to a gain in the number of surgeries completed each hour (White 2012). Adequate staffing minimizes surgeon downtime and decreases the possibility that the surgeon will be required to "scrub out" of surgery and assist in non-surgical tasks in the midst of their surgical time.

Optimal flow also depends upon the size, physical layout, and furnishing of the clinic space. As mentioned in the earlier quote, the most efficient flow requires that each surgeon have more than one surgery table so that they need not wait between surgeries. In some cases (depending on protocols, surgeon speed, and patient species and sex), more than one prep table per surgeon may be required as well to ensure that the surgeon is never left idle between surgeries.

Is High Volume Safe?

At times, the question arises whether high-volume surgical care is safe. The answer is, in short, yes, high-volume spay–neuter can produce morbidity and mortality outcomes as good as or better than those in private general practice (Brodbelt 2009; Gerdin et al. 2011; Miller et al. 2016; Levy et al. 2017).

As with any other surgical practice, development of and adherence to sound standard operating procedures is required in order for high-volume surgical practices to be safe. This is why the task force that chose the designation "HQHVSN" specifically included the term "high-quality." The procedures and protocols described in this book and outlined in the ASV Guidelines document (Griffin et al. 2016) are intended to facilitate the establishment of sound, high-quality protocols and procedures.

Not only are HQHVSN protocols and procedures safe, but it may also be that surgeons who perform more surgeries have better outcomes and lower mortality than those surgeons who perform fewer surgeries. Research on human surgeons reveals lower rates of mortality and surgical complications among patients of surgeons who perform more of a specific type of procedure compared to those who perform that procedure less often (Morche et al. 2016).

What Is "Accessible"?

In the definition of HQHVSN, the ASV describes these programs as "accessible." Accessibility simply means that the service is easy to reach or use. What accessibility means in a practical sense is likely to vary with the type of animals served and the community in which the HQHVSN program is located.

Cost Is Accessibility

Cost is a major factor influencing whether owners elect to have their pets neutered (New et al. 2004; Chu et al. 2009; Benka and McCobb 2016; White et al. 2018), and thus much of what makes a clinic "accessible" is that the cost of its services is within the financial means of a wide range of clients. Pet ownership is nearly as common in households with low incomes as in those with high incomes, and households with lower incomes are more likely to have more than one pet when compared to higher-income households (Access to Veterinary Care Coalition 2018). In addition, animals from low-income households are less likely to be altered than those from higher-income households (Chu et al. 2009), so being able to price services to allow access by low-income owners is a key to accessibility.

Other Factors in Accessibility

Accessibility encompasses more than just the cost of the service. Accessibility may also be influenced or determined by geography and transportation, by cultural norms, by language barriers, or by sense of safety (Aday and Andersen 1974). For HQHVSN clinics, geographic accessibility may include transportation services for pets, or may be achieved by providing a mobile (mobile animal sterilization hospital [MASH] or self-contained mobile) clinic. Cultural and language accessibility may be enhanced by hiring bilingual staff members and by engaging volunteers within the community.

Accessibility also requires that potential clients are aware of the services being provided. The clinic may need to employ diverse advertising strategies to reach the intended clientele, and multilingual advertisements may be necessary.

What Is "Targeted"?

In order to maximize their impact, spay–neuter programs focus or "target" their efforts on known sources of shelter impoundment and surplus cats and dogs in the community (see Chapters 24 and 25). These include those cats and dogs that would otherwise be unlikely to be neutered, including both owned pets from low-income households and community animals. Since intact animals are more likely to be relinquished to shelters (New et al. 2000), targeting spay and neuter services can be helpful

both in preventing unwanted offspring as well as preventing the surrender of existing companion animals. Targeting can be based upon a variety of different characteristics of animals or humans within the HQHVSN program's service area.

Targeting by Income

As mentioned in the previous section on accessibility, low-income pet owners are an important target of HQHVSN programs. Targeting by owner income may not necessarily mean income screening, as other clinic characteristics such as geographic placement and advertising campaigns may also target a lower-income clientele. Even without income screening, the majority of clients who use HQHVSN clinics have below-median income, and choose to use the clinic based primarily on the cost of services (White et al. 2018). Many of the pets visiting these clinics have never seen a veterinarian before (Benka and McCobb 2016; White et al. 2018).

Targeting Community Cats

Of equal importance is the provision of subsidized spay–neuter services for community animals. In the United States, free-roaming and feral cats, or community cats, represent a major source of feline overpopulation and may produce up to 80% of the kittens born annually in the country (Levy and Crawford 2004; see Chapter 25). Targeting these cats (and in places with community or free-roaming dogs, targeting those dogs) is important for population control as well as for the welfare of the individual animals and public health.

Targeting by Geography

Geographic targeting is another strategy that some HQHVSN programs have used, since not all neighborhoods within a program's service area have equal needs. Geographic information system (GIS) mapping technology can allow programs to target services and outreach to areas with high shelter intake (Miller et al. 2014). Simpler techniques for geographic targeting such as zip code targeting can also be useful for reaching the neediest communities (Levy et al. 2014), although zip codes do not allow the same precision as GIS. See Chapter 24 for more information about geographic targeting.

Targeting by Age Group

In addition to targeting efforts to the most vulnerable populations, timing of neutering is also crucial to maximizing its impact. To prevent pregnancy, neutering is most effective when performed before puberty. Given that queens may experience estrus as early as four to five months of age and bitches as early as six months of age, delaying spaying of juveniles beyond this age can easily result in unintentional litters. In fact, many owned pets (especially cats) have one or more unintentional litters prior to being spayed (New et al. 2004; White et al. 2018).

Targeting Shelter Animals

Shelters should strive for 100% neuter before adoption of all cats and dogs, including kittens and puppies as young as six weeks of age. When organizations require neutering but fail to perform the surgery prior to adoption, they inevitably end up adding to the number of litters born in their community. Neutering all cats and dogs prior to adoption ensures control of reproduction and sets an example of responsible ownership for the community.

Fundamentals of an Effective HQHVSN Program

To be an effective HQHVSN provider, planning has to happen within several domains. Some of this planning is big-picture – what kind of HQHVSN program do you want, what changes do you hope to effect, and why? What is the amount of need in your area, and what resources do you have to address it? Other planning is detailed – what protocols will you

use, in what space, with workers acting and interacting in what ways? Without this planning, a program may be doing spay and neuter surgery, but it will not be doing so as efficiently and effectively as it could be.

Belief System, Mission, and Goals

Fundamental beliefs and mission shape and define an organization's priorities and limitations. While it can feel unnecessarily abstract to start planning at such a high level, this understanding will likely shape more concrete plans, including those for facilities, protocols, locations, and patient pool. Chapter 28 describes the process and benefits of drafting an organizational identity document including beliefs, mission, values, and bottom lines.

On a somewhat less abstract level, programs benefit from articulating their goals and then planning to provide spay–neuter services in a way that will reasonably contribute to those goals. This is true whether discussing a spay–neuter program as a whole, or thinking about a new initiative or focus within a larger program. Often, programs have goals that involve decreasing animal shelter intake or decreasing pet homelessness. Chapter 24 describes research on population dynamics, targeting, and measuring impacts. If the goal of the program is to affect community cat populations, Chapter 25 delves into these cats, their life histories, and strategies for addressing their population.

In some cases, the goals of a spay–neuter program are to provide individual health benefits to animals. This may be solely via a one-time spay–neuter–vaccinate visit, or as part of a more comprehensive wellness offering. Chapter 26 discusses the current state of knowledge on the risks and benefits of spay–neuter surgery to animal health and longevity. For programs and individuals wondering about the future of non-surgical contraception, Chapter 27 describes the current state of progress in this field.

Resources and Models

In order to plan an effective program, it is essential to understand the resources that you can access in order to meet the needs in your target community. Resources can include financial resources as well as the human resources (employees, contractors, and volunteers) available to the program. The resources available and the need and targets that have been identified can then help determine which model of HQHVSN program is the best fit.

Funding

One of the most challenging needs to meet for an HQHVSN program is funding. Part of what makes HQHVSN programs accessible is that they provide services at a cost that their target consumers can afford. For some programs such as community cat spay–neuter programs, this may mean offering surgeries at no cost, whereas for other programs, the customers will be expected to pay for the services they receive.

Many HQHVSN programs are nonprofit or are part of government (municipal) entities, which allows them to apply for grants and to ask for tax-deductible contributions or receive direct government funding. Other HQHVSN programs are considered for-profit; these may be completely independent, or may work in conjunction with a nonprofit animal welfare organization that can accept grants and donations and may also provide volunteers. Which type of organization is best in a given circumstance will depend on factors including requirements set in place by state laws and veterinary practice acts, as well as the program's goals and the availability of funding from various sources.

Funding can come from grants, donations, public funding, or fees for service. In some cases, a for-profit HQHVSN clinic may also use personal savings or bank loans, particularly for startup funding. Grant funding may come from other nonprofit organizations, from private foundations, or from government entities.

To receive grants, the requesting organization generally must be a nonprofit or government entity, and must complete an application process for the grant. Nonprofit grants are generally given for specific purposes, for example clinic startup grants, or grants subsidizing spay–neuter surgery for specific target animals, such as community cats or pit bull-type dogs. Funding from governments may vary both in the source of the funds (for example, from a city's animal control budget, from a state's pet-friendly car license plates, or from dog licensing) and in the way that funding is provided to the clinic (White et al. 2010).

Donations from private citizens or from businesses can be an important source of funding for some HQHVSN programs, and a negligible source of income for others. HQHVSN programs that are part of a larger animal welfare organization may benefit from that organization's fundraising efforts. For HQHVSN programs that are associated with animal shelters and that do surgery mostly on shelter animals, the spay–neuter cost may be accounted for in the cost of rehoming these animals. Similarly, shelters whose HQHVSN programs provide spay–neuter services as part of intake diversion (for example, return-to-field and pet-retention programs) may find that the cost of providing spay–neuter surgery is less than the cost of taking the animal into the shelter and will fund the spay–neuter services accordingly.

Fees for service is one of the most important (and obvious) sources of funding for HQHVSN programs. Most programs charge a fee to the clients who use their service. This fee may be the same for all customers with an animal of a specific species, sex, and size, or there may be a sliding scale or the opportunity for additional subsidy for those in special, targeted categories. In order for the HQHVSN program to be accessible, the fees must generally be lower than the prices in general veterinary practices in the area. The difference between the "traditional" general practice price and the lower HQHVSN clinic price can be made up via efficiency, via the use of volunteer labor, or via the other sources of funding mentioned earlier.

Human Resources

Human resources include the employees, independent contractors, and volunteers that allow the HQHVSN program to provide services. Chapters 29 and 30 talk about finding and hiring employees for HQHVSN programs, and may also be useful when considering working with volunteers.

Volunteers are an essential part of some clinic models, and are used minimally if at all in other clinic models. It is important to be realistic about expectations for using volunteers in a clinic setting. Do the available volunteers have the skills needed to contribute meaningfully to the program? Or, if the program is seeking highly skilled volunteers such as veterinarians and veterinary technicians, is it realistic to expect these people to provide their services at no cost? In some circumstances the answer may be "yes" – large monthly MASH-style community cat clinics often rely on an all-volunteer workforce. But in most cases it is more realistic to assume that all highly skilled jobs will need to be performed by paid workers.

Program Models

A variety of program models have been designed and implemented to serve as efficient surgical initiatives providing accessible, targeted sterilization to large numbers of cats and dogs. The model that an HQHVSN program chooses should be shaped by the available resources and need(s) that the program is trying to address. These program models include stationary and mobile spay–neuter clinics, MASH-style operations, feral cat programs, and services provided through private practitioners. See Table 23.1 for a description of these HQHVSN program models and their attributes. Each of these clinic models is covered in its own chapter later in the text.

Stationary clinics (Chapter 32) offer many advantages over mobile clinics, including greater daily surgical capacity compared to most mobile clinics, the ability to establish relationships with local veterinary practices and community members, and the possibility to hospitalize animals if necessary. Disadvantages include time and costs associated with establishing and maintaining a commercial facility and the potential for geographic limitation of the population in need of services. An alternative model of a stationary clinic that may counteract some of these disadvantages is the use of an existing veterinary hospital for regularly scheduled spay–neuter clinics. These "in-clinic clinics" (Chapter 36) are especially valuable for serving the needs of targeted populations in rural communities.

Mobile spay–neuter clinics often take one of two forms: MASH-style clinics (Chapter 34) and vehicles outfitted with surgical facilities (Chapter 33). These models have the advantages of being able to target any geographic area in which services are needed and lower overhead costs. Disadvantages include limited animal housing and time constraints on spay–neuter efforts at a given location, leading to constraints on the number of animals served. Client communication and emergency care protocols must be especially well planned, as mobile clinics often move from an area after completing surgeries for the day, potentially leaving animals without the benefit of veterinary care shortly after recovery and release to their owners. In some states, practice acts prohibit or limit mobile neutering services.

The final type of clinic is a community cat clinic (or feral cat clinic). This type of clinic utilizes any one of the aforementioned models, but focuses exclusively on serving community cats. This type of clinic can offer greater safety and efficiency, with all protocols geared toward cats that cannot be handled, and with all supplies and equipment sized for feline patients. These clinics can be lower stress for cats since they will not be exposed to dogs. Chapter 35 describes the policies and protocols that should be considered when implementing a community cat clinic.

Table 23.1 HQHVSN clinic models.

Clinic model	Description	Startup cost	Surgical capacity	Advantages	Disadvantages	Best uses
Stationary	Clinic operates within a facility dedicated to providing spay–neuter services	High	Highest	Able to operate at the highest capacity Most efficient utilization of veterinarians and technicians Ability to hospitalize patients if needed	Requires adequate nearby population to support full-time service; transport services may be needed to bring in patients from surrounding areas Startup time is greater than other models?	Urban or suburban areas with at least 250 000 human population within 90 miles Programs wishing to target specific geographic areas or neighborhoods that have adequate funding and staffing to run this clinic type
Mobile clinic	Clinic operates in a self-contained mobile unit	High	Medium	Ability to access target communities Visibility: the vehicle is a mobile billboard for the program	Expensive to buy and maintain Lower capacity than stationary clinics due to limited space and travel time Limited animal housing within unit	Locations where MASH clinics are not allowed or where suitable spaces for MASH clinics are not available
MASH clinic (mobile animal sterilization hospital)	Surgical equipment is transported to a space in which a temporary surgery clinic is set up	Medium	Medium	Flexibility Fast startup Ability to access target communities	Time spent driving, unpacking, and repacking Not legal in some states	HQHVSN veterinarian wishing to provide spay–neuter services to multiple local shelters/humane organizations Rural or remote areas with no access to spay–neuter
In-clinic clinic	Clinic operates periodically within a full-service veterinary hospital's space	Low	Low	Startup costs may be very low due to utilization of existing resources	Limited capacity due to full-service hospital's schedule Need to build and maintain working relationships between parties with different goals	Small/rural communities with potentially underutilized veterinary clinics, but without access to low-cost spay–neuter

Protocols and Standard Operating Procedures

Good protocols are essential to effective HQHVSN programs. Protocols codify appropriate care and decrease the odds that aspects of patient care are forgotten or left out. Clear protocols (and good documentation) decrease communication lapses and errors that can arise from unnecessary variability. Protocols reduce uncertainty and the need to make extra decisions, especially at times such as during emergencies or complications when cognitive resources are at a premium.

Protocols are a way to standardize sound practices, but this does not mean that protocols need to be rigid one-size-fits-all mandates. They can include adaptations or variations by species, by health condition, by socialization to humans, or for other specific patient categories. While specific protocols will vary with each program, all should comply with the ASV's 2016 Veterinary Medical Care Guidelines for Spay-Neuter Programs (Griffin et al. 2016).

The Guidelines

The ASV Guidelines (Griffin et al. 2016) describe an achievable high standard of care that can be implemented by HQHVSN programs. Rather than mandating specific protocols, the Guidelines outline recommendations based on current research and expert opinion, and leave the development of specific protocols to each individual program.

There are certain aspects of care that the Guidelines require:

- Medical recordkeeping that complies with all federal, state, and local requirements
- Safe patient handling, housing, and transport
- Attention to effective infectious disease control procedures
- Preparation for emergencies
- Physical examination of each patient
- Anesthesia that incorporates appropriate analgesia throughout and after surgery
- Monitoring during anesthesia
- Appropriate surgical preparation and surgical attire
- Sterile instrumentation and biomedical-grade suture materials
- Safe and effective surgical techniques
- Attentive and responsive post-operative care
- Post-discharge care instructions and plans for post-operative emergencies
- Attention to staff safety and training

The Guidelines are available as a free download from the Journal of the American Veterinary Medical Association (https://avmajournals.avma.org/doi/pdf/10.2460/javma.249.2.165) and are a valuable resource for all HQHVSN programs.

Implementing Protocols

Designing high-quality protocols is only the first step; next, they have to be put into practice. One way to do this is via the clinic's medical record form. A well-designed clinic form can essentially serve as a checklist: it can prompt staff to collect various historical information, determine what the animal needs, deliver appropriate services, and ensure patient data is properly recorded (Haynes et al. 2009; Gawande 2010; Hofmeister et al. 2014).

In other cases, separate checklists or algorithms (apart from the standard medical record) can be useful tools for protocol implementation. In HQHVSN, these may be most valuable for unusual patients or situations. For example, clinics may print a cardiopulmonary resuscitation (CPR) algorithm to be placed in a crash cart and used during a resuscitation effort (Fletcher et al. 2012), or may implement a pregnant patient checklist to ensure that appropriate preparation or monitoring procedures are followed for these patients. For more information about designing and implementing checklists, see the discussions in Chapters 7 and 17 on using checklists to avoid anesthetic and surgical complications, respectively.

Physical Layout and Organization of Space

In addition to written records, checklists, and algorithms, protocol implementation can be enhanced (or hindered) by the physical space and the behavior and interaction of team members. The physical layout of the workspace and the equipment within it shapes and defines the flow of patients and information through that space. The organization of the physical space may enhance efficient flow, or may limit efficiency and increase idle time. Physical spaces determine the surgical capacity of some programs: for example, the number of cages and tables in a mobile spay–neuter unit may define the maximum daily capacity for that unit (see Chapter 33).

When we talk about the physical space shaping and facilitating the ability to provide care, we are talking primarily about efficiency and safety. How far do staff have to travel between tasks? Are the items they need available and nearby, or do they spend a lot of time moving around? Are staff in each area of the clinic aware of safety and flow concerns that arise elsewhere in the clinic? Are sedated or anesthetized animals visible and monitored? To the extent possible, the lines of sight, sound, and flow within the clinic should all facilitate high-quality care.

To make improvements in the layout of a physical space, it is useful to identify the risky processes or locations in the surgical day and focus improvement there (Norris et al. 2014). The points of concern are not going to be the same for every clinic, but may be recognized and identified by staff, or determined by review of the locations in the clinic generating the most adverse events or near misses. Redesign of the physical space is not enough to assure adequate protocols or adequate performance, but it can be a helpful step in facilitating safer and more efficient performance (Hwang et al. 2011).

Staff Roles and Culture

Once the physical space and the protocols are in place, it is up to the people working there to create an effective and safe workplace. The ways in which staff function as individuals and as part of a team and the way they behave and interact within the physical space are what create the clinic's efficiency and effectiveness.

Effective work cultures are likely to be collaborative and not strictly hierarchical (Vaughn et al. 2019). Teamwork allows clinics to perform safely and efficiently: the greater the teamwork, the fewer the complications (Gawande 2010). See Chapter 29 for more information about defining an organization's culture, engaging employees, and hiring people who believe in and embrace the workplace culture.

Staff roles are a combination of defined individual duties and team interactions. On the one hand, each staff member must understand their role in the organization and must be able to perform their duties with minimal wasted time. For example, once in surgery the veterinarian will generally be doing nothing but surgery, moving from patient to patient and only pausing to change gloves in between. On the other hand, staff should be encouraged to respond to the needs of others and to react to circumstances as they occur. This adaptability and teamwork are key to the clinic's reliability and are an important safeguard against complications or patient deaths. Some authors describe reliability and safety as "dynamic non-events," meaning that it is humans' ability to respond and be flexible when needed that creates safety in a complex workplace (Reason 2000).

Taking care of the physical and emotional health and welfare of staff is important for all HQHVSN programs, both in order to create a safe and humane workplace, as well as to ensure the longevity of skilled workers in the field. Chapter 31 discusses health concerns in the HQHVSN workplace and how to address, avoid, or minimize them.

Data: Tracking and Improvement

It is important for HQHVSN programs to be able to track and use data as a way to improve their operations. Two important ways that data tracking can be of use is for monitoring and improving patient *safety* and for evaluating the *effectiveness* of the spay–neuter program in the target community.

Safety

Collection of morbidity and mortality data can allow programs to identify and track problems and improve clinic operations (Gerdin et al. 2011). It is important to understand the circumstances surrounding major adverse events (deaths and serious complications) in order to identify whether an error occurred, when and where an error happened, and what could be changed to reduce the odds of the same error occurring again. This information can be useful for staff training, allowing the surgical team to focus vigilance in areas of greatest likelihood of complications and to change practices that give rise to unnecessary risk.

The use of computerized records can further improve patient care and safety by allowing analysis of trends in patient outcomes. With computerized records, it can be simple to track types of complications by doctor or by animal type, to recognize and evaluate changes in outcomes, and to correlate these changes with any changes in protocols or standard operating procedures.

Effectiveness

Data tracking can also be useful for evaluating the effectiveness of the HQHVSN program. Is it reaching its target population? Is the program affecting local shelters or animals in the community as intended? Program effectiveness can be measured in a variety of ways: via local shelter intake and euthanasia numbers (White et al. 2010; Levy et al. 2014; Miller et al. 2014), by nuisance complaints (Scarlett and Johnston 2012), by cat colony size (Jones and Downs 2011) or kitten production (Hughes and Slater 2002), by disease incidence (Reece and Chawla 2006), or by other meaningful measures. Chapter 24 describes using data to design and evaluate the effectiveness of spay–neuter interventions.

How to Learn More

One of the most valuable things an aspiring or experienced spay–neuter veterinarian, clinic manager, or staffer can do to improve knowledge, skills, and wellbeing is to connect with others in the field. Professional associations, online resources, and in-person training are all available (see Box 23.1).

For those considering starting a clinic or hoping to improve or hone their existing clinic operations or surgical skills or simply to connect with others, there is great value in visiting other HQHVSN clinics or programs. Seeing a clinic in action provides insight into clinic flow and protocols and generates a picture of clinic operations more comprehensive than words and pictures on paper can convey, and watching another surgeon work can be inspiring and educational. Connections with other HQHVSN programs and other HQHVSN veterinarians are also valuable for technical troubleshooting and emotional support in the wake of complications and unexpected events (White 2018).

Conclusion

A successful HQHVSN program is a special organizational and logistical challenge that requires much more than just excellent medical and surgical care and skills. It requires planning, strategies, and protocols to optimize the clinic's operations and impact. This chapter has introduced the core components and considerations for HQHVSN programs and provides a background for those working to establish or improve their HQHVSN program's practices and impact.

Box 23.1 Resources in HQHVSN

Where to Find Other HQHVSN Veterinarians

- Association of Shelter Veterinarians. Online member forum, Facebook group, newsletter, conference tracks, and more: www.sheltervet.org
- HQHVSNvets online group is a resource to facilitate communication and exchange of ideas among HQHVSN veterinarians. Email: HQHVSNvets+subscribe@groups.io
- Facebook groups and other social media connections.
- Attend a conference. Many national and regional veterinary conferences have shelter tracks, some of which include HQHVSN and many of which are attended by veterinarians who do HQHVSN. Likewise, many animal welfare conferences now have veterinary tracks.
- Visit a clinic or a shelter HQHVSN program.

Training in HQHVSN

- The American Society for the Prevention of Cruelty to Animals (ASPCA) Spay/Neuter Alliance offers in-person surgical training in HQHVSN for veterinarians and veterinary students, as well as new clinic startup mentorship and training. Its website also has many free resources for clinic administration and medical and surgical patient care:

https://www.aspcapro.org/about-programs-services/aspca-spayneuter-alliance
- The National Spay Neuter Response Team (NSNRT) is a specific program of the ASPCA Spay/Neuter Alliance that offers startup training and ongoing mentorship to stationary clinics: https://www.aspcapro.org/training-site-training/spayneuter-clinic-mentorships

Training for Leaders and Administrators

- Emancipet offers seminars focused on leadership, management, culture, and impact designed for HQHVSN veterinarians and staff through the Emancipet New School: https://www.emancipet.org/newschool/seminars

International Resources

- The International Companion Animal Management Coalition offers conferences, downloadable reference materials, and literature reviews. Its major focus is on dog population management: https://www.icam-coalition.org
- Katherine Polak and Ann Therese Kommedal (eds) (2018). *Field Manual for Small Animal Medicine*. Hoboken, NJ: Wiley-Blackwell.

References

Access to Veterinary Care Coalition (2018). *Access to Veterinary Care: Barriers, Current Practices, and Public Policy*. Nashville, TN: University of Tennessee College of Social Work.

Aday, L.A. and Andersen, R. (1974). A framework for the study of access to medical care. *Health Serv. Res.* 9: 208.

ASPCAPro (2018). Daily flow. https://www.aspcapro.org/sites/default/files/asna_daily_flow.pdf (accessed 1 March 2019).

Benka, V.A. and McCobb, E. (2016). Characteristics of cats sterilized through a subsidized, reduced-cost spay-neuter program in Massachusetts and of owners who had cats sterilized through this program. *JAVMA* 249: 490–498.

Brodbelt, D. (2009). Perioperative mortality in small animal anaesthesia. *Vet. J.* 182: 152–161.

Chu, K., Anderson, W.M., and Rieser, M.Y. (2009). Population characteristics and neuter status of cats living in households in the United States. *JAVMA* 234: 1023–1030.

Fletcher, D.J., Boller, M., Brainard, B.M. et al. (2012). RECOVER evidence and knowledge gap analysis on veterinary CPR. Part 7: clinical guidelines. *J. Vet. Emerg. Crit. Care (San Antonio)* 22 (Suppl 1): S102–S131.

Gawande, A. (2010). *The Checklist Manifesto: How to Get Things Right*. New York: Metropolitan Books.

Gerdin, J.A., Slater, M.R., Makolinski, K.V. et al. (2011). Post-mortem findings in 54 cases of anesthetic associated death in cats from two spay-neuter programs in New York state. *J. Feline Med. Surg.* 13: 959–966.

Griffin, B., Bushby, P.A., McCobb, E. et al. (2016). The Association of Shelter Veterinarians' 2016 veterinary medical care guidelines for spay-neuter programs. *JAVMA* 249: 165–188.

Haynes, A.B., Weiser, T.G., Berry, W.R. et al. (2009). A surgical safety checklist to reduce morbidity and mortality in a global population. *N. Engl. J. Med.* 360: 491–499.

Hofmeister, E.H., Quandt, J., Braun, C., and Shepard, M. (2014). Development, implementation and impact of simple patient safety interventions in a university teaching hospital. *Vet. Anaesth. Analg.* 41: 243–248.

Hughes, K.L. and Slater, M.R. (2002). Implementation of a feral cat management program on a university campus. *J. Appl. Anim. Welf. Sci.* 5: 15–28.

Hwang, T.G., Lee, Y., and Shin, H. (2011). Structure-oriented versus process-oriented approach to enhance efficiency for emergency room operations: what lessons can we learn. *J. Healthc. Manag.* 56: 255.

Jones, A.L. and Downs, C.T. (2011). Managing feral cats on a university's campuses: how many are there and is sterilization having an effect? *J. Appl. Anim. Welf. Sci.* 14: 304–320.

Levy, J.K., Bard, K.M., Tucker, S.J. et al. (2017). Perioperative mortality in cats and dogs undergoing spay or castration at a high-volume clinic. *Vet. J.* 224: 11–15.

Levy, J.K. and Crawford, P.C. (2004). Humane strategies for controlling feral cat populations. *JAVMA* 225: 1354–1360.

Levy, J.K., Isaza, N.M., and Scott, K.C. (2014). Effect of high-impact targeted trap-neuter-return and adoption of community cats on cat intake to a shelter. *Vet. J.* 201: 269–274.

Miller, G.S., Slater, M.R., and Weiss, E. (2014). Effects of a geographically-targeted intervention and creative outreach to reduce shelter intake in Portland, Oregon. *Open J. Anim. Sci.* 4: 165.

Miller, K.P., Rekers, W., Ellis, K. et al. (2016). Pedicle ties provide a rapid and safe method for feline ovariohysterectomy. *J. Feline Med. Surg.* 18: 160–164.

Morche, J., Mathes, T., and Pieper, D. (2016). Relationship between surgeon volume and outcomes: a systematic review of systematic reviews. *Syst. Rev.* 5: 204.

New, J., John, C., Kelch, W.J. et al. (2004). Birth and death rate estimates of cats and dogs in US households and related factors. *J. Appl. Anim. Welf. Sci.* 7: 229–241.

New, J.C., Salman, M., King, M. et al. (2000). Characteristics of shelter-relinquished animals and their owners compared with animals and their owners in US pet-owning households. *J. Appl. Anim. Welf. Sci.* 3: 179–201.

Norris, B., West, J., Anderson, O. et al. (2014). Taking ergonomics to the bedside – a multi-disciplinary approach to designing safer healthcare. *Appl. Ergonom.* 45: 629–638.

Reason, J. (2000). Human error: models and management. *Br. Med. J.* 320: 768–770.

Reece, J. and Chawla, S. (2006). Control of rabies in Jaipur, India, by the sterilisation and vaccination of neighbourhood dogs. *Vet. Rec.* 159: 379–383.

Scarlett, J. and Johnston, N. (2012). Impact of a subsidized spay neuter clinic on impoundments and euthanasia in a community shelter and on service and complaint calls to animal control. *J. Appl. Anim. Welf. Sci.* 15: 53–69.

Vaughn, V.M., Saint, S., Krein, S.L. et al. (2019). Characteristics of healthcare organisations struggling to improve quality: results from a systematic review of qualitative studies. *BMJ Qual. Saf.* 28: 74–84.

White, S. (2012). Characteristics of spay and neuter employment positions and contributors to efficiency. Midwest Veterinary Conference, Columbus, OH. Shelter Medicine Poster Session.

White, S.C. (2018). Veterinarians' emotional reactions and coping strategies for adverse events in spay-neuter surgical practice. *Anthrozoös* 31: 117–131.

White, S.C., Jefferson, E., and Levy, J.K. (2010). Impact of publicly sponsored neutering programs on animal population dynamics at animal shelters: the New Hampshire and Austin experiences. *J. Appl. Anim. Welf. Sci.* 13: 191–212.

White, S.C., Scarlett, J.M., and Levy, J.K. (2018). Characteristics of clients and animals served by high-volume, stationary, nonprofit spay-neuter clinics. *JAVMA* 253: 737–745.

Section Five

Spay-Neuter Population Medicine

24

Sterilization Programs and Population Control
Margaret Slater and Emily Weiss

There are two main questions that tend to arise when thinking about the topic of sterilizing dogs and cats to control their numbers. The first question is "how many do we need to do?" and the second is "which ones should we do?" It is critical to determine if the goal really is population control or whether the goal is solely individual animal welfare or other concerns like nuisance complaints. In some instances, the impact of the populations on disease, nuisance, or welfare may be of primary or secondary concern, and different types of data and modeling may be needed. This chapter will include some ideas, methods, and data to help make clear which topics should be considered in answering questions about impacting populations, so that a logical plan can be developed to control population size in dogs and cats through sterilization.

There are some general considerations that influence the answer to these questions. First, it depends on what species and sub-group are of interest. Is it owned dogs? Feral cats? Cats and dogs? Owned and unowned? Each of these can influence the answers to the questions above. The answers also depend on the location and its culture. Are you in a warm or a very cold climate? An urban versus very rural area? A country where owned dogs are commonly allowed to roam? The culture and beliefs of the human residents are critical to include in planning for success. Further, it

depends on what the problem is. Are you dealing with litters of puppies or with kittens? Only neonatal kittens with moms? Spay–neuter may have the most impact on population size and on homelessness, particularly for animal shelters when the problem is litters and juveniles rather than adults. Another consideration is that issues like nuisance complaints may require somewhat different solutions than a purely population control goal. For example, male cats may not be a good target for cat population control, but sterilizing them is usually needed for welfare or nuisance abatement.

How Many Cats or Dogs Do We Need to Sterilize?

What Is Population Dynamics?

Population dynamics is "a branch of knowledge concerned with the sizes of populations and the factors involved in their maintenance, decline or expansion" (Merriam-Webster, Inc. 2013). A *population* is typically defined as a group of animals of the same species that live together and reproduce. For the purposes of this chapter, a population can be defined in many potentially useful ways: all owned cats allowed out on a street, all stray dogs entering a shelter from a particular neighborhood, a colony of cats, all intact dogs in a city, and so

High-Quality, High-Volume Spay and Neuter and Other Shelter Surgeries, First Edition. Edited by Sara White.
© 2020 John Wiley & Sons, Inc. Published 2020 by John Wiley & Sons, Inc.

on. Factors influencing the size of the population include the age distribution, reproductive rate, and the frequency of death, for example: (a) are there seasonal or age patterns to births or deaths? (b) how often and how many kittens or puppies are produced? and (c) how often and how many juveniles and adults die?

Targeting a clearly identifiable population that is small enough to sterilize at high levels becomes an essential component of using sterilization to control population size. In thinking about how many animals one needs to sterilize, keep in mind that the number of sterilizations needs to be high enough to exceed the reproductive capacity of the animals (*birth rate, fertility*, or *fecundity*; Gotelli 2001). The ability to get ahead of the breeding curve is also influenced by what age the animals can start bearing offspring, by how long they live (*death rate, survival*, or *mortality rate*), and by how long they are able to reproduce successfully.

While sterilization programs clearly influence the birth rate of the population, they may also influence survival if sterilized adults live longer than intact adults. One study reported that cats who were castrated or ovariohysterectomized lived significantly longer than intact cats or vasectomized male cats (Nutter 2005).

In addition, unless the area is geographically isolated, like an island, dogs and cats from nearby areas are free to move into the area where the sterilization is being done, may be brought in by the people living there, or may be abandoned or lost in that location (*immigration*; Gotelli 2001). Sometimes, cats or dogs leave the area and are adopted into indoor homes, picked up by animal control, or relocate to another location (*emigration*). Immigration and emigration are relative to the defined population. For example, if one is looking at a colony of cats, emigration occurs when a cat moves away to a nearby location. That emigrant becomes an immigrant to a colony in the new location. Populations that have no immigration or emigration are called *closed* (Gotelli 2001). Closed populations are easier to model, but in reality are rare. *Open populations*

allow animals to enter and leave the population through a variety of ways.

The study of population dynamics makes it possible to include whatever knowledge is available about these four vital rates (birth and death rates, immigration, and emigration) in answering the "how many" question. With the right data, population dynamics modeling can not only illustrate how many animals need to be sterilized to stabilize or decrease the population size, but can also compare permanent versus short-term sterilization, how immigration and emigration influence the population of interest, and which vital rate has the most impact on the population being studied.

What Is Population Dynamics Modeling and Why Should I Care?

Understanding the general characteristics of the population of interest is enormously helpful in planning a successful sterilization campaign, and population dynamics modeling is a way to achieve this. A *model* is a way to represent a complex process with a simpler picture or description (Gotelli 2001; Boone 2015). A *dynamic model* is a model that shows the changes that are inherent in animal populations. These changes include not just births, deaths, and the availability of food and shelter, but also may include predation, local animal control laws, and human attitudes, all of which can impact a population. If one takes a verbal, pictorial, or written description of a population model and finds equations to describe it, it becomes a *mathematical model*. The four vital rates (birth and death rates, immigration, and emigration) form the core data that are necessary to develop a mathematical way to describe a population. Important predictions are likely to be how fast the population grows, how big it can get, and, in the context of spay–neuter, how the size of the population can be decreased. While the generation of these models is a specialized task, people with expertise in population dynamics modeling may not be difficult to find. Some zoos, wildlife conservation organizations, government animal regulatory agencies, and colleges/universities may have staff with the needed expertise to assist.

The rate of the population growth is described by mathematical equations. Some species have linear growth rates, but dogs and cats more commonly increase at exponential rates. The growth rate for these exponential populations is the *intrinsic rate of increase* r (sometimes called the Malthusian parameter) or *lambda* (λ; Gotelli 2001). Obtaining values of r greater than 0 from a model means that the population is growing exponentially. Values less than 0 (negatives) mean the population is decreasing, and values equal to 0 mean the population as a whole is stable. A closed, stable population has births and deaths, but those births and deaths tend to counteract each other. An open population with r of about 0 has births and immigration balancing out deaths and emigration overall. Exponential growth rates imply that the population size continues to increase, with no ceiling on the population size.

In reality, most populations do hit a "ceiling" and the growth rate slows as that ceiling is neared. Mathematical models may use some type of logistic formula that accounts for the fact that there are usually finite resources including food and shelter, and that higher populations may lead to easier disease transmission or an increase in human complaints and subsequent trapping for removal. The *carrying capacity* (K) is the ceiling on the population size. One type of logistic model is the Ricker logistic model, which looks at changes from one time step to another. While Ricker models have been used in cats, knowledge about carrying capacity is very sparse for dogs and cats (Slater and Budke 2010).

Birth and death rates may be *density dependent*, so that as the population nears carrying capacity (or zero), these rates change (Gotelli 2001). For birth rates, this means that as the population size gets very small (approaches zero), birth rates may go up due to more available resources and less competition. As the population size becomes large and nears the carrying capacity, the birth rate decreases, possibly due to overcrowding, easier disease transmission, greater predation, less food and shelter availability, or increased nuisance complaints leading to human intervention. For death rates, one expects the opposite: as the population grows toward carrying capacity, the death rate increases. Similarly, as the population size decreases, survival is increased and the death rate goes down. Little is known about density-dependent birth and death rates in cats and dogs, but it is logical that these phenomena occur.

Density-dependent birth and death rate variations are likely part of what helps maintain populations and prevent extinction. However, at very small population sizes, there can be a threshold effect where once the population drops below a certain size, the population cannot recover (the *Allee effect*; Gotelli 2001). This occurs for species where the animals' ability to reproduce, hunt, care for offspring, and avoid predators is dependent on there being large enough groups. In cats, the Allee effect was hypothesized in a model exploring the potential spread of feline immunodeficiency virus, but no real data were used to determine if it actually occurs (Hilker et al. 2007). The Allee effect has not been studied in domestic dogs.

There are also models that take into account animal demographics such as age, sex, and reproductive status, and these are called *demographic models*. These models provide the flexibility to account for different life stages like juvenile (and pre-reproductive), adult-reproductive, or adult-sterilized (Gotelli 2001). Models may also account for the idea that the animals are not spread out evenly across the environment, and that they may not remain in one location (*spatial population structure*; Boone et al. 2014; Beeton et al. 2015). *Simulation modeling* allows for a somewhat more complex model information about the population under study to be incorporated into the model and then to see how closely it matches the real-world system under study (Owen-Smith 2007).

One type of simulation modeling was used to recreate the essential series of events during the life cycles of cats (Miller et al. 2014b). This cat population dynamics model was explicitly modeled at the level of the individual – keeping track of each cat's demographic characteristics throughout his or her life span – and was therefore able to more realistically simulate the application of alternative surgical and nonsurgical treatment methods, with specific application to younger versus older individuals, males versus females, and so on. This approach provided a powerful and flexible tool for analysis that may be absent from other modeling platforms. It is important to note that interpretation of an analysis like this is highly dependent on an understanding of the baseline model structure and the nature of the input data.

An important question that should be documented in any model is which of the vital rates contribute most toward the overall population growth (Owen-Smith 2007). To do this, modelers will run either *sensitivity* or *elasticity analyses*. Any model should have one of these two approaches used to examine the relative importance of each vital rate (Slater and Budke 2010). The choice of approach depends on what is being studied and which method is most appropriate for the model.

Two additional concepts are important in understanding how populations are modeled. The first is whether the model is *deterministic* or *stochastic* (Gotelli 2001). Deterministic models are simpler and use the one best number for each vital rate. The model then calculates one best estimate of the population size. Stochastic models can incorporate natural variation in animal lives as well as environmental influences (Slater and Budke 2010). Figure 24.1 illustrates how predictions vary when the model incorporates stochasticity. The graph shows what 50 population growth curves would look like starting with a mix of five male and female cats in a closed population. For illustration, the maximum number of cats allowed was set at 4000. The mean growth rate was 28.7% per year, but 8% of the time the population went quickly to extinction due to the variability in vital rates.

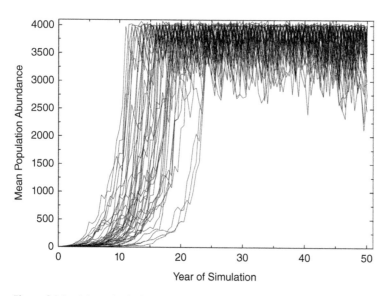

Figure 24.1 A hypothetical example of output from an individual-based simulation model using five cats (two females and three males) reported to have been originally left on Marion Island. Input data included seasonal breeding: 92% high season, 48% off-season (standard deviation [SD] = 3% high season, 15% off-season), kitten mortality (0–6 months old): 75/90% at high densities (SD = 15%), adult mortality per year: 10% (SD = 2%), no immigration or emigration, maximum cat age of 6.5 years. *Source:* Courtesy of Phil Miller.

In the real word, if one is dealing with free-roaming cats or dogs, there are likely nearby populations that interact with the population of interest. *Metapopulation* is the term that describes a set of interrelated populations that might serve as source populations for immigration or emigration of dogs or cats.

How Has Population Dynamics Modeling Helped Us to Understand Dog and Cat Populations?

Dog Population Models While dog populations have long been studied, particularly in regard to controlling rabies, there are few publications that address decreasing population size outside of disease control. Early work on dog and cat populations in urban North America used variations on capture-mark-recapture to count animals (Anvik et al. 1974; Heussner et al. 1978). In the 1980s and 1990s, several publications both presented methods to measure population dynamics in dogs and cats as well as discussed the results (Nassar and Mosier 1982, 1986, 1991; Nassar et al. 1984; Nassar and Fluke 1991; Patronek et al. 1997). A more recent review of companion animal demographics in the United States summarized the data to date and described some of the methods used in regional and national data-gathering efforts (Clancy and Rowan 2003).

Four studies in dogs use simple population dynamics models, one with a visual model in a local situation in the United States (Patronek et al. 1995) and one using a matrix model of owned dogs in a region of Italy to determine how many would need to be sterilized to stabilize the owned dog population size (Di Nardo et al. 2007; Figure 24.2). This study led to an additional project which incorporated cost-benefit analyses for different approaches and considered dog welfare, nuisance, and direct costs to the government (Høgåsen et al. 2013). The last study used a visual and mathematical model examining the influence on spay–neuter, adoption, or decreased abandonment programs on dog euthanasia in a region's shelters (Frank 2004), and reported that spay–neuter was more effective generally than adoption at reducing euthanasia in shelters, but that the full impact may take 30 or more years.

A more recent study performed more complex population dynamics modeling in dogs on the use of immunocontraception with rabies vaccination (Carroll et al. 2010). It compared rabies vaccination alone, rabies vaccination and a contraceptive, and culling. Only the combination of vaccination and contraception controlled rabies due to the otherwise rapid population growth rate and high population turnover. Another recent study in both

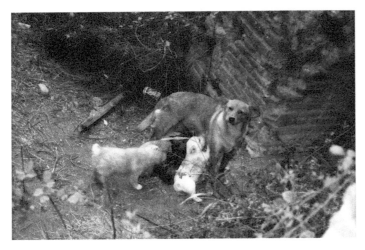

Figure 24.2 Free-roaming dog nursing her puppies in Pompeii, Italy. Due to Italian laws, no dogs or cats can be euthanized unless terminally ill or proven dangerous. *Source:* Photo courtesy of Leo Slater.

Indonesia and South Africa found that free-roaming owned dog populations showed no growth or a decline across three years (Morters et al. 2014). It also discovered that a substantial proportion of the dogs were immigrants brought in by pet owners.

Recent work has begun to combine the concepts of modeling with targeting populations in some way to maximize impact. One recent study in Mexico used population dynamics modeling to understand how existing spay–neuter resources could best be leveraged to control the owned dog population (Kisiel et al. 2018). It was able to determine that targeting young dogs would control the population without increasing existing spay–neuter provision by the government. Another study in Brazil modeled owned and stray dog populations and determined that the carrying capacity was the most important variable in controlling population size, leading to a focus on interventions to reduce capacity by environmental changes such as controlling food sources (Santos Baquero et al. 2016).

Cat Population Models In the past 15–20 years, cat population dynamics modeling has begun to be performed and published. Most studies have examined the effects of trap–neuter–return (TNR) or trap and euthanize using matrix models. At its simplest, TNR includes humane trapping of the cat, sterilization, ear-tipping for permanent identification, and, usually, vaccination against rabies (Figure 24.3). The earliest publication used matrix modeling to compare TNR with trap and euthanize (Anderson et al. 2004). Vital rates were estimated from the published literature. They reported that ≥50% of the population would need to be trapped and euthanized annually or >75% sterilized to control the cat population. Changes in the percentage of the population euthanized resulted in a greater change in growth rate than similar changes in sterilization. Another study used matrix modeling to compare non-surgical three-year contraception with permanent sterilization using literature estimates and a closed population (Budke and Slater 2009). With a short three-year mean life span, >51% of adult and juvenile cats would require permanent sterilization each year to decrease the population size. A three-year

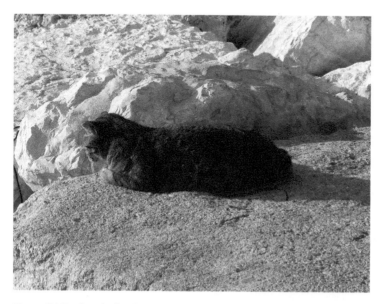

Figure 24.3 Ear-tipping (usually on the left) is an international symbol for a sterilized cat. This cat was sunbathing near the water in Israel near another cat and several people. Israel has recognized a problem with free-roaming cats for decades. *Source:* Photo courtesy of Rama Santchi.

contraceptive in this same population would require >60% to be contracepted annually.

The article by Foley et al. (2005) used a Ricker model and data from two TNR programs in California and from the literature to determine what rate of sterilization would be needed to decrease those specific cat populations. Under current sterilization rates, neither cat population was stabilized or decreased. The annual percentage of cats that would need to be neutered and the overall level of neutering needed to stabilize the population were presented in tables based on the original growth rates of a population and mean life span. To stabilize the estimated cat populations of San Diego and Alachua counties, the annual rate of sterilization would need to be between 14 and 19%, leading to an overall sterilization rate of approximately 71 and 94%, respectively. Another publication used actual data in an open population in Australia to estimate how many cats would need to be removed to eliminate the cat population (Short and Turner 2005). With a population increase of 150% per year, they estimated that between 1.5 and 2.8 cats/km would need to be removed per year for eradication. However, they noted that trapping efforts per cat trapped rose dramatically as cat numbers decreased.

Another model also used some location-specific data from a small town in Texas and included hypothetical immigration rates and their effects on the population (Schmidt et al. 2009). In general, interventions needed to be applied to >50% of the population to decrease the population size. They also reported that "no immigration," "remove and euthanize," "TNR," and "50% removal/50% TNR" showed similar population declines. In the presence of immigration, remove and euthanize tended to show somewhat greater decreases in population size. However, euthanasia required more cats to be trapped than the other interventions.

Nutter (2005) used simulation modeling of individual cats through their lives using data from her colonies in North Carolina. She com-

pared trap and remove with TNR, and immigration and emigration were included. Because of the small starting size of the individual colony modeled (15 cats) and the variability incorporated through a stochastic approach, there was a 29% probability that the colony could go extinct at some point during the 25 years of simulations. However, she also found that due to immigration, those colonies re-established themselves in a few years, emphasizing the importance of immigration in contributing to population size. Annual removal of at least 60% of cats or an annual sterilization of >80% was required for population declines.

Lessa and Bergallo (2012) used the same type of simulation modeling as Nutter, but used data obtained about owned and free-roaming cats on an island in Brazil. They compared no intervention with male only, female only, and both sexes being sterilized as well as annual removal in a closed population. While population sizes for all interventions declined over the 50 years modeled, the most dramatic declines were for the last three interventions, which also had a high probability of the population going extinct. They reported that 70% of female cats or 60% of male and female cats would have to be sterilized or 70% removed for these population declines.

One article examined three potential methods of dispersal (baits, virus, and virus-infected baits) of immunocontraceptives in an island setting (Courchamp and Cornell 2000). It included hypothetical effects of density dependence where either reproduction increases or survival increases as the population declines, and found that both mechanisms led to similar results. They reported that a system using viruses and baits was most effective at decreasing the population size and concluded that immunocontraception was an option for controlling cat populations on islands.

Another article used population dynamics modeling and linked that to costs and benefits comparing TNR and euthanasia in Hawaii (Lohr et al. 2012). The authors used some local data and data from the literature for their vital rates. Hypothesized levels of abandonment had large impacts on population size and time to colony extinction. They estimated costs of TNR and trap and euthanize. However, they also assigned a specific financial cost to a particular bird species death, making these results of limited utility and generalizability.

A simulation model in cats incorporated immigration and emigration and targeting colonies of different sizes with either trap–vasectomize/hysterectomize–return (TVHR) or TNR (Ireland and Miller Neilan 2016). TVHR has been suggested as an alternative to TNR and is based on assumptions about male cat dominance and cat social systems which may not always apply (McCarthy et al. 2013). Ireland and Miller Neilan (2016) incorporated not only the size of the population but also the extent of nuisance reduction as important outcomes. While TNR was substantially better than TVHR at reducing nuisance issues, TVHR was moderately better at reducing population size. This illustrates how modeling can be used for an increasingly wider range of questions.

A more sophisticated population dynamics model used an individual-based stochastic simulation modeling approach to investigate the impact of different population management strategies on free-roaming cats in a variety of environments (Miller et al. 2014b). Populations in resource-rich environments where extra food and sufficient shelter were available (like many urban settings) were modeled as open populations including immigration and emigration, and contrasted to populations in comparatively resource-poor environments (no supplemental feeding, more limited shelter, where no immigration or emigration occurred; like some rural settings). The model also was focused on comparisons of management options included trapping individuals followed by removal, permanent sterilization, or non-surgical temporary contraception.

Sensitivity analysis of the demographic variables used in these models indicated that free-roaming cat population dynamics were more sensitive to changes in survival at different life stages than to fecundity, with adult (more than six months old) survival showing the greatest level of sensitivity (Miller et al. 2014b). Results from simulation models consistently showed that including metapopulations with dispersal between the surrounding neighborhood free-roaming cat populations and through abandonment of litters from households with owned and intact cats could dramatically reduce the effectiveness of population management efforts. In particular, the consistent addition of just a single litter of six-month-old individuals led to a major increase in overall population growth despite intensive management efforts. This insight has profound implications for the design of population management programs.

To reduce the size of the cat populations modeled, the simulation modeling efforts suggested that a sterilization program focused on adults (cats more than six months old), targeting 50% of the intact individuals every six months (or ~75% per year), could be effective in controlling free-roaming cat populations (Miller et al. 2014b). When directly compared against one another, a program of free-roaming cat removal (whether for adoption or euthanasia) demonstrated a larger reduction in population size compared to a sterilization program of equal intensity, consistent with other models (Anderson et al. 2004; Schmidt et al. 2009). This is because the models were all more sensitive to changes in survival than fecundity. Since removal effectively shortens survival while sterilization reduces fecundity, these results are not surprising. Under the structure and assumptions of this simulation model with a 6.5-year cat life span, non-surgical contraceptive methods with about a three-year duration were much less effective in achieving the desired outcome in most situations. Non-surgical contraception was shown to be effective when immigration and emigration were extremely limited and when treatment rates exceeded 40–50% of cats per six-month interval.

How Many Cats or Dogs Do We Need to Sterilize to Decrease the Population?

There is a number in the literature that states that 70% sterilization is needed to stabilize population size. This was popularized by both Merritt Clifton and Marvin Mackie (Clifton 2002; Mackie 2003). They note that spay–neuter programs for owned pets in North America seem to stabilize the populations at about a 70% frequency of sterilization. However, there are wide ranges in reproductive capacity, survival, immigration and emigration, and species differences between dogs and cats, making any single target number unlikely to be quite right in most situations. Differences by age or life stage, nutrition, breeding, human neglect, local laws about picking up strays, and many other factors are potentially important to consider. That is one reason why targeting particular sub-populations of dogs or cats causing the problems will often have the most impact (Hiby 2012). The population of interest and its vital rates must be considered, and understanding which vital rate is most influential on the model outcome (decreasing population size) and how one might creatively influence that rate will be the most constructive way to approach the question.

How Are Dogs and Cat Populations Different?

The numbers of dogs versus cats that must be sterilized to cause a decrease in the population are different, and the problems associated with each species are different as well. In dogs, when considering population dynamics modeling, puppy survival is likely to be lower even than juvenile cats, and therefore overall reproductive success is poorer. Free-roaming dogs tend to gather in small packs and are very visible. They can also be dangerous to runners, bikers, and children as well as livestock. While nuisance behaviors may be a problem even if only one or two dogs are roaming, barking, defecating, and mating, these are rarely primary drivers of dog population control in the United States. On the other hand, cat nuisance problems such as yowling, fighting, urine spraying, and too many cats may be a primary motivator for municipalities in addressing free-roaming cats. In addition, concerns about predation are more commonly expressed about cats; however, dogs can predate wildlife and injure fragile habitats. Both species are implicated in public health complaints, with bites probably the most commonly discussed issue. Many different diseases may be of concern in different locations and some, like toxoplasmosis, are more cat specific. However, rabies is a huge issue in many parts of the world where dogs are the reservoir (WHO Expert Committee 2004). In these countries, public health is often the primary concern relating to free-roaming dogs. In recent years, the welfare of the dogs or cats themselves has been of increasing concern (Slater 2001; Totton et al. 2011). Uncontrolled reproduction, poor juvenile survival, diseases, and injuries all contribute to concerns about free-roaming or intact dog and cat welfare.

The role and capabilities of the male in reproduction and in the modeling process are also different for dogs and cats. Male cats can breed with many females (Kustritz 2005; Natoli et al. 2000). Most female cats do not choose which males to breed with, although a few can have preferences (Natoli et al. 2000). Queens also may share kitten-rearing duties, where litters from several females are mixed and all queens provide care (Deag et al. 2000). These behaviors are in contrast with those of free-roaming dogs. There is often little assistance in rearing the puppies by other dogs (although some owned dogs have been reported to assist by regurgitating food; Kustritz 2005; Boitani et al. 2007). In addition, inexperienced male dogs tend to mount bitches incorrectly, and there may be intermale aggression resulting in fewer matings, particularly when many male dogs are present. Mate preferences are more common, with familiar males being more successful (Daniels and Bekoff 1989; Kustritz 2005).

In cats, therefore, there are usually considered to be enough male cats available except in very unusual circumstances to breed any available females. In the simulation model, sterilizing only males showed no change in population size relative to no sterilization at all (Miller et al. 2014b). Conversely, male dogs may be somewhat more limited in their ability to service all available females due to limitations of viable sperm or mating-related behaviors. No models have been run to examine this hypothesis, and more research is needed to see how male breeding ability could limit population growth in dogs.

What Do We Know about Dog and Cat Populations around the World?

For those who will be conducting modeling or working with modelers, it is vital to have the data about the population in question. Up-to-date references containing such data can be found online using search engines such as Google Scholar. Readers are also referred to the International Companion Animal Management Coalition, which provides a dog population management monitoring and evaluation literature review, available at https://www.icam-coalition.org/download/literature-review (International Companion Animal Coalition 2014).

Which Dogs or Cats Should We Sterilize for the Most Impact?

For a sterilization campaign to be most efficient, one would ideally like to be sterilizing the animals who contribute most to the population growth of the dogs and cats at highest welfare risk. In developed countries, at-risk dogs or cats may be owned or unowned and free roaming and are likely to be identified based on owner surveys or animal shelter data. Interventions may be quite varied and there is

ongoing work to develop effective methods to access these owners and get them to use sterilization services (Pets for Life 2013).

In developing countries there are rarely physical shelters and free-roaming dogs are the issue. Complaints, bite reports, or other methods may be used to locate the higher-risk locations. Conducting dog counts is a common method for enumeration. The typical intervention for dogs that are not in a home or readily leashed or held by their owners is catch–neuter–return (CNR). Like TNR in North America and other countries (Slater 2004; International Companion Animal Management Coalition 2011), programs are in place to capture free-roaming dogs for sterilization (Jackman and Rowan 2007). CNR consists of live capture of the dog, sterilization, permanent identification, and return to the capture location (Reece and Chawla 2006; Hiby 2012). This can lead to a stable and healthy population of dogs if the sterilization rate is high enough. However, when many of the free-roaming dogs are owned or loosely owned, this approach undercuts the culture of asking "owners" to take responsibility for the care of the dog. CNR is also not appropriate unless the free-roaming dogs are a major source of the next generation of roaming dogs (Hiby 2012), and the environment must be such that the dogs can have good welfare. Support of the local and national government is critical too for this approach to succeed. Like TNR in cats, CNR is designed to be an interim solution to the problem by addressing the existing animals until the sources of these dogs can be addressed.

For dogs, recommendations and guidance are available for evaluating the impacts of interventions on population and welfare (International Companion Animal Coalition 2015).

Why and How Should We Target Sterilization?

Most spay–neuter programs work with a goal of "decreasing overpopulation" (Wenstrup 1999). This may be measured, though indirectly, by a decrease in shelter intake or euthanasia or a decline in the number of homeless puppies and kittens, particularly in developed countries. However, most of these programs measure and report their success primarily by the number of sterilization surgeries conducted, not by an assessment of the effects of these surgeries. This disconnect between work and mission could potentially lead to efforts that do not accomplish the intended goals.

If the goal is to decrease shelter intake, not all spays and neuters are created equal. If services were targeted toward those most at risk – be it for entering the shelter or shelter deaths – one would likely do a better job at reaching the animals or the offspring of those animals that would be most likely to enter the shelter system.

Do Most Spay–Neuter Programs Target Who They Serve?

It is unknown what proportion of spay–neuter clinics or programs actually target the services that they offer to specific types of clients or animals, or what proportion of surgeries performed by these programs are targeted surgeries. Many spay–neuter clinics are open to all clients, but offer additional subsidies for clients or pets in certain categories (White et al. 2018). In a survey of 22 stationary spay–neuter clinics in the United States, only 3 (14%) of these clinics restricted their clientele to low-income clients. However, clinics offered additional discounts on spay and neuter services in various categories, essentially targeting animals from those categories, including low-income households, certain breeds of dogs, feral or community cats, residents of target zip codes or locations, juvenile animals, bitches or queens with litters, large dogs, multipet households, and senior citizens. The reasons these clinics chose to target these specific populations for discounted services are unknown and likely varied: while they may have been based on scientific evaluation of local at-risk demographics, they may equally have been based on intuition, tradition, donors' wishes, or other factors.

Income-Targeted Interventions

The programs offered by most spay–neuter clinics are targeted only by income – those with a lower income are targeted with access to the services or with additional subsidies. While there is data supporting that those with a lower income tend to be more likely to have an intact pet (Chu et al. 2009), there are also data pointing to factors unrelated to income. In early studies examining reasons for not sterilizing a pet (Manning and Rowan 1992), cost was rarely cited as an important reason for not sterilizing a pet, with less than 6% of respondents citing cost as a factor. In more recent studies (New et al. 2004; Della Maddelena et al. 2012; Benka and McCobb 2016), cost of surgery is noted among the top two reasons for not having pets sterilized and appears especially important for cats. Some of these studies did not collect data on the income level of respondents (Della Maddelena et al. 2012, New et al. 2004), making it possible that those who reported the surgery was "too expensive" may not be low income, but may simply not believe that the surgery is worth the price. However, the more recent study in Massachusetts (Benka and McCobb 2016) found that total annual owner income was associated with the reason for the cat not yet being sterilized, with respondents with incomes <$25 000 citing cost most often.

In epidemiology there is a bias called an ecological fallacy (Thrusfield 1995). It means that an average characteristic of a group is applied to each individual whether or not that average is correct for that individual. In this case, one is saying that there is a correlation between groups of households with low incomes and not sterilizing pets. However, it is clear that a subset of pet owners in low-income households *do* sterilize their pets (and some owners in higher-income brackets do not), making this generalization incorrect when applied to all individuals.

Are Targeted Programs Effective?

There is limited research on spay–neuter programs' effectiveness at reducing shelter intake and euthanasia. Some of the most persuasive research evaluated a TNR program targeting community cats from a single zip code with proportionally high shelter intake (Levy et al. 2014). At the end of a two-year targeted TNR campaign, 54% of the projected community cat population in the target area had been captured and altered, and shelter cat intake from the targeted zip code decreased by 66%, whereas shelter cat intake from non-target areas decreased by only 12%. Much of the success of this targeted intervention is likely due to the high proportion of the target population that was reached by the intervention.

Other programs discussed in the literature, while targeted, reached only a small proportion of the animals within their target population, and thus have demonstrated limited or mixed results. In New Hampshire, the initiation of a program targeting low-income pet owners and shelter adopters across the entire state was followed by a significant decrease in cat intake and euthanasia during the years after program onset, but the trend of decrease had begun before the start of the program, making causation ambiguous (White et al. 2010). There was no effect on dog intake and euthanasia. In Austin, a spay–neuter program targeting zip codes with high shelter intake found a lower rate of increase for dog and cat intake and euthanasia in the program areas compared to non-program areas (White et al. 2010). However, as baseline data was not readily available, the authors were unable to confirm if the trend started prior to the program's inception. In Transylvania County, NC, the opening of a spay–neuter clinic open to all county residents was followed by a significant decrease in cat intake and euthanasia, but no change in dog intake (Scarlett and Johnston 2012). The authors, however, cautioned a conclusion of causation, as many factors could not be controlled. And finally, a study conducted in 2007 (Frank and Carlisle-Frank 2007) studied data from five US communities and found that while low-cost sterilization increased the total number of surgeries in the communities,

there was no correlation between the sterilization and shelter intake.

This research seems to suggest that simply targeting low-cost surgeries to low-income clients may not lead to high impact at the shelter level. It is possible that this is due to lack of saturation, so that if a higher percentage of the total pet population could be impacted with the sterilization services, intake would be influenced. It could also be that a more specific target may need to be identified.

Targeting by location, by focusing on low-income towns, counties, or zip codes, can have limited success if the spay–neuter program only reaches a small portion of the animals in that geographic area, as seen in several of the studies discussed. However, geographic targeting with greater precision or greater saturation may be able to achieve a larger impact.

GIS Targeting

In 2010, a study was published focused on welfare for cats in neighborhoods in Boston, MA (Patronek 2010). Geographic information systems (GIS) technology was used to map the shelter cat data for over 17 500 cats that had entered the animal shelter organizations over a five-year period. The technology allows the ability to attach data to a specific location, and analysis of human demographics along with shelter animal demographics and specific locations becomes possible. The shelter cat origination address (where s/he was found or where her/his relinquisher lived) along with outcome data for the cat were mapped. When analyzed, a very significant correlation ($R^2 = 0.77$) was discovered between where the cats that died in the shelter (either euthanized or died in care) originated from, and where the highest human premature deaths originated. Where people were most at risk of death in the community was the source of the cats who were most at risk of death in the shelter. The ability to find a strong and plausible correlation as one criterion to support causation was made possible by the use of precise location data.

Recent studies incorporate spatial analysis with GIS techniques. One study in Jaipur, India, compared lethal and fertility control with spatial data from the city to determine the best approach for free-roaming dogs (Yoak et al. 2016). It found that lethal control skewed the population toward younger dogs, which likely would increase the conflicts with people compared to older dogs.

The authors have been exploring the use of GIS technology to map shelter data to identify areas of higher risk. In many cases, sterilization and other services are not being taken advantage of in the areas where the risk for intake is highest (Figure 24.4). The use of GIS technology allows for a more precise target than the use of a zip code, as the high intake within that zip code is likely coming from a subset area within the zip code. Demographic information can help inform outreach methods, and the sterilization can be applied in a more precise manner. One example was reported in Portland, OR (Miller et al. 2014a). Use of shelter data allowed for targeting interventions and documenting which interventions appeared most effective at reducing shelter intake. While use of this technology in the animal welfare field is still limited, the power of visualizing where the animals at risk of euthanasia are coming from, and the opportunity to measure the impact of a more precisely placed spay–neuter program, is already proving to be advantageous to keep the goal of decreased intake top of mind.

The idea of targeting animals at risk of euthanasia at the shelter can be easily extended to other animal-related problems like nuisance complaints, bites, too many free-roaming animals, and so on. Fine-tuning the targeting process will allow for scarce resources to be applied where they will do the most good. Recent work has suggested that knowledge of landscape use of cats and dogs may also be helpful, since species survival and population size are likely influenced by the environment (Guttilla and Stapp 2010; Bengsen et al. 2012).

How Do We Tell How Many Cats or Dogs There Are (before and after Sterilization)?

To be able to plan an intervention or to determine if the effort is working, some estimate of numbers of animals involved before and afterward is needed. How to get those numbers depends on the population of interest. For dogs, there have been several useful publications that summarize the main methods that have been used to ascertain dog ownership and describe exactly how to go about counting free-roaming dogs (International Companion Animal Management Coalition 2007; Hiby et al. 2011). Getting data on owned cats can be done using similar surveys as described for dogs (International Companion Animal Management Coalition 2011; Hiby et al. 2011) and at the same time if needed. Counting cats uses similar principles as dogs, but because cats are much more difficult to see and approach than dogs during daytime hours, they require some special considerations (see later discussion).

Dog and Cat Population Data Sources

In the United States, the owned dog and cat population is surveyed by the AVMA (American Veterinary Medical Association 2012) and the APPA (American Pet Products Association 2018). However, neither of these publications takes ownership numbers to a small enough level of geography like city or county to be applicable to the populations in which spay–neuter professionals are usually interested.

One less well-known source for numbers of households owning one or two or more dogs and cats is through Esri statistical software, which has a set of data called Community Analyst (Esri 2012). Community Analyst is an add-on to the ArcGIS software that maps data. Both ArcGIS and Community Analyst are often available to employees at colleges and universities, sometimes to employees of city or county governments, and at substantial

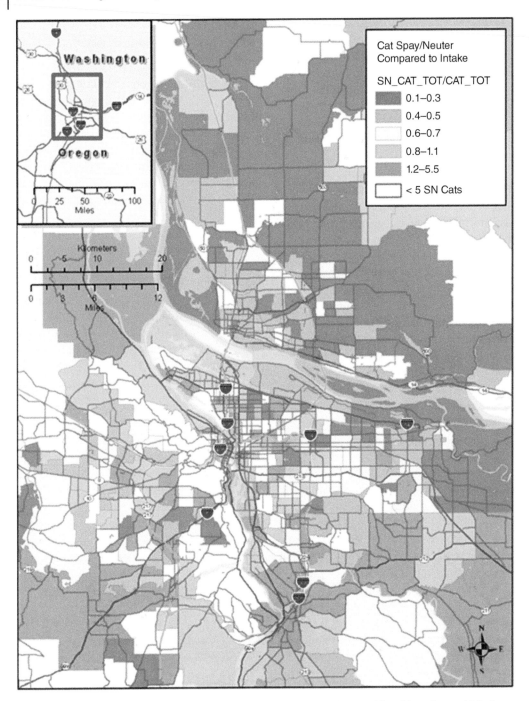

Figure 24.4 Spay–neuter surgery data in this community included the specific address from which the cat came, as did cat intake. This map illustrates spay–neuter surgery numbers divided by total intake numbers to create a ratio from 0.1 to 5.5 neuters per cat intake in a given census block. The red and peach areas indicate potential areas to target with fewer than 0.5 cats neutered per cat entering the shelter in those census blocks. White areas had fewer than 5 cats who were neutered.

of community cats is likely in the same range (Levy and Crawford 2004; Robertson 2008; AAFP 2012) in the United States alone.

Reproductive Biology

Cats have a number of unique features that allow them to reproduce at a high rate. Cats are seasonally polyestrous, induced ovulators. Under optimal conditions they are capable of producing 2–3 litters each year. Significant seasonality in births is seen. Most pregnancies occur in the spring, with a smaller peak in late summer or early autumn. Gestation is relatively short, averaging 63–66 days in length. Lactation does not suppress estrus, and it is not uncommon to find lactating queens already pregnant with another litter. Females reach sexual maturity by 3.5–5 months of age (Griffin 2001), depending on the season and length of day, and early-maturing cats may give birth by six months of age. As a result, spay–neuter performed at the conventional age of six months or older is likely to result in a significant number of accidental litters.

Uncontrolled reproduction of community cats greatly contributes to their numbers. Pet cats that have not been sterilized or that have had a litter prior to being sterilized (Manning and Rowan 1992) do contribute to the population of community cats. However, this is almost negligible compared to the numbers of kittens born to unowned free-roaming cats. The spay–neuter status of pet cats varies geographically and with the socioeconomic background of owners, but national averages are estimated at approximately 80–85% (Levy et al. 2003b; Chu et al. 2009). In contrast, it is typical to find that less than 5% of all community cats in a given area to have been spayed or neutered, unless they are found in a localized area conducting a trap–neuter–return (TNR) program (Scott et al. 2002a; Levy and Crawford 2004; Wallace and Levy 2006). Even allowing for the proportion of pet cats that have given birth prior to being spayed, the community cat population remains the primary source of kit-

tens. Indeed, some authors have estimated that as many as 80% of the kittens born in the United States are to free-roaming queens (Levy and Crawford 2004).

Despite the environmental pressures many community cats face, they remain remarkably capable of reproducing even in environments of limited resources. An average pregnancy rate of 15% was found in feral cats presented for ovariohysterectomy in several studies (Gibson et al. 2002; Foley et al. 2005; Wallace and Levy 2006). However, looking at the peak reproductive times of March, April, and May, that proportion jumped as high as 70–80% in certain geographic locations (Jones and Coman 1982; Nutter et al. 2004b; Wallace and Levy 2006). Other studies have confirmed that pregnant cats could be identified in all months of the year despite cats' seasonally polyestrous nature. With an average of 1.4 litters per year, 4–5 fetuses per pregnancy (Jones and Coman 1982; Brothers et al. 1985; Nutter et al. 2004b; Wallace and Levy 2006), and three live births per litter, an unspayed female cat can easily produce 50–100 kittens in a lifetime. Increasing availability of resources is associated with more frequent births, larger litters, and higher survival rates of kittens (Schmidt et al. 2007). This exponential rate of reproduction results in significant increases to the community cat population, despite high rates (50–75%) of mortality reported for kittens under six months of age (Nutter et al. 2004b); population growth rates as high as 150% have been reported (Short and Turner 2005).

Diet and Environment

Community cats are not confined and roam freely, often living in close proximity to one another. Despite previously accepted notions that cats are solitary creatures, much evidence exists to show that cats will live in matriarchal groups known as colonies, particularly when resources are abundant (Crowell-Davis et al. 2004). These cats form complex social structures and show communal breeding and nursing behaviors (Figure 25.3). Cats can be

(a)
(b)

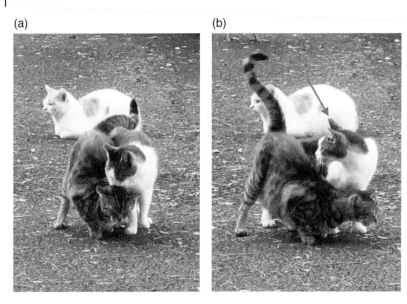

Figure 25.3   (a and b) Affiliative behavior between two feral cats (in the foreground) in a managed colony. Both cats have a slight notch in their right ear (arrow), rather than the more distinct and commonly used ear tip.

found in and often thrive in extremely diverse environments, ranging from rural to urban in subarctic to tropical climates.

The home-range size of a cat may be substantial and can vary significantly among members of a given population. Cats typically show overlap of their home ranges, with few or no cats having exclusive use of an area (Apps 1986). Females generally have smaller home ranges than males. Cats fed by humans have been shown to have smaller movements than those that were not; home ranges and distance roaming was reported to be closer in area to those seen in owned pet cats (Schmidt et al. 2007). Availability of food or other resources, such as suitable shelter in the form of abandoned buildings (Figure 25.4), may also affect cat density and dispersal (Calhoon and Haspel 1989).

The diet of free-roaming cats is varied and is typically dependent on prey abundance and availability in a particular environment. In addition, food provided by humans (e.g. colony caregivers, individuals feeding unowned cats) may represent a significant proportion of the caloric intake of some free-roaming cats. The reader is directed to the section on predation in this chapter for additional information on the dietary habits of free-roaming cats.

Concerns Regarding Community Cats

Welfare Concerns

Welfare concerns regarding free-roaming cats are not insignificant and include concerns regarding the cats' physical condition and health, rates and causes of mortality, quality of life, and eventual outcome. The welfare concerns that are likely to arise for a given population of cats will be influenced at least in part by the environmental conditions and what, if any, management or care the cats are receiving. For example, climate is likely to be of greater concern in extreme northern areas, such as Alaska, than in most parts of the continental United States. The welfare of some community cats may be very good, while that of others may be quite poor; variation is possible across locations

(a)

(b)

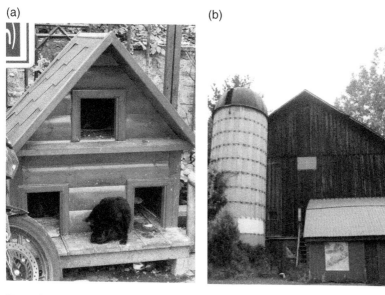

Figure 25.4 Community cats will be found at higher densities where food and sufficient shelter is available. (a) Dedicated cat shelters, such as the one shown here, may be provided for cats by caretakers. (b) Abandoned buildings are frequently occupied by cats. This barn, located on a non-working dairy barn, was utilized as the primary shelter for a colony of approximately 20 feral and semi-feral cats.

as well as among cats within a given geographic area. An individual assessment of each situation and its unique circumstances as well as for each cat is necessary in deciding on the most appropriate management strategy.

Life Span, General Health, and Body Condition

The body condition of younger cats has been reported to be poorer than that of adult cats in the same population (Short and Turner 2005). High mortality rates have been reported for community cats, with up to 75% of kittens confirmed dead or missing before six months of age (Nutter et al. 2004b). Common causes of death include motor vehicle trauma, dog attack, gunshots, infectious diseases, and euthanasia by animal control; predation is suspected to be a likely cause as well (Nutter et al. 2004b; Schmidt et al. 2007). Although these mortality rates are comparable to those seen in other wild carnivores such as foxes and bobcats (Cypher et al. 2000), they are high and of significant concern when considering the welfare of free-roaming cats. Interestingly, a

majority of people feel it is more humane to allow a cat to live out its life and die from traumatic causes in a relatively short period of time than to remove the cat pre-emptively for humane euthanasia (Chu and Anderson 2007).

The current literature suggests that while deaths due to trauma, infectious disease, and various other causes do occur regularly, most free-roaming cats that have made it to adulthood can be expected to do well for several years or longer. Prevalence rates for many infectious diseases and baseline health status are generally similar in free-roaming cats and pet cats (Luria et al. 2004; Nutter et al. 2004a; Stojanovic and Foley 2011). Feeding by humans has been associated with improved survival and longer life spans in community cats (Schmidt et al. 2007). Anecdotally, life spans for cats in managed colonies or otherwise cared for by humans may approach those reported for owned pet cats, with more than 80% of cats in one study still present on-site after six years of observation (Levy et al. 2003a). Disappearances from a colony location or study site do occur, and were reported for

15% of the population over the several years of observation. These may be the result of death, but could also be due to emigration to other locations or removal by humans for adoption or transfer to an animal shelter (Wallace and Levy 2006). Confirmed death rates in free-roaming cats have been reported to be low, with approximately 6% known to have died following return to the capture site in two separate studies (Hughes and Slater 2002; Levy et al. 2003a).

Data regarding euthanasia rates of community cats for illness or injury are seldom reported. The available information suggests that this occurs infrequently and often after a significant period of time, excluding those cats euthanized at the time of capture on the basis of surveillance testing for feline leukemia virus (FeLV) and/or feline immunodeficiency virus (FIV) infection. In one population of cats on a university campus in Florida, only 4% were euthanized for serious medical concerns after a median time on-site of 5.1 years. Data from seven TNR programs in the United States indicates that only 0.4% of cats were euthanized because of the presence of debilitating conditions (Scott et al. 2002a). A retrospective analysis of a single TNR program in Massachusetts estimated that 5–10% of the cats trapped over a 30-year period were euthanized due to serious illness or injury, or a positive FeLV/FIV test result, and that most euthanasias occurred in the early months of the program (Spehar and Wolf 2017).

A cat's sterilization status can be expected to influence its life span and overall physical condition. Spay–neuter is likely to improve cats' health through direct effects of surgery (e.g. elimination of risk of pyometra) as well as resultant behavioral changes that reduce the risk of disease transmission (e.g. reduction in fighting leading to less transmission of FIV). There are also a number of metabolic changes that occur subsequent to sterilization, including a reduced energy requirement compared to both National Research Council recommenda-

tions and pre-surgical requirements in individual cats (Mitsuhashi et al. 2011). Feral cats are reported to often be in lean but adequate body condition prior to surgery (Scott et al. 2002b), with weight gain and improvements in body condition scores reported following spay or neuter (Figure 25.5; Hughes and Slater 2002; Fischer et al. 2007). Longer life spans and increased survival rates of both adults and kittens are also associated with sterilization of community cats. This phenomenon is well enough documented that it has actually been used by some authors as an argument against TNR programs, because survival rates have a greater impact on population size than reproductive rates do (McCarthy et al. 2013).

Quality of Life and Outcomes

Strong differences in opinion often exist as to the quality of life experienced by free-roaming cats and what choice(s) is/are the most humane and appropriate. Some authors have argued that high mortality rates and reduced life expectancy are indicators of a poor quality of life, and that removal of the cats for euthanasia is a more humane choice (Clarke and Pacin 2002), while others have argued the

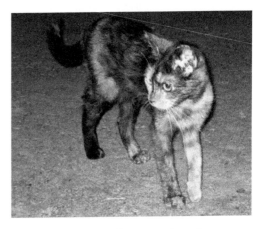

Figure 25.5 Community cats, such as the one seen here, are frequently in lean but adequate body condition. Weight gain and improved body condition scores are typically seen following sterilization.

(a)

(b)

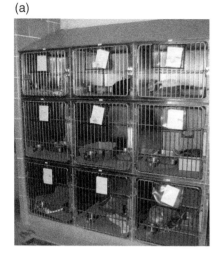
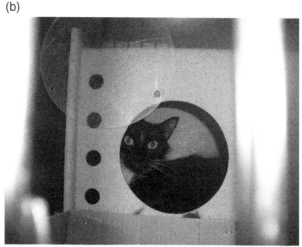

Figure 25.6 (a) Housing in many animal shelters is inadequate to maintain the physical and behavioral health of cats. This is exacerbated for poorly socialized cats that are highly stressed by close proximity to humans. Although modifications can be made to limit this stress, such as the use of a commercially available feral cat den (b), prolonged housing of feral and semi-feral cats is not recommended.

opposite (Chu and Anderson 2007). The importance given to cats' welfare when considering the acceptability of various management strategies varies among surveys, with distinct differences having been shown based on the respondent's location (e.g. urban vs. rural), gender, and age, as well as affiliation with cat or wildlife-based groups. Differences in the importance or priority ascribed to cat welfare have also been shown to differ depending on the specific sub-group (e.g. companion cats, strays, feral cats) of the cats in question (Farnworth et al. 2011).

Availability (or lack thereof) of various options for the management and care of a particular cat or group of cats will almost certainly influence what strategy is judged to be most effective in addressing welfare concerns. Surveys have indicated that people are opposed to trapping and impoundment of free-roaming cats if they will most likely be euthanized, but they are similarly opposed to leaving cats outdoors without a plan for management or care (Dabritz et al. 2006). Sadly, cats' welfare is not necessarily improved by

removal to an animal shelter. Shelter stays are stressful for cats, particularly those who have been poorly socialized to human contact, and positive live release outcomes are far from certain (Figure 25.6). Euthanasia in animal shelters remains a leading cause of death for cats in the United States. In many communities it remains a virtual certainty for feral or semi-feral cats brought to the local animal shelter. Removal of free-roaming cats without health issues for euthanasia raises ethical concerns and does not serve the welfare of the individual or the population.

Infectious Diseases

Another concern frequently expressed regarding community cat populations is their role in the transmission of infectious diseases to other animals (including domestic cats, native wild felids, and other wildlife) and/or people through direct transmission or environmental contamination. However, there is little existing data upon which to base these claims.

Available data indicates that pathogen prevalence rates may vary greatly among different populations of free-roaming cats, as they do for populations of pet cats. One study found that 75% of cats were positive for hookworms (Anderson et al. 2003), while another study found no cats to be infected (Stojanovic and Foley 2011), but neither provided data on the prevalence in pet cats in the same geographic area for comparison. Similar discrepancies in prevalence rates of other pathogens, such as *Toxoplasma gondii*, have been reported (Nutter et al. 2004a) and in some studies the reported prevalence in feral cat populations has actually been lower (Taetzsch et al. 2018). Not surprisingly, significant variation in disease prevalence may also be seen in different colonies within a relatively confined area (Gibson et al. 2002).

While prevalence extremes do exist, available data often show that the frequencies of many infectious diseases and parasitic infections in free-roaming cats are similar to those reported in pet cats. This suggests that the former pose no greater risk to human or animal health than owned cats and do not serve as reservoirs for these conditions (Stojanovic and Foley 2011). For example, free-roaming cats studied in northern Florida had similar or lower prevalence rates compared to pet cats for FeLV, FIV, *Bartonella henselae*, *Dirofilaria immitis*, *T. gondii*, and several other infectious diseases (Luria et al. 2004). A similar study of feral cats trapped for surgery on Prince Edward Island also found prevalence rates to be relatively low. Cats in both of these study populations were tested following presentation by a caretaker for neutering. While they may not be representative of free-roaming cats not receiving such care, they arguably represent the population most likely to come into contact with humans and transmit disease.

Toxoplasma Infection

Infection with *T. gondii*, an obligate intracellular protozoan parasite, is possible in a wide range of species, but cats are the only definitive hosts. Cats typically shed oocysts for a brief period of time following initial infection, but will remain seropositive because of the organism's ability to persist in the form of tissue cysts. Exposure to the parasite is of particular concern for pregnant women, as *T. gondii* infection may lead to abortion, still births, or a myriad of congenital defects, depending on the stage of gestation when the mother became infected. Contamination of soil and water with *T. gondii*-laden cat feces is often noted to be of concern because of potential impacts on public health and, to a lesser extent, on other species (e.g. Miller et al. 2002; Kreuder et al. 2003; Conrad et al. 2005).

Free-roaming cats are often cited as the largest risk with regard to transmission of toxoplasmosis, but the seroprevalence estimates reported have been similar to those for pet cats (Hill et al. 2000; Dubey et al. 2002; Luria et al. 2004; Stojanovic and Foley 2011; Taetzsch et al. 2018). Furthermore, it has been estimated that only ~1% of seropositive cats will be actively shedding oocysts (Dabritz et al. 2007; Stojanovic and Foley 2011) and that community cats are not the principal source of fecal contamination produced by cats (Dabritz et al. 2006). Additionally, human infection is most likely the result of inadvertent ingestion of oocysts that occurs when people fail to adequately wash vegetables, or through the ingestion of tissue cysts from undercooked meat products.

Rabies

Perhaps the most commonly cited public health concern is the role of community cats in the transmission of rabies. Rabies remains a significant disease concern worldwide, with either dogs or wildlife serving as the natural reservoirs for the virus depending on the geographic location. In the United States rabies is detected most frequently in wildlife, representing more than 90% of all animals testing positive (Birhane et al. 2017; Ma et al. 2018). Cats are the most frequently reported domestic animal to test positive for rabies, although the vast majority of these cases have been confined to a relatively small geographic area where the raccoon rabies virus variant is enzootic.

Concern regarding the risk of rabies posed by free-roaming cats is legitimate. However, numerous publications contain misleading, unsubstantiated, or downright erroneous statements regarding the risk of rabies posed by community cats. For example, one review on the ethical and legal dilemmas of TNR programs noted that exposure to a kitten of unknown origin subsequently found to be rabid led to the treatment of more than 600 individuals (Barrows 2004). While this is certainly a cause for concern, the author failed to note that this kitten was actually purchased from a pet store with a health certificate completed by a licensed veterinarian (Noah et al. 1996).

The implications of misleading data can be substantial. In the commentary "Critical Assessment of Claims Regarding Management of Feral Cats by Trap-Neuter-Return," the authors claimed that 80% of the post-exposure prophylaxis (PEP) administered to humans in the United States resulted from contact with stray or feral cats (Longcore et al. 2009). The cited reference provides data for Pennsylvania only (Moore et al. 2000). In that state, 75% of reported exposures involved dogs and 17.2% involved cats, with the remaining 17.8% comprising wildlife and other species. Cat exposures were six times more likely to lead to administration of PEP compared to dog exposures. However, this included exposure to all cats (e.g. pet, feral, stray, and otherwise unowned) and represented only 44% of the total doses administered in the state for the entire year. Of those, 82% were administered as a result of contact with a feral, stray, or unowned cat (Moore et al. 2000).

Precise estimates for annual PEP use are unknown, but it has been estimated that 23 415 courses are used each year (Christian et al. 2009). If 80% of all PEP administered in the United States were the result of exposure to stray or feral cats, this would represent at least 18 732 doses each year. In contrast, 44% of the 556 PEP doses given in Pennsylvania were the result of cat exposure and 82% of those were the result of contact with a stray or feral cat for a total of 200 PEP doses. If this was representative of the national pattern of administration, it would translate to 10 000 doses for exposure to all cats (e.g. approximately half of what was implied as an argument against TNR programs). However, such an extrapolation is likely an overestimate, as Pennsylvania has previously been noted to be the state with the highest number of rabid cats in the entire country (Blanton et al. 2012).

Regardless, rabies is a serious concern, and potential human exposure by cats (including owned, stray, and feral) leads to the administration of thousands of doses of PEP each year. Surprisingly, concerns about rabies transmission are frequently cited as a reason to oppose TNR programs, despite the fact that such programs can reduce the number of at-risk cats through vaccination as well as through a reduction in population. National guidelines for the vaccination of cats include immunization against rabies using a product with a three-year duration of immunity as a core vaccine for all cats in TNR programs, with a recommendation to re-trap cats for administration of booster vaccinations one year later and then triennially thereafter (Scherk et al. 2013). Feral cats have been shown to mount an adequate immune response following administration of a single rabies vaccine at the time of anesthesia and surgery, providing evidence that even a single immunization may provide significant animal and public health benefits (Fischer et al. 2007). An inverse association between free-roaming cat population control interventions (i.e. TNR programs) and the number of animals submitted for rabies testing in Massachusetts counties has been documented. While the magnitude of testing reduction was small, it does indicate that such programs can be successful (McGonagle 2015). It is likely true that vaccination of cats in TNR programs may not change practices regarding human exposure assessment and administration of PEP, because of the difficulty in consistently documenting vaccination of the individual cats in question (Roebling et al. 2014). However, vaccination should still reduce the risk of rabies in these cats and thus the true risk they pose to humans and other animals.

Nuisance Behaviors

The actual incidence of complaints regarding nuisance behaviors of free-roaming cats is not widely reported and likely varies among communities, depending on the population of cats, environment and proximity to people (e.g. rural vs. urban), and the tolerance of the human population. Complaints may be directed to animal shelters or even local law enforcement, and include concerns regarding the physical health and welfare of the cats (e.g. sick, injured, or deceased); yowling, caterwauling, or fighting; and urine spraying or fecal deposition in yards (Figure 25.7). A significant association between cat reproduction and cat-associated nuisances has been documented (Gunther et al. 2015), and many of these complaints stem from hormonally driven behav-

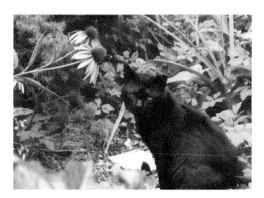

Figure 25.7 Concerns about perceived property damage caused by community cats, such as damage to or fecal deposition in gardens and flower beds, may lead to the filing of a nuisance complaint.

iors that should be substantially reduced following sterilization of some or all of the animals. Published data indicate that fighting and vocalizations are reduced in neutered colony members (Finkler et al. 2011b), and significant (e.g. by 25%) reductions in the number of complaints have been reported in different settings following implementation of a sterilization program (Hughes and Slater 2002; Hughes et al. 2002).

Predation and Environmental Impacts

All cats, regardless of ownership status, socialization, habitat, or relationship with humans, have the potential to kill native and non-native wildlife, including birds, small mammals, reptiles, and invertebrates. Intake data from wildlife rehabilitation facilities indicates that cat predation is not an uncommon occurrence in the population of animals served by such facilities (Jessup 2004; Sallinger 2008; Loyd et al. 2017). Legitimate concerns exist with regard to both individual animal welfare and the population-level impacts on wildlife that may arise from predation.

Hunting Behavior

Cats are opportunistic hunters and will hunt and kill a variety of species, with or without consuming them. Natural prey is typically related to abundance and availability (Liberg 1984). In general, small mammals such as rodents or rabbits represent the vast majority of a cat's diet regardless of study location (Jones 1977; Jones and Coman 1981; Liberg 1984; Churcher and Lawton 1987; Paltridge et al. 1997; Molsher et al. 1999; Woods et al. 2003; Bonnaud et al. 2007). Numerous bird species, reptiles, and invertebrates also may be preyed upon by cats. While this is typically to a lesser extent than predation on small mammals, at least one study found invertebrates, following by amphibians and reptiles, to be the most common type of prey captured (Hernandez et al. 2018a).

The exact proportions of prey type as well as the absolute number of prey killed per cat are likely to vary with the specific area in which the cats were studied as well as the time of year. Cats in rural areas may have different rates of predation than cats in suburban or urban areas, though research on cat populations in those latter areas is limited (Baker et al. 2005). It has been hypothesized that prey species are particularly vulnerable during their reproduction periods and higher rates of predation (e.g. likely from the killing of juveniles) have been documented during these months (Lepczyck et al. 2004; Baker et al. 2005). Thus, extrapolations for annual predation that are based on rates obtained from data collected during the spring are likely to result in erroneously high estimates.

Hunting behavior is highly individual and significant variation in frequency will be seen among cats. This makes it difficult to extrapolate the findings from a small study comprising relatively few cats to larger populations. In one study (Tschanz et al. 2011), a mere 16% of cats accounted for 75% of the prey, and in another more than a third of cats failed to return any prey at all (van Heezik et al. 2010). Older cats and those fitted with collar-mounted warning devices have been found to kill fewer prey (Churcher and Lawton 1987; Woods et al. 2003; Nelson et al. 2005; van Heezik et al. 2010). Supplemental food may also reduce predation rates. Cats have been shown to rely predominantly on meat scraps rather than vertebrate prey when the former is available (Hutchings 2003) and the probability of predation is lower in well-fed cats compared to poorly fed cats (Silva-Rodriguez and Sieving 2011). Cats in one managed colony were found to spend <1% of their time hunting wildlife (Hernandez et al. 2018b). However, even well-fed cats have been shown to hunt, with natural prey reported to make up between 15 and 50% of a house cat's diet when allowed outdoor access (Liberg 1984).

Magnitude and Impact of Predation

Significant disagreement exists regarding the exact magnitude of cat predation and its corresponding impact on wildlife populations, as data on this scale is lacking. Data on predation is often obtained from surveys that ask owners to document how many prey species or items their cat(s) brought home over a particular period of time, with or without attempts to identify the various species presented. The applicability of such data, however, is likely limited. Many authors argue that information obtained from these surveys underestimates the number of wildlife killed by cats, because only a fraction of the prey items are returned to the home for owners to observe. However, there is work to suggest that such surveys may actually result in an overestimation of prey numbers. When owners' estimates of predation rates were compared to the records of prey items actually returned home by their pets, a large proportion of owners considerably overestimated their cat's predation (Tschanz et al. 2011).

Numerous publications make extrapolations from this limited predation data, estimating that billions of living things are killed each year by cats, that this rate of predation exerts a significant and unsustainable toll on populations, and that cats are the leading cause of wildlife population decline in the United States and around the world. Extrapolated estimates of predation rates must be considered in context, however, for the reasons already mentioned and because they do not provide an indicator of the cats' impact on a population level. Even with high rates of predation, the summed effects appear "unlikely to affect population size for the majority of prey species" (Baker et al. 2005) and "there is thus no indication that domestic cats significantly reduce or destabilise vulnerable bird populations in rural landscapes, where the availability and the diversity of other prey are high" (Tschanz et al. 2011). The small size, relatively short life span, and high reproductive rates of many prey species may further limit the impact that predation has on their population dynamics.

It is also important to recognize that the role cats play in an ecosystem is complex and seldom well understood, even in those environments (e.g. islands) that could be considered closed and relatively simple. Eradication of cats is often recommended, and proponents cite examples of rebounding populations when cats are removed from islands, but examples are limited and this is not always the outcome. There are well-documented instances where removal of cats did not increase prey populations, or where eradication actually had a negative impact on wildlife populations and the overall condition of the environment (Hughes et al. 2008; Bergstrom et al. 2009). Mathematical modeling has demonstrated that the presence of cats may have a positive effect on endemic birds in insular ecosystems where rats are also present (Courchamp et al. 1999b). That effect has been borne out in nature as well: the breeding success of Cooks Petrels was approximately 3.5 times higher when cats and rats were present compared to rats alone (Rayner et al. 2007). This has been hypothesized to be due to a phenomenon known as "mesopredator release." Cats are the apex predator on many islands where they were introduced, killing both target prey species as well as other, smaller potential predators (e.g. rats) known as "mesopredators." When the number of apex predators is reduced, mesopredator populations can increase dramatically and lead to higher predation rates on small, vulnerable species like birds, creating a situation where the prey species in question declines dramatically or even becomes extinct (Courchamp et al. 1999a; Zavaleta et al. 2001; Ritchie and Johnson 2009).

Numerous reasons for declining populations exist, including but not limited to habit loss, climate change, and other anthropogenic causes such as collisions with man-made structures or pesticide use (Dauphiné and Cooper 2009). It is important to consider all causes of mortality and population decline of wildlife when determining what can be done to reduce losses and reverse the trend. Even if

one uses an estimate that hundreds of millions of birds are killed by cats each year, it is still likely that window and building collisions remain a greater source of mortality (Loss et al. 2013).

Any analysis of cat-associated mortality, particularly in light of its potential impact at a population level, must also consider the specific animals that are being preyed upon. It is unknown on a larger scale whether predation by cats is additive or compensatory. In the case of additive predation, the animals killed are in addition to those that would have died from other causes, such as starvation. In compensatory predation, the prey killed would have died anyway. A study in Sweden showed that rabbits comprised 93% of cats' diets during a particularly harsh winter in which dead, dying, and weak rabbits were commonly seen (Liberg 1984). Similarly, examination of birds killed by cats found that they were in significantly poorer condition compared to those killed following collisions (Baker et al. 2008). In both of these examples, cat predation was likely compensatory, which could be expected to have minimal additional effect on the population dynamics of the target species.

Neither the relative proportions of the different species killed by cats nor estimates for wildlife population abundance are generally available in predation studies, thus making it difficult to determine which populations and species are most vulnerable (Loss et al. 2013). Many publications on feline predation rely on extensive extrapolations that have been based on information obtained from a single study, which may in turn be based on observations of only a handful of cats from a single colony, or even an estimate based on the available literature at the time. Thus, this data, which often forms the foundation for modeling parameters and broad extrapolations to entire countries, may not be representative of larger populations of cats or wildlife, different geographic areas, variations in climate or season, or numerous other factors influencing the original observations as previously discussed.

Despite these limitations, the information is frequently used as the basis for meta-studies, the publication of which sometimes garners much public discussion and debate regarding the number of animals killed by cat predation each year. For example, Loss et al. estimated that free-roaming cats were responsible for the deaths of 1.4–3.7 billion birds and 6.9–20.7 billion mammals in the United States annually by conducting what the authors described as a data-driven systematic review (Loss et al. 2013). Such numbers are startling, but the findings should be examined with a careful eye, as many limitations exist to arriving at an accurate estimate. Sensitivity analysis in this study indicated that both the population size and predation rates of the unowned cat population explained the greatest variation in total mortality estimates. Unfortunately, the outdoor cat population and predation rates were based on estimates for which reliable data is minimal.

Legal Concerns

Laws governing free-roaming cats are typically local or state based in nature and vary significantly between jurisdictions. Community cats are generally, but not always, protected through anti-cruelty laws. Additional laws regarding their care and management can be much more varied, ranging from prohibitions on feeding cats in public parks or other outdoor locations to clear support with or without funding for TNR programs. In some instances, additional legislation pertaining to the management of free-roaming cats has been adopted to exempt the cats and their caretakers from existing animal legislation. Legislation introduced in Athens, GA, in 2010, for example, allows the registration of cat colonies with the county and provides $10 000 in sterilization vouchers, while exempting caretakers from an existing law that defines anyone feeding stray cats as the owners. Coupled with a policy change at the local animal shelter, this legislative change had the effect of mandating TNR as the only management option for free-roaming cats in that community (Loyd and Hernandez 2012).

In other cases, an increase in ownership laws (e.g. licensing and mandatory spay–neuter) have been recommended to curb the number of free-roaming cats (Dauphiné and Cooper 2009). Legislative attempts have also been considered to remove existing protections for cats as a domesticated species. In New Zealand, feral cats were placed on the list of pest species in 2004, thereby exempting them from the protections of the Animal Welfare Act (Farnworth et al. 2010). Approval of a proposal made by the Wisconsin Conservation Congress would have defined feral cats as an unprotected species, thereby allowing them to be legally hunted within the state (USA Today 2005). Although the measure was never approved by the Wisconsin legislature and signed into law, such extreme measures and their relative popularity with certain segments of the population underscore the contentious nature of community cat management. Some communities have also faced emerging and protracted legal challenges regarding their handling of community cat populations. For example, both the mayor and director of the city's Animal Welfare Department in Albuquerque, New Mexico, were named in a lawsuit alleging animal cruelty and abandonment of stray cats through a TNR program (KOAT 2014). Although the initial suit and a subsequent appeal were both rejected, allowing the TNR program to continue (McKay 2016), another lawsuit was filed approximately five years after the first and is still unresolved at the time of publication (Boetel 2018).

International response to the management of free-roaming cat populations also varies significantly in terms of existing legislation. Australia allows for lethal control of cats threatening native wildlife (Farnworth et al. 2011), while eradication programs are only legal in Israel if there is proof that the animal constitutes a true hazard to public health (Gunther et al. 2011). In Italy there is a complete prohibition of euthanasia of feral cats (Natoli et al. 2006). Further differences regarding management of

(a)

(b)

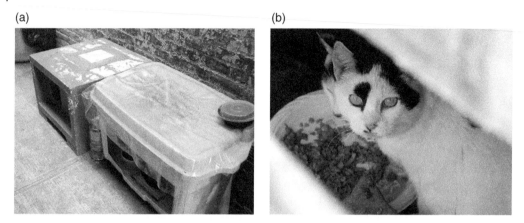

Figure 25.8   (a) Feeding stations provide an enclosed, protected area for cats. (b) A feral cat inside a feeding station during an evening meal. *Source:* Photos courtesy of Maggie O'Neil.

all or a proportion of the community cat populations may also exist depending on the specific language used in the laws. For example, New Zealand law allows lethal control of feral cats, but requires that stray cats be relinquished to a nonprofit organization for assessment prior to placement or euthanasia.

Various laws protect wildlife and birds especially, such as the Migratory Bird Treaty Act and, if applicable, the Endangered Species Act. Additional state and local laws may also exist. What, if any, implications such laws have for caretakers of community cats remains unclear. While it has been suggested that veterinarians and caretakers participating in TNR programs may face legal liability under wildlife protection laws (Barrows 2004), this has not actually occurred to the best of the author's knowledge.

Public Perception of Community Cats

Public perception surrounding community cats varies greatly, as do opinions on the most appropriate methods for their management. For many individuals, community cats represent beloved and valued companions. Studies of feral cat caretakers consistently show a high level of attachment between people and the cats they provide care for, despite the fact that it may not be possible to touch these cats or keep them as pets in a traditional home setting. Surveys have shown that as much as 26% of the population feeds unowned outdoor cats (Centonze and Levy 2002; Lord 2008), even though a large proportion of these individuals are not themselves cat owners (Figure 25.8). Many caretakers provide care well beyond feeding and do so at high financial cost, investing significant amounts of money to sterilize cats even when limited services are available (Natoli et al. 2006). Interestingly, while caretaking generally emerges from the individuals' strong empathy for the cats, some people remain emotionally detached from the cats (Finkler and Terkel 2011).

Available data generally suggests that people recognize the need for effective management of community cats, and in many instances a majority of individuals surveyed are in favor of TNR programs (Dabritz et al. 2006; Chu and Anderson 2007; Loyd and Hernandez 2012). Despite only a minority of respondents indicating that cat welfare or prevention of cat euthanasia was very important, euthanasia was found to be the least acceptable option for management by respondents. TNR was the most popular choice for a management option funded either by tax dollars or charitable donations. Ash and Adams (2003) reported similar findings when surveying university faculty and staff, with more than half of respondents selecting TNR programs over removal or no control for management of cat populations on campus. One survey found that the overwhelming majority of people would rather see a free-roaming cat left outdoors than for it to be captured and euthanized, even if they knew that the cat would die of traumatic injury within two years (Chu and Anderson 2007).

This evidence of positive public opinion should not, however, be misinterpreted as consistent and universal support for the existence of free-roaming cat populations. Public perception may differ with geographic area, socioeconomic group, professional background, personal values and beliefs, and even the language used to frame the particular questions about cat control. New Zealanders were more likely to favor non-lethal control measures and rate welfare concerns more highly when asked about management of stray cats than when asked the same question about feral cats (Farnworth et al. 2011). This may be due, in part, to the laws governing the control methods that may be employed for various groups of cats and the legal designation of feral cats as pests in that country. Categorizing an animal as a "pest" has also been shown in other studies to be associated with lower concern for animal welfare (Taylor and Signal 2009).

Many individuals and organizations are strongly opposed to the presence of any cats outdoors and the management of free-roaming cat populations by any means other than removal. Others likely fall somewhere in the middle of such polarizing debates and may struggle to support one management option over another (Loyd and Hernandez 2012). Organizational membership has been significantly associated with individual opinions regarding the prevention of cat euthanasia, management through TNR programs, or designation of cats as an invasive species (Loyd and Hernandez 2012). Research has shown significant polarization between self-identified bird conservation professionals and cat colony caretakers on opinions regarding the impact of feral cats, efficacy of TNR programs, and which management strategies are most appropriate. Such polarization was found regardless of whether or not these individuals considered themselves to be "cat people," "bird people," or both. It has been hypothesized that the emerging conflicts may be the result of identity politics, data conflict, and/or value conflicts pertaining to cats and wildlife (Peterson et al. 2012).

Even among animal welfare organizations there may be disagreement about appropriate strategies for the management of community cats. Many national animal welfare organizations, such as the American Society of the Prevention of Cruelty to Animals (ASPCA) and the Humane Society of the United States (HSUS), are in favor of TNR programs and do not support efforts aimed at removal and euthanasia (HSUS 2019; ASPCA 2019b). Others, such as People for the Ethical Treatment of Animals (PETA), are of the opinion that the welfare of community cats is poor, TNR programs are inhumane and akin to abandonment, and these cats should be removed from the environment and humanely euthanized (PETA 2019). Similar disparity exists within the veterinary profession, with the American Association of Feline Practitioners (AAFP) being in favor of TNR programs, the Association of Avian Veterinarians (AAV) being opposed, and the American Veterinary Medical Association (AVMA) taking a more neutral position (AAFP 2012; AAV 2019; AVMA 2019).

It has been suggested that public policy decisions regarding cat management have been and will continue to be dictated by "loud and passionate advocacy groups." Individuals and organizations with opposing viewpoints engage in vehement and often emotional debate regarding the best way to manage the existing population of free-roaming cats. In many instances, claims are made that characterize the opposing viewpoints as being mutually exclusive; supporters are in favor of either cat welfare or environmental protection and the welfare of wildlife, but not both. TNR advocates have, in certain instances, been accused of having a commitment to cat population control that ranges from "questionable to entirely lacking" and even been compared to animal hoarders (Dauphiné and Cooper 2009).

Regardless of one's personal feelings on the issue, it is easy to see that such debate is counterproductive. Arguments such as these fail to recognize the mutual goal that animal welfare organizations and wildlife conservation groups both share: a reduction in the number of community cats. By focusing on this common ground rather than on the differences, steps can be taken to develop viable solutions that effectively address concerns regarding the health and welfare of community cats and their impacts on the environment, wildlife, and public health. It should then be possible to design intervention strategies that are cooperative and inclusive in nature, without sacrificing the values of either side. The reality is that no management strategy, whether lethal or non-lethal in nature, will be successful on a large scale without taking public opinion into consideration and securing the cooperation of key stakeholders. Detailed analyses of the social, cultural, and economic costs and benefits are necessary to increase the probability of local community support for whatever program is selected (Oppel et al. 2011).

More recently, some authors have focused instead on ways to improve the effectiveness of TNR (Boone 2015) or to implement it within a wider framework of social engagement (McDonald et al. 2018), as a means to enhance these programs as a population management tool and drive long-term behavioral changes that could better address feline overpopulation.

Management Strategies

There is no single, one-size-fits-all approach that is appropriate for the management of all free-roaming cats in all situations. In general, comprehensive multifaceted programs that consider public opinion and have the buy-in of key stakeholders are most likely to succeed and have a lasting impact. As discussed in the section on public perception, opinions on the most appropriate method(s) for the management of community cats vary significantly, although most people recognize the need for some type of intervention.

Do Nothing or "Wait and See"

Perhaps the longest-standing and most widespread approach to the management of free-roaming cat populations is to "wait and see" or "do nothing." Clearly, this approach is nonproductive and does nothing to address concerns regarding cats (e.g. health and welfare, population size) or their impacts on people, other animals, and the ecosystems in which they live. In some jurisdictions this approach may have arisen from a long-term status quo and inertia or through the default of failing to select an alternate strategy. In other jurisdictions the "wait and see" approach may have resulted from a decision that ignoring the management challenge posed by the free-roaming cat population is the least expensive option, because it does not cost anything to put in place. This rationalization, however, results in a false economy. It fails to consider the variety of expenses that may already be incurred as a result of the unmanaged free-roaming cat population and that inaction will ultimately require greater time and expense to address management of cat populations. As a result of these factors and the common belief that some form of management is necessary for community cats, discussions regarding specific management strategies typically focus on removal or sterilization programs.

Removal-Based Programs

Removal-based programs rely on the permanent removal of some or all of a population of cats from a specific location. This may be accomplished through lethal control, where cats are killed either on-site or removed to an off-site location (typically but not always an animal shelter). Removal may also be accomplished by trapping cats and either relocating them or rehoming them.

On-Site Lethal Control

Lethal control programs rely on a variety of lethal methods to eliminate a population of cats at the location where they live. Various techniques have been tried and, in some instances, are still promoted as a viable option for managing community cat populations. These include introduction of infectious disease (e.g. panleukopenia), poisoning, shooting, hunting with dogs, and the use of leg-hold traps. A variety of techniques are often employed, with hunting and trapping almost universally required to eradicate the last remaining cats in a population. These campaigns are often unpopular and have typically utilized inhumane methods. People may object to eradication programs because of potential health hazards, inconvenience, financial burdens, religious or cultural beliefs, or ethical and welfare concerns (Oppel et al. 2011).

On-site lethal control methods are considered to be unacceptable for widespread use in the management of continental cat populations. They have most frequently been applied in an attempt to eradicate cats from island ecosystems. It has been reported that the vast majority of islands on which eradication has been successful are <5 km^2 (Nogales et al. 2004). Sustained, aggressive methods used in combination are typically required. One campaign often cited as a successful example of cat eradication took place on Marion Island, a small uninhabited island in the Southern Indian Ocean. This "success" required extensive and inhumane efforts over a 19-year period, and included trapping, hunting, poisoning, and disease introduction to eliminate a population of approximately 3600 cats (Bester et al. 2002). Even on small islands the effort expended is tremendous, in one case requiring nearly 4 years to eliminate

a population of just 150 cats (Courchamp and Sugihara 1999).

Many of the methods utilized in island eradication programs are not feasible for use in other locations due to the presence of people and other non-target and domestic species. Severe injuries in native foxes have been reported with use of leg-hold traps (Campbell et al. 2011) and it has been shown that toxic baits will be consumed by non-target species as well as domestic cats (de Torres et al. 2011). The accidental deaths of nearly 40% of pet cats following ingestion of poison bait in a cat eradication program on Ascension Island (Oppel et al. 2011) highlights the risk to owned cats.

It is generally agreed that the efforts required for removal are inversely proportional to the number of cats remaining and tremendous efforts in trapping and hunting are required to capture the last survivors in a population. Thus, the effort to remove a fixed number of animals each year increases substantially as the population declines (Short and Turner 2005). Failure to fully eliminate a population can result in rapid rebound of the population. Preventing the reintroduction of cats is critical if there is to be any long-term effect with eradication. Extensive efforts eliminated feral cats from a fenced conservation reserve in Australia. However, the population was quickly re-established by the immigration of just two cats across an ineffective barrier. Effective control for a sustained period of time was never established in a 14-year period (Short and Turner 2005).

Even if these lethal control methods were considered acceptable by the general public, their use on mainland cat populations is highly unlikely to be effective. This is in large part due to the sheer number of cats that will move in to occupy the temporarily vacated niche, but also due to other factors. For example, disease introduction is particularly unlikely to be effective due to variations in natural immunity between populations of cats on islands compared to continents; modeling has shown that FeLV could be effective on an island, but would be of limited use in the reduction of cat numbers any-where else (Courchamp and Sugihara 1999).

Trap–Remove–Euthanize

The traditional animal control approach of removal for euthanasia (frequently referred to by critics as "catch and kill") is another method for the management of cat populations that has been utilized for significant periods of time in many jurisdictions. Although capture and euthanasia may be the most humane choice for individual cats suffering from significant illness or injury, it is not a viable option on a large or long-term scale for the management of cat populations. Such efforts have been associated with disappointing results, significant expense, and often serious welfare concerns. Trap–removal–euthanize efforts rarely address the various factors that will influence cat density and location, such as a food source or available shelter. In order to be effective, such campaigns must be conducted intensively and consistently in order to remove all of the cats from an area, make the area unattractive to potential new residents, and monitor for any new cats that might arrive or be abandoned and repopulate the location. Similar to eradication campaigns, the effort to remove the last remaining members of a population can be extremely labor intensive. If cats are removed without any efforts made to reduce the carrying capacity of the environment, birth rates and survival rates will typically increase to compensate for the reduction in population.

Efforts to trap and remove cats for euthanasia may also be met with a significant outcry, the impact of which should not be underestimated. Following a decision to begin removal of a colony of cats being fed by volunteers, approximately 50 cats were trapped and brought to a local animal shelter over a two-year period. Some cats had to be trapped repeatedly as volunteers went to the shelter, adopted or reclaimed the cats, and then re-released them on-site (Winter 2004). Public opposition, welfare concerns, and cost makes it extremely unlikely that trap–remove–eutha-nize programs could ever be employed on a large enough scale to have a significant impact on community cat populations.

Trap–Neuter–Relocate

Trap–neuter–relocate programs are similar in most aspects to trap–neuter–return programs as a means of non-lethal management of community cats. Cats are similarly trapped and presented for veterinary care, steriliza-tion, and other medical services before being relocated to another outdoor location, rather than returned to their colonies or the location from which they were trapped (Figure 25.9). While relocation is frequently cited as a desired outcome when nuisance complaints are made, it is not routinely recommended as a management strategy for community cat management because of the time, expense, and myriad of challenges associated with it. Additionally, relocation rarely resolves the concerns surrounding the cats' presence. Because there is likely to be an environmental niche that makes the location attractive to cats, new cats will typically move into the area following removal of the existing popula-tion unless efforts are made to prevent access and reduce desirability.

In some instances relocation is necessary and appropriate. This includes situations where the

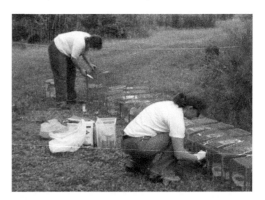

Figure 25.9 Two volunteers prepare humane traps that will be used to capture cats in a trap–neuter–return program. Individuals will often volunteer to assist with trapping for humane management programs, but not for trap–euthanize efforts.

cats' safety is of concern or severe ecologic concerns exist, such as a colony located in an environmentally sensitive area or in close proximity to the habitat of an endangered species. Relocation must be carefully planned in such cases. Finding a suitable location willing to accept the cats in a similar climate, with a reliable food source and suitable shelter, away from heavily trafficked areas, and under the supervision of a caretaker is extremely challenging. Once they have been transported to the new location, the cats must be confined in cages large enough to allow for humane care for several weeks until they habituate to the new location and can be expected to remain onsite once released. Failure to confine newly relocated cats will often result in attempts to return to the original colony location and may result in severe injury or death of the cats.

Adoption and Sanctuary Placement
Rehoming or sanctuary placement may be an option for certain individual cats or particular circumstances, but it is not a viable management strategy for large populations of community cats. Friendly, well-socialized community cats may be candidates for rehoming. However, shelter stays are stressful for cats and positive outcomes are far from certain. Many communities struggle to increase live outcomes as higher adoption rates are offset by increased intake of cats, which would likely be exacerbated if cat intake was greatly increased in an attempt to rehome a sizable portion of the community cat population. Furthermore, the proportion of the free-roaming cat population that is impounded by shelters in most communities is low enough that it is likely to have a negligible impact on the size or wellbeing of the larger population (Hurley and Levy 2014).

Cats that are poorly socialized to people are unsuitable for traditional placement in a home environment. Sanctuary care may be an option for some, provided that sufficient facilities, staffing, resources, and knowledge are available to ensure the humane care of the cats throughout their lifetimes. This is a tall order

and even when such criteria are met, available sanctuary space is extremely limited. This capacity would be quickly overwhelmed before even a fraction of the millions of unsocialized free-roaming cats could be placed in sanctuaries.

Despite these limitations, rehoming or sanctuary placement remains popular in public opinion as a method of control. Farnworth et al. (2011) found that rehoming was strongly supported as the main method of control of free-roaming cats in New Zealand, despite not all cats being adequately socialized to make this a suitable or humane option. Similarly, Loyd and Hernandez (2012) found that placement in sanctuaries was considered by respondents to be the most desirable option to reduce feral cat populations.

Sterilization Programs

These programs rely on veterinary intervention to render some or all of a population of cats incapable of reproducing. This is almost always accomplished through traditional spay–neuter, but vasectomy of male cats has also been proposed and work remains ongoing in the development of a non-surgical sterilant (see Chapter 27). Regardless of the specific means by which sterility is achieved, cats are returned to the same location from which they were trapped or otherwise removed.

There is general agreement that a high proportion of cats (either females only, or both males and females) must be sterilized to stop the continued growth of the population. Estimates as high as 70% or even greater than 90%, depending on the population dynamics and timing and targeting (e.g. juvenile or adult female cats) of the cat population in question, have been suggested as necessary to stabilize and ultimately reduce population size through attrition (Foley et al. 2005; Budke and Slater 2009; Miller et al. 2014). These estimates have been proposed as goals, but the actual percentage necessary remains unknown. Furthermore, this percentage is unlikely to be a constant across populations, given the variation that exists in cat densities, infectious disease pressures, available resources, survival rates, and other similar factors. A limited number of studies modeling the various rates of sterilization required to reduce the population have, however, been published and can provide some indication as to the possible efficacy and scope needed for TNR programs to be successful (Foley et al. 2005). These models are only as good as the data used to generate their results, and accurate information regarding the frequency of immigration and emigration as well as birth and death rates is seldom available. See Chapter 24 for more information on population modeling and the number needed to be sterilized.

Trap–Neuter–Return or Trap–Neuter–Return–Monitor

Trap–neuter–return or trap–neuter–return–monitor programs have become the most common non-lethal control strategy recommended for the management of community cat populations, but they remain controversial. These programs typically use grass-roots volunteers to humanely trap cats and bring them to an animal shelter, high-quality high-volume spay–neuter (HQHVSN) clinic, or veterinary hospital, although paid staff sometimes perform this task as well. Following presentation, the cats are anesthetized, examined, surgically sterilized, and have the distal tip of the ear removed for identification (Figure 25.10). Once recovered, the cats may be observed for a variable period of time before they are returned to the location from which they were trapped, where caregivers continue to monitor and provide basic care.

Beyond these basic tenets, differences exist in the services offered by various TNR programs.

Some programs sterilize and return only feral-behaving cats, removing friendly adults and kittens for adoption. Others alter and return all cats regardless of socialization status and/or age. There can also be variations in the

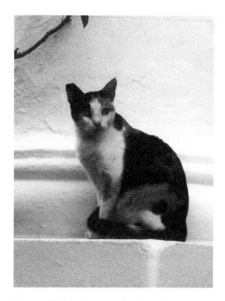

Figure 25.10 Removal of the distal tip of the ear is the recognized form of identification for cats that have been sterilized and returned to their colony or environment. The left ear is most commonly used for this purpose in this author's experience, but the right ear is sometimes used instead.

level of care provided for cats by individual caretakers, which may be influenced by their neighborhood's socioeconomic status (Finkler et al. 2011a). Cats may be treated for internal and/or external parasites and vaccinated against common infectious diseases. Although rabies vaccination is considered a core vaccine for cats undergoing TNR and is usually provided, this is not universal, and administration of other vaccinations, while recommended, may be more variable (Scherk et al. 2013). Some programs screen all cats for FeLV or FIV infection, but this is practice has fallen out of favor; data suggests that screening for retroviral infection with culling of positive cats is less effective than sterilization in reducing disease prevalence. See Chapter 35 for more information on operating a free-roaming cat clinic.

Unlike removal programs, which strive to reduce population below carrying capacity, TNR allows cats to remain in the environment without continuing to reproduce. Cat population size tends to increase until the carrying capacity of the niche is reached, which is largely dependent on an adequate supply of food. In order to control population growth, one of two broad strategies must be used: reduce carrying capacity (generally through reduction of available food sources) or reduce the number of intact female cats (Foley et al. 2005). If efforts are made concurrent with TNR programs to reduce carrying capacity, it may be possible to gradually and humanely reduce the population size through attrition.

TNR programs have been shown to significantly reduce complaints through the reduction of nuisance behaviors like spraying, fighting, and mating. Individuals who perceived cats as a nuisance were more likely to choose removal over TNR as a means of control; it is possible that these individuals would change their opinion as to the more desirable means of cat control if the cats' behaviors changed and they were no longer considered a nuisance (Ash and Adams 2003).

Early publications on TNR programs suggested one reason for the efficacy of sterilization was that an existing cat population would limit immigration of new cats to the area because of their territorial activity (Neville and Remfry 1984). Such claims are often repeated as one of the main benefits of TNR programs, but there appears to be little published data to support this effect on a consistent or significant level. Several case studies have directly refuted it. In a study of cats in a TNR program in Florida, existing cat populations failed to permanently prevent newly arrived cats from joining the colonies (Levy et al. 2003a). Similar findings were reported in Israel: high immigration of sexually intact cats and decreased emigration rates of neutered colony members were seen (Gunther et al. 2011). High rates of immigration have also been reported in colonies with intact males and hysterectomized females, suggesting that preservation of hormone production may provide no benefit with regard to preventing a "vacuum effect" when compared with gonadectomy (Mendes-de-Almeida et al. 2011).

Available data suggest that the cost of TNR programs is lower than traditional approaches that involve impoundment and euthanasia of feral cats, with the former costing only 40% of what would have been spent to respond to a cat-related complaint with impoundment and sheltering costs. In one community, a change in policy from impounding and euthanizing feral cats to TNR resulted in an estimated savings of over $650 000 in just 10 years (Hughes and Slater 2002). However, published claims that TNR is less cost-effective than other control methods do exist. Investigators in one study drew the conclusion that TNR programs were twice as expensive to implement as trap–euthanize programs and did not convey as great a benefit. Their model included a number of questionable assumptions about the fixed costs associated with TNR programs and the rates at which euthanasia could feasibly be performed, but perhaps most startling were the assumptions made regarding the benefits of reduced predation. The model included an estimated predation rate of 21% with a monetary value of $1500 per bird, but no corresponding monetary value for the life of a cat. When the value per bird was reduced to $30, however, there was little difference in cost–benefit ratio between the two programs (Lohr et al. 2013).

The cost effectiveness of various management strategies, including trap–euthanize and TNR, has been shown to be at least partially dependent on the size of the population at the outset of the program (Loyd and DeVore 2010; Lohr et al. 2013). Trapping costs will be specific to individual colonies depending on the traps and bait used, trapping protocol, and available personnel, but use of volunteers to conduct the trapping activities can result in significant savings. Estimates of a per-night trapping cost have been reported to be $0.37/trap/night, with a mean per-cat cost using paid staff ranging from $3.43 to $6.57 depending on the length of the trapping period (Nutter et al. 2004c). While the cost of traps is a significant start-up cost for TNR programs, the cost per cat trapped can be quite low for large-scale programs conducted over a sustained period of time.

Despite their popularity or perhaps because of it, TNR programs remain somewhat of a controversial management strategy for community cats. Much debate exists regarding their efficacy in reducing community cat populations, adequately addressing welfare concerns, and alleviating public health risks and environmental concerns. Research is limited and at times contradictory, and definitions of success vary, with similar reductions in population size alternatively described as a success or failure by different authors.

Data does exist that supports TNR as a management technique. Prior to implementation of a TNR program at the University of Central Florida, cats had been periodically trapped for euthanasia in response to increasing population size or nuisance complaints, with apparently little change in need or long-term impact despite 30 years of the practice. Within four years of the start of the TNR program, no new kittens were born. A 66% reduction in cat population size after a six-year period was noted, including cats removed from the population for adoption or humane euthanasia as well as those known to have died or disappeared (Levy et al. 2003a). A TNR program conducted by the Ocean Reef Cat Club led to the stabilization of a sizable cat population within two years and reduction by 50% within four years of the implementation of intense and targeted efforts (Winter 2004), and a neighborhood-focused TNR program in Chicago, IL, resulted in average declines to colony populations of 54% from entry to the program and 82% from peak levels over a ten-year period (Spehar and Wolf 2018a). A long-standing TNR program in Rome, where euthanasia of free-roaming cats is prohibited by law, is reported to have stabilized or reduced the size of >70% of the colonies studied (Natoli et al. 2006). Not surprisingly, the authors found that sterilization took some time to impact colony size: the larger decreases in cat population were seen in colonies that began sterilization

at the longest time points prior to initiation of the study. Although the success of the program was limited by a high immigration rate (comprised of abandoned cats and spontaneous arrivals), a conspicuous reduction in total cat number was still noted. Similar results have been reported in other instances of TNR (Castillo and Clarke 2003), and the need to address abandonment (regardless of the specific management strategy employed) is often specifically recognized in position statements on community cat management (AAFP 2012; AVMA 2019).

Critics have argued that TNR programs do not lead to the elimination of cat populations on islands, but it is perhaps more likely that such programs have never been attempted in favor of continued use of lethal control strategies; a thorough review of island eradication programs indicates TNR was tried in only one of 111 campaigns discussed (Campbell et al. 2011). Others have suggested that TNR is ineffective at controlling cat populations under prevailing conditions (Dauphiné and Cooper 2009) because of low implementation rates, inconsistent maintenance, and immigration of new cats (Roebling et al. 2014). Several studies have, in fact, shown that the impact of TNR programs was mitigated by the continued addition of new cats abandoned to the area. However, these problems also plague the trap–removal programs to which TNR is most frequently compared. Mathematical modeling suggests that under some conditions the rate of annual capture and removal of cats for euthanasia or sterilization must be the same for either to result in a decrease in population size (McCarthy et al. 2013). Interestingly, trap–remove–euthanize programs continue to be recommended in place of TNR even by authors who point out that this has been the long-term (but unsuccessful) focus of traditional animal control policy for more than 50 years (Roebling et al. 2014).

It has been recommended to focus intense TNR programs on well-defined, geographically restricted populations rather than to spread efforts across a larger population of cats where such diluted neutering rates are likely to be less effective. Analysis of two county TNR programs failed to show a consistent reduction in per capita growth, the population multiplier (which must be <1 for a population to decline), or the proportion of female cats that were pregnant (Foley et al. 2005). Each program had sterilized thousands of cats, but the total numbers of cats trapped represented only 0.63% of the estimated total feral cats in San Diego county and 9.6% in Alachua county. This was far lower than the model-estimated 14–19% annual neutering rate and 71–94% proportion of neutered cats necessary to reduce population growth.

There is widespread recognition, however, that ongoing efforts and education are necessary to address and ultimately control the population of community cats; indeed, some feel that "efforts without an effective education of people to control the reproduction of house cats (as a prevention for abandonment) are a waste of money, time, and energy" (Natoli et al. 2006). It has been documented that immigration of cats can result in the re-establishment of colonies that were previously eliminated if an environmental niche persists that is attractive to the cats (Nutter 2006), and several studies have shown a reduction in the impact of management strategies (including both removal and TNR programs) due to the abandonment of additional cats. Modeling suggests that a colony supplemented with just 1% of the initial population each year can return to carrying capacity within a decade (Lohr et al. 2013). Regardless of the type of intervention employed to manage the cat population, continued surveillance for and attention to new arrivals (e.g. trapping for sterilization and identification) will be necessary for successful outcomes. Numerous organizations, ranging from the AVMA and the AAFP to the American Bird Conservancy, recognize the need to reduce the abandonment of cats. Various studies on the perception of free-roaming cats and their management have also suggested that education is necessary

on cats and their management with a focus on reducing pet abandonment (Loyd and Hernandez 2012).

Return-to-Field and Shelter–Neuter–Return

Historically, TNR programs have focused on returning cats to managed colonies with specific caretakers who provide daily feedings, suitable shelter, surveillance for new cats, and veterinary care for medical conditions that may arise. However, the focus on returning cats to a specific caretaker or colony is changing as animal welfare organizations consider new strategies to improve cat welfare, decrease shelter intake, and reduce euthanasia rates. These programs are generally referred to as return-to-field (RTF), or occasionally shelter–neuter–return (SNR) or Feral Freedom.

An early example of this type of program is one initiated in Jacksonville, FL. Despite years of spay–neuter, the local municipal shelter was still receiving high numbers of unaltered community cats and had a live release rate of less than 10% (Levy and Wilford 2013). In a groundbreaking policy shift, the shelter began transferring these cats, starting with ferals and quickly expanding to all community cats, to the local HQHVSN clinic, where they were sterilized, vaccinated, treated for parasites as needed, and ear-tipped. After a period of overnight observation, cats were then returned to the location from which they had originated and door hangers were left at homes nearby to explain the program.

The community of Jacksonville saw a significant reduction in euthanasia of cats at the municipal shelter by replacing an impound–euthanize control strategy with a TNR program, carried out at no extra expense to the local government with a minimal number of reported complaints (BFAS 2013). Because cats eligible for inclusion in the program were already those "doing well" without a caregiver in an outdoor environment, the expectation is that the cats will continue to do as well or likely better following sterilization, vaccination, and treatment of minor medical conditions.

The popularity of RTF has increased substantially in recent years, though there is significant variability in the recommendations on when and how such programs should be implemented. For example, it is the ASPCA's position that RTF should be reserved for unsocialized, unowned cats unlikely to be eligible in a shelter's adoption program, for whom an exact "found" address is available, and who appear to have been thriving in their previous environment without known threats to their safety (ASPCA 2019b). The Million Cat Challenges include RTF for healthy, unowned shelter cats as an alternative to euthanasia as one of the five key initiatives (MCC 2019), while others have highlighted RTF for friendly and feral community cats as a component of recommended progressive sheltering practices (Pizano 2019).

In contrast to most of the published literature on TNR, the peer-reviewed data on RTF focuses largely on program impact to local shelter intake and euthanasia rates for cats, which can be dramatic and substantial. A retrospective analysis of the records for more than 100 000 cats admitted to a large urban animal shelter in California found that the initiation of an RTF program was associated with a significant decrease in the number of cats admitted to the shelter over an eight-year time period, despite continued human population growth in the area. The proportion of cats euthanized during that same period was reduced almost by half, from 66.6 to 34.9%. There was also a reduction in the percentage of cats received as dead upon arrival to the shelter, and few cats handled through the program were returned to the shelter as either dead or nuisance complaints. The proportion of cats in the program remained fairly stable during the time period evaluated, and the relative distribution between kittens and adults (i.e. kitten intake exceeded adult intake) remained unchanged (Edinboro et al. 2016).

The combination of RTF (~20%) and targeted TNR (~80%) in areas known to have high

feline intake resulted in 37.6 and 84.1% reductions to cat intake and euthanasia rates at a municipal animal shelter, respectively, at a municipal animal shelter in Albuquerque, New Mexico. The number of calls to the city about dead cats was also reported to have declined (Spehar and Wolf 2018b). In Alachua County, FL, a two-year TNR program targeted to an area of historically high cat intake was implemented with the goal of sterilizing at least 50% of the community cats. More than 2000 cats were captured for the program over a two-year period, with 49% being returned to their original locations and 47% (mostly kittens <6 months old) adopted or transferred to rescue groups. During this time feline intake from the target area decreased 66% from baseline, compared to a 12% reduction in the non-target area (Levy et al. 2014). Data on the impact of RTF on overall community cat populations or colony size for this study or others is not available.

Trap–Vasectomy–Hysterectomy–Return

Trap–vasectomy–hysterectomy–return (TVHR) has been proposed as an alternative to castration and ovariohysterectomy for sterilization–return programs. Sterilization techniques that preserve hormone production have been suggested to be more effective than gonadectomy for the reduction of size in community cat colonies, because hormone production is thought to be associated with less frequent immigration of new cats to a colony (Mendes-de-Almeida et al. 2011).

There are a number of concerns with this approach. It is likely that high rates of sterilization would be difficult to achieve with TVHR. Vasectomies and hysterectomies typically take longer to perform than castrations and ovariohysterectomies and fewer veterinarians have received surgical training to perform such techniques, increasing expense and limiting feasibility for large numbers of cats. Even if sufficiently high sterilization rates could be achieved, significant welfare concerns exist. Female cats would still be at risk of mammary

Griffin, B. (2013). Nonsurgical sterilization of cats and dogs. In: *Shelter Medicine for Veterinarians and Staff*, 2e (eds. L. Miller and S. Zawistowski), 689–696. Ames, IA: Wiley-Blackwell.

Gunther, I., Finkler, H., and Terkel, J. (2011). Demographic differences between urban feeding groups of neutered and sexually intact free-roaming cats following a trap-neuter-return procedure. *JAVMA* 238 (9): 1134–1140.

Gunther, I., Raz, T., Berke, O., and Klement, E. (2015). Nuisances and welfare of free-roaming cats in urban settings and their association with cat reproduction. *Prevent. Vet. Med.* 119 (3–4): 203–210.

van Heezik, Y., Smyth, A., Adams, A. et al. (2010). Do domestic cats impose an unsustainable harvest on urban bird populations? *Biol. Conserv.* 143 (1): 121–130.

Hernandez, S.M., Loyd, K.A.T., Newton, A.N. et al. (2018a). The use of point-of-view cameras (Kittycams) to quantify predation by colony cats (*Felis catus*) on wildlife. *Wildlife Res.* 45 (4): 357–365.

Hernandez, S.M., Loyd, K.A.T., Newton, A.N. et al. (2018b). Activity patterns and interspecific interactions of free-roaming, domestic cats in managed Trap-Neuter-Return colonies. *Appl. Anim. Behav. Sci.* 202: 63–68.

Hill, S.L., Cheney, J.M., Taton-Allen, G.F. et al. (2000). Prevalence of enteric zoonotic organisms in cats. *JAVMA* 216 (5): 687–692.

Hughes, B., Martin, G.R., and Reynolds, S.J. (2008). Cats and seabirds: effects of feral Domestic Cat *Felis silvestris catus* eradication on the population of Sooty Terns *Onychoprion fuscata* on Ascension Island, South Atlantic. *Ibis* 150 (s1): 122–131.

Hughes, K.L. and Slater, M.R. (2002). Implementation of a feral cat management program on a university campus. *J. Appl. Anim. Welf. Sci.* 5 (1): 15–28.

Hughes, K.L., Slater, M.R., and Haller, L. (2002). The effects of implementing a feral cat spay/neuter program in a Florida county animal control service. *J. Appl. Anim. Welf. Sci.* 5 (4): 285–298.

Humane Society of the United States (HSUS) (2019). Our position on cats. https://www.humanesociety.org/resources/our-position-cats (accessed 26 April 2019).

Hurley, K.F. and Levy, J.K. (2014). New paradigms for shelters and community cats. https://vetmed-maddie.sites.medinfo.ufl.edu/files/2014/07/New-Paradigms-for-Shelters-and-Community-Cats.pdf (accessed 26 April 2019).

Hutchings, S. (2003). The diet of feral house cats (*Felis catus*) at a regional rubbish tip, Victoria. *Wildlife Res.* 30 (1): 103–110.

Jessup, D.A. (2004). The welfare of feral cats and wildlife. *JAVMA* 225 (9): 1377–1383.

Jones, E. (1977). Ecology of the feral cat, *Felis catus* (L.), (*Carnivora: Felidae*) on Macquarie Island. *Wildlife Res.* 4 (3): 249–262.

Jones, E. and Coman, B.J. (1981). Ecology of the feral cat, *Felis catus* (L.), in South-Eastern Australia I. Diet. *Wildlife Res.* 8 (3): 537–547.

Jones, E. and Coman, B.J. (1982). Ecology of the feral cat, *Felis catus* (L.), in South-Eastern Australia II. Reproduction. *Wildlife Res.* 9 (1): 111–119.

KOAT Albuquerque News (2014). Feral cat trap, neuter, return program met with lawsuit. http://www.koat.com/news/new-mexico/albuquerque/feral-cat-trap-neuter-return-program-met-with-lawsuit/24787264 (accessed 25 April 2019).

Kreuder, C., Miller, M.A., Jessup, D.A. et al. (2003). Patterns of mortality in southern sea otters (*Enhydra lutris nereis*) from 1998–2001. *J. Wildlife Dis.* 39 (3): 495–509.

Lepczyk, C.A., Mertig, A.G., and Liu, J. (2004). Landowners and cat predation across rural-to-urban landscapes. *Biol. Conserv.* 115 (2): 191–201.

Levy, J.K. and Crawford, P.C. (2004). Humane strategies for controlling feral cat populations. *JAVMA* 225 (9): 1354–1360.

Levy, J.K., Gale, D.W., and Gale, L.A. (2003a). Evaluation of the effect of a long-term trap-neuter-return and adoption program on a free-roaming cat population. *JAVMA* 222 (1): 42–46.

Levy, J.K., Isaza, N.M., and Scott, K.C. (2014). Effect of high-impact targeted trap-neuter-return and adoption of community cats on cat intake to a shelter. *Vet. J.* 201 (3): 269–274.

Levy, J.K. and Wilford, C.L. (2013). Management of stray and feral community cats. In: *Shelter Medicine for Veterinarians and Staff*, 2e (eds. L. Miller and S. Zawistowski), 669–688. Ames, IA: Wiley-Blackwell.

Levy, J.K., Woods, J.E., Turick, S.L. et al. (2003b). Number of unowned free-roaming cats in a college community in the southern United States and characteristics of community residents who feed them. *JAVMA* 223 (2): 202–205.

Liberg, O. (1984). Food habits and prey impact by feral and house-based domestic cats in a rural area in southern Sweden. *J. Mammal.* 65: 424–432.

Lohr, C.A., Cox, L.J., and Lepczyk, C.A. (2013). Costs and benefits of trap-neuter-release and euthanasia for removal of urban cats in Oahu, Hawaii. *Conserv. Biol.* 27 (1): 64–73.

Longcore, T., Rich, C., and Sullivan, L.M. (2009). Critical assessment of claims regarding management of feral cats by trap–neuter–return. *Conserv. Biol.* 23 (4): 887–894.

Lord, L.K. (2008). Attitudes toward and perceptions of free-roaming cats among individuals living in Ohio. *JAVMA* 232 (8): 1159–1167.

Loss, S.R., Will, T., and Marra, P.P. (2013). The impact of free-ranging domestic cats on wildlife of the United States. *Nat. Comm.* 4: 1396.

Loyd, K.T. and DeVore, J.L. (2010). An evaluation of feral cat management options using a decision analysis network. *Ecol. Soc.* 15 (4): 10. http://www.ecologyandsociety.org/vol15/iss4/art10.

Loyd, K.A.T. and Hernandez, S.M. (2012). Public perceptions of domestic cats and preferences for feral cat management in the southeastern United States. *Anthrozoos* 25 (3): 337–351.

Loyd, K.A.T., Hernandez, S.M., and McRuer, D.L. (2017). The role of domestic cats in the admission of injured wildlife at rehabilitation and rescue centers. *Wildlife Soc. B.* 41 (1): 55–61.

Luria, B.J., Levy, J.K., Lappin, M.R. et al. (2004). Prevalence of infectious diseases in feral cats in Northern Florida. *J. Feline Med. Surg.* 6 (5): 287–296.

Ma, X., Monroe, B.P., Cleaton, J.M. et al. (2018). Rabies surveillance in the United States during 2016. *JAVMA* 252 (8): 945–957.

Manning, A.M. and Rowan, A.N. (1992). Companion animal demographics and sterilization status: results from a survey in four Massachusetts towns. *Anthrozoos* 5: 192–201.

MCC (2019). Million Cat Challenge. https://millioncatchallenge.org/about/the-five-key-initiatives (accessed 22 August 2019).

McCarthy, R.J., Levine, S.H., and Reed, M. (2013). Estimation of effectiveness of three methods of feral cat population control by use of a simulation model. *JAVMA* 243 (4): 502–511.

McDonald, J.L., Farnworth, M., and Clements, J. (2018). Integrating trap-neuter-return campaigns into a social framework: developing long-term positive behaviour change towards unowned cats in urban areas. *Front. Vet. Sci.* 5: 258.

McGonagle, S. (2015). Effectiveness of trap-spay/neuter-return programs on free-roaming cats as a form of rabies prevention. PhD dissertation. University of Pittsburgh.

McKay, D. (2016). Appeals court upholds ABQ's use of TNR programs for city's feral cats. *Albuquerque Journal* (4 March). https://www.abqjournal.com/735316/appeals-court-upholds-abqs-use-of-tnr-programs-for-citys-feral-cats.html (accessed 25 April 2019).

Mendes-de-Almeida, F., Labarthe, N., Guerrero, J. et al. (2007). Follow-up of the health conditions of an urban colony of free-roaming cats (*Felis catus* Linnaeus, 1758) in the city of Rio de Janeiro, Brazil. *Vet. Parasit.* 147 (1): 9–15.

Mendes-de-Almeida, F., Remy, G.L., Gershony, L.C. et al. (2011). Reduction of feral cat (*Felis catus Linnaeus* 1758) colony size following hysterectomy of adult female cats. *J. Feline Med. Surg.* 13 (6): 436–440.

Miller, M.A., Gardner, I.A., Kreuder, C. et al. (2002). Coastal freshwater runoff is a risk factor for *Toxoplasma gondii* infection of southern sea otters (*Enhydra lutris nereis*). *Int. J. Parasitol.* 32 (8): 997–1006.

Miller, P.S., Boone, J.D., Briggs, J.R. et al. (2014). Simulating free-roaming cat population management options in open demographic environments. *PLoS One* 9 (11): e113553. https://doi.org/10.1371/journal.pone. 0113553.

Mitsuhashi, Y., Chamberlin, A.J., Bigley, K.E., and Bauer, J.E. (2011). Maintenance energy requirement determination of cats after spaying. *Br. J. Nutrit.* 106 (S1): S135–S138.

Molsher, R., Newsome, A., and Dickman, C. (1999). Feeding ecology and population dynamics of the feral cat (*Felis catus*) in relation to the availability of prey in central-eastern New South Wales. *Wildlife Res.* 26 (5): 593–607.

Moore, D.A., Sischo, W.M., Hunter, A. et al. (2000). Animal bite epidemiology and surveillance for rabies postexposure prophylaxis. *JAVMA* 217 (2): 190–194.

Natoli, E., Maragliano, L., Cariola, G. et al. (2006). Management of feral domestic cats in the urban environment of Rome (Italy). *Prevent. Vet. Med.* 77 (3): 180–185.

Nelson, S.H., Evans, A.D., and Bradbury, R.B. (2005). The efficacy of collar-mounted devices in reducing the rate of predation of wildlife by domestic cats. *Appl. Anim. Behav. Sci.* 94 (3): 273–285.

Neville, P.F. and Remfry, J. (1984). Effect of neutering on two groups of feral cats. *Vet. Rec.* 114 (18): 447–450.

Noah, D.L., Smith, M.G., Gotthardt, J.C. et al. (1996). Mass human exposure to rabies in New Hampshire: exposures, treatment, and cost. *Am. J. Public Health* 86 (8, Pt 1): 1149–1151.

Nogales, M., Martín, A., Tershy, B.R. et al. (2004). A review of feral cat eradication on islands. *Conserv. Biol.* 18 (2): 310–319.

Nutter, F.B., Dubey, J.P., Levine, J.F. et al. (2004a). Seroprevalences of antibodies against *Bartonella henselae* and *Toxoplasma gondii* and fecal shedding of *Cryptosporidium* spp, *Giardia* spp, and *Toxocara cati* in feral and pet domestic cats. *JAVMA* 225 (9): 1394–1398.

Nutter, F.B., Levine, J.F., and Stoskopf, M.K. (2004b). Reproductive capacity of free-roaming domestic cats and kitten survival rate. *JAVMA* 225 (9): 1399–1402.

Nutter, F.B., Stoskopf, M.K., and Levine, J.F. (2004c). Time and financial costs of programs for live trapping feral cats. *JAVMA* 225 (9): 1403–1405.

Nutter, F.B. (2006). Evaluation of a trap-neuter-return management program for feral cat colonies: population dynamics, home ranges, and potentially zoonotic diseases. PhD dissertation. North Carolina State University. https://repository.lib.ncsu.edu/bitstream/ handle/1840.16/3891/etd.pdf?sequence=1 (accessed 22 August 2019).

Oppel, S., Beaven, B.M., Bolton, M. et al. (2011). Eradication of invasive mammals on islands inhabited by humans and domestic animals. *Conserv. Biol.* 25 (2): 232–240.

Paltridge, R., Gibson, D., and Edwards, G. (1997). Diet of the feral cat (*Felis catus*) in central Australia. *Wildlife Res.* 24 (1): 67–76.

People for the Ethical Treatment of Animals (PETA) (2019). The great outdoors? Not for cats! http://www.peta.org/issues/companion-animal-issues/overpopulation/feral-cats/ great-outdoors-cats (accessed 26 April 2019).

Peterson, M.N., Hartis, B., Rodriguez, S. et al. (2012). Opinions from the front lines of cat colony management conflict. *PLoS One* 7 (9): e44616.

Pizano, S. (2019). *The Best Practice Playbook for Animal Shelters*. Coral Springs, FL: Team Shelter USA.

Rayner, M.J., Hauber, M.E., Imber, M.J. et al. (2007). Spatial heterogeneity of mesopredator release within an oceanic island system. *Proc. Nat. Acad. Sci.* 104 (52): 20862–20865.

Ritchie, E.G. and Johnson, C.N. (2009). Predator interactions, mesopredator release and biodiversity conservation. *Ecol. Lett.* 12 (9): 982–998.

Robertson, S.A. (2008). A review of feral cat control. *J. Feline Med. Surg.* 10 (4): 366–375.

Roebling, A.D., Johnson, D., Blanton, J.D. et al. (2014). Rabies prevention and management of cats in the context of trap-neuter-vaccinate-release programs. *Zoonoses Public Health* 61 (4): 290–296.

Sallinger, B. (2008). An unorthodox campaign to reduce cat predation on native birds in the Portland metropolitan area. In: *126th Stated Meeting of the American Ornithologists' Union*. Portland: OR.

Scherk, M.A., Ford, R.B., Gaskell, R.M. et al. (2013). 2013 AAFP Feline Vaccination Advisory Panel report. *J. Feline Med. Surg.* 15 (9): 785–808.

Schmidt, P.M., Lopez, R.R., and Collier, B.A. (2007). Survival, fecundity, and movements of free-roaming cats. *J. Wildlife Manag.* 71 (3): 915–919.

Schmidt, P.M., Swannack, T.M., Lopez, R.R. et al. (2009). Evaluation of euthanasia and trap–neuter–return (TNR) programs in managing free-roaming cat populations. *Wildlife Res.* 36 (2): 117–125.

Scott, K.C., Levy, J.K., and Crawford, P.C. (2002a). Characteristics of free-roaming cats evaluated in a trap-neuter-return program. *JAVMA* 221 (8): 1136–1138.

Scott, K.C., Levy, J.K., Gorman, S.P. et al. (2002b). Body condition of feral cats and the effect of neutering. *J. Appl. Anim. Welf. Sci.* 5 (3): 203–213.

Short, J. and Turner, B. (2005). Control of feral cats for nature conservation. IV. Population dynamics and morphological attributes of feral cats at Shark Bay, Western Australia. *Wildlife Res.* 32 (6): 489–501.

Silva-Rodriguez, E.A. and Sieving, K.E. (2011). Influence of care of domestic carnivores on their predation on vertebrates. *Conserv. Biol.* 25 (4): 808–815.

Spehar, D. and Wolf, P. (2017). An examination of an iconic trap-neuter-return program: the Newburyport, Massachusetts case study. *Animals* 7 (11): 81.

Spehar, D. and Wolf, P. (2018a). A case study in citizen science: the effectiveness of a trap-neuter-return program in a Chicago neighborhood. *Animals* 8 (1): 14.

Spehar, D. and Wolf, P. (2018b). The impact of an integrated program of return-to-field and targeted trap-neuter-return on feline intake and euthanasia at a municipal animal shelter. *Animals* 8 (4): 55.

Stojanovic, V. and Foley, P. (2011). Infectious disease prevalence in a feral cat population on Prince Edward Island, Canada. *Can. Vet. J.* 52 (9): 979.

Taetzsch, S.J., Gruszynski, K.R., Bertke, A.S. et al. (2018). Prevalence of zoonotic parasites in feral cats of Central Virginia, USA. *Zoonoses Public Health* 65 (6): 728–735.

Taylor, N. and Signal, T.D. (2009). Pet, pest, profit: isolating differences in attitudes towards the treatment of animals. *Anthrozoos* 22 (2): 129–135.

de Torres, P.J., Sutherland, D.R., Clarke, J.R. et al. (2011). Assessment of risks to non-target species from an encapsulated toxin in a bait proposed for control of feral cats. *Wildlife Res.* 38 (1): 39–50.

Tschanz, B., Hegglin, D., Gloor, S. et al. (2011). Hunters and non-hunters: skewed predation rate by domestic cats in a rural village. *Eur. J. Wildlife Res.* 57 (3): 597–602.

USA Today (2005). Wisconsin is no place for cat-hunting, governor says. http://usatoday30.usatoday.com/news/nation/2005-04-13-cat-hunting_x.htm (accessed 26 April 2019).

Wallace, J.L. and Levy, J.K. (2006). Population characteristics of feral cats admitted to seven trap-neuter-return programs in the United States. *J. Feline Med. Surg.* 8 (4): 279–284.

Winter, L. (2004). Trap-neuter-release programs: the reality and the impacts. *JAVMA* 225 (9): 1369–1376.

Woods, M., McDonald, R.A., and Harris, S. (2003). Predation of wildlife by domestic cats *Felis catus* in Great Britain. *Mammal Rev.* 33 (2): 174–188.

Zavaleta, E.S., Hobbs, R.J., and Mooney, H.A. (2001). Viewing invasive species removal in a whole-ecosystem context. *Trends Ecol. Evol.* 16 (8): 454–459.

26

Influence of Spay–Neuter Timing on Health
G. Robert Weedon, Margaret V. Root Kustritz, and Philip Bushby

Ovariohysterectomy (OHE) and castration are the surgeries most commonly performed by small animal practitioners in the United States (Greenfield et al. 2004). Exhaustive reviews of the benefits and detriments of gonadectomy at various ages have been published (Root Kustritz 2007; Reichler 2009; Root Kustritz 2012; Howe 2015; Houlihan 2017; Root Kustritz et al. 2017).

The optimal age at which to perform OHE or castration of dogs and cats is, however, not defined by the veterinary literature. In the United States, most veterinarians recommend cats and dogs be spayed or castrated when about six months of age, prior to puberty, which is defined as acquisition of normal breeding behavior and semen quality in males and first estrus in females. In other countries, veterinarians recommend that dogs and cats be spayed after their first estrus, or do not recommend elective surgical sterilization be performed at any age. Indeed, in some countries, elective gonadectomy is considered unethical and is either strongly discouraged or illegal (Salmeri et al. 1991; Gunzel-Apel 1998). For this discussion, it is assumed that the veterinarian is comfortable with the ethics of elective gonadectomy and practices in a country in which such surgery is considered acceptable by professional associations and society at large.

The optimal time for spay–neuter depends on species, breed, intended use, financial considerations, and life situation. But it is "life situation" that has the biggest impact. For an individually owned animal living in a home, decisions should be based primarily on factors that impact that animal's individual health and the health and wellbeing of that household, and secondarily on population control. But for the shelter animal facing possible euthanasia if not adopted or potentially producing multiple litters if adopted, decisions should be based primarily on population control.

Population Control

In the United States, a serious problem exists with the supply and demand for pet animals, with a net result of pet homelessness. In some areas of the country, the spay–neuter message has been so successful that shelters have a hard time finding adoptable animals, whereas in other parts of the country the supply significantly exceeds demand. The result of this imbalance is that over a million unowned dogs and cats are euthanized yearly in the United States (Nassar et al. 1992; National Council on Pet Population Study and Policy 1994; ASPCA 2019). Some of these are feral animals, some are abandoned and brought to the animal shelter as strays, and many are relinquished. Intact animals are much more likely to be relinquished than are spayed or castrated animals, and animals that are adopted out from the animal shelter while still intact may either be returned or repopulate that shelter with their offspring (Patronek et al. 1996; New et al. 2000; Mondelli et al. 2004). While in some shelters intact animals are adopted out with a spay–neuter contract, compliance with such contracts has been demonstrated to be less than 60% (Eno and Fekety 1993; Alexander and Shane 1994).

Confounding the situation is a significant lack of knowledge among pet owners regarding normal reproduction. Studies have demonstrated that up to 57% of bitch owners were unaware that bitches cycle at least twice yearly, up to 83% of queen owners were unaware that queens are polyestrous from spring to early fall, and up to 61% of dog and cat owners were unsure or believed that their animal would somehow be "better" after having had at least one litter (Scarlett et al. 1999; New et al. 2000; Scarlett et al. 2002). In one survey of dog- and cat-owning households, 56% of 154 canine litters and 68% of 317 feline litters were unplanned, with the majority of those owners reporting that they did not know the female had been in heat (New et al. 2004). The majority of litters in another study were born to pets that eventually were sterilized (Manning and Rowan 1992).

While increasing pet owner education could lead to more responsible pet ownership and is a worthy goal that should be pursued, gonadectomy of dogs and cats prior to adoption is an important tool in the fight against shelter euthanasia that should be considered best practice. Multiple studies have been published demonstrating the safety of gonadectomy in puppies and kittens as young as six weeks of age (Howe 1992a, b, 1997, 2006; Howe et al. 2000, 2001). To reduce shelter intake and euthanasia, all male and female dogs and cats should be spayed or castrated prior to adoption from humane organizations or animal shelters.

Dogs and Cats with an Owner or Guardian

Male Cats

The normal behavior of most intact male cats is incompatible with their living as house pets (Root Kustritz 1996; Root Kustritz et al. 2017). Breeding behavior in cats is aggressive, and intact male cats show that behavior readily. Urine from intact male cats is used for territorial marking and has a very distinct, strong odor.

The only complications reported with feline castration were scrotal swelling or hematoma, and the rate was low at 2% (Pollari and Bonnett 1996b). Peri-operative mortality was reported at 0.03% in one study (Levy et al. 2017). There are virtually no health conditions reported to be increased or decreased in association with gonadectomy in male cats. Historically, there have been concerns voiced about increased incidence of urinary tract obstruction in castrated male cats due to decreased urethral diameter. However, numerous studies have evaluated the effect of castration at various ages with urethral diameter and none has documented this correlation (Herron 1972; Root et al. 1996a; Spain et al. 2004a). A recent study evaluating several health conditions following gonadectomy found no differences in the incidence of urinary tract obstruction between kittens sterilized at 8–12 weeks and those sterilized at 6–8 months (Porters et al. 2015).

In addition, neutered male cats live much longer than intact male cats. An analysis of records of 460 000 cats at Banfield veterinary hospitals revealed that castrated male cats live an average of 11.8 years, 62% longer than intact male cats (Banfield 2013). To make male cats more acceptable house pets, to give them a longer life expectancy, and to reduce unwanted births, male cats not intended for breeding should be castrated prior to sexual maturity and this can be done as young as six to eight weeks of age.

Female Cats

Benefits of OHE in female cats include increased life expectancy and decreased incidence of mammary neoplasia, ovarian or uterine tumors, and pyometra. Of these diseases, the one with the most significant negative health impact is mammary neoplasia. Mammary neoplasia is the third most common tumor of female cats, and accounts for 17% of feline tumors (Overley-Adamson and Baez 2016). The reported incidence is 25.4 per 100 000 female cats, although geographic variation is likely because of different neutering and care practices (Dorn et al. 1968a; Verstegen and Onclin 2003; Overley-Adamson and Baez 2016). Incidence is increased with number of estrous cycles in the cat's life and is greater in the Siamese and domestic Japanese breeds (Dorn et al. 1968b; Hayes et al. 1981; Verstegen and Onclin 2003). Spayed cats have a 0.6% risk for developing mammary carcinoma compared with intact cats (Birchard and Sherding 2006). More than 90% of cases of mammary neoplasia are malignant adenocarcinoma (Dorn et al. 1968a; Hampe and Misdorp 1974; Hayes et al. 1981).

Spayed female cats live longer on average than intact female cats. In the 2013 analysis of Banfield medical records, life expectancy of spayed female cats was 13.1 years, 39% longer than that of intact female cats (Banfield 2013). In addition, there are no indications that pre-pubertal gonadectomy in cats leads to different occurrence of potentially undesirable behaviors than gonadectomy at a traditional age. Two recent studies (Porters et al. 2014; Moons et al. 2018) concluded that there is no indication that pre-pubertal gonadectomy causes the occurrence of potentially undesirable behavior at a different level than gonadectomy at the age of six to eight months.

Detriments of OHE in female cats include possible complications of surgery, obesity, increased incidence of feline lower urinary tract disease (FLUTD), and increased incidence of diabetes mellitus. Reported incidence of post-surgical complications in cats is 2.6%, with most reported complications mild and self-resolving (Pollari et al. 1996a), and perioperative mortality reportedly 0.063% (Levy et al. 2017). Incidence of obesity after OHE is high, and is due to decreased metabolic rate in cats after gonadectomy, with subsequent changes in metabolic activity of adipose tissue and decline in maintenance energy requirement (Root et al. 1996b; Fettman et al. 1997; Belsito et al. 2007; Mitsuhashi et al. 2011). Obesity, however, can be controlled by proper feeding regimen. Finally, increased incidence of FLUTD and diabetes mellitus has been reported after OHE in queens, with the Burmese breed especially prone to development of diabetes mellitus (Rand et al. 1997; McCann et al. 2007; Prahl et al. 2007). Incidence of these two conditions is 0.6 and 0.5%, respectively (Lekcharoensuk et al. 2001; McCann et al. 2007). There is no significant difference in incidence rates of these conditions between cats spayed at 8–12 weeks and those spayed at 6–8 months (Porters et al. 2015).

In view of the fact that the incidence and morbidity of mammary neoplasia are much higher than are the incidences of FLUTD and diabetes mellitus, morbidity associated with obesity can be controlled by the owner or guardian of the cat, and because spayed cats live significantly longer, female cats not intended for breeding should be spayed prior to puberty (five months of age).

Male Dogs

Benefits of castration in male dogs include decreased incidence of testicular neoplasia and non-neoplastic prostate disease, and possible increased life span. Testicular neoplasia is a common tumor of aged, intact male dogs, with a reported incidence of 0.9% (Hahn et al. 1992). Morbidity generally is low. Benign prostatic hypertrophy (BPH) is a very common disorder of male dogs, with reported incidence of 75–80% in dogs aged 6 years or more (Zirkin and Strandberg 1984; Berry et al. 1986; Lowseth et al. 1990). Again, morbidity generally is low. Finally, several studies have documented increased life span in castrated male dogs compared to intact males (Bronson 1982; Michell 1999; Moore et al. 2001; Banfield 2013; Hoffman et al. 2013). This may be due to greater care by owners after the "investment" of surgery has been made in that animal, or may be due to a decrease in sexually dimorphic behaviors that put the animal at increased risk, such as roaming.

Detriments of castration in male dogs include complications of surgery, increased incidence of prostatic neoplasia (Obradovich et al. 1987; Sorenmo et al. 2003; Bryan et al. 2007), transitional cell carcinoma (Norris et al. 1992; Knapp et al. 2000), osteosarcoma in certain breeds (Priester et al. 1980; Ru et al. 1998; Hart et al. 2016), and perhaps hemangiosarcoma in certain breeds (Prymak et al. 1988; Ware and Hopper 1999; Hart et al. 2014, 2016), increased incidence of cranial cruciate ligament (CCL) injury (Whitehair et al. 1993; Duval et al. 1999; Slauterbeck et al. 2004), obesity (Edney and Smith 1986; Crane 1991), and possible increased incidence of diabetes mellitus (Marmor et al. 1982). Reported incidence of post-surgical complications in dogs neutered at a traditional age (greater than 6 months) is 6.1%, with most reported complications mild and self-resolving (Pollari et al. 1996a). The complication rate of puppy castration is reported lower at 3.5%, with all complications mild and self-limiting (Miller et al. 2018). No mortalities were reported in 20 800 male dogs castrated in one study (Levy et al. 2017). Prostatic neoplasia, transitional cell carcinoma, osteosarcoma, and hemangiosarcoma generally are low in incidence but high in morbidity and mortality (Weaver 1981; Bell et al. 1991; Ware and Hopper 1999; Teske et al. 2002; Poirier et al. 2004). No breed predisposition has been identified for prostatic neoplasia, but it does exist for the other cancers noted (Ru et al. 1998; Chun and DeLorimier 2003; Henry 2003; Smith 2003). The incidence of CCL injury in dogs is relatively high at 1.8%, and

morbidity may be high, although this is generally considered to be a curable condition with surgery (Whitehair et al. 1993; Duval et al. 1999; Slauterbeck et al. 2004). Again, some breeds, most notably large and giant breeds, are predisposed to CCL injury (Duval et al. 1999; Wilke et al. 2005; Harasen 2008; Torres et al. 2013; Hart et al. 2016). Obesity is high in incidence, but morbidity can be controlled by the owner or guardian. Incidence of obesity in castrated dogs does not appear to be dependent on age at castration, and the increased risk of obesity is only significant for the first two years after surgery (Lefebvre et al. 2013).

The appropriate recommendation for castration of male dogs is less readily evident than for male cats. Given that a male dog can be responsible for producing many more offspring than can a given bitch, one can argue that castration is necessary for population control. The morbidity associated with castration as a possible predisposing cause of the conditions described would suggest that castration not be recommended when considering the animal as an individual, although the increased life span noted in numerous studies argues in favor of castration, as does the high incidence of non-neoplastic prostatic disease seen in intact male dogs.

Recommendations on whether or not to castrate and when to castrate should be made on a case-by-case basis, evaluating the breed of the dog, his intended working life or activity level, the ability of the owner to control reproduction in that animal, the owner's wishes regarding use of that animal for breeding, and the owner's level of concern over pet population control. If owners ask for guidance regarding the age at which to castrate their dog, they may wish to consider that of the disorders likely to occur in intact dogs, BPH occurs earlier in life than does testicular neoplasia, is not likely to manifest clinically until the dog is at least 2.4 years of age, and is curable by castration at the time of diagnosis (Zirkin and Strandberg 1984; Berry et al. 1986; Lowseth et al. 1990). An alternative to castration is vasectomy, which sterilizes the dog while sparing testosterone.

The procedure is reportedly quick, less invasive than castration, and not difficult for veterinarians to master (Brent and Kutzler 2018). The downsides to this form of sterilization are that testicular cancer, perianal gland tumor, and enlarged prostate may occur – but if they arise later in life, they are typically treated via castration. Hormones will also influence the male dog's behavior and interest in females in heat. Another concern in animal welfare and rescue/shelter communities is the rationale that dogs may display more intermale aggression, urine marking, mounting, and roaming, which may result in owners abandoning or returning their pets and thus increasing shelter populations. (Brent and Kutzler 2018).

Female Dogs

Benefits of OHE in bitches include decreased incidence of mammary neoplasia, with the greatest benefit if spayed before the first heat, and the essentially eliminated incidence of ovarian or uterine neoplasia and pyometra (Schneider et al. 1969). Mammary neoplasia is the most common tumor of female dogs, with a reported incidence of 3.4%, and some select populations reporting incidence as high as 13% by 10 years of age (Fidler and Brodey 1967; Dorn et al. 1968a; Moe 2001; Richards et al. 2001). It is the most common malignant tumor in female dogs, with 50.9% of mammary tumors reported to be malignant; metastases are found in about 75% of cases of mammary carcinoma, with the lung the most common site of metastasis (Cotchin et al. 1951; Dorn et al. 1968a; Moulton et al. 1970; Brodey et al. 1983). A hormonal basis for malignant transformation of mammary cells and progression of neoplasia is hypothesized based on the decreasing benefit of OHE with increasing number of estrous cycles in the dog's life prior to surgery. The other very common disorder in female dogs when aged is pyometra, reported to occur in 15.2% of dogs by 4 years of age and in 23–24% of dogs by 10 years of age (Egenvall et al. 2001; Fukuda 2001). Morbidity is high, although OHE at the time of clinical presentation is curative; reported mortality ranges from 0 to 17% in dogs (Johnston et al. 2001). Owners should be aware of the acute (often insidious) onset and presentation, and that an emergency pyometra OHE is more challenging and costly when compared to a routine OHE.

Detriments of OHE in female dogs include complications of surgery, increased incidence of transitional cell carcinoma (Norris et al. 1992; Knapp et al. 2000), osteosarcoma in certain breeds (Priester et al. 1980; Ru et al. 1998), hemangiosarcoma in certain breeds (Prymak et al. 1988; Ware and Hopper 1999), and cutaneous mast cell tumor (White et al. 2006), increased incidence of CCL injury (Whitehair et al. 1993; Duval et al. 1999; Slauterbeck et al. 2004), obesity and diabetes mellitus (Marmor et al. 1982; Edney and Smith 1986; Crane 1991), a possible increase in aggression in at least one breed (Reisner 1993; Kim et al. 2006), and possibly increased incidence of urethral sphincter mechanism incompetence (estrogen-responsive urinary incontinence; Stocklin-Gautschi et al. 2001; Angioletti et al. 2004; Holt 2004; Beauvais et al. 2012). Reported incidence of post-surgical complications in dogs is 6.1%, with most reported complications mild and self-resolving (Pollari et al. 1996). One recent study reported the peri-operative mortality rate of female dogs undergoing OHE at 0.018% (Levy et al. 2017).

As in male dogs, the incidence of tumors reportedly associated with gonadectomy is low, but morbidity with these tumor types is high. Breed predispositions exist for all three tumor types. The incidence of obesity is high after OHE, but morbidity can be controlled by the owner. The incidence of obesity after OHE does not appear to be dependent on age at surgery, and the increased risk of obesity is only significant for the first two years after surgery (Lefebvre et al. 2013). The incidence of CCL injury in dogs is relatively high at 1.8%, and morbidity may be high, although this is generally considered to be a curable condition with surgery. Again, some breeds, most notably large and giant breeds, are predisposed to CCL injury. Aggression after OHE has been reported in English Springer Spaniels; there is some suggestion that this effect may be more likely in bitches that demonstrated aggressive tendencies prior to surgery (Reisner 1993). Urethral sphincter mechanism incompetence is a problem of spayed female dogs, especially those weighing more than 20 kg (Holt and Thrusfield 1993). While morbidity is low and this is a disease easily controlled with medical therapy in most female dogs, evidence exists suggesting incidence can be decreased by spaying bitches when greater than three months of age; this has not been rigorously supported by meta-analysis of the veterinary literature (Spain et al. 2004b; Beauvais et al. 2012; Forsee et al. 2013). There is one paper reporting increased life span associated with intact status in a population of exceptionally long-lived Rottweilers (Waters et al. 2009), whereas other studies have shown longer life span in spayed Rottweilers despite higher osteosarcoma risk (Cooley 2002); applicability of these findings to other dog populations is unknown. Several studies report that sterilized female dogs have a longer life expectancy. One study demonstrated a lifespan in spayed dogs 26.3% greater than that of intact female dogs (Hoffman et al. 2013), and the 2013 analysis of Banfield medical records of 2.2 million dogs similarly demonstrated that sterilized female dogs lived 23% longer than intact female dogs (Michell 1999; Banfield 2013).

The appropriate recommendation for OHE of female dogs is less readily evident than for female cats. Certainly, mammary neoplasia and pyometra are of high incidence and high morbidity, and are greatly decreased in incidence by OHE. However, possible predisposition to very high morbidity tumor types or CCL injury must be evaluated. As with male dogs, the recommendation should be made on a case-by-case basis, evaluating the breed of the dog, her intended working life or activity level, and the owner's wishes regarding use of that animal for breeding, but in general it can be recommended that bitches be spayed prior to puberty.

Ovariectomy is an alternative to ovariohysterectomy that offers essentially the same advantages and disadvantages. While some authors (Van Goethem et al. 2006) suggest that OHE is technically more complicated, time consuming, and could be associated with greater morbidity (larger incision, more intraoperative trauma, increased discomfort) compared with OVE, it is unclear whether these differences in surgical time, incision length, and morbidity still hold true when high-volume techniques are employed. The incision lengths and surgery times for both procedures in studies of these techniques are greater than would be expected in a high-quality high-volume spay–neuter (HQHVSN) clinic setting. No significant differences between techniques have been observed for the incidence of long-term urogenital problems, including endometritis/pyometra and urinary incontinence, making OVE and OHE equally acceptable methods of gonadectomy in the healthy bitch.

An alternative option for surgical sterilization of female dogs is sometimes called an ovary-sparing spay or partial spay and involves performing only a hysterectomy, removing the uterus and leaving the ovaries intact. It is important to remove all the uterus to ensure that stump pyometra does not occur (Brent and Kutzler 2018). This complete removal of the uterus requires a longer incision and longer surgery time compared to OHE and OVH, potentially leading to the potential for greater postoperative discomfort. The objective of ovary-sparing hysterectomy is to ensure that the dog is incapable of reproducing while maintaining her natural gonadal hormones. Ovary-sparing hysterectomy is relatively new and as of this writing there is little peer-reviewed information in publication about it. Female dogs with hysterectomy are presumed to have the same disease risks and benefits as unaltered dogs, except for the risks of pyometra and possible complications of pregnancy, which are eliminated by hysterectomy. Dogs who have undergone this procedure will still experience estrus cycles and demonstrate the same behaviors as intact females, a fact for which pet owners must be prepared.

Conclusions

For populations of unowned dogs, for example in animal sheltering organizations, interest in reproductive control outweighs concerns about individual animals. Animals that leave a humane organization intact may repopulate that shelter with their offspring, and may well be returned to the shelter themselves, as it has been demonstrated that being intact is a risk factor for surrender (New et al. 2000). Pets should be considered individually, with the understanding that for these pets, population control is a less important concern than is the health of each animal. Dogs and cats should be maintained as household pets. Responsible owners should ensure that their pets are provided with appropriate and regularly scheduled veterinary care (Root Kustritz 2007).

It is not uncommon for practicing veterinarians to ask for a one-sentence response to the question of the best age at which to spay or castrate dogs and cats. There is no appropriate simple response as there is a large amount of information available, all of which will be assessed slightly differently by each person reading those studies, and non-medical considerations must be taken into account, including population control, effects of gonadectomy on behavior, and the wishes of and ability to provide care by the owner or guardian of the dog (Root Kustritz et al. 2017).

It is clear that obesity is a fairly significant detriment of gonadectomy in both species and sexes. Providing clients with this information helps guide conversations about proper diet and exercise after gonadectomy surgery. Disregarding obesity, it is clear that OHE prior to puberty is beneficial for queens and bitches. For male dogs, the greatest benefits come from prevention of BPH and increased life expectancy. Owners may wait as late as 2.5 years before castration without significantly changing outcomes for their male dog regarding BPH risk. No one has demonstrated the health benefits of castration of male cats, yet pre-puberal castration is recommended to control undesirable aggressive reproductive behaviors and urine spraying and to increase life expectancy.

Much information and misinformation about this topic is available to the owners, guardians, and breeders of dogs and cats. It behooves us, as veterinarians, to practice evidence-based medicine, the conscientious, explicit, and judicious use of current best evidence in making decisions about the care of individual patients (Cockcroft and Holmes 2003). This requires knowledge of the current veterinary literature, including the number of, and quality of, studies supporting or refuting an effect of gonadectomy, the number and breed of animals in that study, and the validity of conclusions drawn. There has been concern that current studies declare all animals as intact or gonadectomized and do not take into consideration how age at the time of surgery may impact the initiation or progression of the changes described (Waters 2011; Waters et al. 2011). A research focus on the timing of gonadectomy and its subsequent impact on biologic processes would help answer this question. Lastly, one must consider that in some reported studies, there may be a hereditary predisposition to the condition in question, making extrapolation to other populations of dogs difficult, and therefore not necessarily generalizable to the canine population as a whole.

References

Alexander, S.A. and Shane, S.M. (1994). Characteristics of animals adopted from an animal control center whose owners complied with a spaying/neutering program. *JAVMA* 205: 472–476.

Angioletti, A., De Francesco, I., Vergottini, M. et al. (2004). Urinary incontinence after spaying in the bitch: incidence and oestrogen-therapy. *Vet. Res. Comm.* 28 (Suppl 1): 153–155.

ASPCA (n.d.). Shelter intake and surrender: pet statistics. https://www.aspca.org/animal-homelessness/shelter-intake-and-surrender/pet-statistics (accessed 18 March 2019).

Banfield (2013). *Banfield state of pet health 2013 report*. Vancouver, WA: Banfield Pet Hospital https://www.banfield.com/Banfield/media/PDF/Downloads/soph/Banfield-State-of-Pet-Health-Report_2013.pdf (accessed 20 August 2019).

Beauvais, W., Cardwell, J.M., and Brodbelt, D.C. (2012). The effect of neutering on the risk of urinary incontinence in bitches – a systematic review. *J. Small Anim. Pract.* 53: 198–204.

Bell, F.W., Klausner, J.S., Hayden, D.W. et al. (1991). Clinical and pathologic features of prostatic adenocarcinoma in sexually intact and castrated dogs: 31 cases (1970–1987). *JAVMA* 199: 1623–1630.

Belsito, K.R., Vester, B.M., Keel, T. et al. (2007). Spaying affects blood metabolites and adipose tissue gene expression in cats. *Proceedings of the Nestle Purina Nutrition Forum*, St. Louis, MO.

Berry, S.J., Strandberg, J.D., Saunders, W.J. et al. (1986). Development of canine benign prostatic hyperplasia with age. *Prostate* 9: 363–373.

Birchard, S.J. and Sherding, R.G. (eds.) (2006). Mammary gland neoplasia. In: *Saunders Manual of Small Animal Practice*, 3e, 311–315. Philadelphia, PA: Elsevier.

Brent, L. and Kutzler, M. (2018). Alternatives to traditional spay and neuter – evolving best practices in dog sterilization. *Innovative Veterinary Care* (26 October). https://ivcjournal.com/spay-neuter-alternatives (accessed 21 March 2019).

Brodey, R.S., Goldschmidt, M.H., and Roszel, J.R. (1983). Canine mammary gland neoplasms. *J. Am. Anim. Hosp. Assoc.* 19: 61–90.

Bronson, R.T. (1982). Variation in age at death of dogs of different sexes and breeds. *Am. J. Vet. Res.* 43: 2057–2059.

Bryan, J.N., Keeler, M.R., Henry, C.J. et al. (2007). A population study of neutering status as a risk factor for canine prostate cancer. *Prostate* 67: 1174–1181.

Chun, R. and DeLorimier, L.P. (2003). Update on the biology and management of canine osteosarcoma. *Vet. Clin. N. Am. Small Anim. Pract.* 33: 491–516.

Cockcroft, P. and Holmes, M. (2003). *Handbook of Evidence-Based Veterinary Medicine*. Oxford: Blackwell.

Cooley, D.M., Beranek, B.C., Schlittler, D.L. et al. (2002). Endogenous gonadal hormone exposure and bone sarcoma risk. *Cancer Epidemiol. Prevent. Biomark.* 11 (11): 1434–1440.

Cotchin, E., Douglas, S.W., and Platt, H. (1951). Neoplasms in small animals. *Vet. Rec.* 63: 67–78.

Crane, S.W. (1991). Occurrence and management of obesity in companion animals. *J. Small Anim. Pract.* 32: 275–282.

Dorn, C.R., Taylor, D.O., Frye, F.L. et al. (1968a). Survey of animal neoplasms in Alameda and Contra Costa counties, California. I. Methodology and description of cases. *J. Nat. Cancer Inst.* 40: 295–305.

Dorn, C.R., Taylor, D.O., Schneider, R. et al. (1968b). Survey of animal neoplasms in Alameda and Contra Costa counties, California. II. Cancer morbidity in dogs and cats from Alameda county. *J. Nat. Cancer Inst.* 40: 307–318.

Duval, J.M., Budsberg, S.C., Flo, G.L. et al. (1999). Breed, sex, and body weight as risk factors for rupture of the cranial cruciate ligament in young dogs. *JAVMA* 215: 811–814.

Edney, A.T. and Smith, P.M. (1986). Study of obesity in dogs visiting veterinary practices in the United Kingdom. *Vet. Rec.* 118: 391–396.

Egenvall, A., Hagman, R., Bonnett, B.N. et al. (2001). Breed risk of pyometra in insured dogs in Sweden. *J. Vet. Intern. Med.* 15: 530–538.

Eno, M. and Fekety, S. (1993). Early age spay/neuter: a growing consensus. *Shelter Sense* (1–7 November).

Fettman, M.J., Stanton, C.A., Banks, L.L. et al. (1997). Effects of neutering on bodyweight, metabolic rate and glucose tolerance of domestic cats. *Res. Vet. Sci.* 62: 131–136.

Fidler, I.J. and Brodey, R.S. (1967). The biological behavior of canine mammary neoplasms. *JAVMA* 151: 1311–1318.

Forsee, K.M., Davis, G.J., Mouat, E.E. et al. (2013). Evaluation of the prevalence of urinary incontinence in spayed female dogs: 566 cases (2003–2008). *JAVMA* 242: 959–962.

Fukuda, S. (2001). Incidence of pyometra in colony-raised beagle dogs. *Exp. Anim.* 50: 325–329.

Greenfield, C.L., Johnson, A.L., and Schaeffer, D.J. (2004). Frequency of use of various procedures, skills, and areas of knowledge among veterinarians in private small animal exclusive or predominant practice and proficiency expected of new veterinary school graduates. *JAVMA* 224: 1780–1787.

Gunzel-Apel, A.R. (1998). Early castration of dogs and cats from the point of view of animal welfare. *Deut. Tierarztl. Woch.* 105: 95–98.

Hahn, K.A., VonDerHaar, M.A., and Teclaw, R.F. (1992). An epidemiological evaluation of 1202 dogs with testicular neoplasia. *J. Vet. Intern. Med.* 6: 121.

Hampe, J.F. and Misdorp, W. (1974). Tumours and dysplasias of the mammary gland. *B. WHO* 50: 111–133.

Harasen, G. (2008). Canine cranial cruciate ligament rupture in profile: 2002–2007. *Can. Vet. J.* 49: 193–194.

Hart, B.L., Hart, L.A., Thigpen, A.P. et al. (2014). Long-term health effects of neutering dogs: comparison of Labrador retrievers with Golden retrievers. *PLoS One* 9: e102241.

Hart, B.L., Hart, L.A., Thigpen, A.P. et al. (2016). Neutering of German shepherd dogs: associated joint disorders, cancers and urinary incontinence. *Vet. Med. Sci.* 2: 191–199.

Hayes, H.M., Milne, K.L., and Mandel, C.P. (1981). Epidemiological features of feline mammary carcinoma. *Vet. Rec.* 108: 476–479.

Henry, C.J. (2003). Management of transitional cell carcinoma. *Vet. Clin. N. Am. Small Anim. Pract.* 33: 597–613.

Herron, M.A. (1972). The effect of prepubertal castration on the penile urethra of the cat. *JAVMA* 160: 208–211.

Hoffman, J.M., Creevy, K.E., and Promislow, D.E. (2013). Reproductive capability is associated with lifespan and cause of death in companion dogs. *PLoS One* 8 (4): e61082.

Holt, P.E. (2004). Urinary incontinence in the male and female dog or does sex matter? *World Small Animal Veterinary Association World Congress Proceedings.* https://www.vin.com/apputil/content/defaultadv1.aspx?meta=Generic&pId=11181&id=3852252 (accessed 20 August 2019).

Holt, P.E. and Thrusfield, M.V. (1993). Association in bitches between breed, size, neutering and docking, and acquired urinary incontinence due to incompetence of the urethral sphincter mechanism. *Vet. Rec.* 133: 177–180.

Houlihan, K.E. (2017). A literature review on the welfare implications of gonadectomy of dogs. *JAVMA* 250: 1155–1166.

Howe, L.M. (1992a). Prepubertal gonadectomy in dogs and cats – part I. *Comp. Cont. Educ.* 21: 103–111.

Howe, L.M. (1992b). Prepubertal gonadectomy in dogs and cats – part II. *Comp. Cont. Educ.* 21: 197–201.

Howe, L.M. (1997). Short-term results and complications of prepubertal gonadectomy in cats and dogs. *JAVMA* 211: 57–62.

Howe, L.M. (2006). Surgical methods of contraception and sterilization. *Theriogenology* 66: 500–509.

Howe, L.M. (2015). Current perspectives on the optimal age to spay/castrate dogs and cats. *Vet. Med. Res. Rep.* 6: 171–180.

Howe, L.M., Slater, M.R., Boothe, H.W. et al. (2000). Long-term outcome of gonadectomy performed at an early age or traditional age in cats. *JAVMA* 217: 1661–1665.

Howe, L.M., Slater, M.R., Boothe, H.W. et al. (2001). Long-term outcome of gonadectomy performed at an early age or traditional age in dogs. *JAVMA* 218: 217–221.

Johnston, S.D., Root Kustritz, M.V., and Olson, P.N. (2001). Disorders of the canine uterus and uterine tubes (oviducts). In: *Canine and Feline Theriogenology* (eds. S.D. Johnston,

M.V. Root Kustritz and P.N. Olson), 206–224. Philadelphia, PA: Saunders.

Kim, H.H., Yeon, S.C., Houpt, K.A. et al. (2006). Effects of ovariohysterectomy on reactivity in German Shepherd dogs. *Vet. J.* 172: 154–159.

Knapp, D.W., Glickman, N.W., DeNicola, D.B. et al. (2000). Naturally-occurring canine transitional cell carcinoma of the urinary bladder. *Urol. Oncol.* 5: 47–59.

Lefebvre, S.L., Yang, M., Wang, M. et al. (2013). Effect of age at gonadectomy on the probability of dogs becoming overweight. *JAVMA* 243: 236–243.

Lekcharoensuk, C., Osborne, C.A., and Lulich, J.P. (2001). Epidemiologic study of risk factors for lower urinary tract diseases in cats. *JAVMA* 218: 1429–1435.

Levy, J.K., Bard, K.M., Tucker, P.D. et al. (2017). Perioperative mortality in cats and dogs undergoing spay or castration at a high-volume clinic. *Vet. J.* 224: 11–15.

Lowseth, L.A., Gerlach, R.F., Gillett, N.A. et al. (1990). Age-related changes in the prostate and testes of the beagle dog. *Vet. Path.* 27: 347–353.

Manning, A.M. and Rowan, A.N. (1992). Companion animal demographics and sterilization status: results from a survey in four Massachusetts towns. *Anthrozoos* 5: 192–201.

Marmor, M., Willeberg, P., Glickman, L.T. et al. (1982). Epizootiologic patterns of diabetes mellitus in dogs. *Am. J. Vet. Res.* 43: 465–470.

McCann, T.M., Simpson, K.E., Shaw, D.J. et al. (2007). Feline diabetes mellitus in the UK: the prevalence within an insured cat population and a questionnaire-based putative risk factor analysis. *J. Feline Med. Surg.* 9: 289–299.

Michell, A.R. (1999). Longevity of British breeds of dog and its relationships with sex, size, cardiovascular variables and disease. *Vet. Rec.* 145: 625–629.

Miller, K.P., Rekers, W.L., DeTar, L.G. et al. (2018). Evaluation of sutureless scrotal castration for pediatric and juvenile dogs. *JAVMA* 253: 1589–1593.

Mitsuhashi, Y., Chamberlin, A.J., Bigley, K.E. et al. (2011). Maintenance energy requirement determination of cats after spaying. *Br. J. Nutr.* 106: S135–S138.

Moe, L. (2001). Population-based incidence of mammary tumours in some dog breeds. *J. Reprod. Fert. Suppl.* 57: 439–443.

Mondelli, F., Prato Previde, E., Verga, M. et al. (2004). The bond that never developed: adoption and relinquishment of dogs in a rescue shelter. *J. Appl. Anim. Welf. Sci.* 7: 253–266.

Moons, C.P., Valcke, A., Verschueren, K. et al. (2018). Effect of early-age gonadectomy on behavior in adopted shelter kittens–the sequel. *J. Vet. Behav.* 26: 43–47.

Moore, G.E., Burkman, K.D., Carter, M.N. et al. (2001). Causes of death or reasons for euthanasia in military working dogs: 927 cases (1993–1996). *JAVMA* 219: 209–214.

Moulton, J.E., Taylor, D.O., Dorn, C.R. et al. (1970). Canine mammary tumors. *Vet. Path.* 7: 289–320.

Nassar, R., Talboy, J., and Moulton, C. (1992). *Animal Shelter Reporting Study 1990*. Englewood, CO: American Humane Association.

National Council on Pet Population Study and Policy (1994). *National Shelter Census: 1994 Results*. Fort Collins, CO: NCCPPSP.

New, J.G., Salman, M.D., Scarlett, J.M. et al. (2000). Shelter relinquishment: characteristics of shelter-relinquished animals and their owners compared with animals and their owners in US pet-owning households. *J. Appl. Anim. Welf. Sci.* 3: 179–201.

New, J.C., Kelch, W.J., Hutchison, J.M. et al. (2004). Birth and death rate estimates of cats and dogs in U.S. households and related factors. *J. Appl. Anim. Welf. Sci.* 7: 229–241.

Norris, A.M., Laing, E.J., Valli, V.E. et al. (1992). Canine bladder and urethral tumors: a retrospective study of 115 cases (1980–1985). *J. Vet. Intern. Med.* 6: 145–153.

Obradovich, J., Walshaw, R., and Goullaud, E. (1987). The influence of castration on the development of prostatic carcinoma in the dog: 43 cases (1978–1985). *J. Vet. Intern. Med.* 1: 183–187.

Overley-Adamson, B. and Baez, J. (2016). Feline mammary carcinoma. In: *August's Consultations in Feline Internal Medicine*, vol. 7 (ed. S. Little), 578–584. Philadelphia, PA: Saunders.

Patronek, G.J., Glickman, L.T., Beck, A.M. et al. (1996). Risk factors for relinquishment of dogs to an animal shelter. *JAVMA* 209: 572–581.

Poirier, V.J., Forrest, L.J., Adams, W.M. et al. (2004). Piroxicam, mitoxantrone, and coarse fraction radiotherapy for the treatment of transitional cell carcinoma of the bladder in 10 dogs: a pilot study. *J. Am. Anim. Hosp. Assoc.* 40: 131–136.

Pollari, F.L. and Bonnett, B.N. (1996). Evaluation of postoperative complications following elective surgeries of dogs and cats at private practices using computer records. *Can. Vet. J.* 37: 672–678.

Pollari, F.L., Bonnett, B.N., Bamsey, S.C. et al. (1996). Postoperative complications of elective surgeries in dogs and cats determined by examining electronic and paper medical records. *JAVMA* 208: 1882–1886.

Porters, N., de Rooster, H., Verschueren, K. et al. (2014). Development of behavior in adopted shelter kittens after gonadectomy performed at an early age or at a traditional age. *J. Vet. Behav. Clin. Appl. Res.* 9: 196–206.

Porters, N., Polis, I., Moons, C.P. et al. (2015). Relationship between age at gonadectomy and health problems in kittens adopted from shelters. *Vet. Rec.* 176: 572.

Prahl, A., Guptill, L., Glickman, N.W. et al. (2007). Time trends and risk factors for diabetes mellitus in cats presented to veterinary teaching hospitals. *J. Feline Med. Surg.* 9: 351–358.

Priester, W.A. and McKay, F.W. (1980). The occurrence of tumors in domestic animals. *Nat. Cancer Inst. Mono.* 54: 1–210.

Prymak, C., McKee, L.J., Goldschmidt, M.H. et al. (1988). Epidemiologic, clinical, pathologic, and prognostic characteristics of splenic hemangiosarcoma and splenic hematoma in dogs: 217 cases (1985). *JAVMA* 193: 706–712.

Rand, J.S., Bobbermien, L.M., Hendrikz, J.K. et al. (1997). Over representation of Burmese cats with diabetes mellitus. *Aust. Vet. J.* 75: 402–405.

Reichler, I.M. (2009). Gonadectomy in cats and dogs: a review of risks and benefits. *Reprod. Domest. Anim.* 44: 29–35.

Reisner, I.R. (1993). Dominance-related aggression of English springer spaniels: a review of 53 cases. *Appl. Anim. Behav. Sci.* 37: 83–84.

Richards, H.G., McNeil, P.E., Thompson, H. et al. (2001). An epidemiological analysis of a canine-biopsies database compiled by a diagnostic histopathology service. *Prevent. Vet. Med.* 51: 125–136.

Root, M.V., Johnston, S.D., Johnston, G.R. et al. (1996a). The effect of prepuberal and postpuberal gonadectomy on penile extrusion and urethral diameter in the domestic cat. *Vet. Radiol. Ultrasound* 37: 363–366.

Root, M.V., Johnston, S.D., and Olson, P.N. (1996b). Effect of prepuberal and postpuberal gonadectomy on heat production measured by indirect calorimetry in male and female domestic cats. *Am. J. Vet. Res.* 57: 371–374.

Root Kustritz, M.V. (1996). Elective gonadectomy in the cat. *Feline Pract.* 24: 36–39.

Root Kustritz, M.V. (2007). Determining the optimal age for gonadectomy of dogs and cats. *JAVMA* 231: 1665–1675.

Root Kustritz, M.V. (2012). Effects of surgical sterilization on canine and feline health and on society. *Reprod. Domest. Anim.* 47 (Suppl 4): 1–9.

Root Kustritz, M.V., Slater, M.R., Weedon, G.R. et al. (2017). Determining optimal age for gonadectomy in the dog: a critical review of the literature to guide decision making. *Clin. Theriogen.* 9: 167–211.

Ru, G., Terracini, B., Blickman, L.T. et al. (1998). Related risk factors for canine osteosarcoma. *Vet. J.* 156: 31–39.

Salmeri, K.R., Olson, P.N., and Bloomberg, M.S. (1991). Elective gonadectomy in dogs: a review. *JAVMA* 198: 1183–1192.

Scarlett, J.M., Salman, M.D., New, J.G. et al. (1999). Reasons for relinquishment of companion animals in U.S. animal shelters: selected health and personal issues. *J. Appl. Anim. Welf. Sci.* 2: 41–57.

Scarlett, J.M., Salman, M.D., New, J.G. et al. (2002). The role of veterinary practitioners in reducing dog and cat relinquishments and euthanasias. *JAVMA* 220: 306–311.

Schneider, R., Dorn, C.R., and Taylor, D.O. (1969). Factors influencing canine mammary cancer development and postsurgical survival. *J. Nat. Cancer Inst.* 43: 1249–1261.

Slauterbeck, J.R., Pankratz, K., Xu, K.T. et al. (2004). Canine ovariohysterectomy and orchiectomy increases the prevalence of ACL injury. *Clin. Orthoped. Rel. Res.* 429: 301–305.

Smith, A.N. (2003). Hemangiosarcoma in dogs and cats. *Vet. Clin. N. Am. Small Anim. Pract.* 33: 533–552.

Sorenmo, K.U., Goldschmidt, M., Shofer, F. et al. (2003). Immunohistochemical characterization of canine prostatic carcinoma and correlation with castration status and castration time. *Vet. Comp. Oncol.* 1: 48–56.

Spain, C.V., Scarlett, J.M., and Houpt, K.A. (2004a). Long-term risks and benefits of early-age gonadectomy in cats. *JAVMA* 224: 372–379.

Spain, C.V., Scarlett, J.M., and Houpt, K.A. (2004b). Long-term risks and benefits of early-age gonadectomy in dogs. *JAVMA* 224: 380–387.

Stocklin-Gautschi, N.M., Hassig, M., Reichler, I.M. et al. (2001). The relationship of urinary incontinence to early spaying in bitches. *J. Reprod. Fertil. Suppl.* 57: 233–236.

Teske, E., Naan, E.C., VanDijk, E.M. et al. (2002). Canine prostate carcinoma: epidemiological evidence of an increased risk in castrated dogs. *Molec. Cell. Endocrin.* 197: 251–255.

Torres, d.l.R.G., Hart, B.L., Farver, T.B. et al. (2013). Neutering dogs: effects on joint disorders and cancers in golden retrievers. *PLoS One* 8 (2): e55937.

Van Goethem, B., Schaefers-Okkens, A., and Kirpensteijn, J. (2006). Making a rational choice between ovariectomy and ovariohysterectomy in the dog: a discussion of the benefits of either technique. *Vet. Surg.* 35: 136–143.

Verstegen, J. and Onclin, K. (2003). Mammary tumors in the queen. *Proceedings of the Society for Theriogenology*, Columbus, OH.

Ware, W.A. and Hopper, D.L. (1999). Cardiac tumors in dogs: 1982–1995. *J. Vet. Intern. Med.* 13: 95–103.

Waters, D.J. (2011). In search of a strategic disturbance: some thoughts on the timing of spaying. *Clin. Theriogen.* 3: 433–437.

Waters, D.J., Kengeri, S.S., Clever, B. et al. (2009). Exploring mechanisms of sex differences in longevity: lifetime ovary exposure and exceptional longevity in dogs. *Aging Cell* 8: 752–755.

Waters, D.J., Kengeri, S.S., Maras, A.H. et al. (2011). Probing the perils of dichotomous binning: how categorizing female dogs as spayed or intact can misinform our assumptions about the lifelong health consequences of ovariohysterectomy. *Theriogenology* 76: 1496–1500.

Weaver, A.D. (1981). Fifteen cases of prostatic carcinoma in the dog. *Vet. Rec.* 109: 71–75.

White, C.R., Hohenhaus, A.E., Kelsey, J. et al. (2006). Cutaneous MCTs: associations with spay/neuter status, breed, body size, and phylogenetic cluster. *J. Am. Anim. Hosp. Assoc.* 47: 210–216.

Whitehair, J.G., Vasseur, P.B., and Willits, N.H. (1993). Epidemiology of cranial cruciate ligament rupture in dogs. *JAVMA* 203: 1016–1019.

Wilke, V.L., Conzemius, M.C., and Rothschild, M.F. (2005). SNP detection and association analyses of candidate genes for rupture of the cranial cruciate ligament in the dog. *Anim. Genet.* 36: 519–521.

Zirkin, B.R. and Strandberg, J.D. (1984). Quantitative changes in the morphology of the aging canine prostate. *Anatom. Rec.* 208: 207–214.

27

Non-surgical Contraception

The State of the Field

Jessica Hekman

Non-surgical contraception is a pressing goal in the veterinary community. Although contraception through spay–neuter surgery has contributed to the reduction of shelter animal populations over recent decades, spay/neuter surgery has not proven an effective tool in other populations of animals. These populations include animals that are sometimes referred to as "unwanted" and are unlikely to present at a veterinary clinic for surgery, such as feral or community cats; feral dogs, or dogs living in regions without a culture of preventive veterinary care; feral horses in the Western United States; wild animals whose natural predators are no longer living in the same region, such as white-tailed deer in the United States; and invasive species, such as the rabbit in Australia or brushtail possum in New Zealand. Additionally, some populations of animal caregivers are interested in temporary contraception. For example, contraception in animal species that readily reproduce in captivity can be vital to maintain zoo populations, but permanent sterilization may not be desirable within the context of maintaining species diversity. Some owners of working or sport dogs have an interest in preventing bitches from going into heat during competition seasons, but prefer to keep them intact for future use as breeding animals. For all of these reasons, interest in non-surgical contraception remains high.

The Ideal Non-surgical Contraceptive

Different animal populations present varied challenges in developing the ideal non-surgical contraceptive. Considerations may include difficulty of capture, whether contraception should be permanent or temporary/reversible, how well adverse effects are tolerated by the animal caretakers, and how many animals to contracept (translating to costs incurred per animal). Just as surgical contraceptive approaches differ markedly between males and females, so do most non-surgical approaches. For any population to be managed through non-surgical contraception, solutions for both sexes must be available. This limits the use of some approaches, such as chemical castration via injection, which requires easy access to the gonads and is therefore not a viable approach in females. Additionally, different approaches may be required for different species. For example, immunocontraceptives that are successful in some species may be less successful in others (Kirkpatrick et al. 2011).

For feral or wild animals, the ideal contraceptive would be both long lasting (for the life of the animal, or, for many species, at least 10 years) and easy to administer in a field setting, preferably by a non-veterinarian. Capture of free-roaming animals may be more or less time consuming depending on the species of animal, and often constitutes a significant hurdle in

High-Quality, High-Volume Spay and Neuter and Other Shelter Surgeries, First Edition. Edited by Sara White.
© 2020 John Wiley & Sons, Inc. Published 2020 by John Wiley & Sons, Inc.

contraceptive delivery. Therefore, a long-lasting contraceptive is ideal, as a contraceptive that needs to be reapplied at regular intervals may be no more effective at population control than a surgical intervention. Additionally, interventions that require a visit to a veterinary clinic are less desirable, as transportation logistics can significantly increase the cost of a sterilization campaign. Administration by a veterinarian also increases cost. In the case of community cat populations, for example, administration of a contraceptive in the field by volunteers could result in a significant increase in the number of animals contracepted, with a concomitant effect on population reduction. In populations of large wild animals, such as deer and horses, remote delivery of small volumes of the contraceptive is an important criterion for an approach's success (Kirkpatrick et al. 2011), due to the need for a contraceptive method that is easy to distribute and does not require application by a veterinarian.

The ideal non-surgical temporary contraceptive for owned animals would last a shorter period of time, allowing a return to fertility for potential future breeding, and be non-invasive to administer. Expense is less of an issue in this population; while most owners prefer less expensive alternatives, managing intact animals through other means is an option when the expense is considered onerous. Owners of competitive sports dogs, for example, are typically prepared to devote considerable funds to increasing their animal's competitiveness. Some dog owners also use temporary contraception to assess how their animal's behavior might change in the face of reduced levels of reproductive hormones, prior to committing to an irreversible surgery. These types of owners also tend to be more willing to commit funds to their dog.

Approaches to Non-surgical Contraception

While surgical approaches to contraception have traditionally focused on removal of the gonads, non-surgical approaches can poten-

tially target different levels of the reproductive system. This system, known as the hypothalamic–pituitary–gonadal (HPG) axis, originates in the hypothalamus, which releases gonadotropin-releasing hormone (GnRH) in a pulsatile fashion (see Figure 27.1). GnRH is transmitted directly to the anterior pituitary gland through a venous portal system, where it stimulates the release of the gonadotropin hormones, follicle-stimulating hormone (FSH), and luteinizing hormone (LH). These two protein hormones are released into the systemic circulation by the anterior pituitary and stimulate release of the steroid reproductive hormones from the gonads – androgens and estrogens. Negative feedback from androgens and estrogens, as well as from progesterone (released by the corpus luteum), suppresses release of GnRH, FSH, and LSH (Mastorakos et al. 2006). Therefore, interference with the axis at any of its three levels (hypothalamus, anterior pituitary, and gonads) has the potential to disrupt fertility.

Contraceptive approaches have targeted different levels of the HPG. The hypothalamus is a particularly challenging target – it is difficult to approach directly via injection, as is any brain region; it is also difficult to approach via the bloodstream, as it lies behind the blood–brain barrier. However, GnRH may be targeted after it has left the hypothalamus and crossed the blood–brain barrier. Gonadal targets include the zona pellucida, proteins expressed on the ovulated egg to facilitate sperm recognition, and the thecal support cells of the ovaries and testes.

As previously discussed, ease of delivery to the gonads differs markedly between sexes. Delivery by injection directly to the testes has been successfully applied with chemical contraceptives such as zinc gluconate. Whether safe and humane injection in this region of the body requires chemical restraint has been a matter of debate among practitioners. Direct injection to the ovaries is indisputably impractical. However, both male and female gonads are accessible via the systemic circulation. Blocking access to the gonads may be an alternative approach, as with an intrauterine

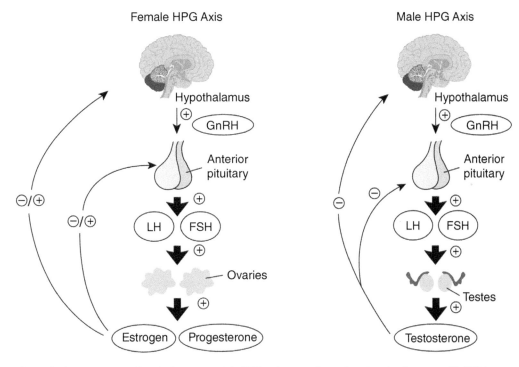

Female HPG Axis

Male HPG Axis

Figure 27.1 Hypothalamic–pituitary-gonadal (HPG) axis: gonadotropin-releasing hormone (GnRH) is secreted from the hypothalamus, triggering release of luteinizing hormone (LH) and follicle-stimulating hormone (FSH) from the anterior pituitary. These hormones trigger release of estrogens or androgens from the gonads, which in turn regulate hormone release at the level of the anterior pituitary and hypothalamus through negative feedback. *Source:* Adapted from Hiller-Sturmhöfel & Bartke (1998). Reproduced with permission of Alcohol Health & Research World.

device (IUD). In veterinary species, this approach is only practical for females.

Solutions to Non-surgical Contraception

Contraceptive approaches include immuno-contraceptives, which use the animal's immune system to attack a specific cell type at one or more levels of the HPG axis; chemical contraceptives, which destroy tissue and reduce or eliminate the function of a particular organ, most commonly the gonads; hormonal contraceptives, which provide negative feedback at a variety of levels of the HPG axis; physical devices blocking reproduction, such as IUDs; and gene delivery, typically via viral vectors, to increase or decrease expression of a specific gene in order to change the function of

a given cell type, again at one or more levels of the HPG axis.

Immunocontraception

Immunocontraception uses the animal's own immune system to destroy cells or proteins that are necessary for the function of the reproductive system. Early successes targeted the zona pellucida. Porcine zona pellucida (PZP) is typically used in this vaccine, as it may be inexpensively obtained (Aitken et al. 1996). The PZP vaccine is only effective in females, but has the advantage of taking effect downstream in the reproductive system, with fewer concomitant changes in hormone levels and behavior, which is a goal in the management of some populations, and possibly fewer health consequences than a vaccine with a target higher in the HPG axis (Kirkpatrick et al. 2011). Because ZP proteins are not highly conserved across species, a consideration of this vaccine target is that a vaccine developed against proteins from one species might work poorly when used in a different species (Eade et al. 2009). Another target is GnRH, the hormone released by the hypothalamus, as in this hormone's absence, both testicular function and ovulation decrease (Einarsson 2006). A vaccine against GnRH would therefore be effective in both males and females, unlike PZP vaccines.

Vaccines against GnRH (GonaCon™, USDA APHIS, Riverdale, MD) and PZP have been used successfully in populations of large, free-roaming animals such as white-tailed deer, feral horses, and elephants. In most of these populations, immunocontraceptive vaccines require booster administration annually for continued effectiveness (Kirkpatrick et al. 2011). Injection site reactions vary by population and by vaccine; local reactions with some progressing to chronic abscesses occurred in multiple studies (Kirkpatrick and Turner 1990; Curtis et al. 2007; Gionfriddo et al. 2009).

PZP and GnRH vaccines have also been tested in dogs and cats, with less success. PZP vaccination was ineffective in queens, though feline ZP, as opposed to PZP, appeared to be a potential vaccine target in this species (Eade et al. 2009). PZP vaccine administration in bitches resulted in abnormal estrous cycles and injection site reactions (Mahi-Brown et al. 1985). A recombinant canine ZP approach has been debated in this species (Shrestha et al. 2015). Development of species-specific canine or feline ZP vaccines may prove prohibitively expensive for the available market. Canine use of GnRH vaccines was deemed neither safe nor effective due to severe injection site reactions and lack of change in sperm population and morphology post-vaccination (Griffin et al. 2005). In cats, GonaCon does not appear to elicit serious injection site reactions (Vansandt et al. 2017). Though an initial captive population study suggested that the vaccine may be effective in this species (Levy et al. 2011), a subsequent study in a colony setting

found that pregnancy rates were not sufficiently reduced in this species to warrant use of this vaccine (Fischer et al. 2018). Therefore, immunocontraception at this point is mostly used in free-roaming large animal species rather than in small animal species, due to both efficacy and adverse effects.

Chemical Contraception

Chemical contraceptives are injected into the target tissue – typically the testes – and render it permanently non-functional. The most widely used chemical contraceptive currently is zinc gluconate, which is used as an intratesticular injection in dogs. After injection, the testes sclerose, resulting in permanent azoospermia or oligospermia and reduction of circulating testosterone levels (Oliveira et al. 2012). Injection must be performed with care, as subcutaneous injection may result in necrotizing injection-site reactions, necessitating complete scrotal ablation (Forzán et al. 2014). Therefore, while injection may be performed in awake dogs, chemical restraint may be advisable; additionally, complication rates of zinc gluconate injection depend on practitioner skill level and may rival the complication rates and seriousness of traditional orchidectomy (Levy et al. 2008).

Zinc gluconate has been marketed as Neutersol™ and as Zeuterin™ in the United States, where it is no longer available, and is currently marketed as Esterisol™ (Ark Sciences, New York) in South and Central America. Use of zinc gluconate is attractive for large-scale population management in areas where surgeons, surgery suites, or skilled staff are difficult to obtain, and in areas where physical removal of the testicles is culturally unacceptable (Levy et al. 2008). In areas where surgical intervention in canines is widely accepted, however, it has failed to find a market. Anecdotally, veterinarians hesitate to turn to this solution for neuter of male cats, as feline orchidectomy is much less time consuming than canine orchidectomy.

Calcium chloride can also be used to sterilize male dogs via intratesticular injection (Jana and Samanta 2007). As few efficacy and safety studies have been performed on this substance for this use, anecdotally many veterinarians hesitate to use it.

A novel approach to injection of a sterilant involves the use of saponin, a substance that is harmless in the bloodstream but toxic once taken into a cell. Injected distally, saponin may be carried in a lipid-based nanoparticle and guided to the gonads by an anti-Mullerian II receptor antibody. Once taken up by the gonadal support cells, it will trigger apoptosis. This process has resulted in reduction in sperm number and motility in male rats and in reduced estrous cycling in female rats (Ayres et al. 2018). Studies in companion animals have yet to be performed.

In summary, chemical contraceptives are currently in use as Esterisol in South and Central America in male dogs, but are otherwise not currently widely used due to lack of market demand.

Hormonal Contraception

Hormonal contraception in veterinary species typically functions through negative feedback to the HPG. Deslorelin, a GnRH superagonist, functions to reduce reproductive hormones and suppress fertility. After initial implantation, deslorelin will initially stimulate, then suppress, the release of androgens and estrogens. As the implant's effectiveness wanes, reproductive hormone levels will again increase. This leads to an estrous cycle shortly after implantation and at the end of effectiveness in females, and can lead to behavior changes in males. Because HPG axis function is highly conserved across species, this approach has wide cross-species efficacy (McKinnon et al. 1993; Bertschinger et al. 2001; Munson et al. 2001). While not approved in the United States for use in dogs or cats, deslorelin is currently marketed in Europe as Suprelorin™ (Virbac, Glattbrugg, Switzerland), in both 6- and 12-month prod-

ucts. While advertised as being able to be injected subcutaneously without anesthesia, the process appears to be painful for the animal. Suprelorin is used off-label in the United States in zoo species for contraception, and to manage ferret adrenal hyperplasia.

As a timed-release formulation of Suprelorin lasting longer than one year has not yet been developed, this approach is not appropriate for permanent sterilization. However, it functions well as a temporary contraceptive, and has been used in companion animals in Europe.

Intrauterine Device

A canine IUD is currently marketed as Dogspiral (Veterinary Research Centre, Rijkevoort, Netherlands). In humans, IUDs change the environment of the uterus to prevent implantation of fertilized eggs, and are widely used. No peer-reviewed safety or efficacy studies have been performed on IUDs in dogs. Theriogenologists have expressed concern about canine IUD insertion, given the shape of the canine cervix, as well as the device's safety once inserted (ACC&D 2017).

Gene Delivery

Alteration of targeted genes in an animal's genome, or introduction of transgenes, could be used to disrupt reproductive function. Alteration of genes may mean changes in gene sequence, leading to proteins with disrupted function; it could also mean changes in regulatory sequence, leading to increased or decreased expression of targeted genes. For example, an increase in gene expression could lead to increased production of a particular antigen, which could lead to a stronger immune response and result in improved immunocontraception.

Gene delivery has been used on GnRH, a target also used in contraceptive vaccines, in cats. An adeno-associated virus (AAV) vector was used to deliver anti-GnRH antibodies. Antibody titer levels increased, but then returned to baseline within one month of injection, presumably due to immune system attack of the foreign anti-GnRH antibody (Vansandt 2018). A novel target of gene delivery is Mullerian-inhibiting substance (MIS), a ligand produced by the ovaries which inhibits primordial follicle activation. Lifelong super-physiological expression of MIS would lead to permanent contraception in females. This approach has been tested in cats, also using an AAV vector, and resulted in brief (several-month) ovarian suppression followed by a return to cyclicity. Research on MIS as a target is ongoing (Pepin 2018).

Gene delivery is not yet in use as a veterinary contraceptive, but shows promise for the future.

Marking of Contracepted Animals

In the US, many shelters mark dogs and cats who have been surgically altered with a tattoo to signal their non-reproductive state. Community cats are frequently subjected to removal of one ear tip (ear-tipping) for easy identification of surgically altered cats from a distance. These approaches may not be appropriate for non-surgical contraception, however. In the case of temporary contraceptives, such as current immunocontraceptives, marks must also be temporary. In the case of owned animals in locations without traditions of veterinary care, ear-tipping may not be societally acceptable, either by the animals' caretakers or by the funders of a contraceptive outreach program. The ideal marker would be non- or minimally invasive, easy to apply in a field setting, visible from a distance so that it could be used in capture decisions in wild or feral animals, and either last approximately as long as contraception is expected to last, or contain encoded information about contraception type and when it was applied. Ear-tagging has been explored (Benka 2015), but does not appear to be an appropriate solution for dogs or cats due to the short time that tags remain on the ear (Benka and Getty 2018). Another approach may be the application of a tattoo using ultraviolet ink delivered through a microneedle patch. This approach may prove challenging in animals with particular morphologies, such as dogs with flopped ears or cats with dark coat colors (Benka and Getty 2018).

Looking to the Future

While immunocontraceptives have proven useful in the control of wild or feral populations of large animal species, convenient and long-lasting contraceptives for small animals remain elusive. Delayed-release hormones are also not a long-lasting option for these populations, and are difficult to administer in a field setting. Novel approaches, however, hold out promise for the future. Delivery of antibody-guided toxins to gonadal cells may provide lifetime contraception. Current gene delivery research suggests that the immune system is competent at overcoming introduced foreign proteins, resulting in only brief contraception over several months. However, ongoing research is addressing this problem. The goal of producing long-lasting injectable solutions to the problem of animal overpopulation is still in sight.

References

Aitken, R.J., Paterson, M., and van Duin, M. (1996). The potential of the zona pellucida as a target for immunocontraception. *Am. J. Reproduct. Immun.* 35 (3): 175–180.

Alliance for Contraception in Cats & Dogs (2017). Dogspiral: Product profile and position paper. http://www.acc-d.org/docs/default-source/Resource-Library-Docs/dogspiral-final-for-web.pdf (accessed 1 November 2018).

Ayres, S., Meadows, K., and Xu, Q. (2018). A new approach for non-surgical sterilization: targeting gonadal support cells. *Proceedings of* the 2018 Alliance for Contraception in Cats and Dogs (ACCD) International Symposium on Nonsurgical Methods of Pet Population Control, Boston, MA.

Benka, V.A.W. (2015). Ear tips to ear tags: marking and identifying cats treated with non-surgical fertility control. *J. Feline Med. Surg.* 17 (9): 808–815.

Benka, V. and Getty, S. (2018). Marking and identifying free-roaming dogs and cats. *Proceedings of the 2018 Alliance for Contraception in Cats and Dogs (ACCD) International Symposium on Nonsurgical Methods of Pet Population Control*, Boston, MA. https://www.acc-d.org/docs/default-source/6th-symposium-proceedings/benka-getty-marking-accd-symposium-ppt.pdf (accessed 5 November 2018).

Bertschinger, H.J., Asa, C.S., Calle, P.P. et al. (2001). Control of reproduction and sex related behaviour in exotic wild carnivores with the GnRH analogue deslorelin: preliminary observations. *J. Reprod. Fertil. Suppl.* 57: 275–283.

Curtis, P.D., Richmond, M.E., Miller, L.A., and Quimby, F.W. (2007). Pathophysiology of white-tailed deer vaccinated with porcine zona pellucida immunocontraceptive. *Vaccine* 25 (23): 4623–4630.

Eade, J.A., Roberston, I.D., and James, C.M. (2009). Contraceptive potential of porcine and feline zona pellucida A, B and C subunits in domestic cats. *Reproduction* 137 (6): 913–922.

Einarsson, S. (2006). Vaccination against GnRH: pros and cons. *Acta Veterinaria Scandinavica* 48 (1): S10.

Fischer, A., Benka, V.A.W., Briggs, J.R. et al. (2018). Effectiveness of GonaCon as an immunocontraceptive in colony-housed cats. *J. Feline Med. Surg.* 20 (8): 786–792.

Forzán, M.J., Garde, E., Pérez, G.E., and Vanderstichel, R.V. (2014). Necrosuppurative orchitis and scrotal necrotizing dermatitis following intratesticular administration of zinc gluconate neutralized with arginine (EsterilSol) in 2 mixed-breed dogs. *Vet. Path.* 51 (4): 820–823.

Gionfriddo, J.P., Eisemann, J., Sullivan, K. et al. (2009). Field test of a single-injection gonadotrophin-releasing hormone immunocontraceptive vaccine in female white-tailed deer. *Wildlife Res.* 36 (3): 177–184.

Griffin, B., Baker, H., Welles, E. et al. (2005). Response of dogs to a GnRH-KLH conjugate contraceptive vaccine adjuvanted with Adjuvac®. *Proceedings of the 2004 Alliance for Contraception in Cats and Dogs (ACCD) International Symposium on Nonsurgical Methods of Pet Population Control*, Denver, CO.

Hiller-Sturmhöfel, S. and Bartke, A. (1998). The endocrine system: a review. *Alc. Health Res. World* 22 (3): 153–164.

Jana, K. and Samanta, P.K. (2007). Sterilization of male stray dogs with a single intratesticular injection of calcium chloride: a dose-dependent study. *Contraception* 75 (5): 390–400.

Kirkpatrick, J.F. and Turner, J.W. (1990). Remotely-delivered immunocontraception in feral horses. *Wildlife Soc. B.* 18 (3): 326–330.

Kirkpatrick, J.F., Lyda, R.O., and Frank, K.M. (2011). Contraceptive vaccines for wildlife: a review. *Am. J. Reprod. Immun.* 66 (1): 40–50.

Levy, J.K., Crawford, P.C., Appel, L.D., and Clifford, E.L. (2008). Comparison of intratesticular injection of zinc gluconate versus surgical castration to sterilize male dogs. *Am. J. Vet. Res.* 69 (1): 140–143.

Levy, J.K., Friary, J.A., Miller, L.A. et al. (2011). Long-term fertility control in female cats with GonaCon™, a GnRH immunocontraceptive. *Theriogenology* 76 (8): 1517–1525.

Mahi-Brown, C.A., Yanagimachi, R., Hoffman, J.C., and Huang, T.T. Jr. (1985). Fertility control in the bitch by active immunization with porcine zonae pellucidae: use of different adjuvants and patterns of estradiol and progesterone levels in estrous cycles. *Biol. Reprod.* 32 (4): 761–772.

Mastorakos, G., Pavlatou, M.G., and Mizamtsidi, M. (2006). The hypothalamic-pituitary-adrenal and the hypothalamic-pituitary-gonadal axes interplay. *Pediatr. Endocrin. Rev.* 3: 172–181.

McKinnon, A.O., Nobelius, A.M., del Marmol Figueroa, S.T. et al. (1993). Predictable ovulation in mares treated with an implant of the GnRH analogue deslorelin. *Equine Vet. J.* 25 (4): 321–323.

Munson, L., Bauman, J.E., Asa, C.S. et al. (2001). Efficacy of the GnRH analogue deslorelin for suppression of oestrous cycles in cats. *J. Reprod. Fertil. Suppl.* 57: 269–273.

Oliveira, E.C.S., Moura, M.R., de Sá, M.J. et al. (2012). Permanent contraception of dogs induced with intratesticular injection of a zinc gluconate-based solution. *Theriogenology* 77 (6): 1056–1063.

Pepin, D. (2018). Gene therapy with AAV9 delivery of an MIS transgene inhibits estrus in female cats. *Proceedings of the 2018 Alliance for Contraception in Cats and Dogs (ACCD) International Symposium on Nonsurgical Methods of Pet Population Control*, Boston, MA.

Shrestha, A., Srichandan, S., Minhas, V. et al. (2015). Canine zona pellucida glycoprotein-3: up-scaled production, immunization strategy and its outcome on fertility. *Vaccine* 33 (1): 133–140.

Vansandt, L. (2018). AAV-vectored generation of GnRH-binding immunoglobulins for non-surgical sterilization of domestic cats. *Proceedings of the 2018 Alliance for Contraception in Cats and Dogs (ACCD) International Symposium on Nonsurgical Methods of Pet Population Control*, Boston, MA.

Vansandt, L.M., Kutzler, M.A., Fischer, A.E. et al. (2017). Safety and effectiveness of a single and repeat intramuscular injection of a Gn RH vaccine (GonaCon™) in adult female domestic cats. *Reprod. Domest. Anim.* 52: 348–353.

Section Six

Human Resources and Management

28

Starting with Why

Know Your Purpose and Name Your Bottom Lines
BJ Rogers

Perhaps one of the biggest mistakes mission-based organizations make time and again is charging head first into a program or practice without having taken the time to clearly and accurately articulate their purpose.

As you set out to start a new organization, program, or initiative, it's critical that the key stakeholders (founders, board members, key investors or funders) have a voice in drafting a shared understanding of organizational or program *purpose*. From the start – and down the road – this will be the guiding light of your work; don't short-change this effort, it's among the most important conversations you can have. According to author and speaker Simon Sinek, it will also inform and drive the likelihood of your success. In his best-selling book *Start With Why: How Great Leaders Inspire Everyone to Take Action*, Sinek (2009) posits: "People don't buy WHAT you sell, they buy WHY you do it."

According to this understanding, as you set out to provide a service or sell a product, it's vital not only that you know *why* you're doing what you're doing, but that you're able to communicate that purpose to those people you hope to reach and serve.

Foundational Belief Statement

The most explicit and powerful mechanism to communicate your organization or program's purpose is through the creation of a *foundational belief statement*. Not to be confused with a mission statement (that's *what* you do and we'll get there in a bit), a foundational belief statement speaks to *why* you exist. It answers the question: "What do you believe – so fervently and so specifically – that it's compelled you to give of your time, energy, and resources to embark on this effort?"

If your foundational belief statement doesn't start with the words "We believe…" then it's just another sentence. At Emancipet, an Austin, TX-based organization with low-cost spay–neuter and wellness clinics located around Texas (and in Philadelphia, PA), the foundational belief statement is a driver for values identification, establishing bottom lines, clinic operations, hiring decisions, customer service; it doesn't just drive *what* gets done, it profoundly informs *how* things get done. It simply reads:

> We believe that people love their pets and will do what is best for them when given the opportunity.

Opportunity can mean all sorts of things – affordability, geographic access, a welcoming environment, and so on – but the foundation of the foundational belief statement is the belief that people love their pets and will do what's best for them. While the work isn't necessarily *easier* as a result of a well-articulated foundational belief, it's unquestionably clearer.

High-Quality, High-Volume Spay and Neuter and Other Shelter Surgeries, First Edition. Edited by Sara White.
© 2020 John Wiley & Sons, Inc. Published 2020 by John Wiley & Sons, Inc.

A clear and precise foundational belief statement is also a filter – for program decisions, hiring decisions, resource allocation, and a host of other considerations. As you go about crafting your statement – and certainly once it's been formalized – it should be something that everyone involved on your team buys into, hook, line, and sinker. If someone doesn't ascribe to that belief, chances are there'll be persistent friction – and likely division that will impact culture, organizational/program success, and the overall efficacy of your work.

Mission Statement

Once a foundational belief statement has been finalized, an organization should take the time to translate it into the ever-monolithic "mission" statement. More often than not, this happens the other way around, or a mission statement is drafted but a foundational belief statement is never articulated. A well-crafted mission statement should be a sentence – truly, just one sentence – that tells people clearly (and reminds everyone in your organization) what it is you aim to do. In other words, "Our mission is to...," fill in the blank, or "We're on a mission to..." At Emancipet, the translation of the foundational belief statement into a mission reads:

> Emancipet is on a mission to make high-quality spay/neuter and veterinary care affordable and accessible to all pet owners.

As you can likely see, the translation is fairly direct: if one believes people love their pets and will do what is best for them when given the opportunity, then it follows that one may endeavor to provide at least one "opportunity" (in this case, the provision of high-quality, affordable, and accessible spay–neuter and veterinary care). Of course, there is also an assumption in this translation – albeit one based on years of both hard data and experiential learning – that at least one thing that keeps people from doing what is best for their pets is a lack of access to affordable spay–neuter and veterinary care/services. As you craft both a foundational belief statement and a mission statement, be sure to check those assumptions – and make sure they're well founded.

Once approved (by an organization's founders, board, or leadership team), both the foundational belief statement and the mission statement should figure prominently – literally and figuratively – in decision-making and organizational efforts moving forward.

Drafting Your Statements: Starting with Discovery

While it's often apparent on one level or another what has driven people to convene around a particular cause (a neighborhood struggling with an overwhelming number of strays, overtaxed shelter systems, etc.), a catalyst or an initial motivation isn't the same as a clear purpose. Sometimes, the best way to get to an articulation of that purpose is through a deliberate and facilitated discovery process. Whether lengthy and involved or brief and succinct, the process should be thorough, thoughtful, and rooted in the asking and answering of a series of probing questions that are aimed at getting to the core of why a program or organization matters. In his book *Ask More: The Power of Questions to Open Doors, Uncover Solutions and Spark Change*, Frank Sesno (2017), former journalist and current director of the School of Media and Public Affairs at George Washington University, not only makes a compelling case for the power of asking intentional questions, but outlines 11 types of powerful questions – among them, diagnostic and mission questions, both of which have a powerful role to play in the discovery process. Far from complex, the types of questions you might consider in the process of discovery intended to produce foundational belief and mission statements might sound like this:

- What problem(s) are we trying to solve?
- What do we care about most?
- What's calling for this effort at this particular time?
- What things are non-negotiable or unwavering for us?
- What do we believe about the nature of the problem that others might not understand, believe, or be aware of?
- What is our particular value proposition; what makes us uniquely positioned or qualified to embark on this effort?

In asking – and gathering answers to – these questions, we begin to amass words, themes, and understanding that speak to the heart of our intention, desire, and dreams. Well captured, these keywords can and should find a home in your organization's communications across departments – in fundraising material, job postings and descriptions, employee handbooks, and so on. With a little wordsmithing and, to use a word favored by researcher and author Brene Brown, "rumbling," you should be a whole bunch of steps closer to being able to draft your foundational belief and mission statements.

At the same time, this process can and should also include the identification and refinement of your organization's core values. While slightly more fluid in how they are "lived," an organization's core values – like the bottom lines that we'll discuss below – should be universally understood by members of your team and, ideally, should be concepts that they identify with personally.

Emancipet has four core values. They are:

- Excellence
- Teaching and Learning
- Optimism
- Compassionate Service

Translated behaviorally, these values mean that we work hard in pursuit of the best possible outcome; that we seek and seize opportunities to both learn and share information in ways that respect the experience and dignity of each person we interact with; that we believe unwaveringly – and behave accordingly, if with modesty – that our work is changing the world; and that we approach each other and our clients with kindness, generosity, and an assumption that people both *are* good and want to *do* good.

Our values are those things we hold dear and they inform how we both receive and respond to the world around us. They are an organizational agreement that describes how we'll "show up" at work.

Our values drive our behavior and, when we fail to take the time to articulate what they are, we run the very real risk of our behavior being driven by an individual's personal values. More often than not, the group will adopt the personal values of the "loudest" member of the team. This particular liability is what people commonly mean when they refer to a "toxic" person on staff. While the term toxic is problematic when referring to a human being, what people mean to say is that the values of a given individual are out of alignment with the desired culture of the organization, and they are influencing the behavior of others in negative ways.

The simple lesson? Take the time to discover and articulate your values; it's what makes living them possible.

The Bottom Line: Operationalizing Your Beliefs and Mission

Tough as it can and may be, putting your *what* and your *why* into words is often the easy part (which makes the frequency with which so many forgo it all the more perplexing). Once you've achieved clarity about what you believe and what you aim to do, the next important – and often more difficult – step is to establish exactly what your operational bottom lines are. These are the filters you will use – and the commitments to which you will remain unwavering – in both your day-to-day operations and your assessment of new opportunities and ideas. Just as your mission statement should directly derive from your foundational belief, so too should your bottom lines flow from, and feed, your mission statement. Bottom lines are uncompromising: they are the standards to which you hold yourself when considering "What's next?" or "What now?" In effect, they also communicate part of your *how*; that is, the things you do, that you'll *only* do, if they meet these bottom lines. They are standards to which you believe everything must rise to make it possible for you to realize your stated mission.

Emancipet has three bottom lines, all equal in weight and powerfully interdependent. They are:

1) **Quality Medical Care**

   We practice the highest quality medicine possible and minimize pain and anxiety in every patient.

2) **Transformative Service**

   We facilitate positive personal transformations for our clients, donors, and staff.

3) **Sustainable Finance**

   We care for our financial health because it allows us to fulfill our mission and to do more good.

Each of these bottom lines drive both what we do and how we do it. When we consider adding a new module to a clinic's menu of services (say, low-cost dentals), we require an answer in the affirmative to each of the following questions before moving forward.

> Can we offer and deliver this service in a manner that is both high-quality and minimizes pain and anxiety in every patient?
>
> In offering and delivering this service, can we facilitate positive personal transformations for the people involved (our clients, donors, and staff)?
>
> Can we offer and deliver this service in a way that meets our previous two

bottom lines while also being both affordable to clients and fiscally responsible to our organization?

Of course, answering these questions is rarely (or never) as simple as yes or no. When we consider quality medical care, we need to explore protocols, understand best practice, and consider staff expertise and training needs. When we consider sustainable finance, we need to draft realistic budgets that take into account equipment costs, patient volume, and an understanding of what is both affordable and sustainable. In other words, getting to yes or no for each of these questions requires a bit of homework, it requires that we do our due diligence and have confidence that our answer is on solid ground and well informed.

The other thing to know about these bottom lines is that they are intentionally designed to exist with a certain amount of tension between them. In other words, they form a sort of equilateral triangle, and the idea is for that tension to hold enough at each point to maintain that shape. If we pull too hard on sustainable finance, we may pull things out of shape (say, compromising quality medical care). The tension is there so that pulling in one direction activates enough resistance for us to remember we've got more than one bottom line to consider.

Putting It All Together: Your Organizational Identity Document

Once you've done the hard and rewarding work of discovering and articulating your foundational belief statement, mission, core values, and bottom lines, it's not a bad idea to put them together in one powerful identity document (Figure 28.1). Shareable with staff, donors, clients, and the public in general, one should be able to read this document and come away with a clear (and powerful! and compelling!) understanding of why your organization exists, what you believe, and what you care

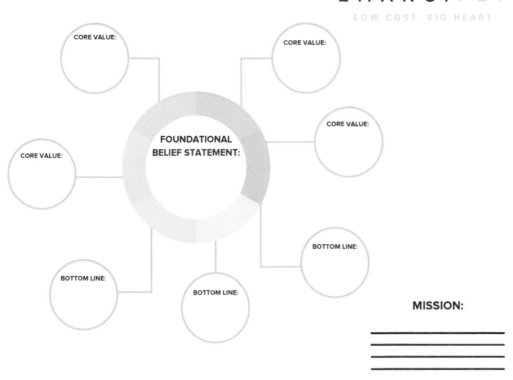

EMANCIPET
LOW COST. BIG HEART.

CORE VALUE:

CORE VALUE:

CORE VALUE:

FOUNDATIONAL
BELIEF STATEMENT:

CORE VALUE:

BOTTOM LINE:

BOTTOM LINE:

BOTTOM LINE:

MISSION:

Figure 28.1   Template for identity document.

about most. Staff, volunteers, and board members should be well versed in each element.

Perhaps most importantly, when an individual interacts with your organization – regardless of the context, the medium, or the time – they should recognize these key elements of your organizational character and identity. In other words, if asked "Did you walk away with the impression that this organization works hard in pursuit of the best possible outcome?" or "Does it seem to you that this organization strives to deliver the very best in veterinary care?" an individual should be able to answer "Yes!" without pause.

The translation of the concepts that you explore and articulate while crafting the elements we've discussed is paramount. If you don't *live* your values and beliefs, then they're just meaningless words on a page – and that will become quickly apparent to those you serve and those who work for you. These identity commitments set the stage for your organizational culture, and for how you recruit and retain team members who will behave in ways that exemplify what your organization stands for and believes.

References

Sesno, F. (2017). *Ask more: The power of questions to open doors, uncover solutions, and spark change*. New York: Amacom.

Sinek, S. (2009). *Start with why: How great leaders inspire everyone to take action*. New York: Penguin.

29

Hiring for Impact, Hiring for Culture
BJ Rogers

If you work at a large organization, there's a chance that the very mention of engaging Human Resources in a hiring process gives you pause – not because of the people in HR, but because, in many cases, the systems that are meant to facilitate successful hires can also be time consuming and slow when put up against a team's urgent need to fill an opening. If you're a brand-new organization, then the good news is that you've got some license to decide how you'll go about hiring. Either way, it's our experience that hiring well means hiring for culture – and by *hiring for culture* we mean taking into account an individual's alignment with your organization's core values, beliefs, and mission, and with how people in your organization behave when they're at their very best.

Put simply, when you make a concerted effort to hire for culture, the likelihood of a good match for both parties increases. Understanding the culture of your team or organization, then, is a critical asset in developing job postings and profiles, screening candidates, and making successful hires.

Though skills and experience will always be both necessary considerations and key requirements, to the extent possible, they should never come at the expense of culture fit. Hiring a poor culture fit inevitably leads to losses in productivity, cohesion, and morale, either because of the strife that comes from the mis-

alignment or the time you spend "managing" someone's behaviors (or ultimately, "managing them out"). And remember, unless you're hiring for a hard-to-find and specific skill set, there's a good chance you can teach a new hire what they need to know (which is *much* easier than trying to shape a person's values or beliefs to align with the team or organizational culture). Though that training may seem like a big investment up front (and training is and *should* be a big investment!), you'll realize the savings later, in increased output and impact and in a happier and more unified team.

Hiring for culture is multiphased, collaborative, and intentional by design. Sometimes, that means it can take a little longer – at least up front. Once you get the hang of it, though, this process can actually be *faster* than others, and will consistently yield better results. It's not fool-proof, but it's worth whatever extra time it might take to get into a groove.

On-boarding and Training

Most of us tend to think that the hiring process runs up to and including a signed offer letter – and it's that thinking that's to blame for failed starts and the loss of precious resources (namely time, productivity, and money). On-boarding is the final phase of hiring, not only

High-Quality, High-Volume Spay and Neuter and Other Shelter Surgeries, First Edition. Edited by Sara White.
© 2020 John Wiley & Sons, Inc. Published 2020 by John Wiley & Sons, Inc.

because it's how we transition individuals from applicants to employees, but because it's also a bit of an insurance policy. Though most new hires are on their best behavior when they start, sometimes a mishire shows itself early on. When it does, there's some wisdom to the hire slow/fire fast adage. That's not to encourage snap judgments, only to remember that we sometimes get it wrong, and acknowledging and acting on that mistake with some speed can save us from suffering future losses.

If you commit yourself to hiring for culture, sometimes you'll bring folks on whose skill levels need some brushing up. Whether you're hiring internally, because you already know someone is a great culture fit, or you've found a real outside gem who seems like an ideal match, one of the things that the luxury of hiring for culture mandates is a commitment to skill development and training. Whether you deliver that yourself through an in-house program or outsource through professional development training or seminars, robust training is the other side of the thoughtful on-boarding coin.

Your success in hiring for culture depends on three key factors:

- How well you understand and can describe your own culture.
- How much you can learn about a candidate's values, beliefs, and behaviors.
- How accurately you judge the alignment between your culture and those values, beliefs, and behaviors.

Seek First to Understand: Know Your Culture

Before you even begin the hiring process, you must start with a look inside your own culture and ensure you fully understand it.

You may already be able to describe your own culture pretty well. Still, using tools like the Culture Questionnaire (Figure 29.1) can give you an eye-opening reality check to ensure that your perception and reality are in sync. Though intended for staff, this tool could be adapted for volunteers, board, and other stakeholders if you're a new or all-volunteer organization.

Once you've got some data, look for those keywords and phrases that seem to appear again and again across responses. These are the words that describe what it's like to work at or be a part of your organization, what someone can expect when joining your team, and the type of person you're looking for. Remember, this is about culture fit – the "hard" skills you need someone to have are another consideration.

Creating a Job Profile

A job profile is neither a posting nor a job description. Instead, it is a one-page capture that indicates the skills, abilities, and qualities that would make for a successful candidate. Job profiles allow you to think through all aspects of the position, assess the skill and experience fit, and ascertain the culture fit. Effective job profiles also allow you to assess what skills you can train for and what skills you need someone to have on day one.

The following are definitions of each section of the template in Figure 29.2:

- *Job relationships.* This field details all team members the position works with regularly.
- *Reporting relationships.* These fields describe all *direct* supervisory relationships (both who the role reports to and who the role supervises, if anyone).
- *Collaborators.* This field is intended to describe other positions within the organization with whom the individual will interact or work on a regular or frequent basis.
- *Strengths.* This field should capture – in a brief and concise manner – the key high-level characteristics of someone who would excel in this role.
- *Position summary.* Starting with a brief statement of impact (what this position will

EMANCIPET

CULTURE QUESTIONNAIRE

Primary Questions:

1. What are the skills or qualities that seem to be the most valued and rewarded in employees at work?
    _____
    _____

2. Describe the qualities of the employee you most admire at work?
    _____
    _____

3. In general, what happens when someone makes a mistake at work?
    _____
    _____

4. What are the issues that everyone at work agrees on?
    _____
    _____

5. What are the issues that divide us, or people disagree about at work?
    _____
    _____

6. What are the unwritten rules at work–the three most important rules of working here?
    _____
    _____

Alternative/Additional Questions:

1. How would you describe the culture at work?
    _____
    _____

2. What would another company need to offer you to make you leave us and go to work for them?
    _____
    _____

3. What role do you play in helping to fulfill the mission of the organization?
    _____
    _____

Figure 29.1   Culture questionnaire.

achieve if executed successfully), the position summary is a bulleted list of key responsibilities articulated as achievement-based objectives; that is, they start with a verb and represent the primary activities that an individual in this role will be expected to engage in on behalf of the organization and its mission.

- *Key experience and requirements*. This field should capture, again in a bulleted list, the

Job Profile Template	
Reports to:	**Direct Reports:**
Collaborators:	**Strengths:**
Position Summary:	
Key Experience & Requirements	**Culture & Accountability**
Technical Capabilities/Skills/Experience:	**Core Values Alignment:** **Bottom Line Responsibilities:**

E M A N C I P E T

Figure 29.2   Job profile template.

position requirements (e.g. education or degree requirements, years of experience, technical skills or proficiencies, etc.). In addition to the personal traits that are most essential for success *specifically* for this position, be sure to also include the skills or traits that are critical to the success of any person working anywhere in your organization.

- *Core values alignment.* This is simply a place on the job profile (which is or should be a document you can share with candidates as a one-page snapshot of the role) where you name your core values as a way of highlighting what they are and that they matter. You may consider also including your organization's foundational belief statement (see Chapter 28) if you do, in fact, plan to share this profile with candidates.
- Bottom-line responsibilities. While many roles may be accountable to all of your bot-

tom lines (see Chapter 28), there are circumstances in which a position may only be accountable to one or two. For example, if high-quality medical care is a bottom line and you're hiring a marketing professional, it may be that their role will be held accountable for other bottom lines (say, transformative service and sustainable finance in relation to Emancipet's bottom lines). but not that or those related to the delivery of medical care.

Creating Effective Job Postings

Once you've got your profile constructed, you're ready to draft a posting and begin the recruiting process. In fact that's easier said than done; after all, making your opportunity stand out – while also attracting candidates who have the skills and culture fit you're looking for – is not always a simple task.

Effective job postings should:

- Describe the organization and the phase you are in – make it exciting!
- Include all *required* skills (the ones you can't or won't train for).
- Frame skills as what the person should *love* to do, not what they can do.
- Convey your culture and values clearly (remember those key words).
- Include "Is it you?" statements or questions. These allow you to share the key elements of the job while appealing to the kind of person that fits in best with your culture and the people they will be working with most often. Sometimes framed as if/then statements ("If you love interacting with people then..."), this part of your posting has the most potential to be playful and creative.
- Ask for a cover letter specifically detailing why the candidate is a perfect fit.

Hiring Teams

Since hiring for culture means *knowing* your culture – and seeking a good fit – it's critical that your hiring teams reflect your culture well. To that end, your hiring team should have at least three members, and diversity is key: you don't want all members to come from one department or have a single perspective.

The members should include:

- The direct supervisor of the position you are hiring.
- A peer of the position you are hiring.
- A team member from a different department or different job function (when possible).

When deciding who should be on the hiring committee, look for team members who:

- Are genuinely curious about other people.
- Are respected and admired by staff (and embody the culture).
- Understand the organization's culture and feel protective of it.

Employment Information Sessions

At Emancipet, we require attendance at an information session to apply for open line staff positions. The goals and benefits of these sessions are that potential candidates learn about your organization:

- Less time is spent going over basics and answering frequently asked questions (FAQs) in interviews.
- Candidates can self-select out if they don't fit.
- Building a community of advocates who love your work and your culture.

Also, you learn about them:

- You have a chance to observe behavior to assess culture fit (rather than relying on a resume only).
- You can engage in some relationship building prior to interviews.
- You can include a larger group of staff to weigh in on the potential fit/hire.

This is what an information session should cover:

- Introduction to the organization – mission, values, beliefs, programs, etc.
- Description of the organizational culture and what a "fit" looks like.
- Description of "a day in the life" of the open position(s).
- HR details about the positions that are open (compensation, benefits, etc.).
- Details about the hiring process and timeline.
- Facility tour.
- Question and answer (Q&A) time at the end (post-presentation and tour).

Behavior Indicators

During every information session, staff observe the behavior of the candidates to watch for evidence of culture fit. The staff take notes and check off specific behaviors as they see them (Figure 29.3).

The behaviors you watch for should be based on your own culture and the qualities you know you need for a strong culture fit.

At Emancipet, the behavioral indicators used for assessment are:

- Friendliness – look for smiling, eye contact, laughing.
- Empathy – look for helping behaviors, yawn contagion, nodding along, leaning in.
- Mission enthusiasm – look for high energy, engagement during the tour and Q&A.

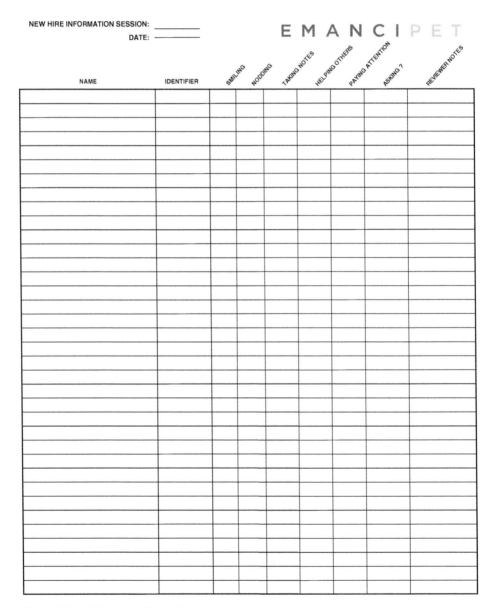

Figure 29.3   Behavior indicator form.

- Learning – look for asking questions, taking notes.

After the information session, participating staff compile individual lists that are then combined to create a final ranking. Using a tier system, the lists might include:

- First tier – Candidates whose behavior indicates high culture fit *and* whose resumes indicate strong skill/experience fit.
- Second tier – Candidates whose behavior indicates high culture fit but whose resumes lack strong skill/experience fit (based on our ability to train for the specific position).
- Third tier – Candidates whose resumes are stellar but who didn't have high culture fit scores.

Your first-tier candidates are those you want to schedule interviews with pronto! These are folks who seem like *just* the people you want on your team. Get those interviews scheduled and don't let them get away!

Second-tier candidates may still be individuals you want to interview (particularly depending on the size of your first-tier group). These are people you think will fit great *and* may require a more significant investment in terms of training and time to get up to speed.

Third-tier candidates are potentially highly skilled but not great when it comes to your perceived culture fit. You *might* want to interview individuals from this group to give them a phone or face-to-face opportunity to shine. This is the group with which it makes sense to be particularly thoughtful; it can be easy to be tempted by the pedigree or skills someone could bring to your team. Just make sure you're not jeopardizing anything else by way of a poor culture fit.

Next Up: Interviews

Interviewing candidates at least twice (regardless of whether you hold an information session or not) is a great practice, and allows you the space to have one conversation centered around culture fit and one around skills/experience fit.

Interviewing for Culture Fit

- When possible, the whole hiring team should participate in the interview.
- The tone of the interview should be:
  - Personal
  - Conversational
  - A genuine dialog.
- The questions are focused on learning about the candidate's:
  - Values
  - Beliefs
  - Behavior in certain situations.
- Leave at least 30 minutes for their questions.

Sample questions
- How would your best friend describe you?
- Tell us about a time you were caught up in a conflict with a co-worker – what was it about and how did you resolve it?

Interviewing for Skills/Experience Fit:

- When possible, the whole hiring team should participate in the interview.
- Start by sharing (in detail):
  - What the position will entail
  - What skills and abilities are most important to you in this position.
- The questions should be focused on learning about the candidate's:
  - Skills
  - Approach to work.

Sample questions:
- The most important thing this position will have to achieve in the first 30 days is X. What would be your approach to tackling that?
- What aspect of this position do you think you will excel at, and which will be the most challenging for you?

Once you've made offers, on-boarded, and trained staff, the sky's the limit if you can keep staff engaged.

Employee Engagement

Engaged employees are employees who feel a connection to the work they do that leads to fulfillment, connection, and satisfaction. Based on data points numbering in the many millions, the Gallup Organization defines engaged employees as "those who are involved in, enthusiastic about and committed to their work and workplace" (Harter 2018). It has gone on to develop and test a series of 12 questions by which an organization can assess engagement in an efficient and accurate way. Emancipet uses this tool, known as the Q12, on an annual basis to assess engagement, address areas of concern, and take the organization's temperature when it comes to healthy culture, employee opportunity, and the strength of connection to colleagues and mission. It's a critical tool to ensure that the time and energy spent making thoughtful hires for culture pay off in the long run, by keeping in touch with how engaged teams are (and, as a result, how likely they are to stay).

Building a great team is step one – keeping them engaged and in place requires living organizational values, regularly revisiting purpose, and maintaining allegiance to thoughtful bottom lines. When this is done well, there are few challenges that can't be tackled and the capacity for positive and meaningful impact increases almost infinitely.

Reference

Harter, J. (2018). Employee engagement on the rise in the U.S. *Gallup.com* (26 August). https://news.gallup.com/poll/24169/ employee-engagement-rise.aspx (accessed 22 August 2019).

30

Recruiting and Hiring HQHVSN Surgeons

James Weedon

Many organizations struggle to find the surgeon they need for their high-quality high-volume spay–neuter (HQHVSN) program. In fact, filling these essential positions may be the single biggest challenge such programs face as they try to end animal overpopulation with all its tragic consequences.

The current number of veterinarians in the United States is relatively small and they would all fit in a major university's football stadium. The majority of veterinarians are employed in private practice, but many are also employed by universities, pharmaceutical companies, the military, city, county, state, and federal government agencies. The demand is great in many areas. In this highly competitive environment, HQHVSN programs face some additional challenges. It is demanding work and many veterinarians do not consider it to be as exciting or prestigious as private practice or specialization in a specific area of interest. In addition, many veterinarians are under the impression that such programs cannot or will not offer competitive compensation. The challenge is to overcome often negative perceptions and find creative ways to meet financial expectations, so HQHVSN programs can recruit the quality people needed to do this very important work.

The Challenge

It helps to look at the situation from the veterinarians' point of view. There are several perceptions of HQHVSN – some of them accurate and some of them not – that need to be kept in mind to fashion job descriptions and recruitment messages that will attract the veterinarians needed.

1) *Quality concerns.* Any veterinarian should be very concerned about quality of care. Unfortunately, some veterinarians believe that the only way large numbers of spay–neuter surgeries can be performed is by cutting corners. HQHVSN programs cannot stress enough the fact that higher volume and lower costs are never achieved at the expense of quality. Ensuring and making it clear that HQHVSN programs adhere to recognized high standards will eliminate one of the major obstacles to attracting quality veterinarians.

2) *Fear of the numbers.* Some veterinarians are intimidated by the numbers of surgeries done on a daily basis at HQHVSN facilities. While an experienced surgeon at such a facility may do as many as 50 or 60 surgeries in a day, most veterinarians have never

High-Quality, High-Volume Spay and Neuter and Other Shelter Surgeries, First Edition. Edited by Sara White.
© 2020 John Wiley & Sons, Inc. Published 2020 by John Wiley & Sons, Inc.

done close to that number. The recruiting organization needs to be clear about expectations, but reassure prospective candidates that, if the desire is there, surgical speed will come with training and practice. Providing an opportunity to observe a good team in action will allow prospective candidates to see at first hand what can be achieved with a trained surgical team and proper procedures in place.

3) *The one-trick pony.* Veterinarians considering full-time work as HQHVSN surgeons may be concerned that they will become or be perceived as unable to function in a clinical practice situation. Address this concern by offering continuing education and encouraging involvement in local veterinary associations. They should be reminded that HQHVSN surgeons still examine animals, diagnose diseases and conditions, monitor patients, and improve lives. HQHVSN surgeons develop exceptional soft tissue surgery, anesthesia, and time-management skills, all of which are valuable in the veterinary market.

4) *Professional reputation.* Some veterinarians may worry about how their colleagues will view them if they work in a HQHVSN program. They may have heard the comments: "Reduced-cost or free surgical sterilizations cheapen the value of such surgeries," or "Veterinarians in those jobs can't make it in private practice." While such comments are unfair and untrue, they cause some to worry about their reputation or future employment opportunities. This situation has improved greatly in recent years with the advances and interests in shelter medicine and HQHVSN. Still, it is important that veterinarians working in HQHVSN programs stay involved with organized veterinary medicine so the profession recognizes that price does not determine quality and that they are current and competent. All veterinarians should understand that efficiencies and volume of procedures make the economies of HQHVSN programs very different from those in a typical private practice.

5) *Unfair competition.* Some private practitioners and veterinary associations argue that nonprofit HQHVSN programs take business from private practices and are unfair because of tax advantages. While there might be some truth to this, such operations generally provide a one-time service for clients who would most likely never have their pets altered in a private clinic. Additionally, such operations provide a service in sharing information with clients and encouraging them to take their pets to private veterinary clinics for routine care.

Job Description

Creating a written job description will help define the needs and expectations of the position. The resulting document will become an important part of the interview process, giving both the interviewer and the prospective candidate specifics to discuss and reducing the possibility of misunderstandings. As the job description is developed, the following should be considered:

1) *Organizational mission.* It is critical to make sure that any candidate for the position understands and is aligned with the mission of the organization (see Chapters 28 and 29).

2) *Type of clinic.* The veterinarian's role should be defined in the specific context of the type of clinic operation.

3) *Client/patient profile.* Most veterinarians have experience only with companion animals. If the clinic serves feral and/or shelter animals, it will be important, during the hiring process, to make this clear and to provide the candidate with resources to learn about the unique challenges of dealing with these special populations.

4) *The team.* It is very important to most veterinarians to have a strong support team in place that functions well together to get the job done. A strong team culture with capable support staff allows both veterinarians

and staff to apply their specialized knowledge and experience and to trust in and rely on the expertise of others on the team.

5) *Chain of command.* It is important to be clear about whether the position will report to an Executive Director, Director of Operations, Chief of Surgery, or directly to a Board of Directors. When the veterinarian reports to a non-veterinarian supervisor, it is important to clarify the factors that impact clinic decisions, to what extent the veterinarian is in control, and who has the final say. Specific considerations include whether current protocols are guidelines or must be strictly followed; who makes changes to protocols and the procedure for making such changes; who selects, evaluates, and disciplines the clinic staff; and the process for selection and purchase of medical equipment and supplies.

6) *Scope of services summary.* The job description should provide a summary statement to provide a general overview of responsibilities. Will the position be limited to HQHVSN or will additional veterinary services be required?

7) *Essential duties and responsibilities.* This is the heart of the job description. A list of specific duties and responsibilities assigned to the veterinarian should be included.

8) *Additional skills.* If the job requires certain language, computer, or other skills, they should be identified.

9) *Certificates, licenses, registrations.* In addition to a state veterinary license, list other requirements such as Drug Enforcement Administration (DEA) registration, malpractice insurance, etc.

10) *Work environment.* Noise levels, exposure to anesthetic gases, and other environmental factors intrinsic to the job should be listed.

11) *Physical demands.* The job might require that the veterinarian be able to perform such physical tasks as lifting patients, equipment, and supplies up to 50 lb in weight.

While many veterinarians want to help homeless animals and end animal overpopulation, the reality is that the job description and recruiting message must do more than tug at the heart strings or play to the conscience. Although the organization may be driven by mission, it must operate in a business-like manner. The goal is to attract veterinarians to HQHVSN by demonstrating that they will be fairly compensated (salary and benefits), treated professionally, and given the ability to have a real impact.

Compensation

The cost of a veterinary education is huge and most veterinarians graduate with debt. The payback for typical educational debt takes several years. The American Veterinary Medical Association (AVMA) routinely reports average debt and the average starting salary for graduating veterinarians. It also issues an annual report on the market for veterinarians (Hansen et al. 2018), giving the average salaries for veterinarians with varying years of experience in different areas of employment. While averages are good to know, it is more important to be competitive with total compensation for the position and location. There is great variation in the cost of living for different areas even within the same state. Knowing competitive salaries and benefits for the specific area is very important.

Salaries

Salaries for veterinarians are offered in several different methods. It may be a fixed salary, a percentage of revenue generated, or a combination. An example of such a combination would be when the veterinarian is given the greater of a "base rate" and/or a percentage of production. This assures the veterinarian of a reasonable salary, but also incentivizes them to be more productive. Other salary methods for HQHVSN surgeons could be pay by the day or by the surgery.

Benefits

Competitive benefits may include the following:

- Insurance (medical, life, disability)
- Reimbursement for state license, DEA, professional liability insurance, etc.
- Dues for veterinary associations and/or organizations
- PTO (paid time off) for holiday, personal, continuing education, and sick leave
- Continuing education allowance
- Retirement plan such as 401 k

It is important that all employees understand the benefit package and its value. Providing a list of the offered benefits and their cost/value is recommended. Benefits are a tax-advantaged way to compensate employees.

Professional Employer Organizations

It can be difficult for a small organization to offer the kind of benefits that a corporate or large private clinic can provide. A solution might be to use a professional employer organization (PEO). This works by becoming the legal employer of the staff for the purposes of payroll, employee benefits, workers' compensation, and human resources. By aggregating the employees of many businesses, a PEO can offer better rates on health and workers' compensation insurance, while giving employees better benefits. For the business owner, PEOs take on the headache of payroll taxes, regulatory compliance, and a gamut of human resources (HR) issues, from hiring to drafting an employee handbook to mediating conflicts. Using a PEO allows the organization to compete more effectively for employees. The organization manages the day-to-day activities of the employees and can concentrate on providing services rather than HR, insurance, and legal compliance with myriad state and federal regulations. PEOs have been around since the early 1980s. Because they help businesses comply with state laws, it is important to choose one that operates in the state where the business is located. The

National Association of Professional Employer Organizations' website (www.napeo.org) provides a list of member PEOs by state. Typically, PEOs require a one-time startup fee and then an ongoing percentage of the payroll, which can fluctuate depending on the services and the average worker salary.

Schedule/Lifestyle Issues

At some time in their careers, some veterinarians may be seeking a balance between their professional lives, personal lives, and/or family responsibilities. HQHVSN programs may be in a better position than a private practice to help them achieve that balance. Here are some things to be considered when crafting job descriptions and ads to appeal to these veterinarians:

- Surgery hours that enable the veterinarian to have shorter work days
- Job-sharing
- Part-time positions
- Flexible schedules
- Eliminating evening, weekend, and/or emergency duties
- Childcare assistance
- Absence of or fewer administrative and supervisory responsibilities
- Working with animals rather than with the guardians of animals
- Less "downtime"
- Feeling good about helping homeless animals, animal overpopulation, etc.
- Enjoying surgery and the feeling of accomplishment they get from altering enough animals to make a difference

Be proactive in communicating these very significant possible lifestyle advantages when possible.

Part-Time Veterinarians

One way to create positions with wider appeal and avoid the cost of benefits is to hire part-time veterinarians. Part-time employees who work fewer than two shifts per week typically do not receive benefits. Part-time employees working a minimum of two shifts a week may receive a percentage of the benefits, and those working 32 hours and above typically receive full benefits.

In addition to veterinarians only wanting to work part-time, there might be able surgeons performing all types of surgeries at private practices willing to work for HQHVSN programs one or two days a week. Another option might be veterinarians wanting to supplement their income by working on their days off from their primary employer. Part-time veterinarians may be paid by the hour, by the surgery, or by the shift.

Recruiting

There are several methods for recruiting veterinarians.

1) *Advertising*. While placing employment opportunities in veterinary journals is still a common practice, it is slow, costly, and usually lacking in results. Most veterinary schools have a website for postings. Local, state, and national veterinary associations and some national animal welfare organizations have electronic classifieds that are faster and cheaper than print ads. The goal is to reach a large number of potential candidates in a short period of time.

2) *Veterinary schools*. If the HQHVSN program has a good training veterinarian on staff who can mentor a new graduate and immediate high productivity is not an issue, the program might target the veterinary schools. They are generally very helpful in assisting senior students in finding positions prior to graduation. With many of the schools now having shelter medicine programs, many new graduates are interested and eager to become HQHVSN surgeons. Make sure that your organization has a mentorship program in place and is prepared to provide intensive surgery training to new graduates, as it can be a frustrating experience for both the

employee and the employer if appropriate expectations and training are not established beforehand.

3) *State board and local associations*. Most state boards of veterinary medical examiners will provide a list of all currently licensed veterinarians for that state along with their addresses. Many will provide the information in an electronic form for a very reasonable fee. With this information, a recruitment letter can be sent to every veterinarian licensed in the state or the list can be sorted to target specific zip codes for specific cities. Asking a member of the local association to take fliers to a meeting or requesting time to speak to the membership about the work of the organization are other good ways to get the word out. Careful attention to tone in recruiting letters or fliers may be necessary to avoid backlash or controversy if the local veterinary community harbors doubts or concerns about the HQHVSN clinic.

4) *Networking*. Networking with other HQHVSN programs can be an effective way to recruit. These organizations likely work with veterinarians in private practice and might know of someone thinking about making a change. Colleagues and veterinary distributor representatives may also be sources of candidates for the position. Networking and word of mouth work best alongside a good reputation for quality work and being a good employer. Past and currently employed veterinarians can often help recruit classmates and colleagues.

5) *Veterinary reception*. One might consider hosting an event for veterinarians at the HQHVSN facility. Not only might this attract veterinarians interested in the position, but it may also be a good way to educate local veterinarians about quality operations and help to dispel some misconceptions.

Selling the Position

In order to attract the attention of potential candidates for a position, it is necessary to highlight the positive attributes of the position. Here are some examples:

1) *Recruiting message.* A professional-looking message for ads or postings will be needed. It should provide positive highlights of the position, organization, and area. It is important to portray and be a good place to work and live.
2) *Be upbeat.* Don't depress candidates by dwelling on the enormity of the overpopulation problem or the number of homeless animals. Instead, tell the candidates how they can have a positive impact by working with the existing dynamic support team.
3) *Tout strengths.* If in a rural area with a lower cost of living, recreational activities, and good schools, use that as a selling point. If in an exciting city with great cultural opportunities, use that. The point is that every location and organization should offer some special qualities. Find those and highlight them.
4) *Accentuate the positive.* If the position offers part-time work with flexible hours and no emergency duties, mention that and get the attention of candidates looking for such opportunities. If the position offers great benefits in addition to a competitive salary, that would be an attention grabber.

The Interview

Before you do any interviewing, take some time to come up with a short list of non-negotiables for the position. Look at veterinarians that are/were successful at your organization and identify what they had that made them work so well. It can be things like high energy level, excellent communication skills, flexibility, and so on. Strong mission fit should always be one of the non-negotiables. Do not compromise on these traits when looking at candidates. Set up some questions or situations that will help you assess these traits. For example, if you want someone who is comfortable around clients and patients, walk them through the

lobby during check-in and see how many pets and people they engage with. Or if you want to assess their commitment to the mission, ask a question like: "How do you feel about owners that do not have enough money to have their pet on heartworm prevention?" Pay attention to "red flags"! For example, if a candidate expresses disapproval and concern about the conventions and standards of HQHVSN, this person will not be comfortable with the high pace that HQHVSN demands. You will end up having to spend a lot time convincing them to do things the way that you need them to.

It is important to have an organized and systematic plan for the interview. The interviewer should thoroughly review the candidate's resume before the interview. This will help in developing interview questions and demonstrate that the interviewer has taken the time to prepare for the interview. The interviewer should ask open-ended questions and listen carefully to the responses. Since it is illegal to ask any question that does not pertain to the applicant's ability to perform the job, the interviewer should confine the questions to the following topics:

- Why they want to work at your organization
- Background
- Education
- Skill
- Insight
- Personality
- Current situation
- References

During the interview, the interviewer should ask the following questions:

- What shifts or hours is the candidate willing to work? Are they willing to work on weekends or take emergency work (if necessary)?
- What is their minimum salary requirement? Some applicants are reluctant to give this for fear of underselling their skills or exceeding the hiring salary limits. The interviewer should make them comfortable with a starting point for negotiations.

- How far does the applicant live in relation to the job for commuting or will they be moving to the area?
- Will they be working for another organization if given the position?

The interviewer should remember that both parties are evaluating each other and should treat the candidate accordingly. They should offer professional courtesies such as touring the facilities, the opportunity to speak to prospective team members, and the chance to ask questions. It is also professional courtesy to follow up with all interviewed candidates to let them know whether they got the job and to give closure to the process.

There should also be a surgical interview whenever possible. The key indicators here are a willingness to learn new techniques and accept feedback. It is also important that the candidate has a talent for surgery and already has good tissue and instrument handling.

If the interview is successful and the interviewer determines that they want to hire a candidate, the negotiation process begins. The interviewer needs to determine what the candidate requires to accept the position. Often, with a little creativity, a position offer can be put together that is mutually acceptable. It may mean that the salary is increased and the candidate works more shifts in order to make a required compensation level. Or, it may mean that a moving allowance is needed to help defray the cost of relocation. It is very important that both parties enter the arrangement on a positive note.

The Offer

An offer letter is recommended so that the prospective employee understands the terms and conditions of the offer. The offer letter should cover the following:

1) *Compensation.* The letter should state the rate and method of pay. For example, is it $400 per shift, 22% of production, or the greater of two? Will they be paid weekly or every two weeks?

2) *Exempt position.* The letter should indicate if the position is considered an exempt position for purposes of federal wage and hour law, which means that the employee will not be eligible for overtime pay for hours worked in excess of 40 in a given week.

3) *Conditions of employment.* If employment is contingent upon passing a drug test within 24 hours of receipt of the letter and a background check, then the letter should state such conditions of employment. The prospective employee should be told not to give notice to a current employer until they have received confirmation that they have met the required conditions.

4) *Documentation for employment.* The letter should instruct the individual to bring appropriate documentation for completion of new hire forms, including proof they are eligible to work in the United States for I-9 purposes (or the equivalent in other countries).

5) *Contract or at will.* The letter should state if employment is "at will" or a term contract.

6) *Summary of benefits.* A summary of the benefits offered should be included in or attached to the offer letter.

7) *Acceptance of the offer.* The letter should state that the offer will expire in seven days if not accepted in writing.

Turnover

Recruiting and hiring the right surgeon for the position is such an important process because turnover can be a very costly event. If the person selected is not a good fit for the position and leaves, the entire process must be repeated, causing stress, loss of production, and considerable expense related to recruiting, hiring, and training the next person. The goal is to not only to hire a veterinarian who is a good fit for the organization, but also to retain that person as a valued employee. Helping the new employee adjust to the new position with feedback and coaching is important, as is valuing their ideas and allowing their input in decision-making. A formal performance and development review in the first three months and annually thereafter is a good policy to insure formal communication.

Bottom Line

Veterinarians must be viewed as highly skilled professionals with personal lives, bills to pay, career goals, a need to be respected, and a desire for personal satisfaction. Finding the right veterinary surgeon to meet the needs of an organization requires a recruiting plan that attracts qualified candidates, an interview process that identifies the best candidate, a mutually agreeable offer, and real effort by both parties to make the employment agreement a success.

Reference

Hansen, C., Salois, M., Bain, B. et al. (2018). *AVMA report on the market for veterinarians. Veterinary Economic Reports*. Schaumberg, IL: AVMA Veterinary Economics Division https:// www.aavmc.org/data/files/annual%20reports/ avma%20market%20for%20veterinary%20 education.pdf (accessed 20 August 2019).

31

Health Considerations for the HQHVSN Surgeon

Sara White

High-quality high-volume spay–neuter (HQHVSN) and shelter surgery can be rewarding, but at times it can also be physically, emotionally, and mentally challenging. Health and wellbeing are important not only for surgeons' quality of life, but also for their longevity in the field of HQHVSN, and the quality of patient care that they can provide. In this chapter general safety, physical ergonomics, and mental health, stress, and wellbeing are discussed, and information on how to minimize associated risks for surgeons and staff is provided.

General Safety Concerns

There are numerous hazards associated with animal care and surgical workplaces, and excellent resources are available that describe these hazards and provide precautionary measures to minimize their harm (see Box 31.1). These hazards may be chemical (waste anesthetic gases, disinfectants), biologic (zoonoses, allergies), or physical (patient handling concerns, equipment malfunction, sharps injuries). Because of the ready availability of these resources, discussion of general safety in this chapter will be limited to waste anesthetic gas exposure and animal handling safety.

Controlling Risks in the Workplace

The general approach to addressing risks in the workplace can be visualized as a risk control hierarchy pyramid (see Figure 31.1). The most effective techniques for reducing risk are at the top of the pyramid, while the least effective are at the bottom.

Not all problems will be amenable to all of these controls, nor are all levels of control practical: for example, it is impossible to eliminate risk of injury from animals in an animal care setting. But the higher up the hierarchy (eliminating the hazard or substituting a less hazardous alternative), the better and safer the solution. Relying on the bottom controls (administrative rules and protective gear) will not produce a robust safety environment.

Different workplace hazards may generate different solutions from different places on the hierarchy. In many cases, the staff involved in the task will be the ones who can devise the most usable solutions to the problem if given the permission and freedom to do so. This type of *participatory ergonomics* (Hignett et al. 2005) is capable of producing creative solutions as well as offering employees a sense of engagement in the process of finding solutions. Ultimately, this sense of engagement can be key to staff adopting and using new equipment, protocols, and procedures.

High-Quality, High-Volume Spay and Neuter and Other Shelter Surgeries, First Edition. Edited by Sara White.
© 2020 John Wiley & Sons, Inc. Published 2020 by John Wiley & Sons, Inc.

Box 31.1   Where to Learn More

Where to find other HQHVSN veterinarians

Association of Shelter Veterinarians (ASV). Online member forum, Facebook group, newsletter, conference tracks, and more: www.sheltervet.org

HQHVSNvets online group is a resource to facilitate communication and exchange of ideas among HQHVSN veterinarians. To subscribe email HQHVSNvets+subscribe@groups.io

Information specific to ergonomics in veterinary surgery and HQHVSN

Ergovet: www.ergovet.com

Surgical area and hospital hazards

OSHA's Hospital E-Tool. Applicable to human healthcare and veterinary care:

http://www.osha.gov/SLTC/etools/hospital/surgical/surgical.html
http://www.osha.gov/SLTC/etools/hospital/hazards/hazards.html

Workplace hazards in the veterinary profession

Centers for Disease Control and Prevention (CDC) Veterinary Safety and Health. Includes links to information about physical, biological, and chemical hazards in veterinary practice: http://www.cdc.gov/niosh/topics/veterinary

American Veterinary Medical Association (AVMA) Professional Liability Insurance Trust. Information about many aspects of occupational health and safety in veterinary practice: http://www.avmaplit.com/education-center/safety

SafetyVet. A consultant website with summaries and interpretations of Occupational Health and Safety Administration (OSHA) guidelines for veterinary practices: http://www.safetyvet.com/OSHA/OSHAdefault.html

Patient handling

American Association of Feline Practitioners (AAFP) Feline-Friendly Handling Guidelines: https://www.catvets.com/guidelines/practice-guidelines/handling-guidelines

Fear Free: https://fearfreepets.com

Low Stress Handling: Restraint and Behavior Modification of Dogs & Cats by Sophia Yin. Useful for decreasing stress on patient and stress and risk to handlers: http://drsophiayin.com/lowstress

Zoonotic diseases in shelters

American Humane, *Animal Shelter Operation Guide: Companion Zoonotic Diseases*:

https://www.americanhumane.org/publication/animal-shelter-operation-guide-companion-animal-zoonotic-diseases

Center for Food Security & Public Health, *Maddie's® Infection Control Manual for Animal Shelters Resources*:

http://www.cfsph.iastate.edu/Products/maddies-infection-control-manual-for-animal-shelters-resources.php

Mental health, crisis intervention, suicide prevention

ASV's crisis intervention resource list:

https://www.sheltervet.org/crisis-intervention

AVMA Wellness resources:

https://www.avma.org/professionaldevelopment/peerandwellness/pages/default.aspx
https://myvetlife.avma.org/rising-professional/your-wellbeing

Compassion Fatigue Strategies, online course at University of Florida, taught by Jessica Dolce:

https://sheltermedicine.vetmed.ufl.edu/education/courses/compassion-fatigue-strategies
https://jessicadolce.com/compassion-fatigue-strategies-ufl

Vetlife, a UK resource for veterinarians: www.vetlife.org.uk/mental-health

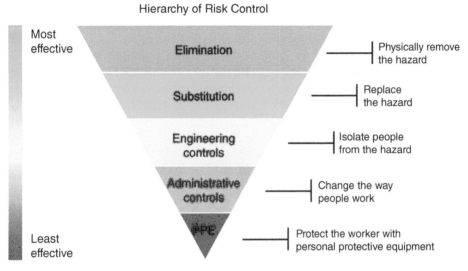

Figure 31.1 Hierarchy of risk control. Control methods higher on the hierarchy are potentially more effective and protective, leading to inherently safer systems with reduced risk of illness or injury. *Source:* Reproduced with permission of National Institute for Occupational Safety and Health (NIOSH).

Anesthetic Gases

Waste anesthetic gases are a potentially common chemical exposure in HQHVSN workplaces. There is conflicting evidence for the types and severity of health risks from trace levels of anesthetic gases in the work environment (ACVAA 2013; Molina Aragones et al. 2016). In many cases, studies showing potential health risks from occupational anesthetic gas exposure have looked at circumstances without waste gas scavenging (Nilsson et al. 2005) or using older anesthetic agents, including methoxyflurane, halothane, nitrous oxide, and enflurane (Shirangi et al. 2009). Health risks reported to be associated with waste anesthetic gases

(albeit with these older agents and inadequate scavenging) may include miscarriage (Molina Aragones et al. 2016), pre-term delivery (Shirangi et al. 2009), difficulty with balance and proprioceptive control (Vouriot et al. 2005), hematologic and blood chemistry changes (Casale et al. 2014), and genotoxicity (damage to DNA) (Yılmaz and Çalbayram 2016).

In addition to the possibility of individual health risks to workers, halogenated anesthetic agents contribute to ozone depletion, and isoflurane has a global warming potential over a thousand times that of carbon dioxide (Ishizawa 2011). Since most anesthesia scavenging systems simply exhaust the anesthetic gas unchanged to the outdoors, these systems do nothing to reduce the global environmental impact of these gases.

The only commonly used scavenging option that does not release gas into the atmosphere is activated charcoal canisters, which adsorb the anesthetic gas rather than releasing it; however, these canisters are one of the least effective methods of protecting staff from waste gas. Charcoal canisters are inconsistent in their performance, with certain brands adsorbing waste gas more effectively than others (Smith and Bolon 2003). If canisters are used, canister weight gain should be monitored and usage recorded daily so that canisters may be exchanged when exhausted (ACVAA 2013).

It is essential that all practices that use volatile anesthetic gases have a plan in place to minimize staff exposure to these gases. Reducing exposure to waste anesthetic gas should be accomplished by use of scavenging systems and safe protocols, rather than relying on personal protective equipment (PPE) (OSHA 1999). Surgical masks or charcoal masks are not effective at protecting workers from anesthetic agents (Centers for Disease Control 2017), nor are negative-pressure high-efficiency particulate air (HEPA) filters (ACVAA 2013). Effective protection could be achieved by use of respirator with a self-contained air source (Centers for Disease Control 2017), but these devices are expensive and awkward and are unlikely to be a practical alternative (ACVAA 2013). See Box 31.2 for techniques for decreasing anesthetic waste gas exposure in the HQHVSN workplace.

Box 31.2   Recommended Methods for Decreasing Anesthetic Waste Gas Exposure

- Reduce the clinic's use of anesthetic gases:
  - Choose anesthetic protocols that minimize or eliminate the use of inhalant anesthetics.
  - Choose the lowest appropriate gas flow rates consistent with patient safety and with the proper function of flow meters, vaporizers, and breathing systems.
- Use engineering controls to minimize anesthetic gas contamination of the work environment:
  - Ensure proper maintenance of anesthesia machines and anesthetic circuits.
  - Leak test anesthesia machines and breathing circuits daily.
  - Use a scavenging system (active or passive).
  - Consider the use of a keyed vaporizer filling system for liquid anesthetic, or use a drip-free bottle adapter to minimize spills during vaporizer filling.
  - Non-recirculating room ventilation systems can help decrease the concentration of waste gases inadvertently released into the room.

- Minimize or eliminate procedures that increase personnel exposure to anesthetic gas:
  - Avoid chamber induction of patients.
  - Minimize use of masking with anesthetic agents, or ensure tightly fitting mask.
  - Minimize use of uncuffed endotracheal tubes.
  - Avoid disconnecting patients from anesthesia circuit while flowmeter or vaporizer is on.
  - Avoid turning on vaporizer before patient is connected.
- Implement procedures to limit gas escape into the work environment:
  - Use a well-fitting endotracheal tube and inflate the cuff before turning on the vaporizer:
    - Add air to the cuff until there is no audible leak at a pressure of 10–12 cm of water.
    - Or, use a Posey cuff inflator.
  - Eliminate residual anesthetic gas from the breathing circuit prior to disconnecting patient. This may include:

- Turn off the vaporizer prior to completion of the anesthetic procedure. Ideally, the vaporizer should be turned off for five minutes prior to disconnection.
- For rebreathing systems, empty the breathing bag through the pop-off valve into the scavenger system periodically after the vaporizer has been turned off. Always empty the rebreathing bag before disconnecting the patient.
- For rebreathing systems, increase oxygen flow rate after the vaporizer has been turned off.
- Allow the patient to remain attached to the anesthesia machine and scavenger as long as possible without interrupting surgical flow.
  - Fill vaporizers when as few staff as possible are present:
    - In most stationary clinics, evenings are an appropriate time for vaporizer filling.
    - In mobile and mobile animal sterilization hospital (MASH) clinics, mornings prior to the beginning of anesthesia may be most appropriate in order to minimize driving with full vaporizers.
    - Pregnant personnel or personnel trying to conceive should not be present during filling. Staff should audibly announce that they are filling vaporizers so those who want to avoid exposure can leave the area.
  - Be prepared in case of a spill:
    - Spills of small amounts (several milliliters) will likely evaporate before cleanup is possible.
    - Larger spills such as a broken bottle require ventilation and cleanup:
      - Ventilate the area (open windows and doors if possible).
      - Use absorbent material such as cat litter to soak up the spill.
      - Sweep the used absorbent material into a container that can be sealed and disposed of.
      - If a spill occurs in the operating room and suction is available, it is acceptable to use suction to collect the spilled liquid.
- Create administrative procedures to monitor exposure:
  - Periodically, use anesthetic monitoring badges for individual staff members. Mail-in halogenated anesthetic gas monitoring badges are available from many veterinary distributors as well as other online sources.
- Utilize personal protective equipment (PPE):
  - Generally, PPE is not recommended during routine use of anesthetic gases.
  - Respirators are effective, but impractical and expensive.

Patient Handling

Patient handling presents one of the greatest risks to HQHVSN clinic staff. The most frequent employee injuries in veterinary practices include animal bites, strains from lifting animals, and slips and falls (often occurring during animal handling; Cima and Larkin 2018). Educating staff in appropriate animal handling is essential: low-stress animal handling techniques using appropriate restraint methods and equipment can decrease stress and risks to staff as well as patients (Yin 2009; Chapter 6 in this book). Lifting patients, whether awake and struggling or anesthetized and limp, is a common strain. Use of equipment such as lift tables and stretchers, where available, can reduce the strain of lifting. In situations without lifting equipment, a two-person lift, using bent knees and a straight back, may reduce risk of injury when lifting large dogs (AVMA-PLIT 2015). There is strong evidence that lumbar belts or supports do not prevent or reduce work-related low back pain (Waddell and Burton 2001).

Physical Ergonomics

Surgeons use their bodies to perform work. Like athletes and musicians, surgeons engage their entire body along with their mental concentration to produce skilled motor movements to accomplish a goal. Unlike athletes and musicians, surgeons are rarely taught the biomechanics of the movements and postures used in their work, and are often unaware of the way they use their bodies to perform.

Musculoskeletal Discomfort

Musculoskeletal loads during work – including static postures, awkward postures, repetition, and force – are related to musculoskeletal discomfort (MSD) in the areas subjected to the loads (McAtamney and Corlett 1993). Some HQHVSN surgeons have worked in the field for decades without experiencing work-related pain, but most experience some MSD that they attribute, at least in part, to their work (White 2013). The most common body regions in which HQHVSN surgeons experience discomfort are the lower back, neck, and shoulders. Hand regions with the greatest pain prevalence are the right thumb and wrist (White 2013). Low back pain is extremely common in the general population (Waddell and Burton 2001) and occurs at similar rates in HQHVSN veterinarians. Neck and shoulder discomfort is more common in HQHVSN veterinarians than in the general population (Hogg-Johnson et al. 2008), and is likely exacerbated by the forward bending of the neck during surgery (Esser et al. 2007; Szeto et al. 2010).

Discomfort tends to be greater in those surgeons who spend more hours in surgery each week, and in those who work in HQHVSN for more years. The actual *number* of surgeries each week is relatively unimportant; what matters is the amount of *time* the surgeon

spends in surgery (White 2013). This argues for efficiency – including skilled use of efficient surgical techniques and streamlined workflow – as well as for considering decreasing the number of hours per week in surgery for those who find themselves experiencing MSD.

Low job satisfaction and high work stress are important risk factors for MSD in veterinarians working in HQHVSN (White 2013) as well as in other practice areas (Smith et al. 2009; Scuffham et al. 2010). It is important to remember that pain is not entirely due to biomechanical factors. The experience of pain may be influenced by psychosocial factors, including job characteristics such as workload and lack of social or managerial support (Baird 2008), and by individual factors such as life stress, coping, and beliefs about and fear of pain (Asmundson et al. 2004). This chapter will return later to the subject of workplace stress.

Physical activity outside of work is known to be associated with lower prevalence of pain (Morken et al. 2007; Holth et al. 2008), and surgeons who are physically active experience less fatigue due to work (Rodigari et al. 2012). For people experiencing low back pain, maintaining daily activities as much as possible is associated with quicker recovery from symptoms (Waddell and Burton 2001). Staying physically fit, maintaining friendships outside of work, eating well, and maintaining a work–life balance are all ways to reduce work-related MSD and stress.

Veterinarians who experience MSD that concerns them should seek medical attention early in the course of the problem, rather than allowing pain to become chronic. Some cumulative trauma disorders are completely reversible if addressed early, but much more difficult to address once they have persisted for months or years (Proctor and Van Zandt 2008). Medical providers and physical therapists can perform diagnostics, provide physical activity recommendations and, if necessary, medications, and may be able to determine workplace factors that should be modified.

Physical Environment

Several factors in the physical environment that are easy to change can influence the surgeon's posture and comfort and can reduce the strains placed on the surgeon's body during work.

Surgery Table Height

At an appropriate-height surgery table, the surgeon's hands should generally be about 5–10 cm below elbow height (Pheasant and Steenbekkers 2005). In human medicine, failure to adjust the height of the operating table for each operation is associated with increased incidence of surgeon pain after performing surgery (Rodigari et al. 2012). In veterinary surgery, instead of adjusting between each patient, it would likely be sufficient to adjust the table between each patient size or category (for example, between large, medium, and small dogs, and cats). A table that is too low may result in the surgeon bending forward at the waist, upper back, and neck, leading to back pain and fatigue (see Figure 31.2). A table that is too high may result in the surgeon having raised shoulders and abducted elbows and upper arms, leading to neck, shoulder, and arm fatigue (see Figure 31.3).

For surgeons working in facilities with non-adjustable or inadequately adjustable table heights, the surgeon may need to increase their own effective height by standing on a stool or on exercise steps (such as for step aerobics), or to raise the patient height by placing the surgery table on blocks or risers, or placing a platform or foam support atop the existing table.

Patient Position on Table

The placement of the patient on the table is also important to shaping surgeon posture. A small patient placed in the center of a standard surgery table will require that the surgeon reach forward to access the surgery site (see Figure 31.4). This long reach leads to unnecessary strain and fatigue (Esser et al. 2007). Instead, small patients can be placed

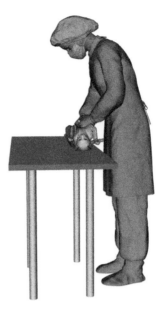

Figure 31.2 This surgery table is too low, so the surgeon bends forward at the at the waist, upper back, and neck.

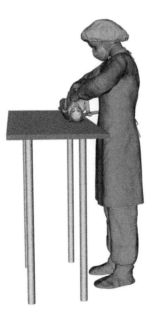

Figure 31.3 This surgery table is too high, so the surgeon raises her shoulders and abducts her elbows, leading to neck, shoulder, and arm fatigue.

to the side of the surgery table closer to the surgeon to minimize the need for reach (see Figure 31.5).

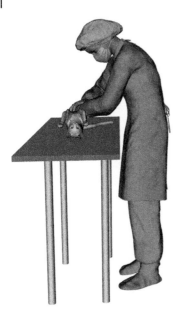

Figure 31.4 Placing this cat in the center of a standard-sized surgery table causes the surgeon to lean forward and reach to access the surgery site, leading to strain and fatigue.

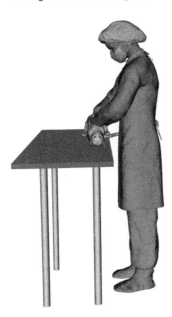

Figure 31.5 Appropriate table height and appropriate patient placement result in correct posture in this surgeon.

Sitting versus Standing

Most HQHVSN surgeons stand during surgery (White 2013), but research with surgeons operating on humans found that sitting for surgery, or alternating between sitting and standing, resulted in less general fatigue and less fatigue specifically in the spine and lower limbs (Rodigari et al. 2012). Sitting for surgery is most easily accomplished with a surgery table that allows the surgeon to sit close to the table with the surgeon's legs beneath the table. The table height will be lower than for standing surgery. Both of these demands may be difficult to meet with many standard pedestal surgery tables paired with a standard stool or chair. Optimal height of the surgery site relative to the surgeon's upper body is fairly easy to achieve while sitting for surgery with small patients (see Figure 31.6a). However, with larger, deep-bodied dogs, a surgeon sitting on a standard stool will find that the surgery site is too high, so that the surgeon's shoulders are raised and elbows abducted (see Figure 31.6b). In this scenario, the table cannot be lowered further due to interference with the surgeon's thighs.

A solution to the problem of the incorrect table height for large patients, as well as the problem of the table pedestal, can be the use of a saddle-shaped seat (see Figure 31.7). These seats produce a greater trunk-to-thigh angle, generating a more upright posture than a standard seat (Annetts et al. 2012), and allow the surgeon to position themselves close to the table without interference of the table pedestal or the table against the surgeon's thighs (see Figure 31.6c). Saddle seats allow for more appropriate lumbar and pelvic positioning than standard seats and may be helpful for those with low back pain (Annetts et al. 2012). Not all users find saddle seats comfortable, and others find that they are comfortable for short sitting periods but not for continuous use (Gadge and Innes 2007). Some HQHVSN surgeons with two surgery tables use a saddle seat at one table for the larger patients, and either stand or use a standard stool at the other table, alternating tables between each surgery. This allows the surgeon greater opportunity to change positions throughout the day and minimizes fatigue on any specific body regions.

(a)   (b)   (c)

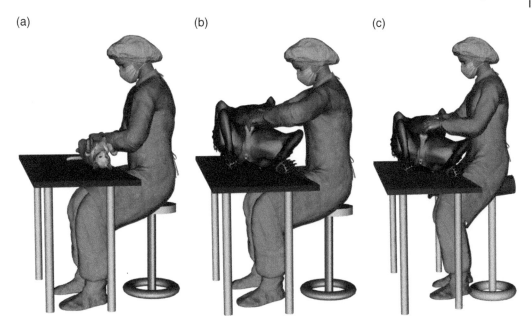

Figure 31.6   When sitting for surgery with a small patient (a) the surgeon is able to sit close to the table and maintain relaxed upper body positioning, but with a large dog (b) the surgeon sitting on a standard stool raises her shoulders and abducts her elbows to clear the patient's body. She is unable to lower the table or raise her stool, since her thighs are already in contact with the underside of the table. Using a saddle-shaped stool when operating on a large dog (c) allows the surgeon to achieve appropriate upper body position while still remaining close to the surgery table.

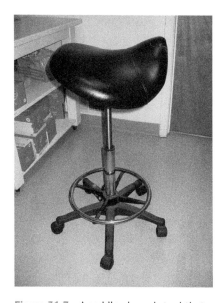

Figure 31.7   A saddle-shaped stool that can be purchased from a hairdressing supply store. This stool is adjustable in height and has brakes that engage when a person is seated, preventing it from rolling away from the table during surgery. *Source:* Photo courtesy of Bernie Robe.

Flooring and Footwear

Standing surgeons may experience less discomfort and fatigue in the back and lower limbs with the use of a floor mat (see Figure 31.8). The best mats tend to be thick but firm and elastic (Cham and Redfern 2001). Cushioned shoes (Lin et al. 2012) and insoles (King 2002) can also decrease fatigue during prolonged standing, while a combination of cushioned footwear and floor mat provides the best results.

Surgical Techniques and Movements

Surgical tasks in HQHVSN require a combination of repetitive movements that can at times require force, or may be performed with awkward positioning of the hands and wrists. Alone, each of these factors (repetition, force, posture) is only moderately associated with MSD of the hand and wrist; when combined, the association with MSD is strong (Bernard 1997).

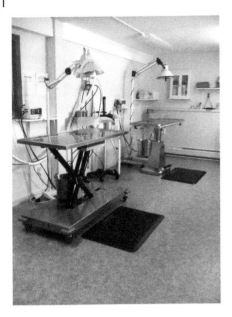

Figure 31.8 A surgical area with anti-fatigue floor mats and adjustable height tables. *Source:* Photo courtesy of Pamela Krausz.

To some extent, human bodies can adapt to these strains, given adequate time for rest, recovery, and adaptation. Ligaments will increase in strength, size, and collagen content with use (Solomonow 2009), so that the HQHVSN surgeon in regular work may have greater resilience than the new recruit. Performing repeated, unaccustomed movements with the hands can be a risk factor for hand and wrist disorders (Proctor and Van Zandt 2008), so it may be valuable to introduce new surgeons to HQHVSN with a lighter schedule, then work up to a full schedule once their bodies have become conditioned to the work. It is also worth remembering that there are safety risks associated with more mundane tasks like computer work. Repetitive motions and sustained postures used while on the computer or while texting or using a tablet may exacerbate the risk of activities in surgery, so should be considered when looking at an individual surgeon's risk profile.

This section will describe some of the ways in which surgeons may reduce the risks from these factors.

Repetitive Motions

Repetitive motion is inherent in any high-volume workplace that has a limited variability in tasks. Fortunately, spay and neuter procedures contain multiple steps – such as autoligation (see Chapter 12), suture knot tying, and suturing – each of which requires different hand motions. The use of efficient high-volume techniques will minimize the need for excessive repetition of any of these motions in each procedure. Short incisions require less suturing, and autoligation in cats and male puppies will require less suture knot tying. In addition, efficient techniques and shorter incisions result in fewer overall movements per procedure, reducing the cumulative number of repetitions required for a given number of procedures. This may be why MSD appears to be more related to hours in surgery rather than numbers of surgeries. The number of movements per hour may be the same for "fast" and "slow" surgeons, but the "slow" surgeons require more movements to complete each surgery.

Instrument Grips

In addition to reducing the overall number of movements in a surgery, surgeons can reduce repetition by varying their techniques during and between surgeries, such as by using hand ties for some suture ligations and instrument ties for others. Another way to limit repetition is to use different grips when holding instruments, such as by choosing a tripod grip for some portions of the surgery, and a palm grip for others (see Figure 31.9). The tripod grip is generally considered to be more precise because the digits are used to control the instrument (Toombs and Bauer 1993), whereas the palm grip relies more upon movements in the hand and forearm to provide control, although some research suggests that palm grasp may actually be more accurate (Seki 1988). Some HQHVSN surgeons report decreased hand discomfort with the use of palm grip, and others report increased strain and discomfort in the area of the flexor tendons of the wrist when using the palm grip.

(a)

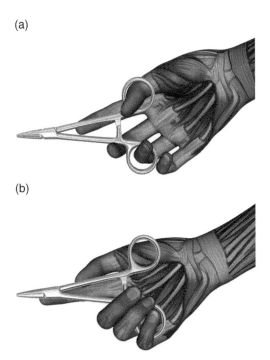

(b)

Figure 31.9 Methods for grasping the needle holder. (a) The tripod grip allows finer control and uses muscles of the fingers and hands to manipulate the instrument, and (b) the palm grip relies more upon muscles of the hand and arm than upon the fingers.

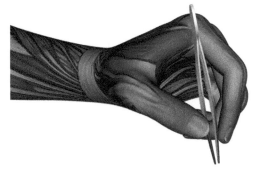

Figure 31.10 The pinch grip is used for thumb forceps. This grip can be fatiguing and may exacerbate discomfort in people with hand pain.

Awkward Hand and Wrist Positions

Awkward hand and wrist postures include pinch grip, ulnar or radial deviation of the wrist, and extreme wrist flexion or extension (Bernard 1997). An example of a pinch grip is the use of thumb forceps (see Figure 31.10). Some surgeons minimize the use of thumb forceps, particularly when performing skin closure, both in order to reduce tissue trauma to the patient's skin as well as to reduce the hand strain from the sustained pinch grip.

In most cases, awkward postures with extreme flexion, extension, or ulnar or radial deviation are not necessary to perform HQHVSN, but surgeons may inadvertently use awkward grips and techniques. Since it can be difficult to observe one's own movements during surgery, it can be useful to record video or take photographs during surgery in order to evaluate hand motions and postures. Many mobile phones have the capability of recording video and may be mounted and secured in a location to allow recording of the surgical procedure. Alternatively, a second person may be able to record video while the surgeon works.

Forceful Motions

Fortunately, spay and castration procedures do not often require the application of high forces by the surgeon. The two main times when force is required is while tying knots with large suture, and during adult dog castration.

Suture Size and Knot Tying Force   Secure knot tying (see Figure 31.11) requires that the surgeon apply forces to the ends of the suture equivalent to 80% of that suture's breaking strength (Mazzarese et al. 1997). For 3-0 absorbable monofilament suture, breakage occurs at 3.9 lb of force, whereas with size 1 suture, breakage occurs at 11.2 lb (USP 2006). Thus, a secure knot with 3-0 suture will require the surgeon to apply just over 3 lb of force with each throw, but a secure knot using size 1 suture requires nearly 9 lb of force on every throw. Human ligaments are affected by cyclic loading, and a repeated load of 9 lb has been associated with ligament inflammation and muscle excitability (Solomonow 2009). Without adequate rest, this chronic use and inflammation can lead to ligament damage and pain.

By selecting appropriately sized suture, surgeons can avoid the need to apply unnecessary

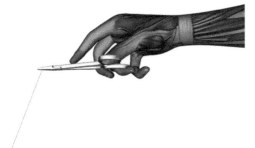

Figure 31.11 Use of force when tying knots in large-gauge suture with the tripod grip places strain on the tendons and ligaments of the thumb and wrist.

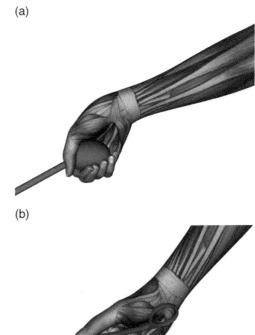

Figure 31.12 Exteriorization of the testicle during closed castration of large dogs requires force. Grasping the testicle by hand (a) leads to an awkward hand posture with ulnar deviation of the surgeon's wrist, and requires considerable grasping strength in the fingers due to the testicle's shape and slippery texture. Using a hemostat across the spermatic cord (b) allows the surgeon to maintain a straight position through the wrist, and enables a more secure grip.

force during knot tying. Some veterinary surgeons tend to choose inappropriately large suture sizes (Boothe 1993). Suture that is larger than necessary does not decrease the possibility of dehiscence. Also, avoiding inappropriately large suture sizes minimizes the amount of suture that must be absorbed by the animal's body.

Applying Force in Dog Castration Many surgeons find that considerable hand and arm strength is required to grasp and exteriorize the testis during closed castration of large, mature dogs. Various techniques may decrease the force required to accomplish exteriorization of the testes in these dogs. An open castration may be performed instead of a closed castration, as the tissues present very little resistance during open castration. If closed castration is preferred, the fibrous attachments between the vaginal tunic and the subcutaneous tissue may be sharply dissected rather than broken by traction. Further, once the spermatic cord is exposed, the surgeon may use a hemostat to clamp the cord just proximal to the testis to provide a more favorable grip for applying traction, rather than grasping the testis itself (see Figure 31.12).

Movement during the Surgery Day

Being able to change position during an operation or, by extrapolation, between successive short operations, is associated with decreased fatigue. Fatigue during surgery leads to pain after surgery (Rodigari et al. 2012). "Micropauses" of 15–30 seconds taken multiple times per hour (for example, between each surgery, or for long surgeries, during the course of the surgery) are shown to reduce MSD, especially if combined with stretches or exercises (Barredo and Mahon 2007). Some HQHVSN veterinarians do this by listening and moving to music, stretching during or between surgeries, and taking brief breaks between surgeries for stretching, yoga, or dancing (White 2013).

Posture and Technique

Some surgeons may find themselves adopting less than ideal postures when using certain suture patterns or surgical techniques. In some cases, modifications to surgical routine can drastically change postural demands. For example, when performing a continuous subcuticular suture, right-handed surgeons suturing from left to right may adopt a posture with twisted torso and abducted arm (see Figure 31.13a). If instead the continuous suture is performed right to left in right-handed surgeons (from left to right in left-handed surgeons), the need for twisting and arm abduction is eliminated (see Figure 31.13b). However, the new posture may create the need for greater wrist extension and lateral wrist deviation, which may be uncomfortable for surgeons with pre-existing hand or wrist problems.

Brief and intermittent twisting, bending, limb abduction, or wrist deviation is unlikely to result in pain or fatigue. However, if these postures are difficult or uncomfortable to perform, or cause post-operative discomfort, the simplest solution may be to adopt alternative surgical techniques where appropriate, such as using a buried simple interrupted subcuticular suture pattern rather than continuous pattern for short incisions.

Surgical Instruments and Needles

Surgical instruments are central to the task of surgery, but poorly designed or maintained surgical instruments can cause unnecessary musculoskeletal strain on the surgeon. Hemostats and needle holders should not require excessive force to operate the jaws. Some needle holders require several kilograms of force to close the ratchet, and over 1 kg of lateral push to disengage the ratchet (Patkin 1970). More appropriate force would be 3–5 lb to close, and less than 1 lb to open the ratchet.

Instrument sizes should be appropriate to the task and sized comfortably for the surgeon's hands. Appropriate instrument cleaning,

(a)   (b)

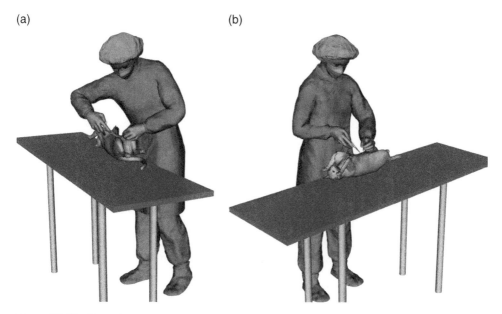

Figure 31.13 Sometimes poor posture can be solved by improving surgery technique. When a continuous subcuticular closure is performed from left to right by a right-handed surgeon (a), the surgeon's posture is twisted and her arm is abducted. However, when the surgeon sutures the same incision from right to left (b), she remains upright, with her only postural concern being the wrist extension and ulnar deviation of her right wrist.

lubrication, repair, and sharpening will maintain instrument quality and reliability, and avoid placing increased strain on the surgeon using them. If reusable needles are used, they should be disposed of when no longer sharp to prevent the need for the surgeon to apply increased amounts of force to patient tissues (Patkin 1970) and to reduce tissue trauma.

Surgical Environment

Noise, ambient temperature, and lighting are environmental factors that can affect staff comfort and stress level, as well as the stress and comfort level of patients (particularly cats). Minimizing noise from dogs in the surgery area can be accomplished by separating the kennel area from surgical areas whenever possible. Temperature in surgery should be kept at a comfortable room temperature, and lighting should be adequate for clear visualization without producing excessive glare.

Vision and Lighting

Lighting in the Surgical Suite
Lighting in the surgical suite should be adequate for staff to observe and monitor patients during induction through recovery. Task lighting over surgical prep areas may be beneficial. More muted lighting in kennels or post-recovery areas may help reduce stimulation and agitation among kenneled patients and may assist in smoothing recovery.

The surgery lighting should be adequate to illuminate the surgical field without excessive glare. Surgical lighting is accomplished in most stationary clinics by using ceiling or floor-mounted surgical lights, while MASH clinics and some stationary and mobile clinics may use a table-mounted lamp or headlamps for this purpose. If a lamp is used, compact fluorescent or light-emitting diode (LED) lights are recommended, as they produce less heat (and thus are less uncomfortable to stand near) than incandescent lights with similar brightness.

It is worth noting that the light required by a person to perform a given task increases with age (Schlangen 2010). This increased need for light may exacerbate vision trouble due to the onset of presbyopia (see next section). Some HQHVSN surgeons may find that surgical lighting that was once adequate must be updated or supplemented as they age in order to attain the levels of contrast they need to perform surgery.

Be aware that the specifications of a light and the spectrum of wavelengths emitted may affect color perception and may thus affect patient assessment and care. This is applicable to room lighting as well as surgical and task lighting. "Warmer" lights with a lower Kelvin value produce yellow or orange color perception and "cooler" lights with a higher Kelvin value can create a bluish cast and even an appearance of cyanosis in patients. Either extreme may cause inaccuracies in patient assessment. Recommended lighting in the surgical suite should have a color rendering index (the ability to render color accurately) over 90 and should include a broad spectrum of wavelengths, including those in the red spectrum over 600 nm, where the difference in spectral transmittance between oxyhemoglobin and reduced hemoglobin becomes maximal (Schlangen 2010) in order to allow accurate assessment of cyanosis.

Corrective Lenses for Surgery
Some surgeons require the use of corrective lenses (glasses or contacts) throughout their career, while others only begin to need visual correction as they age. At around age 40, most people begin to lose the ability to focus on near objects, a condition called presbyopia (du Toit 2006). At some point in their 40s, many surgeons find that they can no longer focus clearly on the surgical field and that they require corrective lenses during surgery. Surgeons who use eyed needles and suture from a cassette may notice the need for corrective lenses sooner than those who use swaged-on suture, as needle-threading is often performed at a shorter focal distance than the surgery itself.

Many HQHVSN surgeons use over-the-counter reading glasses for presbyopia correction during surgery. Those who need corrective lenses and for whom over-the-counter glasses are unsuitable, inadequate, or uncomfortable should work with an optometrist to select the appropriate vision correction. Some HQHVSN veterinarians wear progressive lenses for surgery, but not all are happy with their everyday progressive lenses for use during surgery. An optometrist can help select the appropriate lens refractive power and regions of refractive power for the individual's specific workplace needs (Long 2003).

Some surgeons use contact lenses for vision correction during surgery. For some, these are their everyday contact lenses that allow for near and far vision. This may be accomplished using multifocal contacts, or with contacts with one eye for near vision and one eye for far vision. These configurations may be combined with reading glasses for particularly fine tasks like ophthalmic surgery. Other surgeons choose to have a set of contacts optimized for near vision for use during surgery and similar tasks, and a different set of contacts for near and far vision for driving and everyday use.

If an HQHVSN surgeon is contemplating having a vision correction surgery (such as LASIK) or cataract surgery, they should be sure to discuss their particular needs and preferred focal distance(s) with their surgeon prior to the surgery. While cataract surgery is not primarily performed to correct near- or far-sightedness, this surgery involves the implantation of a new intraocular lens and thus can affect the ability to focus at different distances. Some veterinarians have reported dismay at discovering that their post-cataract surgery focal distance is inappropriate for their work, and would have benefited greatly from prior discussion with their surgeon about job tasks. Various types of intraocular lens implants are available and it should be possible to find one that suits one's needs.

Ergonomics and Glasses From an ergonomics perspective, it is important to ensure that the use of glasses, whether over the counter or prescription, does not adversely affect the surgeon's posture by influencing head and neck position (see Figure 31.14). Glasses frames that block the lowest portion of the visual field, or that do not reach the lowest portion of the visual field, will require the surgeon to work with a greater head and neck angle, since the eyes can no longer be inclined downward at as great an angle as without glasses (White 2018a). Wearing glasses low on

(a)   (b)

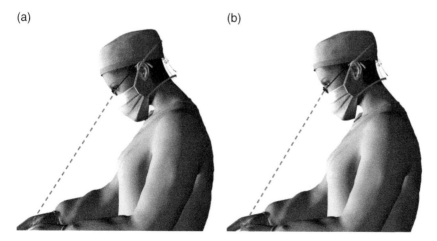

Figure 31.14 Neck position during surgery may be influenced by the fit of glasses. (a) When glasses block the lowest portion of the visual field, the surgeon's neck angle is 40°, but (b) when the glasses are designed to sit low enough on the nose to include the lowest portion of the visual field, the surgeon's neck angle decreases to 32°.

the nose if they are not designed to be worn this way is likely to be uncomfortable and may lead to the glasses slipping or falling off during surgery. Half-glasses with a thin, lightweight frame that sit low on the nose or progressive lenses with a thin frame can allow the surgeon to use the lowest portion of the visual field and thus allow for a less extreme neck angle.

Fogged Lenses and Surgery Masks Those who wear glasses and a face mask for surgery may have experienced fogging of the lenses. Several suggestions for decreasing fogging exist in the literature and anecdotally, and work either by redirecting the breath away from the top of the mask, or by changing the surface properties of the lenses. To redirect the breath, some have suggested using a piece of adhesive tape over the bridge of the nose to divert breath away from the lenses (Karabagli et al. 2006). Anti-fog surgical masks work on a similar concept and use adhesive, foam, or film to keep condensation from escaping out the top of the mask. Other authors suggest crossing the mask's ties behind the head, such that the upper ties are tied at the base of the skull, and the lower ties are tied atop the head, redirecting the breath out the sides of the mask (Jordan and Pritchard-Jones 2014). This technique is not applicable to ear-loop masks. Other authors have suggested washing the lenses with soap and water prior to each donning, leaving a surfactant layer that prevents fogging (Malik and Malik 2011); some HQHVSN vets suggest the use of cleaning/defogging solutions designed for scuba masks.

Mental Health, Stress, Wellbeing

In addition to attending to physical workplace health, the HQHVSN veterinarian, staff, and management should be aware that there are psychosocial aspects that affect workplace health as well. These psychosocial factors are,

on their own, important to the wellbeing of the veterinarian and staff. They are also important in that they impact the severity and prevalence of musculoskeletal pain, as described previously.

The HQHVSN Workplace

There is no single type of HQHVSN job or workplace, but many share common features. HQHVSN surgeons often practice in relative isolation from other veterinarians, making it challenging for them to exchange concerns, advice, and information. Their work requires speed and precision. There are often resource limitations paired with high work demands. And, as in any workplace, there may be conflicts with other staff, with management, and with clients.

Stress

"Stress" is an interaction between the pressures and demands placed upon a person (stressors) and the person's assessment of their own ability to cope with those demands (Baird 2010). For some veterinarians HQHVSN is not at all stressful, whereas others experience it as extremely stressful (White 2013). HQHVSN surgeons may avoid some stressors noted in general practice veterinarians, such as client interactions, but may have greater exposure to other stressors such as consciousness of time pressure (Smith et al. 2009).

In any workplace, high work demands paired with low control or decision latitude is a recognized source of strain (Bartram et al. 2009). In some cases, HQHVSN veterinarians may feel as though they do not have adequate control in their job, and may be frustrated in situations in which their managers are non-veterinarians. Veterinarians may find it particularly stressful if they feel pressure to provide care to more animals than they believe they can safely serve, or they feel that they are unable to provide high-quality care with the resources they have available. Good communication between manager and veterinarian is key, and each should work to recognize the pressures, demands, and point of view of the other.

Mental Health

Veterinarians overall appear to be no more at risk for mental illness than those in the general population, but certain sub-groups of veterinarians – young, female veterinarians, and those who work alone rather than with others – are at higher risk than other veterinarians for suicidal thoughts, mental health difficulties, and stress (Platt et al. 2012). While there is no published data about mental health in HQHVSN veterinarians, shelter veterinarians (many of whose work consists primarily of spay–neuter) do appear to be at higher risk for serious psychological distress (Nett et al. 2015). Also, many shelter and HQHVSN veterinarians are young and female (White 2013) and work apart from other veterinarians, placing them in a higher-risk demographic. The suicide rate published for the veterinary profession is approximately four times that of the general population, and twice that of other health professionals (Bartram and Baldwin 2010). While no one is certain of the reasons for this, most authors propose that it is due to a combination of personal characteristics, feelings of stress, and having medical knowledge and access to medications.

Any veterinarian who is experiencing anxiety, depression, thoughts of suicide, or other mental health problems should seek the care of a health professional. Box 31.1 contains resources for crisis intervention and links to more information about veterinarians, mental health, and suicide. Anecdotally, many HQHVSN surgeons report experiencing anxiety, stress, and/or depression at some point in their professional career, and many have been able to receive support and advice from their peers in the field.

Complications and Stress

Performing surgery can be stressful, and events that occur while in surgery can increase the amount of intraoperative stress experienced. Unlike workers in other industries in which the safety of others is at stake, surgeons are not typically trained in stress management or how to mitigate the effects of stress on surgical performance (Arora et al. 2010).

All veterinary practices that perform surgery experience peri-operative complications and deaths. In HQHVSN, the high volume of surgeries performed means that, even in clinics with exceptionally low mortality rates, some peri-operative deaths will occur. Peri-operative deaths can lead to feelings of guilt, responsibility, and self-blame, as well as grief and sadness (Lin et al. 2012; White 2018b). When a patient death occurs, fear, grief, or self-doubt can make it difficult to continue with the day's scheduled surgeries, but the schedule of many HQHVSN clinics makes it difficult or impossible to interrupt the work schedule for debriefing and time away.

After a serious adverse event or patient death, HQHVSN veterinarians have described a variety of ways of coping with and moving past the incident. Once the acute emotional reactions subside, four factors appear important for successful coping (White 2018b). *Technical learning* can help veterinarians decrease future occurrences of similar adverse events and can improve the veterinarian's and team's skills and boost confidence. Finding *perspective* by placing the event in a larger context (such as the value the HQHVSN program provides to the community, or the context of one's religious faith) can help to mitigate the trauma of the event without minimizing its importance. Seeking and receiving *support* from colleagues can help in many ways, providing technical help, psychological support, and the knowledge that others have experienced similar events. And finally, *emotional learning* can help veterinarians learn how to handle and support themselves through an adverse event. Mindfulness training, psychotherapy, and compassion fatigue training are all examples of ways veterinarians can learn to understand, accept, and manage their own reactions and build resilience.

Managers and institutions also have a role in fostering open communication and creating a workplace that allows for discussion of complications and error without blame, shame, and fear. Candid discussion of deaths, errors, mistakes, and mishaps can be taboo in medicine: surgeons often have the expectation that they should perform flawlessly (Wu 2000). In HQHVSN, there appears to be more open discussion of complications and near misses than in many medical fields; however, HQHVSN veterinarians may still benefit from increased discussion of early recognition of danger, errors, decision-making, expertise, and error recovery (Patel et al. 2011). For those who work in facilities without access to peers, electronic listservs and other online forums can be valuable resources that allow communication with other HQHVSN surgeons (see Box 31.1 for resources).

Conclusion

HQHVSN is an exciting and rewarding field that presents physical, emotional, and mental challenges. With careful attention and good management, veterinarians, staff, and supervisors can minimize the risks presented by work in HQHVSN and provide a high-quality, caring, and humane environment for both animals and staff.

References

ACVAA (2013). Commentary and recommendations on control of waste anesthetic gases in the workplace. American College of Veterinary Anesthesia and Analgesia. http://www.acvaa.org/docs/2013_ACVAA_Waste_Anesthetic_Gas_Recommendations.pdf (accessed 10 November 2018).

Annetts, S., Coales, P., Colville, R. et al. (2012). A pilot investigation into the effects of different office chairs on spinal angles. *Eur. Spine J.* 21 (Suppl 2): S165–S170.

Arora, S., Sevdalis, N., Nestel, D. et al. (2010). The impact of stress on surgical performance: a systematic review of the literature. *Surgery* 147: 318–330, 330 e1-6.

Asmundson, G., Norton, P., and Vlaeyen, J. (2004). Fear-avoidance models of chronic pain: an overview. In: *Understanding and Treating the Fear of Pain* (eds. G. Asmundson, J. Vlaeyen and G. Crombez), 3–24. Oxford: Oxford University Press.

AVMA-PLIT (2015). Preventing back injuries. *Safety Bulletin*, p. 23. https://www.avmaplit.com/education-center/library/preventing-back-injuries (accessed 22 August 2019).

Baird, A. (2008). Teaching about musculoskeletal disorders – are we barking up the wrong tree?

In: *Contemporary Ergonomics 2008: Proceedings of the International Conference on Contemporary Ergonomics (CE2008), 1–3 April 2008, Nottingham, UK* (ed. P.D. Bust), 441. Boca Raton, FL: CRC Press.

Baird, A. (2010). Ergonomics and occupational 'stress' – where do we stand? In: *Contemporary Ergonomics & Human Factors 2010* (ed. M. Anderson), 350–359. London: Taylor & Francis.

Barredo, R.D.V. and Mahon, K. (2007). The effects of exercise and rest breaks on musculoskeletal discomfort during computer tasks: an evidence-based perspective. *J. Phys. Ther. Sci.* 19: 151.

Bartram, D.J. and Baldwin, D.S. (2010). Veterinary surgeons and suicide: a structured review of possible influences on increased risk. *Vet. Rec.* 166: 388–397.

Bartram, D.J., Yadegarfar, G., and Baldwin, D.S. (2009). Psychosocial working conditions and work-related stressors among UK veterinary surgeons. *Occup. Med. (Lond.)* 59: 334–341.

Bernard, B.P. (ed.) (1997). *Musculoskeletal Disorders and Workplace Factors: A Critical Review of Epidemiologic Evidence for Work-Related Disorders of the Neck, Upper Extremities,*

32

Stationary Clinics
Karla Brestle

Stationary high-quality high-volume spay–neuter (HQHVSN) clinics are located in a facility that is dedicated to providing spay and neuter services. These clinics may or may not provide a regional animal transport to their facility. Stationary clinics may work with a wide variety of shelters, humane societies, and other animal welfare organizations in their communities to provide affordable surgeries to economically disadvantaged clients.

The American Society for the Protection of Cruelty to Animals (ASPCA) Spay/Neuter Alliance (ASPCAPro 2018) mentorship program provides guidance for the establishment of full-time stationary clinics, and this model will provide the basis for this chapter. However, other models for stationary HQHVSN locations exist, and these models may have different financial, capacity, and staffing requirements from those of a full-time HQHVSN clinic. Stationary clinics within shelters may operate only part-time by sharing staff and equipment between shelter medicine, shelter surgery, and HQHVSN services. Alternatively, a "mini-clinic" model has been proposed and implemented in some locations, in which a smaller, donated, or low-cost dedicated spay–neuter clinic space operates part-time with part-time or per diem staff (Spay FIRST! 2017). However, these hybrid and mini clinic models are beyond the scope of this chapter and will not be covered further.

Stationary Clinic Requirements and Structure

In general, the success of the full-time stationary clinic model depends upon its financial sustainability, which in turn is dependent upon having sufficient local need to allow the clinic to operate at full capacity.

Capacity and Need

To be financially sustainable, a full-time stationary HQHVSN clinic must be able to fill its schedule. Typically, this requires that the clinic perform 35 surgeries per vet per day, 5 days per week, 48 weeks per year. In order to achieve this volume of surgeries, the ASPCA Spay/Neuter Alliance recommends that clinics be located in an area with a human population of at least 250 000 in a 60-mile radius of the clinic. The actual human population required to support a full-time stationary HQHVSN clinic may vary depending on geographic accessibility, region and regional need (for example, northern vs. southern USA), and grant or donor funding to subsidize surgeries for clients with no ability to pay.

There must be a considerable need for the service in the proposed region. If there is an existing spay–neuter program nearby that is

High-Quality, High-Volume Spay and Neuter and Other Shelter Surgeries, First Edition. Edited by Sara White.
© 2020 John Wiley & Sons, Inc. Published 2020 by John Wiley & Sons, Inc.

capable of meeting the need, energies and resources may be better spent in a collaborative effort. At the very least, an open discussion between the proposed and existing organizations is in order.

Budget

When starting a stationary clinic, an organization must have the ability to raise funds to support the procurement and remodel of a suitable building and to purchase the necessary equipment and supplies. Additional funds will be required for staff training, and it is advisable that the organization acquires a minimum of $35 000 reserve on opening day.

Budgeting for Transport

In the initial planning phases of a stationary clinic, a determination must be made as to whether the clinic will provide services solely as a stand-alone facility or will include a regional transport service. Transport is the act of going into surrounding communities, picking up the animals scheduled for sterilization surgeries, transporting them to the stationary clinic, and then returning them to the pick-up site to be reunited with their caretakers or owners. See later in this chapter for details on transport protocols.

Transport programs require the additional initial expenses of procuring a suitable transport vehicle and hiring a staff member to drive that vehicle. Ongoing expenses include vehicle expenses (ongoing fuel costs to provide the transport, insurance, registration, maintenance, and eventual replacement), as well as staff expense for a driver and, in larger programs, a transport manager.

The advantages of transport include the ability to serve a larger area and to reach clients with limited transportation access while also maximizing the use of their veterinarians' and technicians' time. Unlike mobile units and mobile animal sterilization hospital (MASH) spay–neuter programs in which veterinarians

and technicians must spend part of their workday traveling, stationary clinics with transport are able to serve a large area by allowing veterinarians and technicians to remain in a centralized location while animals are transported to them. This greater efficiency is an advantage both for budget and for the number of surgeries in a given workday.

Initial Funding

Many stationary HQHVSN clinics operate under a nonprofit structure, while others are operated by government entities such as municipalities, and still others operate under a for-profit structure. For nonprofits and government entities, grant-writing and community fundraising are common sources of initial funding, whereas in for-profit clinics, initial funding may be drawn from personal savings or bank loans.

Financial Sustainability

Meeting the budget is a challenge for any company and is especially so when attempting to keep the cost of services dramatically lower than those of full-service for-profit clinics. However, meeting this challenge is feasible due to the "high-volume" nature of these services. Furthermore, the fact that spay–neuter clinics provide a service that is highly focused allows for a significant reduction in the amount of overhead compared to a full-service practice. There is no need to carry the product inventory, invest in the array of equipment, or retain the large staff that a private general practice requires. Thus, the HQHVSN clinic is capable of functioning in a very efficient, cost-effective manner, and is capable of being self-sustaining.

In order for the organization to be self-sustaining, the total yearly operating cost for the program should be determined, being sure to include wages and salaries (including for relief veterinarians), benefits, taxes, insurance, licenses, vehicle expenses, supplies, rent or mortgage, utilities, care at outside veterinarians, and equipment and property repair and maintenance. The clinic can then calculate the average surgery fee required in order to cover the operating cost. For example, if it costs $400 000 per year to operate a clinic performing 8400 surgeries and the clinic is open 48 weeks/year (240 days), the cost for each surgery would need to be approximately $47 to break even (see Table 32.1). Computation of this figure enables the clinic to prepare for the amount of funds that need to be raised to help further subsidize the cost for those individuals who cannot afford that charge. A sample budget worksheet can be found in Figure 32.1.

Facility

Although some clinics have elected to construct a building, it is always not necessary to do so. Completion of a remodel on an existing building can very easily meet the needs of an HQHVSN clinic by keeping a few key points in mind. Location of the facility in close proximity to a major thoroughfare is exceedingly beneficial both for the public and transport arms of the program. Other important features to consider include ample parking and a safe area to walk dogs.

Table 32.1 Sample budget – one-veterinarian stationary clinic.

Total Operating Expenses & Cost of Services		$400 000.00
Days open/week	5	
Weeks open/year	48	
Days open/year	240	
Revenue needed/year		$400 000.00
Revenue needed/week		$8 333.33
Revenue needed/day		$1 666.67
Number of surgeries/day	35	
Number of surgeries/week	175	
Number of surgeries/year	8400	
Revenue needed/surgery (average service fee)		$47.62

Facility Legal and Regulatory Issues

Prior to selecting a site for a stationary clinic, city and county code and zone restrictions must be researched to verify that a veterinary facility may be sited in the prospective location. It is also important to review the veterinary practice act for the state in which the facility is to be located, to ensure that all requirements for facility inspection and permitting are properly addressed. A facility in the United States must comply with regulations set forth under the federal Americans with Disabilities Act (ADA) in order to provide accessibility or accommodations for people with disabilities (United States Department of Justice Civil Rights Division 2010). Additional areas that may be subject to regulation by veterinary practice act or by municipal code include air exchange and ventilation, as well as solid waste disposal and drain requirements.

Facility Size and Design

The ASPCA Spay/Neuter Alliance recommends 2000–3000 sq. ft. for a one-vet practice, and 3500–5000+ sq. ft. for a two-vet practice. Overall, the floor plan must be designed in such a way as to allow for the most efficient flow of patients through the clinic. As much as possible, flow should be one way to avoid inefficiency as well as unnecessary cross-contamination. It is highly recommended that interested groups visit as many high-volume clinics as possible to see floor plans in functioning clinics and how patient "flow" within the facility is achieved (see sample floor plans in Figure 32.2). For more detailed information about selecting, designing, and remodeling a clinic space, see https://www.aspcapro.org/sites/default/files/asna_building_resource_guide.pdf.

Particular areas require consideration during construction or remodel. Clinics must comply with appropriate ventilation and air exchange according to the veterinary practice act and city/county government code requirements for their

NSNRT Budget Worksheet - Month 1

Organization Name: Sample 1-Vet Clinic

Completed by: 0

Date completed:

Cells shaded in green have formulas. DO NOT EDIT CELLS SHADED IN GREEN. ONLY EDIT CELLS SHADED IN WHITE.

Revenue	
Income - Clinic Fees	$23,546
Fundraising	$1,250
Grant Income	$0
Income - Misc.	$0
Total Revenue	**$24,796**

Clinic Information	
Average service fee/patient	$61.96
Enter average cost/animal here	$15.00
Ave. number of weeks/mo.	4.0
Number of days open/week	5
Estimated # of surgeries per day	19
Surgeries per month	**380**

Cost of Services		
Cost of Goods - Transport Gas	$250	0.7%
Cost of Goods - Med Vet Drugs	$5,700	15.4%
Outside Vet Services	$250	0.7%
Surgical Payroll	$14,333	38.8%
Staff Incentives	$0	0.0%
Taxes (15%)	$2,150	5.8%
Health Insurance (med. Staff)	$1,083	2.9%
Total Cost of Services	**$23,767**	**64.4%**
Gross Profit (Loss)	**$1,030**	

Surgical Payroll	
# Veterinarians	1.0
Vet salary	$6,500
Total Vet Cost	**$6,500**
# Technicians	1.0
Tech salary	$2,667
Total Tech Cost	**$2,667**
# Assistants	2.0
Asst. salary	$1,833
Total Asst. Cost	**$3,667**
# Other	1.0
Other salary	$1,500
Total Other Cost	**$1,500**
Total Surgical Payroll	**$14,333**

Operating Expenses		
Office Payroll	$6,500	17.6%
Taxes (15%)	$975	2.6%
Health Insurance (admin staff)	$542	1.5%
Printing Expense (inc. admit forms)	$167	0.5%
Rental of Equipment	$0	0.0%
Repairs to Trucks/Autos	$42	0.1%
Advertising Expense	$208	0.6%
Recruitment of Staff	$0	0.0%
Web Hosting	$8	0.0%
Clinic Software	$63	0.2%
Fundraising Expenses	$83	0.2%
Travel Expenses	$0	0.0%
Bank Charges	$167	0.5%
Office Supplies	$125	0.3%
Postage Expense	$42	0.1%
Telephone Expense	$167	0.5%
Dues and Subscriptions	$42	0.1%
Insurance - BOD, vehicle, liability, proper	$167	0.5%
Insurance - Workers Comp	$583	1.6%
Legal and Professional Fees	$167	0.5%
Building Lease and/or Mortgage	$2,000	5.4%
Repairs to Building	$167	0.5%
Utilities Expense	$667	1.8%
Waste Management	$42	0.1%
Other Taxes and Licenses	$42	0.1%
Miscellaenous Expense	$167	0.5%
	$0	0.0%
	$0	0.0%
	$0	0.0%
	$0	0.0%
Total Operating Expenses	**$13,129**	**35.6%**

Office Payroll	
Office Manager	0.0
Office Manager salary	$0
Total Office Manager Cost	**$0**
Director of Clinic Operations	1.0
DCO salary	$3,750
Total DCO Cost	**$3,750**
Other Admin	1.5
Other Admin salary	$1,833
Total Other Admin Cost	**$2,750**
Total Office Payroll	**$6,500**
Total Payroll	**$20,833**

TOTAL EXPENSES $36,896 | 100.0%

NET INCOME (LOSS) ($12,099)

Figure 32.1 Monthly budget worksheet for a stationary clinic.

(a)

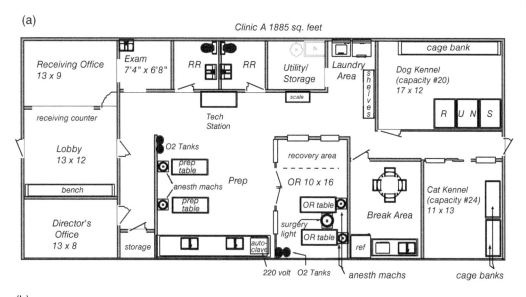

(b)

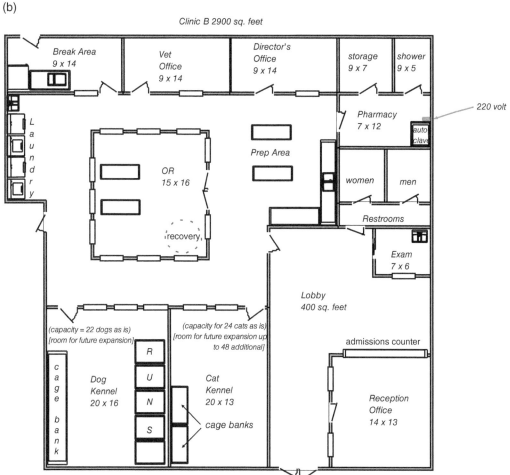

Figure 32.2 (a) Sample floorplan for a 1-veterinarian, 1800 sq. ft. stationary clinic. (b) Sample floorplan for a 1–2-veterinarian, 2900 sq. ft. stationary clinic.

area, if any. Clinic designers should also be mindful of zones for heat, ventilation, and air-conditioning (HVAC), as kennels, surgery, and administration areas may need to be on separate controls.

Proper and safe individual housing accommodation for each patient must be provided (i.e. stainless-steel cages, runs). Kennels should be positioned in a manner to separate dogs and cats as much as possible, with special attention to community/feral cat holding. Code requirements on drains (if used) should be reviewed and implemented. A secure area should be identified for housing of the controlled substance safe(s).

Also during clinic construction or remodel, a decision must be made regarding oxygen delivery (central oxygen, portable tanks, oxygen generator), as well as which gas scavenging system will be utilized.

While small, portable "E" tanks are the least expensive oxygen setup option initially, they are the most expensive over time. For this reason, E tanks are not generally recommended for full-time stationary clinics. A more cost-effective option is central oxygen provided via large, refillable "H" tanks. The initial cost of these systems is higher because central oxygen lines to connect the tanks to the anesthesia machines must be installed by a licensed company. However, ongoing oxygen purchase expenses are reduced compared to E tanks.

Oxygen generators are most expensive initially, but in the long run save money, as there is no ongoing need to purchase oxygen. One caveat to the use of oxygen generators is that if power is lost, oxygen will not be available. Thus, if using oxygen generators, it is prudent to have a small amount of bottled oxygen (such as E tanks) available as an emergency backup option.

Waste anesthetic gas scavenging may be passive or active. Passive scavenging may be accomplished by directly exhausting waste gas to the outdoors or via activated charcoal canisters. Direct exhaust can be safe and very cost-effective, but requires that the anesthesia machines are located near an outside wall or

window through which waste gas can be piped via transfer tubing. Passive exhaust ports should be below the level of the anesthesia machine pop-off valve to facilitate flow of the heavier-than-air anesthetic gases.

Activated charcoal canisters (such as F/Air) are a second method of passive waste gas scavenging. These canisters are affordable and do not require access to an outside wall. However, the canisters must be monitored and replaced on a routine basis, are variable in their performance, and are not as effective at removing waste gas as active or passive scavenging systems that exhaust waste gas to the outdoors (Smith and Bolon 2003).

Active scavengers rely on vacuum evacuation to move waste gas from the anesthesia exhaust tubing to the outdoors. Advantages of active scavenging systems are that waste gas may be collected from multiple anesthesia machines and exhausted together in a single location that may be distant from the anesthesia machines and does not rely on gravity and gas flow rates to push gas out of the building. Active scavenging units are useful for clinics with anesthesia machines located away from outside walls and where direct passive outdoor exhaust is impractical. These systems are fairly permanent with no need for routine maintenance or replacement, but the initial cost is relatively high and connecting pipes must be installed to connect the scavenging unit to each anesthesia machine.

For both active and passive systems that rely on outdoor exhaust, ensure that the waste gas is not being exhausted near open windows, doors, or air intake vents which may direct the waste gas back into the building. For more information on waste gas health and safety, see Chapter 31.

Transport

As discussed earlier in this chapter, transport is the act of going into surrounding communities, picking up the animals scheduled for sterilization surgeries, transporting them to the stationary clinic, and then returning them to the pick-up site to be reunited with their caretakers or owners. Transport to and from a facility can be accomplished by either the host facility or the animal welfare groups that use the clinic's spay and neuter services.

Transport Vehicle

Transport requires its own set of policies to ensure that the animals conveyed in the transport unit will receive the same quality of care during that phase as during their time in the clinic. The transport unit must be tailored to ensure animal safety. The truck in Figure 32.3 is actually the same type as a "box" ambulance. The rear compartment houses a separate climate control unit to provide ventilation, as well as heat and air-conditioning for patient comfort on the trip. The animals travel in standard travel crates that are secured to the wall of the unit by use of a rack system (Figure 32.4). The driver is able to monitor the animals during the trip via a "pass-through" door that connects the cab to the back.

Transport Infection Control and Safety

The driver is the first line of defense in monitoring of patient health. Prior to loading the patients, the driver will do an inspection of the patient inside its kennel. Should that animal in any way appear to be unhealthy to the driver, he or she has the authority to decline transport of that animal. This allows for the entire transport population to be safeguarded by eliminating a potentially detrimental exposure.

Equally essential is strict adherence to an established schedule for cleaning and disinfection of the transport vehicle. In addition, travel kennels must be in good condition and must be cleaned and sanitized between uses. These kennels must allow the animal to be transported safely, prevent escape, and provide accurate patient identification on both the animal and the crate.

If a transport partner group experiences a disease outbreak in its shelter or humane society, it is essential that it notify the HQHVSN clinic so transport from that facility can be canceled until the outbreak is under control.

Transport Partner Requirements

A local "Transport Coordinator" should be identified who will take responsibility for organizing all necessary components of the process on-site (at the pick-up/drop-off location). This individual is the primary contact with the clinic and books the actual appointments for the travel day. Transport partners should contact the HQHVSN clinic three business days prior to the travel date to confirm the number of patients they have booked. This allows the clinic to add more appointments

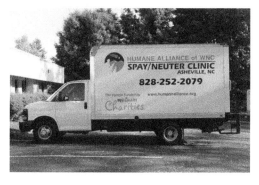

Figure 32.3   Humane Alliance transport vehicle. This vehicle is a custom-fitted box ambulance with climate control in the animal compartment.

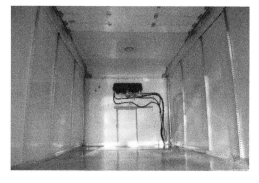

Figure 32.4   Climate control unit and rack system for securing crates in the transport vehicle.

in-house or stop booking depending upon the expected patient load.

The distance the facility is from the clinic dictates the number of patients required to justify sending the truck. The transport manager at the HQHVSN clinic determines the minimum number of patients necessary to book the truck, and creates a transport calendar that is circulated among the groups one to two months in advance to allow those groups to secure the appropriate number of animals. Shelters or rescue groups in the same general region may join together to reach the minimum number. Some groups coordinate a travel date for animals from low-income households in their local communities as well. Screening processes to qualify those individuals vary depending upon requirements established by the individual transport partner groups.

In addition to booking, the transport partner group is responsible for providing a medical record for each patient, and to ensure that each patient has identification both on the animal and on the crate. Regardless of the type of group picked up, all admission forms must be completed, including answers recorded for medical history questions and verification of compliance with pre-operative instructions.

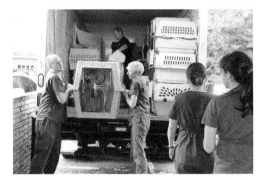

Figure 32.5   Unloading of patients upon arrival at the clinic.

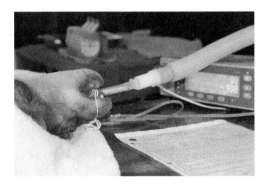

Figure 32.6   Good patient care includes appropriate monitoring and record-keeping.

Transport Arrival and Return

Upon arrival at the HQHVSN facility, the patients are unloaded from the transport vehicle and checked in by the clinic medical staff (Figure 32.5). Each patient receives a physical examination by the veterinarian as they are admitted into the clinic. The sterilization surgeries are completed that day and the patients are returned on the transport the following day.

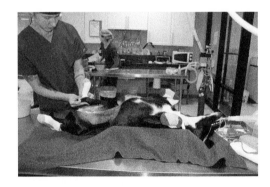

Figure 32.7   Patient care. Here, booties have been placed on the pet's feet to prevent hypothermia.

Patient Care

The Association of Shelter Veterinarians' (ASV) Spay Neuter Guidelines (Griffin et al. 2016) and the chapters in this textbook provide excellent sources to draw upon to guide patient care. Patient care encompasses all aspects of

dealing with the patient, including but not limited to anesthesia, analgesia, surgery, medical records, physical examination, client communication, infectious disease control, and pre-, intra-, and post-operative care (Figures 32.6 and 32.7). Box 32.1 describes a typical day at a stationary clinic.

Box 32.1	Timeline for a Typical Day
7:00 a.m.	Staff arrive and begin patient re-evaluation, incision inspection, and loading transport animals from previous surgery day.
7:30 a.m.	Clinic opens to public, verbal and written post-op instructions are given to owners, and public animals from previous surgery day are released.
8:00 a.m.	Public animal intake for the day. Pre-op physical examinations are performed by clinic veterinarian(s).
9:00 a.m.	Surgery schedule begins.
10:30 a.m.	Transport arrives and is unloaded. If more than one vet, surgery continues while the other vet(s) do intake and physical examinations. If only one vet, that individual will stop surgeries and do physical examinations.
11:30 a.m.	Return to surgery.
1:00 p.m.	If only one vet, lunch break for 30 minutes; if more than one vet, staff cycle through lunch break.
1:30 p.m.	Return to surgery.
3:30 p.m.	Surgery schedule complete, patients recovered, snack provided. Any rechecks or other duties can be completed at this time.

Policies

As well as quality of care and professionalism, an integral part of any thriving clinic is its careful attention to detail. Standard operating procedures are valuable in providing a guide for existing staff and as a tool in training of new staff, and should be developed for both medical and administrative procedures. Standard operating procedures should be established in the early stages of the clinic, and all staff members must have access to this manual and be aware of the guidelines described therein.

Relationships with Area Veterinarians

Relationships with area veterinarians can be one of the most challenging aspects of working in this field. Relationships between spay–neuter programs and private practice veterinarians can at times be adversarial. Unfortunately, the only loser in those types of battles ends up being the animals we all

endeavor to help. The best avenue to pursue to avoid these conflicts is open appreciation, open communication, and an open-door policy:

- *Open appreciation.* Private practice veterinarians provide an invaluable service to the communities that we all serve. Many private practices provide free and discounted services to many animal welfare groups. They have a bottom line to meet and bills to pay, as do we all. The private practice efforts should be publicly acknowledged.
- *Open communication.* It is always best to make the veterinary community aware of your clinic's policies and protocols so they understand how your organization functions. Let them know instances when you will refer clients to private practices, and share your policies on incision checks, complications, and after-hours care for your patients (see Figure 32.8).
- *Open-door policy.* Another important aspect of facilitating a good working relationship with the local veterinary community is to make them aware that they are invited to visit your facility, take a tour, and meet the

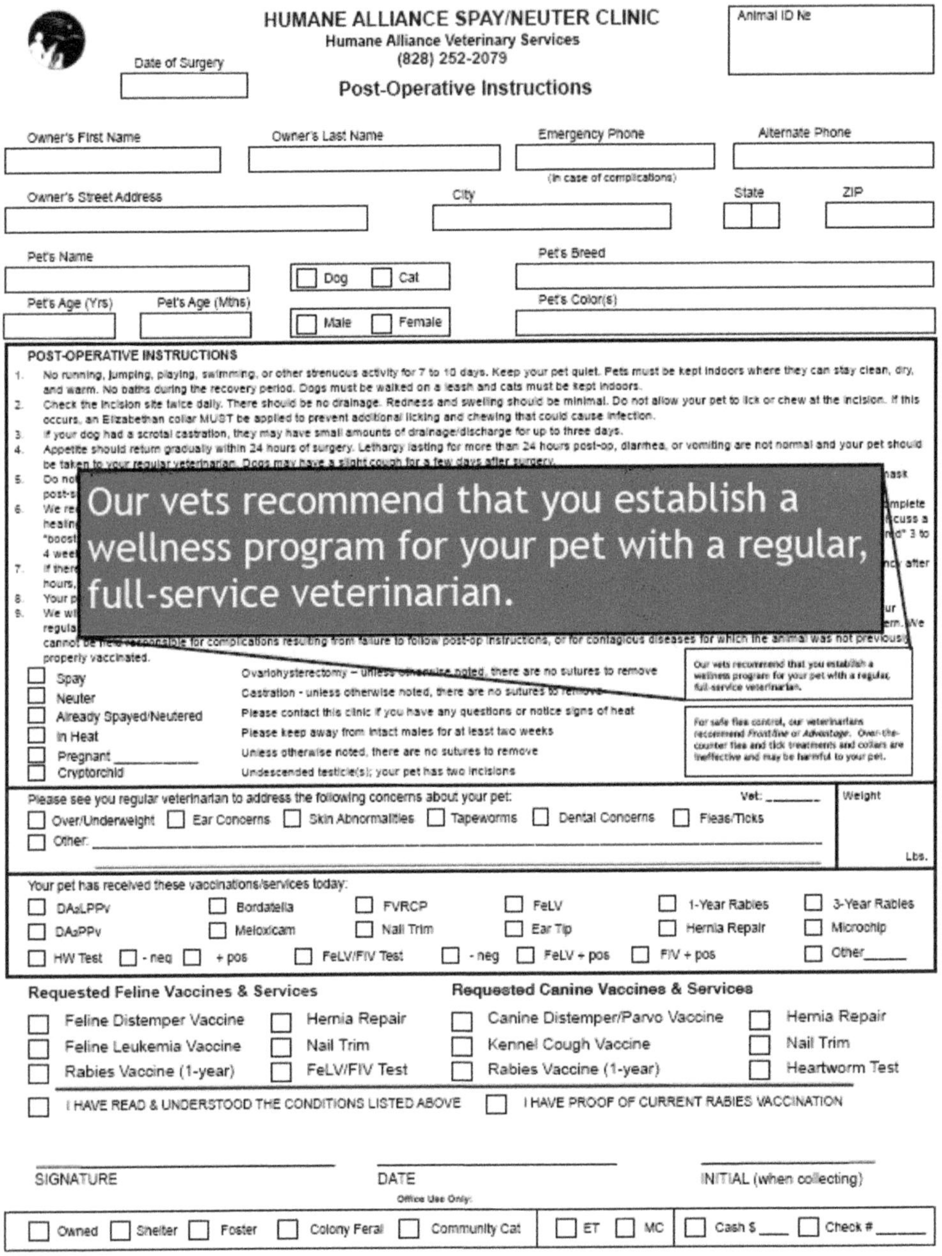

HUMANE ALLIANCE SPAY/NEUTER CLINIC
Humane Alliance Veterinary Services
(828) 252-2079
Post-Operative Instructions

Date of Surgery ______ Animal ID № ______

Owner's First Name ______ Owner's Last Name ______ Emergency Phone ______ (In case of complications) Alternate Phone ______

Owner's Street Address ______ City ______ State ______ ZIP ______

Pet's Name ______ ☐ Dog ☐ Cat Pet's Breed ______

Pet's Age (Yrs) ______ Pet's Age (Mths) ______ ☐ Male ☐ Female Pet's Color(s) ______

POST-OPERATIVE INSTRUCTIONS

1. No running, jumping, playing, swimming, or other strenuous activity for 7 to 10 days. Keep your pet quiet. Pets must be kept indoors where they can stay clean, dry, and warm. No baths during the recovery period. Dogs must be walked on a leash and cats must be kept indoors.
2. Check the incision site twice daily. There should be no drainage. Redness and swelling should be minimal. Do not allow your pet to lick or chew at the incision. If this occurs, an Elizabethan collar MUST be applied to prevent additional licking and chewing that could cause infection.
3. If your dog had a scrotal castration, they may have small amounts of drainage/discharge for up to three days.
4. Appetite should return gradually within 24 hours of surgery. Lethargy lasting for more than 24 hours post-op, diarrhea, or vomiting are not normal and your pet should be taken to your regular veterinarian. Dogs may have a slight cough for a few days after surgery.
5. Do no… mask post-s…
6. We re… complete healin… discuss a "boost… red" 3 to 4 wee…
7. If there… ncy after hours,…
8. Your p…
9. We wi… ur regula… rm. We cannot be held responsible for complications resulting from failure to follow post-op instructions, or for contagious diseases for which the animal was not previously properly vaccinated.

Our vets recommend that you establish a wellness program for your pet with a regular, full-service veterinarian.

☐ Spay — Ovariohysterectomy – unless otherwise noted, there are no sutures to remove
☐ Neuter — Castration - unless otherwise noted, there are no sutures to remove
☐ Already Spayed/Neutered — Please contact this clinic if you have any questions or notice signs of heat
☐ In Heat — Please keep away from intact males for at least two weeks
☐ Pregnant ______ — Unless otherwise noted, there are no sutures to remove
☐ Cryptorchid — Undescended testicle(s); your pet has two incisions

Our vets recommend that you establish a wellness program for your pet with a regular, full-service veterinarian.

For safe flea control, our veterinarians recommend *Frontline* or *Advantage*. Over-the-counter flea and tick treatments and collars are ineffective and may be harmful to your pet.

Please see you regular veterinarian to address the following concerns about your pet: Vet: ______ Weight ______ Lbs.
☐ Over/Underweight ☐ Ear Concerns ☐ Skin Abnormalities ☐ Tapeworms ☐ Dental Concerns ☐ Fleas/Ticks
☐ Other: ______

Your pet has received these vaccinations/services today:
☐ DA₂LPPv ☐ Bordatella ☐ FVRCP ☐ FeLV ☐ 1-Year Rabies ☐ 3-Year Rabies
☐ DA₂PPv ☐ Meloxicam ☐ Nail Trim ☐ Ear Tip ☐ Hernia Repair ☐ Microchip
☐ HW Test ☐ - neg ☐ + pos ☐ FeLV/FIV Test ☐ - neg ☐ FeLV + pos ☐ FIV + pos ☐ Other______

Requested Feline Vaccines & Services
☐ Feline Distemper Vaccine ☐ Hernia Repair
☐ Feline Leukemia Vaccine ☐ Nail Trim
☐ Rabies Vaccine (1-year) ☐ FeLV/FIV Test

Requested Canine Vaccines & Services
☐ Canine Distemper/Parvo Vaccine ☐ Hernia Repair
☐ Kennel Cough Vaccine ☐ Nail Trim
☐ Rabies Vaccine (1-year) ☐ Heartworm Test

☐ I HAVE READ & UNDERSTOOD THE CONDITIONS LISTED ABOVE ☐ I HAVE PROOF OF CURRENT RABIES VACCINATION

SIGNATURE ______ DATE ______ INITIAL (when collecting) ______

Office Use Only:
☐ Owned ☐ Shelter ☐ Foster ☐ Colony Feral ☐ Community Cat ☐ ET ☐ MC ☐ Cash $____ ☐ Check #______

Figure 32.8 Post-operative instructions encourage clients to establish care with a full-service veterinary practice.

veterinary staff. Many clinics do an open house when they begin, but it is a good idea to continue to keep the invitation perpetual.

It is vital to continue to foster these relationships in order to further the HQHVSN mission of reducing the unwanted companion animal population through means other than euthanasia. Any aspiration of this scope and magnitude can only be accomplished by securing the cooperative efforts of the veterinary community as a whole. With that intention, the hope is to create a mutual spirit of cooperation with the veterinarians in the region to encourage clients to develop an ongoing veterinarian–client–patient relationship. After all, the collective goal is to end animal suffering.

Conclusion

The strategies described in this chapter have been developed over a number of years, with experience gained in mentoring more than 168 clinics. The ability of an organization to follow these steps has been paramount in determining the new clinics' success and sustainability. Prior to establishing a full-time, stationary clinic, it is crucial to ensure that this model is the right fit for the given organization and community. If the basic requirements for capacity, need, and fundraising listed in this chapter cannot be met, another service model such as a MASH clinic, mobile unit, or in-clinic clinic might be a more appropriate alternative based upon resources, community needs, and opportunities available.

References

ASPCAPRO (2018). ASPCA Spay/Neuter Alliance. https://www.aspcapro.org/about-programs-services/aspca-spayneuter-alliance (accessed 7 July 2018).

Griffin, B., Bushby, P.A., Mccobb, E. et al. (2016). The Association of Shelter Veterinarians' 2016 veterinary medical care guidelines for spay-neuter programs. *JAVMA* 249: 165–188.

Smith, J.C. and Bolon, B. (2003). Comparison of three commercially available activated charcoal canisters for passive scavenging of waste isoflurane during conventional rodent anesthesia. *J. Am. Assoc. Lab. Anim. Sci.* 42: 10–15.

Spay FIRST! (2017). Mini clinics. http://www.spayfirst.org/programs/remote-area-programs/spay-pods (accessed 7 July 2018).

United States Department of Justice Civil Rights Division (2010). Americans with Disabilities Act: Public Accommodations and Commercial Facilities (Title III). https://www.ada.gov/ada_title_III.htm (accessed 18 November 2018).

33

Profile of the Mobile Spay–Neuter Clinic
Kathleen V. Makolinski

Mobile clinics are self-contained units that travel to or within various communities to perform spays and neuters for cats and dogs. Surgery is performed on the unit and animals are discharged on the same day following spay–neuter. Mobile clinics are utilized in rural, suburban, and urban environments. Some mobile clinics perform spay–neuter for one day at a particular site, while others remain on-site for multiple days in a row. A major advantage of mobile spay–neuter clinics is that they travel to targeted locations to provide veterinary care to underserved animal populations and eliminate "transportation issues" as a barrier to obtaining spay–neuter.

Mobile Clinic Requirements and Structure

Legal/Regulatory Issues

Before considering implementation of a mobile spay–neuter clinic, both state and local veterinary laws and regulations should be reviewed to ensure that operation of such a clinic is permitted. One also needs to determine if any specific requirements need to be met. For example, does a veterinarian need to own the mobile spay–neuter clinic? Is a premise permit necessary to operate the clinic? Additionally, the mobile unit will require inspection, registration, and insurance. Some units, depending on size, weight, or presence of air brakes, may require the driver to possess a commercial driver's license (CDL).

Organizational Structure

Some not-for-profit organizations exist exclusively to operate a mobile spay–neuter clinic, while other mobile clinics are operated by humane societies, municipal animal shelters, societies for the prevention of cruelty to animals (SPCAs), stationary spay–neuter clinics, or veterinary schools. Veterinarians may also provide spay–neuter in addition to other veterinary services aboard for-profit mobile veterinary clinics.

Financial Considerations

When starting a mobile spay–neuter clinic, an organization needs to raise funds to purchase the unit and, if necessary, a truck to pull the unit (or arrange for financing for these items). Since a new program may not function at full capacity for the first few months, the program should have adequate funds to cover operational costs (such as supplies and wages) during this time.

High-Quality, High-Volume Spay and Neuter and Other Shelter Surgeries, First Edition. Edited by Sara White.
© 2020 John Wiley & Sons, Inc. Published 2020 by John Wiley & Sons, Inc.

At the initiation of a mobile spay–neuter clinic and routinely thereafter, it is prudent to determine:

- Yearly operational cost of program
- Number of surgeries (and their associated pricing) that must be performed in order to cover operational costs
- Sources of funding that can be used to subsidize spay–neuter for targeted animal populations (examples: grants, government contributions, fundraisers, income from associated wellness clinic)
- Best use of any subsidies received to lessen client cost for spay–neuter

Additionally, the number of days per year that the clinic operates will very likely be affected by adverse weather conditions, mechanical issues, and staff absences. Some mobile clinic programs choose to operate on a seasonal basis due to the risk of driving the vehicle in inclement weather. These factors need to be considered when determining the clinic's yearly budget.

Generally, the operation of a mobile spay–neuter clinic tends to be more expensive than the cost of performing spay–neuter in other types of programs. This is due to costs associated with maintenance and fuel for the vehicle as well as insurance and registration. Additionally, a mobile spay–neuter clinic may have fewer kennels than a stationary spay–neuter clinic and therefore generate less revenue on a daily basis, since fewer surgeries are performed. However, when mobile clinics are managed properly they have the potential to decrease fertility in targeted animal populations (A. Mills, personal communication, 2013).

Facilities

Mobile spay–neuter clinics vary greatly in their size as well as in the number and configuration of on-board cages. Clinics may be contained within a trailer that is pulled behind a truck or have a truck cab incorporated into the clinic (see Figures 33.1–33.3). One advantage of a pull-behind clinic is that if the truck needs

servicing, a different vehicle can be utilized to pull the unit to the site of a scheduled clinic.

Since bathrooms take up a considerable amount of mobile unit space, many programs opt not to have an on-board bathroom and instead park near a facility that contains a bathroom that staff/volunteers can utilize.

Size and Cost

The length of mobile clinics generally ranges from 20 to 33 ft.; however, larger units are available (38 ft. gooseneck trailer and 53 ft. tractor trailer). Mobile clinics can be purchased from companies that specialize in building such vehicles, may be custom designed, or be purchased second-hand. The reported base price for a new clinic with an incorporated cab ranges from $144 824 for a 26 ft. unit and $213 855 for a 33 ft. unit. Each clinic includes a surgical area and an examination table (La Boit 2019).

Mobile spay–neuter clinics should be constructed with the following base items:

- Fresh and gray water tanks
- Power cord hook-up to external source of electricity
- Heating/air-conditioning units
- Water heater
- Refrigerator/freezer

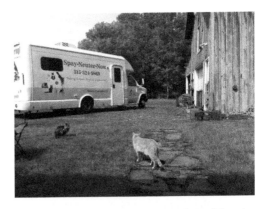

Figure 33.1 Mobile spay–neuter clinic of Spay/Neuter/Now, Hammond, NY. Total length of clinic is 27 ft., maximum number of cages is 12. Spays–neuters owned cats/small dogs and free-roaming cats. Utilizes off-board recovery as needed. *Source:* Photo courtesy of Kevin Mace.

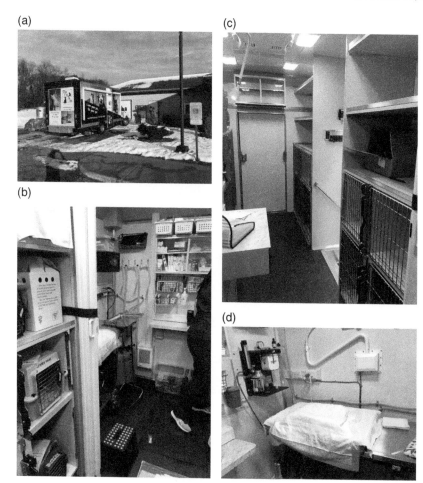

Figure 33.2 Mobile spay–neuter clinic of The Fix Is In Spay/Neuter Clinic in Wisconsin. (a) The unit is a 26 ft. converted box truck from Magnum Mobile in Phoenix, AZ. (b) It has 4 shelves for cat carriers and 13 kennels. (c) Four pairs of kennels have a removable wall between them, so they can be converted to larger cages for medium-sized dogs. (d) This mobile unit utilizes two surgery tables (one regular surgery table and one adjustable-height utility cart) and saves space in the surgery area by positioning one side of each surgery table against the wall. The mobile unit aims to perform 40+ surgeries per day and, due to size constraints, works mostly with cats and small or medium dogs. *Source:* Photos courtesy of Brooke Groskopf.

- Gas or diesel-powered generator
- Cabinets and drawers that securely latch

Home Base

When not in use, it is ideal for the mobile clinic to be parked in a locked garage. The parking site for the clinic may also be used for:

- Delivery and storage of equipment, consumable items, and pharmaceutical agents
- Laundering of towels/blankets and surgical drapes/pack wraps

- Cleaning, lubricating, wrapping, and sterilizing surgical instruments (if an on-board autoclave is not available)

Hybrid Model

Some clinics utilize smaller mobile units that are large enough to house a surgical area, a place for animals to be prepped for surgery, and a few cages. Here, an adjacent building is utilized for intake, monitored recovery, and discharge of animals. A temperature-controlled

(a)

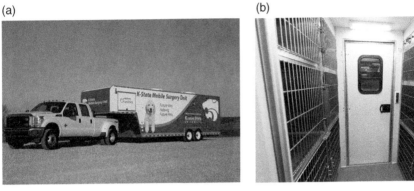

(b)

(c)

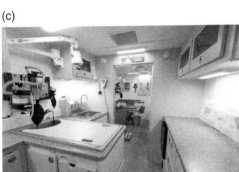

(d)

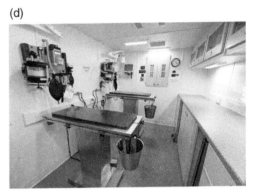

Figure 33.3 Mobile unit utilized by Kansas State University College of Veterinary Medicine. (a) The unit is a 32 ft. trailer pulled by a F350 truck. The unit travels with one faculty member, one registered veterinary technician, and three students at a time, and serves shelter animals and community cats. (b) The trailer contains a total of 12 cages, 6 on either side, stacked 3 high and 2 across. One side (6 cages) has the ability to be heated. The bottom kennels on both sides can have the divider removed to be larger. Patients are rotated on and off the trailer through the day, with early post-operative recovery on board. (c) The unit contains two surgery tables and a wet-to-dry prep table. Note the ample supply of latched drawers/cabinets and the separate surgical suite. (d) The surgery tables are oriented to allow access to both sides of the table for teaching purposes, and there is adequate space so that both tables may be used simultaneously. *Source:* Photos courtesy of Kansas State University College of Veterinary Medicine.

building with electricity and running water is necessary. Such programs are considered to be a hybrid between mobile spay–neuter and mobile animal sterilization hospital (MASH) programs. They allow veterinary staff to work in a familiar and consistent setting while avoiding the loading/unloading of heavy medical equipment. Here, the program can purchase a less expensive, cargo-style trailer. Such units should be insulated and retrofitted to include lights, a breaker box, and plumbing. An example of an organization that utilizes this model is Spay FIRST! (Figure 33.4).

A disadvantage of this type of program is the need for animals to be moved between the adjacent building and the clinic. Animals need to be sufficiently recovered on board before they can be moved. Trained volunteers are often utilized to move animals and provide adequate monitoring of animals who continue their recovery in the off-board location. If the host organization does not provide crates for housing animals in the off-board location, the hybrid program will need to travel with such crates. (For instructions on how to clean and disinfect such crates, see Chapter 5).

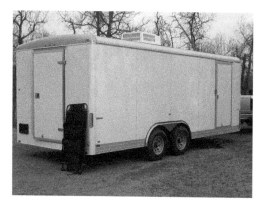

Figure 33.4   Cargo-style spay–neuter trailer of the Oklahoma Spay Network. This mobile unit is utilized with an off-board recovery site. This trailer is 20 ft. long by 8 ft. wide, with 2 doors, each 36 in. wide. The unit does not contain cages, but cages can be built into the unit if desired. A stretcher is used to help transport large dogs from the clinic to an adjacent recovery site. *Source:* Photo courtesy of Ruth Steinberger.

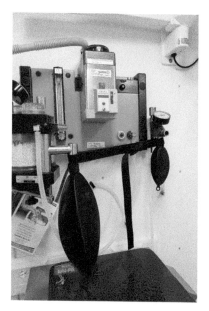

Figure 33.5   Wall-mounted anesthesia machine secured for transport. *Source:* Photo courtesy of Kansas State University College of Veterinary Medicine.

Equipment

Anesthesia Machines

It is advised that durable, wall-mounted anesthetic machines be utilized in the mobile clinic (Figure 33.5). At least two anesthetic machines are necessary, one for the animal preparation area and one for the surgical area. In order to avoid small cracks in the tubing, breathing circuits should be removed from the anesthetic machines prior to travel.

Surgery Tables

In an effort to optimize efficiency in high-quality high-volume spay–neuter (HQHVSN) programs, it is ideal to have two surgery tables (Figures 33.2d and 33.3d). When two tables are available, the veterinarian can re-glove after completion of a spay or neuter and immediately start surgery on the next animal patient. However, mobile units may be too small to accommodate two surgery tables. In such cases, efficiency in animal flow may be improved by having the next animal transported to the surgery table immediately following completion of the preceding spay–neuter.

Oxygen

Many mobile spay–neuter clinics use portable oxygen tanks or oxygen concentrators (Figure 33.6). Oxygen tanks come in a variety of sizes and must be adequately secured to an interior clinic wall or inside a compartment so that they do not pose a safety hazard during transport of the clinic. Oxygen tanks should be turned off prior to transport.

Surgical Instruments and Autoclave

Some mobile clinics have an on-board autoclave (Figure 33.7) and staff members are responsible for cleaning, lubricating, wrapping, and sterilizing surgical instruments throughout the day. Other mobile programs immediately soak the surgical instruments after use to remove organic debris, but finish

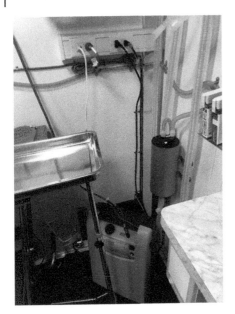

Figure 33.6 Oxygen concentrator and active anesthetic gas scavenger on a mobile unit. *Source:* Photo courtesy of Brooke Groskopf.

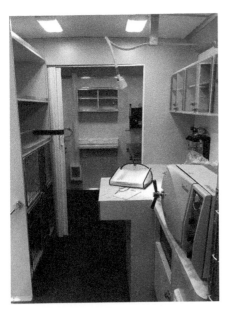

Figure 33.7 Autoclave located in a mobile unit. Also notice the efficient use of space and the latching cabinets. *Source:* Photo courtesy of Brooke Groskopf.

processing and sterilizing the instruments in an off-board location. In case the autoclave becomes non-functional, it is ideal to have at

least enough surgical instrument packs to do the expected number of spays–neuters for a typical day. It is unacceptable to use surgical instruments that have not been sterilized or that have been used on a previous animal.

Scales

Obtaining an accurate weight for cats and dogs will allow staff to determine appropriate anesthetic/analgesic drug volumes. A mechanical baby scale may be used to weigh cats and a digital platform scale is often used to weigh dogs. In order to protect the weight receptors in platform scales, they should be transported on their side, adequately affixed to a wall, or upside down lying on a blanket (Figure 33.8).

Supplies

All mobile clinic supplies need to be well organized, stored in a location close to where they are

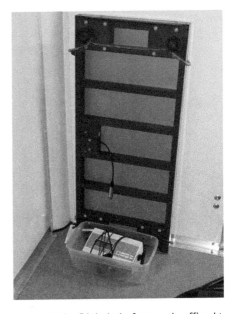

Figure 33.8 Digital platform scale affixed to wall with bungee cords at top and bottom for appropriate transport. The platform is facing the wall to protect the weight receptors. *Source:* Photo courtesy of Ruth Steinberger.

utilized, and secured within latched cabinets or drawers during transport. Additionally, it is helpful to label cabinets and drawers to describe their contents. Since on-board storage is limited, at the end of each day a list of items that need to be re-stocked should be maintained. Staff members need to determine which supplies can stay on board while the unit is parked overnight and which supplies need to be returned to the program's centralized location for storage at optimum temperature and in a secured location. Veterinarians who work on mobile spay–neuter clinics should consult the Veterinary Medicine Mobility Act of 2014 (Congress.gov 2014) and, as needed, their local Drug Enforcement Administration (DEA) office to determine how controlled substances are best transported and stored.

Personnel

Staff Training

It is essential that staff receive training in the proper:

- Operation of the heating/air-conditioning unit, generator, and anesthetic scavenger
- Transport of equipment including anesthetic machines, patient monitors, autoclave, and scales
- Overnight housing of the clinic, especially during cold and hot temperatures

Additionally, key staff members may need to receive training in order to safely drive and park the mobile clinic.

Standard operating procedures (SOPs) that are easily accessible to clinic personnel and updated regularly can greatly assist in staff training and aid in performance of employee reviews. As with all types of clinics, SOPs should cover customer service expectations as well as medical protocols for intake and discharge of patients, safe and efficient flow of animals, vigilant patient monitoring, medical record-keeping, and handling of emergencies.

Ratio of Veterinarian to Medical Support Staff

When one veterinarian is performing spay–neuter on board a mobile clinic, it is essential to have at least two highly trained medical support staff members. Some clinics find that the addition of a third medical support staff member is beneficial. However, depending on the size of the mobile clinic, this extra person may create an overcrowded work environment.

Workday Considerations

Based on staff availability, clientele served, and cost effectiveness, mobile spay–neuter clinics need to determine the length of their workday and how many days they will work each week. Example work weeks include 4 10-hour days and 3 12-hour days. Maintaining an 8-hour workday, 5 days a week may be difficult due to extended travel times and the need to set up and close the clinic. A typical workday in a mobile clinic is shown in Box 33.1.

Staff Safety

In a mobile spay–neuter clinic, patients recover in close proximity to staff members. Staff members may be exposed to excessive waste anesthetic gas as it is exhaled from patients (see also Chapter 31 for more information on waste anesthetic gas). The level of anesthetic gas on board the mobile clinic should be routinely monitored and additional ventilation systems should be utilized as needed to decrease waste anesthetic gas. Figure 33.6 depicts an active anesthetic gas scavenger system mounted in a mobile unit. It is also recommended that mobile clinics utilize a carbon monoxide detector, especially if the unit is powered by a gas or diesel generator.

Volunteers

Trained volunteers are often valuable in performing clerical and customer service tasks,

---

Box 33.1 Mobile Spay–Neuter Clinic: A Typical 10-Hour Day (Approximately 25 Animals Spayed–Neutered)

7:30 a.m.–8:00 a.m.	Mobile spay–neuter clinic and staff arrive on site, greet clients, set up clinic
8:00 a.m.–10:30 a.m.	Patient admissions, physical examinations performed by veterinarian, prepare drugs/medications
10:30 a.m.–11:00 a.m.	Break
11:00 a.m.–3:00 p.m.	Spays–neuters
3:00 p.m.–3:30 p.m.	Monitor recovery, complete medical records, clean unit/equipment
3:30 p.m.–4:00 p.m.	Break
4:00 p.m.–5:30 p.m.	Discharge adequately recovered animal patients, finish cleaning/ disinfecting, run autoclave (if present on board mobile clinic)
5:30 p.m.	Leave site

Note: The veterinarian should not leave the clinic until all patients are adequately recovered. If the driver is a clinic staff member, he or she may be paid extra for driving the unit. Extra staff members may be necessary for additional cleaning, laundry, and re-stocking of the clinic.

---

cleaning kennels, and transporting animals. Highly skilled volunteers may assist in the monitoring of animals in off-board recovery. Due to limited space within a mobile spay–neuter clinic, it is often very difficult to have volunteers work on board the unit.

Clinic Operations

Clinic Location Sites

Mobile spay–neuter programs often choose clinic location sites based on poverty level and population density. This information can be obtained from the United States Census Bureau (2019). Locations may also be chosen because they lack veterinary hospitals, other animal service providers, or transportation options. Local neighborhood associations within targeted areas can assist in communicating the mobile clinic's role and schedule.

Depending on the type of mobile clinic being utilized, the parking site may need water/electricity hook-ups, a bathroom for staff, and facilities for off-board recovery. The use of leveling jacks or blocks upon which the unit rests

may be necessary to maintain an optimum clinic position when parked on-site. Common clinic locations include pet stores, community centers, animal shelters, fire halls, parks, apartment complexes, libraries, and shopping centers. It is important to avoid selecting clinic sites where disease transmission to humans could be a concern (for example a school cafeteria). It is important to gain approval for the site to be utilized as a place to park the mobile clinic well in advance of the planned clinic day.

A geographic information system (GIS) is a tool that allows shelters to map the location of incoming shelter animals (ASPCApro 2019). This information can help determine mobile spay–neuter clinic locations that will target animal populations that are most at risk for relinquishment to a shelter.

The distance from the home base must also be considered when choosing a clinic site. The farther the location, the greater the fuel cost. Additionally, the time it takes staff members to travel to the clinic site needs to be added to their already busy workday. In order to avoid unnecessary travel, sometimes it may be best for the mobile clinic to be secured at a particular site for several days.

Animals Served

Mobile clinics may spay–neuter shelter animals, publicly owned animals, community cats/dogs, or animals from rescue organizations. Some groups choose to serve only cats, while others are equipped to serve cats and various sizes of dogs.

Animal Admissions

The mobile clinic's size and individual cage capacity as well as the veterinarian's skill and efficiency will determine how many animals can be admitted for spay–neuter. Species, sex, and size of animals also need to be considered.

In order for a mobile spay–neuter clinic to be sustainable, the organization needs to determine their "break-even" number of spays–neuters per day and ensure they reach that goal. With one veterinarian and two highly skilled veterinary support staff, many mobile clinics can spay–neuter at least 25 dogs and/or cats per 10-hour workday.

Appointments

Some mobile programs make appointments for animals for spay–neuter. Appointment-based programs require a telephone line and staff member or volunteers to schedule animals, deliver pre-operative care instructions, and answer client questions. In an effort to have an optimal number of animal patients per day, mobile clinics often find that they need to over-book in order to compensate for the average "no-show" rate of approximately 15–20%.

First Come, First Served

Other mobile clinics admit animals on a first-come, first-served basis. In this case, a comprehensive website that lists clinic locations and pre-operative instructions is essential (ASPCA 2019). Having a staff member or volunteer on-site before the mobile clinic arrives to explain the admissions process to those who are lining up for service is extremely valuable. At least

one organization uses a lottery system to determine which animals will receive service.

With a first-come, first-served process, well-attended clinic sites have the advantage of routinely admitting the maximum number of surgical patients. However, having people wait an extended amount of time and be disappointed that their animal will not receive services on that day is a disadvantage.

Mobile Clinic Hosted by Shelter or Rescue Organization

Mobile clinics may also encourage shelters or rescue organizations to reserve and pay for the clinic's use. Here, the shelter or rescue organization is responsible for booking appointments and collecting fees.

Informed Consent for Surgery

It may be most efficient to explain spay–neuter and discuss the risks of anesthesia and surgery with groups of clients who bring animals to the clinic. Individual clients can then read and sign an informed consent statement indicating that they understand and accept the associated risks with anesthesia and surgery. However, state veterinary regulations will dictate exactly how clients must grant informed consent within each particular state.

Examination of Animals

Medical staff should triage animals to determine if overt clinical signs of illness are present before admission of the animal to the clinic. If such signs are present, they may preclude admission for spay–neuter. A veterinarian or supervised veterinary student should examine tractable patients prior to administration of any anesthetic/analgesic agents and spay–neuter surgery. Intractable animals can be visually examined prior to anesthesia; however, they too should be examined by a veterinarian prior to spay–neuter.

Anesthetic/Analgesic Considerations

It is ideal to maintain a relatively quiet, stress-free environment for animals aboard the mobile clinic. Although a number of adequate anesthetic/analgesic protocols exist for spay–neuter, when such procedures are performed on a mobile unit, the following should be considered:

- Administration of pre-medication to groups of animals in the order in which they will undergo surgery. This may help decrease the number of barking dogs and maintain a relatively quiet environment.
- Spay–neuter the animals who are likely to have a longer recovery period early in the day.
- Use of reversible anesthetic agents so that if necessary, patient sedation can be minimized in the post-operative period.
- Minimize masking of animals with inhalant anesthetic agent in an effort to decrease the presence of environmental waste gas.

Patient Discharge

If allowed by state regulations, it is most efficient to explain general post-operative animal care instructions to groups of people as they come to pick up the animals. Each client is to receive written discharge instructions, preferably in the client's primary language. Any specific animal concerns must be noted on the patient's medical record and be addressed on an individual basis with clients, caregivers, or shelter staff. Recommendations regarding any required veterinary care should be made at the time of discharge. Also, clients should be strongly encouraged to establish a relationship with a local veterinary hospital to provide routine care for their pet in the future.

Client Communication and Care of Patients in the Post-operative Period

Clients, caregivers, and shelters should be given instructions on where to call with post-operative questions or concerns. In many cases, these calls are to be directed to the mobile program. Since a mobile clinic will likely not be present in the community in the days following an animal's discharge, if the staff believe that an animal needs to be evaluated by a veterinarian, it is essential that a plan be in place for the animal to receive such care. Mobile clinics will need to make arrangements with a nearby veterinary hospital or emergency clinic for this purpose.

Maintenance of Vehicle and Clinic

After a day of regular clinic use, the following will need to be completed:

- Refill fresh water tank
- Empty gray water tank
- Provide fuel for generator (if used)
- Provide fuel for vehicle

Water tanks should be cleaned and disinfected as needed. The vehicle and all accessory items should be maintained according to the manufacturer's recommendations. The heat/air-conditioning unit, refrigerator, and generator may best be maintained by a company that provides service for recreational vehicles. For drivable units, this same type of company can often provide routine maintenance for mechanical (truck) components. Before purchasing a mobile clinic, be sure that the unit can be adequately maintained by a local company and investigate the costs related to routine maintenance. Additionally, local companies that provide maintenance services for medical equipment should be identified. Due to travel, such equipment (especially anesthesia machines) will endure greater wear and tear than comparable equipment in a stationary clinic.

Conclusion

Mobile clinics have many advantages when delivering spay–neuter services to animal populations in need. Although certain challenges have been identified in this program model, proper management of the mobile clinic and appropriate staff training will allow for its success.

References

ASPCA (2019). ASPCA mobile spay/neuter clinic. http://www.aspca.org/nyc/spay-neuter-services/mobile-spay-neuter-clinic (accessed 23 February 2019).

ASPCApro (2019). Preparing to use GIS to save more lives. http://www.aspcapro.org/webinar/201206-7/gis (accessed 23 February 2019).

Congress.gov (2014). Veterinary Medicine Mobility Act of 2014. https://www.congress.gov/bill/113th-congress/house-bill/1528/text (accessed 21 August 2019).

La Boit (2019). Mobile veterinary clinics. http://www.laboit.com/animal-health/veterinary.html (accessed 23 February 2019).

United States Census Bureau (2019). United States census. www.census.gov (accessed 23 February 2019).

34

MASH Clinics

Sara White

Mobile animal sterilization hospital or MASH clinics are a type of mobile spay–neuter program in which clinic staff transport surgical equipment to a venue and set up a temporary surgical space in that location. Surgeries are not performed in the MASH vehicle, but instead an existing space in the community is used. Examples of locations utilized by MASH clinics in various communities include animal shelter buildings, church basements, animal care (grooming and boarding) facilities, fire stations, town offices, school gymnasia, senior centers, and many more.

MASH programs vary in the number of surgeons, technicians, and support staff, the frequency of surgery days, the number of consecutive days at a single venue, and the mission and organizational structure. Some MASH programs work independently of other humane organizations (independent MASH programs), while others conduct all their work in collaboration with other humane organizations (collaborative MASH programs).

MASH Clinic Requirements and Structure

Legal

Before considering a MASH clinic, be certain to check any relevant state or provincial veterinary practice acts and local regulations to be sure that MASH clinics are permitted. Some states and provinces require premise permits for any practice location, which may preclude MASH clinics. However, in some cases, states or provinces that require premise permits may allow exemptions for MASH clinics if asked in advance.

Location and Organization

MASH clinics are adaptable and there are not specific prerequisites for regional population density or shelter animal intake. They are suitable for rural areas where low population density does not easily support a stationary clinic, as well as for densely populated urban areas. MASH clinics are valuable for local shelters that wish to provide in-house high-quality high-volume spay–neuter (HQHVSN), but either cannot afford to build and equip their own surgical suites, or have surgical areas but lack veterinary staff. MASH clinics are also suitable for international and remote-area spay–neuter programs.

For a veterinarian with surgery skills seeking spay–neuter work, establishing a MASH clinic can be one of the fastest and lowest cost ways of starting a HQHVSN clinic. In most cases, veterinarians who choose this route should be willing to operate the business aspects of the clinic and be able and willing to

High-Quality, High-Volume Spay and Neuter and Other Shelter Surgeries, First Edition. Edited by Sara White.
© 2020 John Wiley & Sons, Inc. Published 2020 by John Wiley & Sons, Inc.

work with shelters and humane organizations in their target region.

In some cases, programs with limited startup funds may wish to offer surgery services before fundraising is complete or before a clinic site is located for a future stationary clinic. In this case, a MASH clinic may serve as a temporary, economical option during the development of the HQHVSN program. Since any equipment purchased for MASH can be used in other models, the MASH clinic provides the opportunity for quicker startup without loss of equipment investment.

While MASH programs are diverse, this chapter will focus on programs that utilize paid veterinarian(s) and technician(s) and operate within a prescribed region (as opposed to national or international scope). However, many of the descriptions in this chapter may be adapted to MASH programs that operate internationally and/or use volunteer veterinarians and technicians. For information on setting up international or remote-area MASH clinics, the reader is referred to Susan Monger's chapter on operating a field spay–neuter clinic in the *Field Manual for Small Animal Medicine* (Monger 2018).

Independent versus Collaborative MASH Programs

MASH programs can operate their clinics independently of other humane organizations in a region or may collaborate with other humane or community organizations to host their clinics. Some MASH clinics may use a combination of these two approaches. There are advantages and disadvantages to each of these models.

Collaborative MASH Programs

Collaborative MASH programs are generally small organizations that collaborate with various local humane or community groups that act as their hosts in the communities within their service area. These host groups (or "ground teams") must provide the venue and personnel, consisting of two to five staff members or volunteers, while the MASH program (or "surgery team") provides the veterinarian, the technician, and all surgical supplies and equipment. The host organization is responsible for scheduling, admitting, and discharging patients, and for printing, preparing, and distributing clinic paperwork such as medical record forms, liability releases, discharge instructions, rabies certificates, and neuter certificates. Host groups are often required to provide non-medical supplies such as tables, chairs, animal bedding, extra pet carriers, and trash receptacles. In these collaborative programs, the MASH group generally works with several different host organizations throughout its service area to host clinic days. At times, more than one local humane group may work together to host a MASH clinic.

Collaborative MASH programs empower small humane organizations and shelters to host their own "Spay Days," affording them the chance to enhance their community relations and outreach. The opportunity to host and assist with a MASH clinic enables staff and volunteers at host shelters to do something "fun" and different, compared to their usual shelter duties. These collaborations also allow opportunities for MASH clinic staff to share information and best practices for shelter medicine and HQHVSN with their host organizations.

Generally, it is the responsibility of the MASH organization to provide training and mentorship to new or potential new host organizations. Before hosting their first clinic, host organizations will need to know how to schedule the appropriate surgical load and how to determine the number and skill level of volunteers required. They need to understand the paperwork and be able to provide appropriate pre- and post-operative instructions to clients. An in-person meeting between the MASH organization and potential new hosts, along with written instructions on hosting protocols and expectations, is recommended prior to the first clinic.

Once a MASH organization has established relationships and carried out clinics with one or more host organizations, potential new host organizations can benefit greatly by visiting and observing existing host organizations during MASH clinic days. This peer-to-peer mentorship helps new host organizations develop their own protocols and systems, and allows them to see clinic flow and ask questions before their first clinic. In some cases, this mentorship may even continue, with representatives from existing host organizations attending the first few clinics sponsored by new host organizations, smoothing their transition into their role as host.

Advantages of the collaborative MASH model include flexibility and decreased operating costs. Staffing costs are decreased for the MASH organization because of the symbiotic relationship between the MASH organization and its hosts. The MASH organization pays only one veterinarian and one technician per day, in addition to an after-hours surgical pack preparation staff, and relies upon the host organization to provide additional resources (two to five staff or volunteers, and a venue). The hosts are motivated to provide this because they need the MASH program's staff, equipment, and expertise in order to offer affordable HQHVSN clinics.

In contrast to an independent MASH clinic, the collaborative MASH clinic requires a relatively small vehicle given the small staff and minimal equipment required. Purchasing a smaller vehicle results in a lower initial purchase price, as well as lower ongoing fuel and maintenance costs. This decreased operating cost often means that a collaborative MASH clinic is able meet its budget entirely via low-cost fees for service, without additional fundraising.

Independent MASH Programs

Independent MASH programs have sole responsibility for scheduling the venue, booking patients, securing volunteers and staff, and admitting and discharging patients. The independent MASH model is more likely to be adopted by large, pre-existing organizations, by new HQHVSN programs planning to transition to stationary clinics in the future, or by organizations doing MASH clinics intermittently. This is because developing and training the network of collaborating host organizations that is required for a collaborative MASH clinic take time and effort. For large, established organizations that have the resources to perform ground team tasks in addition to surgical team tasks, this extra task of collaborator development may be unnecessary. For MASH clinics that operate intermittently, the collaborative relationships may languish and be harder to maintain.

In an independent MASH clinic, staffing and finances are likely to be similar to a stationary clinic or self-contained mobile surgery unit, unless adequate, reliable volunteer staffing is available. Minimum required staff would consist of a veterinarian, a veterinary technician, one or more veterinary assistants, and administrative staff for record-keeping, patient booking, and reception.

Independent MASH clinics may require larger vehicles than collaborative programs to transport staff, surgical equipment, and some non-medical items such as animal bedding and extra pet carriers or crates. Since the staffing for this model of clinic is similar to that of a stationary clinic, the costs are higher as well, making this model harder to sustain financially than collaborative MASH clinics. However, independence can offer the advantage of more predictability by utilizing more consistent clinic staff and by not needing to rely on other humane groups to schedule clinic dates and locate suitable staff and volunteers.

Facilities

Venues for MASH clinics may be diverse and creative (see Figure 34.1). Examples of venues that have been used to house MASH clinics are included in Box 34.1. Despite these diverse locations, with few exceptions MASH clinics require an enclosed space of a minimum of 1000 sq. ft. (preferably 2000 sq. ft. or greater) that can be

(a)

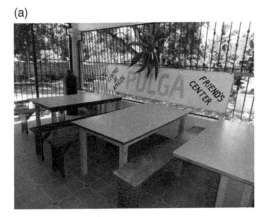

(b)

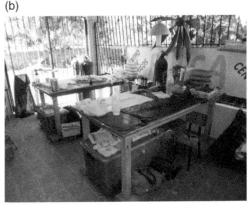

Figure 34.1   The arts and crafts area at a local elementary school (a) is transformed into a surgical suite (b) in Cabrera, Dominican Republic. *Source:* Photo courtesy of Cristie Kamiya.

Box 34.1   Examples of MASH Clinic Venues

- Shelter surgery suite
- Other shelter space (multipurpose/ activity room, dog training room)
- Pet boarding and grooming facility
- Fire station
- Church basement
- Town hall
- School gym
- American Legion post
- Senior center
- Low-income apartment complex's activity room
- Knights of Columbus hall

---

maintained at a safe, comfortable temperature, and access to hot and cold water and electricity. In cases where running water is not available, hot and cold water may be brought to the venue. Facilities may be able to provide large non-medical objects such as folding tables, chairs, and trash receptacles; if not, these items should be provided by the host organization.

"Home Base"

MASH clinics require a small area (minimum 10 × 10 ft.) for receiving and storage of supplies and medications. The ideal space is easy to access with a convenient geographic location and a convenient physical location (first floor, near supply delivery area), and is temperature controlled for safe medication storage. If the MASH program is part of an existing organization with a physical building, the MASH clinic can use this space. If the MASH is a new organization or has no suitable site, possible sites include the home of a staff member or a rental space. Renting space from an existing animal care organization such as a veterinary clinic offers the advantage of on-site staff to receive deliveries of temperature-sensitive items such as vaccines or medications.

If the home base is to be used for surgical pack preparation, it should contain or allow access to laundry facilities (unless all drapes and pack wrappers are disposable) and electricity, and should be large enough to accommodate pack assembly and an autoclave.

Animal Housing

Since many MASH clinics do not take place in animal care facilities, animal housing often consists of pet carriers or folding wire cages (see Figure 34.2). In these cases, host groups should be prepared to provide crates and bedding for housing dogs, as many owners will not have or will not be able to transport appropriate crates or cages for their dog. Cats and rabbits are generally housed in the carriers in which they arrive at the clinic, and community cats remain

(a)

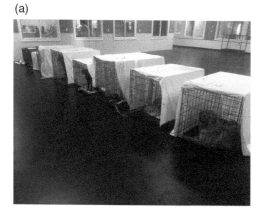

(b)

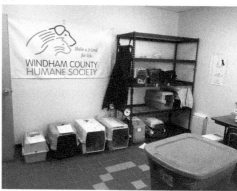

(c)

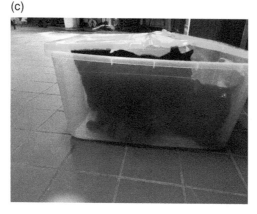

Figure 34.2 Animal housing at MASH clinics. (a) Dogs are housed in wire crates provided by the host organization at a MASH clinic in New Hampshire. (b) Cats are housed in the carriers in which they arrived. A shelter in Vermont has constructed a shelving unit to save floor space while housing cats. (c) Cats may arrive in inappropriate containers and should be transferred to appropriate housing for the day.

in their traps. It is wise to have additional crates available in which to house cats who arrive in inappropriate or inadequate housing.

Organizational Structure

MASH clinics may be established within any organizational structure, including nonprofit, for-profit, and government or tribal entities. In some cases, MASH clinics may represent a single program within a large, diverse existing organization. For example, an animal shelter with an in-house spay–neuter clinic may develop a MASH program to reach certain communities in its service area. In others, a new organization is formed for the purpose of offering MASH clinics, and this organization exists solely for the purpose of offering MASH clinics.

Financial Investments and Ongoing Costs

Financial requirements for a MASH clinic are generally much lower than for a stationary clinic or self-contained mobile unit. There will also be some differences in the initial investments between MASH clinics following a collaborative model versus an independent model. In all MASH clinics, the major initial costs will include acquisition of a vehicle, surgical and anesthetic equipment, initial consumable supplies (for example, drugs, vaccines, syringes and needles, gauze sponges, antiseptics, and suture material) and an autoclave. In cases in which the MASH clinic already has access to a suitable vehicle, or if the MASH vehicle is purchased with a car loan, the initial investment to start a collaborative MASH clinic will likely range from $20 000 to $35 000.

Ongoing costs for MASH will include personnel costs (salaries, wages, benefits, payroll taxes, workers compensation), consumable supplies, and vehicle gas and maintenance. Most MASH clinics will also need to rent a small, climate-controlled "home base" physical space for safe storage of consumable supplies (see earlier in this chapter).

Because overhead costs are low, it is possible to sustain a collaborative MASH clinic with low-cost fees for services, without additional fundraising. In cases where extremely discounted or free surgeries are to be offered, additional fundraising and grant-writing by the MASH clinic or by one or more host organizations will be required to subsidize program costs.

Personnel

Minimal personnel requirements for a collaborative MASH clinic generally consist of one veterinarian and one veterinary technician. Some MASH programs employ additional staff for instrument care or for management. In many collaborative MASH programs, the veterinarian and technician handle instrument care and management responsibilities without additional staff. For example, the veterinarian serves as the program director/manager, and the technician assumes the responsibility for preparing surgical packs.

Independent MASH programs require additional personnel, including veterinary assistants and administrative staff. The staffing model for these clinics is similar to that for a stationary or mobile self-contained clinic (see Chapters 32 and 33).

Surgical Capacity

Surgical capacity for a MASH clinic should be comparable to other HQHVSN models, although in many MASH clinics only one surgery table is available, so surgical flow and resulting speed are somewhat slower than in a fully equipped stationary clinic. However, unlike in some self-contained mobile units, physical space for animal housing need not be a limitation for MASH clinics. Approximately five hours of surgery time is a full day for a MASH clinic, and this may consist of as few as 15–20 dogs or as many as 50–60 cats for one veterinarian, depending on surgical speed and species and sex composition of the patient load.

Timeline

Startup time for a MASH program can vary. In the case of collaborative MASH programs, startup may be delayed if collaborating organizations need to be identified and persuaded. However, if collaborating organizations are prepared to host clinics immediately, a MASH program can start up in less than three months once finances are obtained.

Protocols and Equipment

Protocols

As with all HQHVSN clinics, MASH clinics should adhere to the Association of Shelter Veterinarians' (ASV) Guidelines for Spay-Neuter Programs (Griffin et al. 2016). Surgery techniques, patient selection, and disinfection and sterilization of equipment are no different than in other HQHVSN clinics. Anesthesia and analgesia protocols are similar to those in stationary clinics, although care must be taken to select protocols that are suitable for same-day discharge of patients. As with all clinic types, proper medical record-keeping is essential, and clients must be provided with written and verbal post-operative instructions.

Post-operative Care

As with other clinic types, there is a need to develop a post-operative care plan for emergencies and client questions. In most cases, this is achieved by providing a phone number to clients to contact MASH clinic staff in case of questions or emergencies. This phone may be carried by a veterinarian or a technician who can answer client questions and concerns and triage cases requiring veterinary care. For independent MASH clinics, administrative staff may carry this phone, triage calls, and refer medical questions to a veterinarian. Emergencies and rechecks will generally need to be seen by outside veterinary hospitals, as the MASH staff may be distant from the animal in question and may have no available facility in which to see patient rechecks. It is up to the MASH program to set policies with regard to client reimbursement or payment to outside veterinary hospitals seeing MASH clients. In many MASH clinics, as with other HQHVSN clinics, outside care is reimbursed if related to the surgical or anesthetic procedure, and if the client has generally followed post-operative instructions.

Some MASH programs have established relationships with specific local veterinarians or emergency clinics within their service areas who are willing to provide emergency care, and in some cases the clients may be provided with this contact information instead of or in addition to contact information for the MASH clinic. Other MASH programs establish relationships with local practices as needed, as the geographic areas covered by some MASH programs are large enough that specific local relationships may be difficult to establish. Regardless, it is essential that the MASH clinic has a plan in place for how it will address follow-up or emergency care for its patients.

Equipment

Equipment requirements for a MASH clinic are similar to those in other clinic types, but all items must be compact and packable, and must have the durability to withstand transport, as well as packing and unpacking daily. Choices for surgery table, surgery light, and anesthesia machines will be influenced by this need for packability and durability.

Vehicle

For a collaborative MASH clinic, the vehicle must have space for two people and the necessary equipment (see Figure 34.3). A small minivan, a compact sport utility vehicle (SUV), a station wagon, or a boxy passenger car can be adequate for a collaborative MASH program. Small, mass-market vehicles have the advantage of low purchase price, good fuel economy, and low maintenance costs.

For independent MASH programs, a somewhat larger vehicle such as a full-sized minivan may be necessary to contain and transport the surgical equipment plus the additional supplies (such as animal bedding, extra crates, and paperwork) required in this model.

With either model, for MASH programs operating regularly (weekly or more frequently), it is ideal to obtain a vehicle to be used exclusively for the MASH program, to eliminate the need to unload and reload equipment between surgery days.

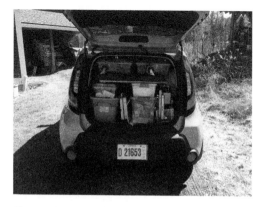

Figure 34.3 MASH vehicle. This Kia Soul is used exclusively for MASH spay–neuter and transports veterinarian, technician, and equipment to venues.

Anesthesia Equipment

Many MASH clinics use inhalational agents for patient anesthesia. If these agents are used, two anesthesia machines (one for the surgical preparation area and one for surgery) are recommended. Tabletop anesthesia machines are easy to carry and need not be disassembled to pack in a small vehicle (see Figure 34.4a). A Tec 4 vaporizer (see Figure 34.4b) is recommended over Tec 3-type vaporizers, as the Tec 4 contains internal baffles that limit the movement of the anesthetic agent and continues to deliver appropriate anesthetic concentrations even if the vaporizer is temporarily tipped or upended (Scott 1991). Oxygen may be obtained in portable E cylinders (see Figure 34.4c) and placed in two-wheeled oxygen cylinder carts and attached to the anesthesia machine via a regulator and an oxygen hose. Oxygen cylinders should be immobilized in the vehicle for transport.

Anesthetic gas scavenging may be achieved by active scavenging, if the MASH site is an existing surgery venue, or more commonly via passive scavenging. Passive options include exhaust through a window, through a hole made in the wall, or using an activate charcoal absorbent canister (brand names include F/Air, AneSorb, Clean Air, Breath Fresh, and others; see Figure 34.5). For more information on staff safety and anesthetic scavenging, see Chapter 31.

(a) (b) (c)

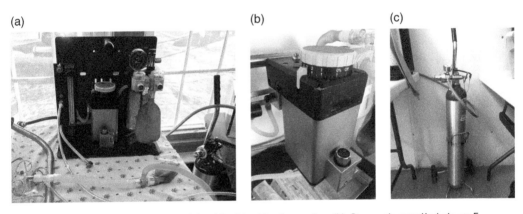

Figure 34.4 Tabletop anesthetic machine (a) with a Tec 4 vaporizer (b). Oxygen is supplied via an E cylinder (c) in a wheeled oxygen cylinder cart, attached with a regulator and oxygen hose.

(a) (b) (c)

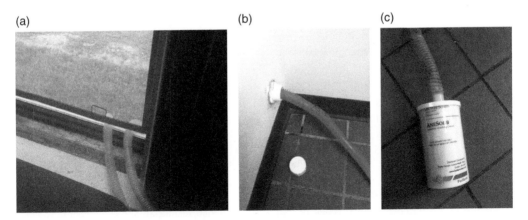

Figure 34.5 Passive anesthetic gas scavenging options (a) through a window; (b) through a hole made in the wall; (c) via a charcoal absorber canister.

Equipment Bins

Small equipment and supply items used during the MASH surgery day are packed in bins or totes to facilitate organization and transport (see Figure 34.6). Examples of bin storage are described in Box 34.2. As for all clinic models,

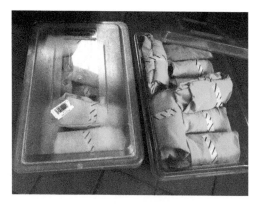

Figure 34.6 Bins contain smaller equipment and supplies to ease organization and transport, such as the 3.5 gallon food service bins used here as durable storage for surgical packs.

Box 34.2 Equipment Bins

- Anesthesia tubing/bags
- Surgical instruments (use smaller bins that hold 12–14 packs apiece)
- Electronics (light, clippers, vacuum, extension cords, laryngoscope)
- Syringes and needles
- Surgeon supplies (suture, masks, blades, glue)
- Liquids (items that freeze should be brought indoors in cold climates)
- Medications (items that freeze should be brought indoors in cold climates)
- "Crash cart" emergency medications (items that freeze should be brought indoors in cold climates)
- "Wake-up" table items (nail trimmers, flea combs, flea treatment, rabies tags and certificates, ear-cleaning supplies, ear mite treatment)
- Squeeze cage that collapses to become a container, and contains sharps containers, surgery gloves, Kevlar gloves

---

a "crash cart" or emergency bin should be designated and equipped (see Chapters 10 and 11 for more information on dealing with anesthetic emergencies).

Tables and Lighting

Some MASH programs require that host organizations provide appropriate-height surgery and prep tables and a surgery light at each venue. This is most easily achievable if clinic venues are used repeatedly and are owned by the host organization. In these cases, steel food service tables or appropriate-height tables constructed by volunteers offer alternatives to commercial surgery tables.

Other MASH programs have a portable surgery table or tabletop, allowing for greater flexibility in temporary surgery venues. A portable tabletop may be constructed using a piece of countertop with folding legs at a fixed or adjustable height that can be placed atop a standard-height table (see Figure 34.7). A small bin, such as a surgical instrument bin, may be used as an instrument stand. Other portable table alternatives include a small or standard folding table with bed risers (available online or in discount stores; see Figure 34.8). Low-cost, adjustable-height folding tables are also available from various retailers (see Figure 34.9). Further height adjustment can be made by using a surgical step stool to change surgeon height. Alternatives to a surgical step stool include an aerobics exercise step or a stack of click-together foam mats. The surgical prep table may be elevated to the appropriate height for the veterinary technician using bed risers or blocks (see Figure 34.8).

Portable surgical lighting may be achieved using an architect's lamp (see Figure 34.7) with a compact fluorescent bulb of 23 watts or greater, or a light-emitting diode (LED) bulb of 16 watts or greater (equivalent to a 100-watt incandescent bulb). Alternatively, a head lamp may be used (see Figure 34.10).

Patient Warming

Selecting a surgical patient-warming device for MASH can be challenging, as some are too

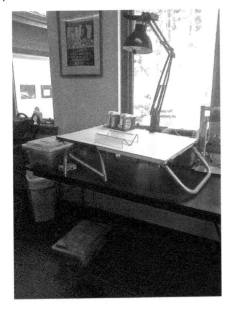

Figure 34.7 A piece of countertop with aluminum legs is placed upon a standard-height table. A small bin is used as an instrument tray. Lighting is provided using an architect's lamp with a compact fluorescent bulb.

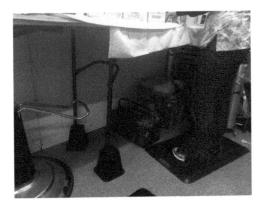

Figure 34.8 A surgery prep table is elevated using bed risers under the legs to achieve a comfortable working height for the veterinary technician.

bulky to transport in small MASH vehicles, and those containing water may be difficult to transport due to spilling or freezing water during transport and storage. A low-voltage conductive polymer fabric heating pad (such as Hot Dog or ChillBuster) can be used, as they are compact and fairly durable. In collaborative

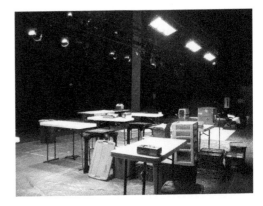

Figure 34.9 A MASH venue using adjustable-height folding tables for surgery and prep tables. This clinic is located onstage at a performing arts center in the Navajo Nation in Shiprock, New Mexico. *Source:* Photo courtesy of Cristie Kamiya.

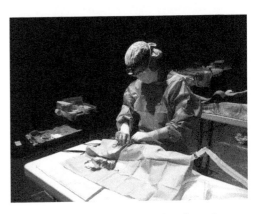

Figure 34.10 A surgeon uses a headlamp for illumination at a MASH clinic in Shiprock, New Mexico. *Source:* Photo courtesy of Cristie Kamiya.

MASH clinics, any post-operative warming devices to be used, such as heating pads, rice socks, or electric blankets, are generally supplied by the host organization, and should be used with caution (i.e. no skin contact, and only with direct human supervision) to avoid thermal burns.

Other Equipment

Additional equipment transported by the MASH clinic includes a scale to weigh surgery patients, anesthesia monitor(s) such as a pulse oximeter or capnograph, anti-fatigue floor mats, and an insulated container for vaccines.

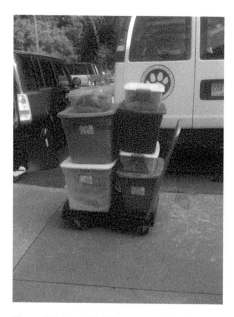

Figure 34.11 A folding cart assists in moving equipment bins between vehicle and surgery venue.

A folding cart to move bins between the vehicle and the surgery building speeds up loading and unloading and decreases lifting and carrying (see Figure 34.11). Safety equipment such as a cat net, animal handling gloves, syringe pole, squeeze cage, and dog muzzles should be included, as many venues will not have adequate handling equipment. An additional useful piece of handling equipment is a snappy snare, which is a 3–5 ft. stiff leash that can be placed on the dog from a distance, and is useful for safely applying a leash to a frightened dog in a crate or kennel.

Surgical Instruments and Their Care

In most cases, MASH clinics have no on-site autoclave. Most surgical instrument care, including ultrasonic cleaning, pack preparation, and autoclaving, takes place after hours or between clinic dates. Thus, many small, collaborative MASH clinics maintain enough sterile surgical packs for multiple (two to three) days' worth of surgery or schedule time between

surgery days for packing and sterilization. This may be especially important if the pack preparation is performed by staff who are also members of the traveling MASH clinic team.

Surgical instruments should be soaked to remove organic debris and cleaned by hand by volunteers at the surgical venue, then rinsed and returned to the transport vehicle to be transported back to the home base with the surgical team. Further instrument cleaning, laundering of drapes and pack wrappers, pack preparation, and sterilization may occur at the MASH clinic's home base, or alternatively may take place in a staff member's home. This at-home pack preparation and autoclaving may be advantageous if the staff member lives far from the home base, or if the staff member has household obligations (such as small children) that make after-hours travel to the home base difficult.

MASH: The Day of Surgery

MASH clinics are typically located in different venues with a different layout each day. Collaborative MASH clinics work with different assistant staff each day, as provided by the host organization. These changes can affect clinic flow and efficiency, and they require the MASH veterinarian and technician to adapt to a variety of new situations and circumstances.

Setting Up the Clinic

In a collaborative MASH clinic, the host organization's staff admits patients before the veterinarian and technician arrive, or while the veterinarian and technician are unpacking and setting up (see Figure 34.12). In each new clinic venue, the MASH veterinarian and technician must plan the layout and flow for the clinic. The veterinarian's and technician's workspaces are re-created as consistently as possible, but must be adjusted to accommodate the locations of windows, electrical outlets, and doors. Flow through the clinic should

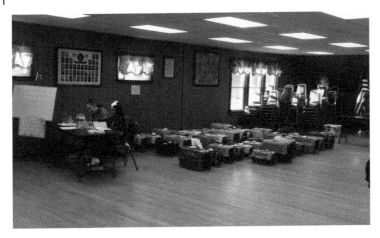

Figure 34.12 Volunteers admit patients to a MASH surgery day for cats at an American Legion Post in New Hampshire. Most MASH clinics use the carriers in which the animals arrive at the clinic as animal housing for the day, as built-in clinic cages are generally not available.

be optimized, although not every venue will lend itself to smooth flow between pre-op, prep, surgery, recovery, and post-op areas.

Clinic Flow

Clinic flow in a MASH program may be somewhat slower than flow in a stationary clinic. Typically, a MASH clinic has one surgery table per surgeon, such that the surgeon must wait while patients are exchanged on the table. To improve flow while working on cats, the surgeon may alternate male and female cats, castrating male cats on a side table or countertop while female cats are exchanged on the surgery table (see Figure 34.13). MASH clinics also usually have only one prep station, which may be the rate-limiting step during fast surgeries. Also, since clinic layout and staffing vary between locations, ideal flow may not be achievable at each clinic site.

Clinic Day

The MASH clinic day includes travel, setup, and re-packing, in addition to the usual tasks related to operating a HQHVSN clinic such as performing patient exams, anesthetic procedures, and surgery. As can be seen in the

example in Box 34.3, the total day length for the veterinarian and technician may be 11 hours, whereas the surgery time is only 4–5 hours. Thus, more than half the staff's time is spent driving, setting up, and re-packing the surgery area. This time budget may be improved somewhat by changing clinic policies: driving time may be reduced by restricting the travel radius, and setup and takedown time may be reduced if the clinic is located in the same venue for multiple days.

The time required for these additional tasks of driving, setting up, and packing means that MASH clinics are not the most efficient clinic model in regard to use of the veterinarian's and technician's professional time. A MASH that employs only one veterinarian and one technician may be operating "full-time" (36–40 hours a week) with just 3 clinics – or about 100 surgeries – per week, if the technician is also preparing packs between surgery days, and the veterinarian is acting as administrator and business manager. However, despite achieving fewer surgeries per full-time veterinarian, the lower overhead costs mean that the cost per surgery is equivalent to that of a stationary clinic. This allows MASH clinics to pay hourly wages to the veterinarian and

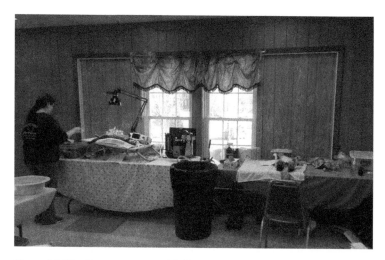

Figure 34.13 Surgery area at a MASH surgery day for cats at an American Legion Post in New Hampshire. Female cats are placed on the surgery table to the left in the photo, and male cat neuters take place on the table on the right. At this clinic, the surgeon stands for cat spays and sits for cat neuters.

Box 34.3   MASH Spay–Neuter Clinic: A Typical Day

7:30 a.m.: Vet and tech meet up to travel together

7:30–9:00 a.m.: Drive to clinic location, up to 1.5 hours away

9:00–9:30 a.m.: Unpack and set up surgery area

9:30–10:30 a.m.: Physical exams

10:45 a.m.: First animal goes to surgery

12:45 p.m.: Lunch break

1:30–3:30 or 4:30 p.m.: Surgery

4:00–4:45 p.m.: Clean up and pack vehicle

5:00–6:30 p.m.: Drive home

---

technician that are on a par with, or in some cases greater than, stationary or self-contained mobile HQHVSN clinics.

Conclusion

MASH clinics provide a flexible, low-cost, high-quality method for delivering spay–neuter services. The MASH clinic's versatility, adaptability, relatively low capital investment, and short time to startup are the particular strengths of this clinic type, and make these clinics useful both as short-term solutions as well as long-term, sustainable HQHVSN providers.

References

Griffin, B., Bushby, P.A., McCobb, E. et al. (2016). The Association of Shelter Veterinarians' 2016 veterinary medical care guidelines for spay-neuter programs. *JAVMA* 249: 165–188.

Monger, S. (2018). Operating a field spay/neuter clinic. In: *Field Manual for Small Animal Medicine* (eds. K. Polak and A.T. Kommedal). Hoboken, NJ: Wiley https://doi.org/10.1002/9781119380528.ch5.

Scott, D.M. (1991). Performance of BOC Ohmeda Tec 3 and Tec 4 vaporisers following tipping. *Anaesth. Intens. Care* 19: 441–443.

35

Feral and Free-Roaming Cat Clinics
Christine Wilford

Feral and free-roaming cat clinics are clinics that offer spay–neuter for cats that have no clear ownership in the community (see Chapter 25). In more recent years, these clinics are increasingly referred to as community cat clinics, because cats brought for spay–neuter are typically a mix of feral, stray, abandoned, and lost pet cats. Because the tractability, health, and rabies vaccination status of these community cats are unknown, the clinics must follow specific policies and procedures for the safety of the people and cats involved. Once they are anesthetized, sterilization surgery on a feral cat is much the same as any other cat, but to organize a safe and successful clinic, important pre- and post-operative differences require planning/consideration and accommodation.

A popular and humane approach to population control of community cats is trap–neuter–return or TNR, which involves trapping, surgical sterilization, rabies vaccination, and return of cats to where they were trapped. TNR is palatable for people who feed community cats compared to trap and kill programs. Without access to spay–neuter through community cat clinics, TNR could not succeed.

Clinic Requirements, Structure, and Costs

Legal Requirements

The same legal requirements for any spay–neuter clinic apply to community cat clinics. In some areas, local ordinances may restrict trapping or legislate the management and disposition of unowned cats. Each clinic must check the regulations in its area.

Independent versus Collaborative Structure

Community cat clinics can be independent or may collaborate with local rescue groups and trappers. The structure of independent community cat clinics resembles standard spay–neuter clinics. The clinics offer surgery and leave the responsibility of collecting cats to individual clients. Caregivers – the people who feed, monitor, and manage community cats – are responsible for trapping, transport, and return, thus limiting the clinic's role to surgical sterilization. In independent clinics, the reservations process can be cumbersome, especially when many inexperienced trappers require instruction for

High-Quality, High-Volume Spay and Neuter and Other Shelter Surgeries, First Edition. Edited by Sara White.
© 2020 John Wiley & Sons, Inc. Published 2020 by John Wiley & Sons, Inc.

successful trapping and support for humane, safe care during transport and recovery after surgery. Clinics may accept the responsibility for training, or they may refer people to the many resources available via the internet.

Collaborative clinics partner with rescue groups and experienced hobby trappers who trap cats for other people. Hobby trappers typically have better success and fill more surgery spaces than people who are new to trapping. In addition, rescue groups may train volunteers to trap cats. With this structure, the clinic simply allots a block of reservations per group or trapper. This simplifies reservations, streamlines the check-in and check-out process, and reduces no-shows.

Financial Investments and Ongoing Costs

The financial investment for community cat clinics is similar to any other feline spay–neuter clinic. If the clinic also loans traps (discussed later), then the financial investment in high-quality traps can be substantial. The purchase of a squeeze cage and a couple of capture nets is advisable, but does not constitute a large investment. The ongoing cost that differs from typical spay–neuter clinics is rabies vaccine, which is administered free of charge to all community cats.

Mission Control

Taking the time to identify the clinic's mission *before* embarking on a community cat clinic saves time, money and headaches. The mission functions as the clinic's compass, offering guidance to stay on course. The mission is the ultimate goal and must be central to all clinic functions and decisions (see Chapter 28 for more on purpose and mission).

Feral versus Tame

Because community cats usually range from truly feral cats to pet cats, the first decision

regarding the mission is whether to limit surgeries to feral cats, or whether to accept all free-roaming cats for surgery. Because all feral cats ultimately come from unaltered pet cats, the general wisdom is to achieve feral cat prevention by accepting all community cats for spay–neuter. Furthermore, since a fractious pet cat is indistinguishable from a feral cat, restricting a clinic to feral cats is logistically impossible.

Core Services

The most basic community cat clinic must provide certain core services: safe and sufficient anesthesia, high-quality surgical sterilization with absorbable suture, rabies vaccine, ear-tipping, appropriate recovery monitoring and care, and euthanasia when indicated.

Individual Health versus Population Control

Because cats may arrive at sterilization clinics with additional health issues, the clinic's mission needs to be clear as to whether the goal is to improve the individual lives of all community cats or to maximize surgical sterilization for population control. It is not possible for the mission to be both unless human and financial resources are unlimited. The more services performed per cat, such as retroviral testing, vaccines, and flea control, the fewer resources remain for spay–neuter. Consequently, clinics that maximize population control will minimize additional services. A middle ground is to offer a few additional services, such as FVRCP vaccines and flea control, at a nominal fee either to cover the clinic's cost or with a profit margin to subsidize surgery costs.

Surgery Only versus Trapping Assistance

Community cat clinics can be limited to surgical sterilization without becoming involved in trapping. At the other extreme, clinics may purchase traps, train trappers, organize trapping, and handle every aspect of TNR. Between these extremes lies the surgical clinic that limits trapping assistance to loaning traps and training people in how to use them.

Clinics that offer trapping assistance need human and financial resources sufficient to support trapping in addition to maximizing surgery. The organization must consider the responsibility and liability of sending volunteers to trap cats on private or public property.

Create Clear Policies

Once the mission is defined, clear policies help prevent mission drift. Exceptions are expected, but policies provide the structure needed to maintain the mission.

Retroviral Testing

Screening every cat for feline leukemia and feline immunodeficiency virus is costly and detracts from the mission to reduce overpopulation. If a community's infection rate is 2%, then the cost of identifying one positive cat equals the cost of 50 tests. Furthermore, low disease prevalence combined with the specificity and sensitivity of retroviral tests leads to false positives and potential euthanasia of healthy, uninfected cats. The original feral cat clinics in the 1980s and 1990s viral tested early in their programs and later discontinued testing, due to high cost and low disease prevalence. Experts agree with the current strategy that resources should be prioritized for surgical sterilization.

Euthanasia

According to a large-scale study of over 100 000 cats, an average of 0.4% cats presented to community cat clinics required euthanasia (Wallace and Levy 2006). When a cat's condition appears too poor to survive surgery and live a humane lifestyle in its free-roaming home, euthanasia must be considered. Retroviral testing cats in poor condition is often suggested, but in reality euthanasia should be based on health. A debilitated cat with a negative retroviral test result should still be euthanized, if it cannot be treated.

Euthanasia decisions must be delegated to a trusted, qualified person, because the decision is more often unclear than straightforward. Questions to consider are: Can this cat find shelter? Find food? Escape predators? Survive without suffering? These are the quality-of-life requirements for any community cat. Consulting caregivers about the recent history of difficult cases may offer valuable insight to simplify the decision.

Ear-Tipping

Ear-tipping, the surgical removal of approximately 1 cm from the tip of one ear (see Chapter 16), is a worldwide, universal mark of a surgically sterilized cat (Figure 35.1). It should be noted that an ear tip does not mean the cat is behaviorally feral or that it ever was, nor does an ear tip indicate the cat has ever been rabies vaccinated or that a rabies vaccine is current. A visible ear tip is meant to prevent future trapping and unnecessary surgery; in essence, the ear tip protects the cat. Ear tips also keep clinic reservations and resources directed toward unsterilized cats.

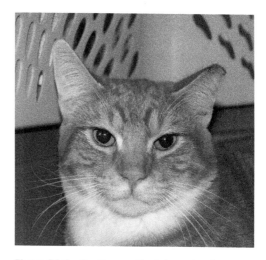

Figure 35.1 Ear tips are the international standard verifying surgical sterilization, but do not indicate the cat is feral or ever was.

Several ear-tipping dilemmas should be addressed in the ear-tipping policy. One is whether to ear tip feral kittens that may become adoptable after fostering. If the ear-tipped kittens become adoptable, the ear tip becomes unnecessary. In the author's experience, ear tips do not make kittens or cats less adoptable and are worth performing during surgical sterilization in case the kittens must return to their colony.

Another policy issue is whether to ear tip tame community cats believed not to have owners. If they are unaltered, then ear-tipping seems a clear choice, but already altered tame cats without a microchip or collar might have an owner.

Ear-tip size must be policy. All ear tips should be 1 cm, and proportionately less for kittens. Caregivers often request small ear tips, but minimizing an ear tip for cosmetic purposes risks negating the entire goal: to protect the cat from repeated trapping, transport, anesthesia, and surgery. Small ear tips are much more likely to be overlooked once the ear heals and the hair regrows.

Rabies Vaccination

Because of public health implications, all cats presented to community cat clinics should be vaccinated for rabies unless an owner is located. Use of a three-year vaccine is recommended, if it complies with local and state legal requirements. Manufacturer's recommendations should be followed according to the minimum age. Kittens too young to vaccinate may stay in foster until old enough to vaccinate.

Additional Services

In addition to core services, which additional services to provide depends on the financial and human resources as well as the primary mission: individual health or population control. When the health of each cat is the primary mission and resources are finite, this paradigm spends more money per cat and performs fewer surgical sterilizations. Some clinics provide dentals, all vaccines, viral testing, parasite treatment, grooming, and more. Ear mite treatment, flea control, deworming, and vaccination for panleukopenia, upper respiratory viruses, and retroviruses are considered optional, because they target individual health.

Limiting additional procedures translates into more surgical sterilizations; however, even a basic spay–neuter clinic can perform some basic services in special circumstances without significantly impacting resources or efficiency. For example, benefits from the occasional tail amputation, enucleation, abscess flush, basic wound care, deeply positioned polydactyl nail declaw, or flea control for severely infested kittens or cats require minimal resources in addition to surgical sterilization.

Although there is an emotional reward for treating external parasites, these infestations are not cured with one treatment, and reinfestation occurs after return to a colony; consequently, resources allocated for these services would be better redirected toward spay–neuter.

Bite Injuries to People

Protocols must be in place to prevent cat bite injuries, but nonetheless, bites will occur. Bite victims should always seek medical care. The local public health department can assist with developing a protocol regarding the cat, which would either consist of quarantine or euthanasia and rabies testing. Bites are typically provoked; that is, a conscious cat is frightened and defensive, or the cat is not fully sedated when being handled. Clinics should consider restricting involvement of volunteers or staff that repeatedly break protocols and put themselves and cats at risk.

Containment

Clinics must set a policy for whether cats can be brought only in traps or in any other type of containers or carriers (plastic, cardboard, wooden, metal). Prohibiting containers other than traps allows for safe and simple anesthetic induction. However, traps are unwieldy, occupy more space, and may limit how many cats fit inside a clinic or can be transported. Good-quality traps cost more than carriers. Many trappers and caregivers can bring more cats if carriers are permitted. Cats transfer from a carrier to a squeeze cage fairly easily, though there is a minimal risk of escape. Inducing anesthesia in a squeeze cage is as simple and safe as in a trap.

Microchip

Every cat should be carefully scanned with a universal scanner during the pre-operative exam. If a chip is revealed, clinic policy must consider ethical and legal implications while providing the best outcome for the cat. The clinic can accept full responsibility for following up or relinquish this work to the caregiver. In the author's experience, some caregivers ignore the chip information and simply return a cat to a colony, while others do whatever it takes to locate an owner. Deciding how to handle all the contingencies in advance saves chaos and confusion when a chip is found.

Sick but Treatable Cats

Inevitably, cats arrive with conditions that are potentially curable but too serious to allow immediate, humane return to the colony. The options are euthanasia or captivity and treatment. Clinics that cultivate good relationships with caregivers can identify individuals who responsibly and correctly care for sick community cats at home. Some cats need referral to a veterinary practice for further care. Clinic veterinarians must screen cases on an individual basis to avoid releasing a sick or suffering cat to a hoarder or insufficient care. If a clinic cannot ensure good care, then euthanasia is the better choice.

A related issue is the value of pre-operative care to improve patient condition. In many circumstances, caregivers bring sick cats for spay–neuter and plan on nursing care afterward. Instead, caregivers should be taught to provide nursing care *prior* to surgery rather than after, when possible.

Kittens

Policy should state what age and size kittens are allowed. Many caregivers place kittens into foster for socializing and adoption after spay–neuter. However, in the kittens' best interests, caregivers should be instructed to vaccinate, observe, and treat for health problems prior to surgery, when feasible.

Ventral Abdominal Scars

Handling ventral abdominal scars, misnamed "spay scars," requires a clear policy. While many spays cause scars, not all scars are from spays. In the author's experience, most perfectly straight ventral abdominal scars in the exact region of a spay surgery are, in fact, spay scars. However, the author has personally seen pregnant and intact female cats with scars that others deemed spay scars. Had these cats not been explored, they would have returned home with ear tips and subsequently given birth to kittens. The only method to verify sterilization is to explore all female cats that have ventral abdominal scars but do not have tattoos or ear tips. Ear-tipping and releasing an intact or pregnant female negate the entire mission and undermine the reputation of a community cat clinic.

Ear-Tipped Cats

Occasionally, ear-tipped cats are not recognized and show up at the clinic. When noticed prior to anesthesia, they can simply be returned home. Some clinics take advantage of having the cat and boost the rabies vaccine. These cats can easily be vaccinated in a trap or squeeze cage without sedation.

Patient Considerations

Trap Etiquette

Captivity causes extreme stress for feral cats as well as many tame cats. Covering traps and carriers allows cats to hide, thereby reducing stress. Covers also reduce transmission of contagious disease and help cats maintain adequate body heat. Traps and carriers should be covered at all times prior to anesthesia, from the time cats are first trapped, during transport, and until anesthetic induction. Once cats have safely recovered from anesthesia and no longer need observation, they should be covered again until return to their homes. (See Chapter 6 for more information about reducing stress in the spay–neuter clinic.)

Transport Standards

Transport can present risks of its own (see Chapter 33 for more information about patient transport). Transport must be safe, comfortable, and humane, with particular attention to temperature, space, and ventilation. Covers are imperative for humane transport. Traps should not be stacked on top of each other to avoid eliminations descending from higher traps to cats in lower traps.

Pre-anesthetic Fasting

Many cats are trapped the day, night, or morning before surgery, thus fasting pre-operatively is not always possible. Because trapping is often hit or miss, any trapped community cat should be accepted for surgery regardless of fasting. To maximize fasting, cats that present without food can be anesthetized ahead of cats with food in their traps.

Safety Measures

The primary difference between a community cat clinic and a standard feline clinic is cat handling. Handling a conscious feral cat almost guarantees serious injury to the handler and risks potential exposure to rabies. Using the proper tools (see the additional equipment section later in this chapter) and adhering to protocols are vital for preventing injury to people and cats.

Rabies

In most regions, rabies exposure is a potential risk when handling any free-roaming animal of unknown history, including cats. Community cats without ear tips have no known history of previous ownership or rabies vaccination. Hence, with regard to safety, clinics must treat all community cats as feral and unvaccinated. Every individual with direct exposure to cats should be rabies vaccinated prior to working in a community cat clinic.

Anesthetic Induction

Using only an intramuscular injectable anesthetic protocol prevents handling of conscious cats and the associated risk of injury. Cats may be restrained in a trap with a trap divider or transferred from a carrier to a squeeze cage for injection without risk of injury to the anesthetist (Figures 35.2 and 35.4). Under no circumstances should a cat be handled without sedation.

Exam Gloves

Exam gloves should be worn by anyone having any direct contact with cats or their tissues, as well as anyone carrying cats in traps, to prevent contact with body fluids and eliminations.

Bite Incidents

Anyone sustaining a bite or scratch should immediately seek medical attention. Typically, the local health department dictates whether a cat should be quarantined or euthanized and

(a)

(b)

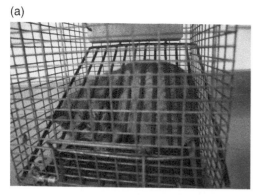
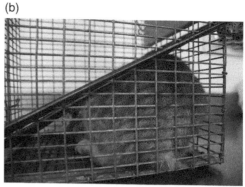

Figure 35.2 (a) The trap tipped on end and (b) using a trap divider to restrain the cat for injection.

(a)

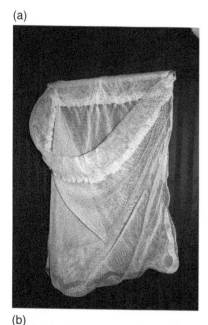

(b)

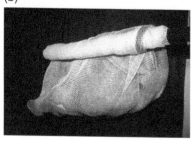

Figure 35.3 A capture net, such as the Freeman Cage net, should be on hand for escaped cats. (a) The net opens and closes by sliding the plastic handle up and down the pole. (b) Once the cat is inside, rolling the net around the pole provides restraint.

rabies tested. All staff and volunteers should be regularly reminded that well-meaning efforts that involve breaking safety protocols not only put themselves at risk for a bite wound, but also put the cat at risk for euthanasia or the stress of quarantine, at the very least.

Additional Equipment

Only a few unique items are necessary to properly equip a community cat clinic.

Capture Net

While many protocols aim to prevent loose cats, invariably a cat escapes. Using bare hands, gloves, or a towel does not protect against injury. Capture nets specific for catching cats, such as the Freeman Cage net (freemancanada.com), prevent injury to cats and people. When one is used correctly, one person can catch and restrain the cat, and administer an anesthetic injection. Fishing nets should not be used, because they are insufficient for ideal restraint and the nylon netting can injure the cats (Figure 35.3a and b).

Squeeze Cage

If cats are not presented in traps, then a squeeze cage is very useful. With experience and skill, transferring a cat from a carrier to the

(a)

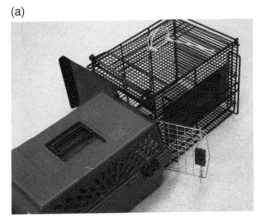

(b)

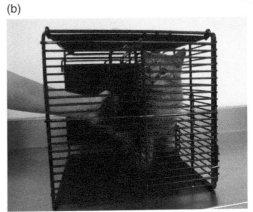

Figure 35.4 Transferring a cat from a carrier to a squeeze cage (a) provides safe restraint (b) for the anesthetic injection.

squeeze cage can be done with minimal risk of escape (Figure 35.4a). Once inside the squeeze cage, anesthetic induction is simple and safe for cat and human. The OmniCage (http://campbellpet.com) is the author's favorite because of its smooth operation, ease of use by a single person, and durability (Figure 35.4b).

Trap Divider/Comb

Trap dividers or combs are used to restrain the cat for anesthetic induction (http://livetrap.com). Dividers also contain the cat in order to remove food.

Traps

If a clinic elects to purchase traps for loaning or for a trapping program, there are many brands and styles available, all at different costs. Some function more smoothly or are more durable. Styles with a guillotine door on one end are most useful for removing sedated cats and transferring conscious cats into carriers (Figure 35.5).

Trap Covers

Trap coverings should be inexpensive, washable, and easy to put on and take off. Sheets and towels are sufficient. In colder climates, blankets

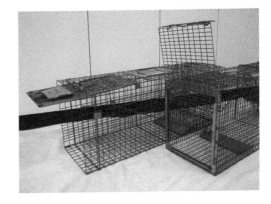

Figure 35.5 Trap types: the trap on the left has one trap door and one closed end. The style on the right with one guillotine door and one trap door is preferable.

and comforters work well. Fitted trap covers are available commercially.

Protocols

Anesthesia

Anesthetic Cocktails

To avoid handling a conscious cat, an intramuscular injectable regimen is required. A long-acting combination of Telazol® (Zoetis, Parsippany, NJ; tiletamine 50 mg/ml and zolazepam 50 mg/ml when reconstituted) reconstituted with 4 ml ketamine and 1 ml xylazine

(100 mg/ml) instead of sterile water is used as the sole anesthetic regimen (see Chapter 8) for clinics with lengthy processing of cats through all procedures. A shorter-acting combination of Telazol reconstituted with 4 ml ketamine and 1 ml xylazine (20 mg/ml), nicknamed TKX20 by the author, works well for clinics in which cats are processed more quickly. The TKX20 cocktail is also ideal for induction followed by mask isoflurane. TKX20 for compromised cats may promote more rapid recovery, as well as for lactating queens when prompt return to kittens is needed. Other injectable cocktails are widely used in typical spay–neuter clinics, but TKX is more cost effective and is well established for its safety in community cats whose medical histories are unavailable (Williams et al. 2002). In a study of over 100 000 community cats, the death rate with TKX protocols averaged 0.4% or 4/1000 cats (Wallace and Levy 2006).

Anesthetic Dosing

Since handling conscious cats is prohibited, the anesthetic dose is an estimate, not a calculation based on actual body weight. Many clinics simply categorize patients into small/kitten, medium/average, and large/tomcat and pre-draw the anesthetic into three doses of 0.125, 0.25, and 0.3 ml, respectively. The relatively low incidence of adverse reactions after estimated doses attests to the relative safety of TKX at both concentrations. An alternative method is TKX20 dosed at 0.02 ml/lb estimated body weight by 0.5 lb. People who estimate cat weights consistently develop skill and become quite accurate.

Alternatively, some clinics know the actual or approximate weight of the traps, so are able to weigh the cat in the trap and then subtract the weight of the trap to determine the weight of the cat for drug dosing purposes.

Anesthetic Injection Technique

When using a trap or squeeze cage, anesthetic administration is straightforward. By tipping the trap on end, the cat is moderately confined.

Using a trap divider or comb further restrains the cat for the injection. (see Figures 35.2). The squeeze cage has one movable side used to compress the cat against the opposite wall. This provides humane and safe restraint for injection (see Figure 35.3).

Any accessible muscle mass can be used for injection; paralumbar and thigh muscles are typically simplest. Before inducing anesthesia, all cats must be scrutinized for an ear tip on either ear. If they are ear tipped, anesthesia is not needed.

Vomiting

Xylazine can induce vomiting, thus close monitoring can literally be life-saving, particularly at induction. If vomiting begins, conscious cats should not be removed from the trap because of bite risk. Instead, lowering the cat's head by tipping the trap or cage is safest. If the cat is too conscious to remove but too sedate to clear its own mouth, a long spoon can be inserted through the trap to remove food from the cat's mouth. Once safely sedated, the cat can be removed and the mouth cleared with a spoon, not fingers! Many bite wounds that occur in community cat clinics are from people inserting their fingers into a cat's mouth.

Supplemental Anesthesia

For fast-paced clinics, the TKX20 is ideal, because cats recover sooner for earlier discharge. If cats need additional anesthesia, then supplemental masking with isoflurane works well without putting staff at risk of being bitten when intubating. If nasal breathing is compromised, then endotracheal intubation should be considered.

If gas anesthesia is unavailable, then one-quarter to one-third of the original dose of TKX20 or TKX100 given subcutaneously or intramuscularly is a good starting point to lengthen anesthesia. Careful monitoring is advised whenever subsequent injections are required. Yohimbine can be used for reversal, as needed.

Induction Monitoring

Inattention and complacency toward observation and monitoring are often the greatest danger to cats. Onset of anesthesia can be rapid, within minutes in some cats, so very close monitoring of body position and respiration is vital for patient safety. The airway may become obstructed when a cat bends its neck as it becomes sedate. Tilting the trap to reposition a semiconscious cat will straighten the neck. Apnea is not rare, but is easily resolved if recognized promptly. Once cardiac depression and arrest begin, resuscitation is less successful (see Chapter 11).

Shush!

Clinics should be quiet. Noise increases stress for most cats, but especially feral cats. Loud music and conversation typically lead to louder music and louder conversation. When an urgent situation erupts, noise delays the response and increases chaos. Silence is not necessary, but soft voices and perhaps soft music are better for cats and people. See Chapter 6 for more information about stress reduction in the spay–neuter clinic.

Loose Cat

Two or three individuals should be designated as the capture team for any loose cat. The chaos that develops when a cat escapes is magnified when too many people attempt to catch it. Ideally, when a cat gets loose, only the capture team should mobilize. Approaching a cat quietly and slowly is more successful than chasing and yelling. Everyone else should stand still, monitor any cats in their care, protect the surgeons, and face the cat! Terrified cats attempt escape by climbing up anything and everything, including a person whose back is turned. No one should ever try to grab the cat with their hands, a towel, or leather gloves. Using a capture net is safest. Everyone on the capture team should practice and become proficient with using the net before ever needing it (Figure 35.3a and b).

Pre-operative Examination

A full pre-op exam can be performed in less than two minutes during surgical preparation. Most cats are in good health. Besides confirming sex and lack of ear tip, the examiner assesses the cat's general health and looks for conditions that require additional medical attention or euthanasia. The more common abnormal findings include external parasites, upper respiratory infection, wounds, flea dermatitis, and dehydration. Less common findings include healed fractures, diarrhea, mats, pododermatitis, dental disease, self-mutilation secondary to ear mites, ruptured eyes, mastitis, chronic aural hematomas secondary to mites, ingrown polydactyl nails, and tail injuries warranting partial amputation. Identifying and documenting pregnancy or lactation is also important. Careful scanning for a microchip with a universal scanner is strongly recommended. Weighing cats after induction is useful for dosing additional medications, such as buprenorphine and antibiotics.

All cats should be carefully scrutinized for ear tips during their pre-op exam in case it was overlooked prior to anesthesia. Small ear tips are difficult to recognize. In regions with severe cold, frostbitten ears can look exactly like ear tips, so other means of confirming previous sterilization are warranted. The absence of penile spines indicates sterilization has been performed on male cats. A ventral abdominal tattoo is the only means of confirming previous sterilization of female cats during a pre-op examination.

Ear Tip

The ear tip declares the cat surgically sterilized in order to avoid transport, holding, anesthesia, and unnecessary surgery in the future. If ear tips are made too small, they are easily missed. Ear-tip technique is discussed in Chapter 16.

Spay

For the most part, community cat spays differ very little from routine cat spays. Many community cats will be pregnant, in heat, or postpartum. Community cats require absorbable sutures. A ventral midline incision is appropriate. Some veterinarians prefer a flank approach for lactating cats to avoid the engorged mammary glands. When pyometra is discovered, the cats typically recover well with only surgery and a long-acting antibiotic injection.

Neuter

Large tomcats are commonly presented. While the castration technique is the same as for younger male cats, the tunics and vessels in a large tomcat are more prone to loosening and bleeding. When using self-tie techniques, surgeons must ensure the knots are very tight, and the cords are not cut too close to the knots. For cryptorchid cats, absorbable suture is used for skin closure.

Pain Relief

Buprenorphine is a pain relief medication that meets all the requirements of community cat clinics because of its efficacy and safety in cats with unknown medical histories. Buprenorphine may be administered by intramuscular injection.

Non-steroidal anti-inflammatory drugs (NSAIDs) are not advised for dehydrated patients, thus their use in community cat clinics is undesirable or should be implemented with caution. Some community cat clinics have successfully incorporated Onsior® (robenacoxib; Elanco Animal Health, Greenfield, IN) injections into their community cat clinic protocols.

Recovery

Anesthetic Reversal

Clinics using the longer-acting TKX may reverse all cats with yohimbine post-operatively. The dose of yohimbine is based on the dose of TKX. When using the shorter-acting TKX, reversal is reserved for prolonged recovery or anesthetic complications, such as respiratory arrest. Yohimbine may also be used for frail or compromised cats with greater anesthetic risk, in order to hasten their recovery before discharging to the caregiver. Lactating queens similarly benefit from reversal, to facilitate earlier return to kittens.

Post-operative Monitoring

Cats recover from TKX very well as a rule, but post-op monitoring must be rigorous. Delayed recovery is most commonly caused by low body temperature and/or higher relative dose of anesthesia. Close monitoring of breathing and consciousness reveals problems sooner, when treatment is more likely to be successful.

Recovering cats can be safely assessed and stimulated without direct handling by moving the cage/trap or prodding with a dowel. If a cat cannot be aroused, then it should be removed from its trap/cage and evaluated, paying particular attention to body temperature, mucous membrane color, and pulse rate and quality. Providing supplemental heat and stimulation, for example by moving the legs, flipping the cat over, patting its chest, and so on, usually enhances recovery in the absence of more serious complications, such as hemorrhage.

Re-anesthetizing

If a cat needs to be re-anesthetized, a second dose of TKX can be used at one-quarter the original dose, or more depending on the cat's level of consciousness. Netting the cat and masking with gas anesthesia is an alternative; however, the risk of injury to people can be greater, and exposure to waste anesthetic gas is also increased. Each case must be evaluated on an individual basis, but human safety must be a priority.

Euthanasia

If issues develop warranting euthanasia after a cat is conscious or semiconscious, the cat should be re-sedated before being euthanized. This ensures human safety during handling as well as preventing stress for the cat. Euthanasia solution can be administered intravenously once the cat is fully anesthetized.

Return

Cats are discharged from the clinic on surgery day. Caregivers typically return the cat home the next day after surgery. Every cat must be fully recovered from anesthesia, with no visual evidence of complications before release. Most community cats will eat and drink in captivity, particularly in a quiet environment, during the night, and when covered. Cats in substandard condition may benefit from recovering in captivity for a longer period.

Anorexia/Hyporexia

The simple stress of captivity causes some cats to refuse food and water. They appear bright and alert but scared, often hiding in a corner with a very tense posture. These cats may benefit from being returned to their free-roaming homes as soon as possible. If the cat appears depressed or lethargic, or if it had been eating well at first but the appetite declined, then further evaluation by a veterinarian is warranted before release.

Lactating Queens

Lactation indicates kittens. A caregiver may promptly try to locate kittens, if notified soon enough that a cat is lactating. If kittens are not found, releasing the queen the night of surgery may increase the survivability of the kittens. Extremely thin lactating queens can incite thoughts of euthanasia, but fortunately these cats quickly gain weight in captivity, especially if kittens are weaned.

Enucleated Cats

One-eyed cats survive very well when returned to their colonies. The traumatized eyes are blind before enucleation, so the cats are already adapted to having only one visual eye. Because many of these eyes are infected, cats undergoing enucleation benefit from a longer recovery in captivity. Observation can ensure the surgical site is healing and that infection is resolving.

Complications, Pyometra, Debilitation

Cats recovering from serious conditions benefit from longer care post-operatively. Surprisingly, many cats with serious infections may eat antibiotics mixed in food. Cats with complications or debilitation from any condition should not be returned until they are past the potential for suffering. Caregivers experienced with using a capture net may be able to administer subcutaneous fluids and injectable medications with minimal risk of injury.

With proper equipment, protocols, and planning, community cat clinics are a rewarding experience and a valuable contribution to population control.

References

Wallace, J.L. and Levy, J.K. (2006). Population characteristics of feral cats admitted to seven trap-neuter-return programs in the United States. *J. Feline Med. Surg.* 8: 279–284.

Williams, L.S., Levy, J.K., Robertson, S.A. et al. (2002). Use of anesthetic combination of tiletamine, zolazepam, ketamine and xylazine for neutering feral cats. *JAVMA* 220 (10): 1491–1495.

36

In-Clinic Clinics
Ruth Steinberger

Introduction

What Is an In-Clinic Clinic?

An in-clinic clinic is a clearly defined cooperative effort between a private practice and an animal welfare organization or a dedicated group of volunteers, in which the two come together to facilitate regularly scheduled spay–neuter services. Essentially, the private practice becomes a low-income clinic for a limited amount of time on a regular basis, using an allotted time to provide services at prices comparable to spay–neuter programs within the region. This model takes components of a public health approach (i.e. high volume, easy access, and low cost) into the private veterinary practice and, through a partnership with an animal welfare organization, creates an income-targeted program that generates a positive revenue stream for the veterinary hospital. Since this unique partnership relies on existing resources, it is the easiest and least costly spay–neuter program to initiate.

What Is Wrong with Old Ways of Using Private Practices?

The private practice has often been overlooked as a partner in the effort to address pet overpopulation. The traditional way in which private practices have collaborated with animal welfare organizations has been through a voucher system. In the voucher system, a reduced-cost surgery is provided by the private practice during a regular appointment slot, with a humane society or municipal agency making up part of the cost difference. Due to voucher clients' often limited income, limited access to transportation, and lack of prior relationship with the practice, the risk of no-shows among these clients may be far greater than that of clients paying full price. If scheduled during the regular workday, each no-show represents a loss, and because these no-shows are unpredictable, "extras" cannot be scheduled in the same time slot in anticipation of no-shows.

Why Is an In-Clinic Clinic Better?

Making high-quality high-volume spay–neuter (HQHVSN) financially rewarding for the veterinary hospital is the only sustainable way to fit low-cost spay–neuter services into the private practice. By isolating the time block for these surgeries so that the reduced-cost surgery does not compete with regular client time slots, an in-clinic clinic program can work for the community and the private practice as well.

In-clinic clinics maximize the use of the veterinarians' and the technicians' or assistants' time. And because in-clinic clinics rely on existing resources, they significantly reduce the financial demand on the animal welfare organization, although some fundraising is still needed.

High-Quality, High-Volume Spay and Neuter and Other Shelter Surgeries, First Edition. Edited by Sara White.

Where Are In-Clinic Clinics Best Suited?

Many rural communities have a high proportion of low-income households, yet lack the population or financial resources needed to support full-time HQHVSN programs. In areas with low population density or in communities in which a limited number of services are needed (such as around college student housing), in-clinic clinics can be an ideal way to eliminate pet overpopulation, change pet-care habits, and generate revenue.

In-clinic clinics are ideal for:

- Communities with populations under 25 000 people
- Providing spay–neuter prior to adoption or release from local shelters
- Programs that target specific populations, for example feral cats.

How In-Clinic Clinics Work

The key to this clinic model lies in isolating the time block for reduced-cost surgeries from the practice's regular work time. In-clinic clinics operate during a dedicated time block that otherwise would be idle or slow time, or during which the veterinary hospital would normally be closed, and thus do not compete with the veterinary hospital's regular workload. During this dedicated time block, in-clinic clinics operate, as much as possible, in a high-volume model, and extra surgeries can be scheduled to compensate for probable no-shows.

In-clinic clinics have most of the same components as other spay–neuter programs. Overall, these tasks include outreach to clients, outreach to the community (advertising), and the surgeries themselves, with the tasks divided between the veterinary hospital and the organization. Each part of the team (the veterinary hospital and the animal welfare organization) has set responsibilities. Each must have a clear understanding of what is expected of them and must be able to communicate well with the other.

In-clinic clinics are best suited to private practice veterinary hospitals that are reasonably well equipped for small animal surgery, with a good surgery team, and with staff that are on board and comfortable with animal welfare programs. Physical considerations include whether the facility can handle the additional animals one morning a week or on a day off, and whether existing equipment will work, at least during start-up.

An animal welfare organization that is a nonprofit (as recognized by the Internal Revenue Service) is the best partner. While volunteer teams can raise funds through bake sales and car washes, gaining nonprofit status should be the goal of an animal welfare partner that does not already have that status.

If there is a stand-alone spay–neuter clinic within the region, a visit to that clinic can help the veterinarian and their staff get some ideas for increasing their efficiency and implementing high-volume flow as they move forward.

Benefits of In-Clinic Clinics

The benefits for the animal hospital include using isolated "downtime" to capture revenue not coming into any veterinary practice, to provide a positive community service, and possibly to gain some future clients.

Benefits to the animal welfare organization include:

- The surgery program is run by the veterinary hospital itself, so it is easy for inexperienced volunteers to do their part.
- No major capital fundraising is needed for start-up. Funds raised by the welfare group mainly provide a sliding scale to clients unable to afford the costs of the surgeries.
- Eliminates competing for weekends (or other time slots) from a visiting mobile unit, if such services are even available in the community.

Whole Day or Partial Day?

The two models of in-clinic clinics are:

- Holding a clinic on a day in which the veterinary hospital is otherwise closed (usually monthly) and planning to do 35 surgeries on that day.
- "Bunching" a few slower hours together (usually one morning a week) and performing up to 15 surgeries in that time.

All-Day Clinics on "Closed" Days

Operating on a day that the veterinary hospital would otherwise be closed enables busy veterinary hospitals that cannot make time within their regular schedule to participate. The drawbacks to holding clinics on a day the veterinary hospital is otherwise closed include that staff members lose a day off that they may count on for family time, that at least one experienced staff person must be hired for the day, and that volunteers must be on-site throughout recovery, check-out, and clean-up. This type of program relies on heavily on volunteers, so committed and consistent volunteers are required.

Since all-day clinics are often held monthly, this lower frequency makes it necessary to make separate plans for pregnant animals. Also, the longer people wait for services, the more likely they are to be a no-show, no longer have the money, or no longer own the pet.

Partial-Day Clinics during the Work Week

Scheduling smaller blocks of time during the regular work week (two to three hours) can be less disruptive than full-day clinics. Although the in-clinic clinic is held during the week, regular clients are not scheduled during those hours. While volunteers may be needed at check-in, the rest of the day is handled by the regular staff that are already on-site.

Benefits to holding weekly clinics during regular hours include that a veterinary hospital with some "downtime" can make use of a short time block within the normal day, so it is less disruptive to everyone's schedule. Most veterinary hospitals can provide five to eight surgeries in a two-hour block. The humane organization does the scheduling, income screening, and outreach. Although staff time is used, it is during the regular workday so overhead is not increased.

A potential drawback to this model is that because it is on weekdays when the veterinary hospital staff are likely to be responsible for check-in, some staff may resent what they perceive as "extra" work and/or feel challenged by a different clientele. If the staff are not on board, a weekend all-day in-clinic clinic program that relies more heavily on volunteers should be considered (see previous section).

Organization

No two veterinary hospitals are exactly alike and each in-clinic clinic must be tailored to its home base.

The duties in running an in-clinic clinic program are basically the same as in any other type of spay–neuter program. What is most important is that the tasks must be clearly defined between the veterinary hospital and the volunteer base, with special attention paid to communication between the two. The volunteer organization should assign one person to be the program coordinator; this person will be the primary "go-to" person for the veterinary hospital's communication needs. While the entire volunteer team should be familiar with the program, the point person should be available for the veterinary hospital to reach regarding necessary supplies, client issues, and so on. Also, the veterinary hospital may find it helpful to have one person who oversees the supplies that are used for the in-clinic clinics and primarily communicates with the volunteer point person. The greater the level of organization, the fewer misunderstandings there will be.

Task Partitioning between Private Practice and Humane Organization

Some of the tasks (i.e. "who does what") change depending on whether the clinic is held during the work week or on a day the veterinary hospital is closed. For example, in a clinic that is held one morning a week, volunteers would not be expected to be on-site to wash instruments or complete other on-site tasks.

However, the animal welfare partner is always responsible for advertising, contacting social service and/or animal control agencies, receiving calls and scheduling the surgeries, income screening, and making reminder calls with the pre-op instructions. The animal welfare partner is also responsible for fundraising for any sliding scale that is offered to clients.

The veterinary hospital is always responsible for developing the pre-op instructions, exams, the surgery, check-out information, and after-care if needed.

Coordinating Client Booking

An online document system enables multiple volunteers to schedule the clinic days without overbooking and enables the veterinary hospital staff to see the appointments that are booked for the upcoming clinic. In the absence of such an electronic system, the humane organization will email or fax a list of clients to the receptionist the evening before the clinic.

Income Screening

Many in-clinic clinics elect to screen client income. Income screening over the phone is simple and straightforward. Income screening can be based on a household income level (such as $35 000 per year) or those receiving Food Stamps, or eligible for the Special Supplemental Nutrition Program for Women, Infants and Children (WIC), Medicare, or Department of Housing and Urban Development (HUD) public housing. Using an overall household income level enables the program to include low-income working people who receive no public benefits. For the programs in which the hospital staff check in the clients, clients are reminded to bring proof of income.

The procedures should be streamlined when it is possible to do so. For example, in an animal hospital that is fully computerized, the animal welfare partner may complete the clients' intake "form" over the phone and email it to the animal hospital receptionist the night before surgery. The client then simply brings the pet and their proof of income. If the system is on paper, the check-in can take place in the animal hospital or at off-site locations such as a social services office.

Budget

A very limited amount of funding is needed to start an in-clinic clinic. Funds are needed for a dedicated phone line, advertising, postering, and paperwork. Having a separate phone number for spay–neuter appointments enables the humane organization to advertise the program and prevents the veterinary hospital receptionist from having to discern which callers are seeking the low-income services. This is vital unless the animal hospital itself is dedicated to taking over a portion of the animal welfare tasks.

The income from providing 10 surgeries per week at $45 per surgery is $22 500 over the course of 50 weeks. Most clinics limit payment for these services to cash, money orders, or credit cards. If a sliding scale is provided, the remainder is raised by the animal welfare partner.

Organizing Animals and Medical Records

Clear patient identification is vital, as it is easy to have confusion between patients (especially cats) when a greater number of patients enter the clinic than the staff is used to handling. One way to achieve this is via a standard numbering system. The chart or intake paperwork and carrier of each cat should be assigned a number upon entry and the number will be marked in the cat's ear when it is sedated. Starting with a low number is important, as it is difficult to write a multidigit number in a cat's ear.

Organizing Supplies

Keeping all intake supplies in a large plastic tub is helpful (Figure 36.1). The tub will hold forms, aftercare instructions, pens, paper collars, other marking supplies, and so on. Ultimately, if the animal hospital determines that this model is a good fit, adding surgery packs, V-trays (Figure 36.2), and a few other items later may be helpful.

Common Pitfalls

Communication Breakdowns

Communication breakdowns are the primary challenge to in-clinic clinics and they cause many to fail. This type of program brings together two entities that may have little understanding of how the other functions. Genuine misunderstandings can be avoided by having detailed written procedures and protocols, and by each group spending some time visiting and understanding each other's procedures. Typical problems include unresolved issues between the veterinary hospital and the humane organization (scheduling too many large dogs in a day, for example), veterinary hospital staff resenting the extra work or

(a)

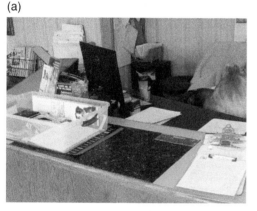

(b)

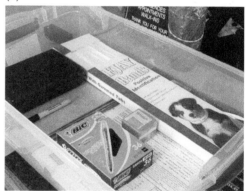

(c)

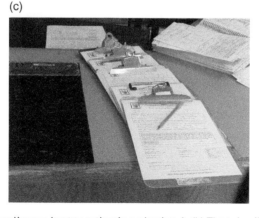

Figure 36.1   (a) Intake supplies are kept together in a plastic tub. (b) The tub will hold forms, aftercare instructions, pens, paper collars, and other marking supplies. (c) Clipboards with intake forms are also made available at the intake desk.

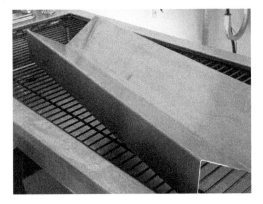

Figure 36.2 A V-tray atop a clinic tabletop can create an additional prep station. Ultimately, adding surgery packs, V-trays, and a few other items may be helpful in increasing capacity and facilitating flow.

perceiving the clients as misusing the program (feeling that someone has too much money to use the program), and/or the humane organization asking for discounts on additional services. Staff dissatisfaction is the single greatest obstacle to these programs. The animal welfare partner can help diffuse some of the perception of extra work by recognizing the staff's effort and planning a way to say thank-you, for example providing lunch for the veterinary hospital staff on the last Friday of every month. This does not need to be an expensive lunch, but it tells the staff that they are indeed appreciated. Making sure they are aware that the number of surgeries they did has an impact is also important.

Judgments and Stereotypes

Negative judgments or stereotypes about low-income homes can create major pitfalls for in-clinic clinics. Unlike nonprofit spay–neuter clinics, private practice animal hospitals are not established primarily in order to assist the poor.

Everyone, including veterinary hospital staff and the animal welfare volunteers, needs to become educated about poverty in order to avoid making judgments that damage the program.

Pricing Transparency

Added or hidden charges are another major pitfall for in-clinic clinics. The total amount of money that the client should expect to pay should be included up front in the price that is advertised. Clients who were asked to prove that they have a low income and are then hit with extra charges often perceive this as a "bait and switch," something that results in bad word of mouth. For the program to succeed, low-income clients must recommend it to friends. Poor attitude from staff or upselling to get a few extra dollars from the clients will damage the program. The revenue should be generated by volume and increased by increasing volume only.

Conclusion

In-clinic clinics provide a model for cooperation between local private veterinary hospitals and animal welfare organizations, and are well suited to low-population communities that would be unable to support a full-time HQHVSN clinic. In-clinic clinics provide low-cost services using existing resources and can be a win–win for both the veterinary hospital and the animal welfare group. With the use of an in-clinic clinic, a privately owned veterinary clinic, in combination with a group of volunteers or a small humane organization, can lead the local effort to get pets spayed or neutered, while capturing income that might otherwise leave their community.

Index

High-Quality, High-Volume Spay and Neuter and Other Shelter Surgeries, First Edition. Edited by Sara White.
© 2020 John Wiley & Sons, Inc. Published 2020 by John Wiley & Sons, Inc.